GERONTOLOGY

To the reader:

The collage depicted on the cover and threaded throughout the design of this text is intended to represent the common theme of lifespan; the past, present and future that is part of all of our lives no matter our age.

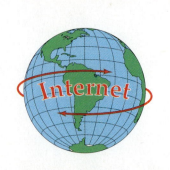

GERONTOLOGY
NURSING CARE OF THE OLDER ADULT

Mildred O. Hogstel, PhD, RN, C

Professor Emeritus
Harris School of Nursing
Texas Christian University
Fort Worth, Texas
Gerontological Nurse Consultant

Managing Editors

Cora D. Zembrzuski, RN, MSN, CS, PhDc

New York University
New York, New York
The Connecticut Visiting Nurses Association

Meredith Wallace, PhDc, RN, CS-ANP

Assistant Professor, Nursing
Southern Connecticut State University
New Haven, Connecticut

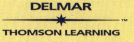
DELMAR

THOMSON LEARNING™

Australia   Canada   Mexico   Singapore   Spain   United Kingdom   United States

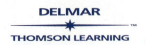

DELMAR
™
THOMSON LEARNING

Gerontology: Nursing Care of the Older Adult
by Mildred O. Hogstel, PhD, RN, C

Business Unit Director:
William Brottmiller

Channel Manager:
Tara Carter

Executive Editor:
Cathy L. Esperti

Project Editor:
Patricia Gillivan

Developmental Editor:
Patricia A. Gaworecki

Production Coordinator:
John Mickelbank

Editorial Assistant:
Elizabeth M. O'Keefe

Art/Design Coordinator:
Jay Purcell

Executive Marketing Manager:
Dawn F. Gerrain

For permission to use material from this text or product, contact us by
Tel   (800) 730-2214
Fax   (800) 730-2215
www.thomsonrights.com

Library of Congress Cataloging-in-Publication Data
Gerontology : nursing care of the older adult / [edited by] Mildred O. Hogstel ; managing editors Cora D. Zembruski, Meredith Wallace.
    p. cm.
  Includes bibliographical references and index.
  ISBN 0-7668-0729-0
  1. Geriatric nursing.   I. Hogstel, Mildred O.
RC954 .G485 2000
610.73'65—dc21

00-050898

NOTICE TO THE READER

Publisher does not warrant or guarantee any of the products described herein or perform any independent analysis in connection with any of the product information contained herein. Publisher does not assume, and expressly disclaims, any obligation to obtain and include information other than that provided to it by the manufacturer.

The reader is expressly warned to consider and adopt all safety precautions that might be indicated by the activities herein and to avoid all potential hazards. By following the instructions contained herein, the reader willingly assumes all risks in connection with such instructions.

The Publisher makes no representation or warranties of any kind, including but not limited to, the warranties of fitness for particular purpose or merchantability, nor are any such representations implied with respect to the material set forth herein, and the publisher takes no responsibility with respect to such material. The publisher shall not be liable for any special, consequential, or exemplary damages resulting, in whole or part, from the readers' use of, or reliance upon, this material.

Dedication

*In loving memory of
my mother, my father,
my grandparents, and so many
other older adults who have
touched my life and taught
me so much.*

CONTENTS

PREFACE

Issues related to the nursing care of older adults will be major factors in the evolving health care systems throughout the world in the twenty-first century. The population of older adults in almost every country is rapidly increasing. In fact, 1999 was designated the International Year of the Older Adult with increasing emphasis on older adults throughout the world. Nurses have a major responsibility to identify and coordinate care to meet the holistic needs of their clients and family members through a continuum of care in a complex and fragmented health care delivery system.

The primary purpose of this book, therefore, is to help nursing students of all kinds, both undergraduate and graduate, to meet that challenge. This book also will help to update licensed nurses who are just beginning their nursing practice as well as nurses who have been in the field for many years. Parish/congregational nurses, social workers, hospital and community case managers, rehabilitation therapists, and health insurance company staff members, including those in managed care organizations, will benefit from this book by helping them to understand how to work with and care for and about older people using a holistic approach.

Gerontological nursing is one of the more recent specialties in nursing (the first major nursing textbook was published in the late 1970s). It was slow to develop at first because of the lack of research and availability of specific courses and degrees in the specialty. Gerontological nursing is now a growing specialty meeting the needs of the increasing population of older adults.

Conceptual Framework

Because gerontology is becoming a more recognized specialty in nursing, this text presented the opportunity to respond to the market need for an extensive revision and greatly expanded version of *Nursing Care of the Older Adult*, 3e.

Now considered a first edition, *Gerontology: Nursing Care of the Older Adult* presents a broad and holistic view of the needs of older adults through a continuum of care and in all settings. It is essential that nurses and others who work with older adults know and appreciate how their care might differ from that of other age groups. Older adults need to be respected and honored, regardless of their age or physical and/or mental status. That does not always occur in our current health care delivery system, possibly because of stereotyping and lack of knowledge by some about normal aging issues, concerns, and care.

Organization

The text is divided into eight units and 28 chapters. **Unit 1** introduces the major issues of aging, the emerging and current status of gerontological nursing, and how geriatric care is becoming a major factor in the health care delivery system. Current facts and trends related to payment methods for geriatric care (for example, Medicare, Medicaid, and long-term care insurance) are discussed. **Unit 2** presents the developmental, biological, physiological, psychological, and social theories and effects of aging, which provides a theoretical framework for understanding the principles of holistic geriatric care.

Unit 3 focuses on health promotion and wellness because it is never too late to improve one's health status. The components of successful aging, including nutrition, mental and physical activity, types of support systems, spirituality, and sexuality are discussed. Health promotion, including recommended types of screening and immunizations, is covered. Chapter 8 focuses on health education, including principles and methods of geragogy, those practices and processes used in educational settings for older learners.

Geriatric health care is covered in **Unit 4** beginning with assessment, diagnosis, and planning. Some of the most common medical diagnoses of older adults together with the related nursing diagnoses and interventions are discussed. Health problems presented are cancer, cardiovascular disease, diabetes, chronic obstructive pulmonary disease, cerebrovascular accident, common infections, and Parkinson's disease. Acute care issues such as emergency care and surgery as well as the major chronic illnesses such as arthritis, osteoporosis, and sensory deficits are presented. Acute and chronic pain in older adults is another important issue discussed. Unit 4 concludes with special chapters on mental health issues and geriatric pharmacology.

One of the major dilemmas in the U.S. health care delivery system is long-term care, which is covered in **Unit 5**. Chapter 19 focuses on nursing facility care, Chapter 20 on home health care, and Chapter 21 on hospice and palliative care, which is often not used as much as it could be. The continuum of health care continues in **Unit 6** with discussion of a variety of community health care resources such as outpatient clinics designed especially for older people. These types of clinics are expanding rapidly and need qualified nurses, nurse practitioners, and case managers to staff them. Discussion focuses on the shift from inpatient to outpatient care in hospitals, including day surgery, wound care centers, and sleep clinics. This unit concludes with discussion in Chapter 24 of a variety of community organizations, agencies, and services that focus primarily on older adults maintaining an independent lifestyle for as long as possible.

Ethical, legal, and financial issues in the care of older adults are very important and are discussed in **Unit 7**. Issues such as quality of life, access to health care, and end-of-life decisions and choices will continue to receive increasing emphasis as the population ages and health care resources become more expensive and complicated. Availability and management of finances in diverse populations are also discussed.

Unit 8 summarizes key issues and emerging trends, including nursing implications, legislation and public policy advocacy, and research needs for the future.

Special Features

There are numerous special features in *Gerontology: Nursing Care of the Older Adult* designed to stimulate critical thinking and self-exploration, and enhance professional advancement. These features also encourage learners to synthesize and apply critical knowledge in this text. All of these features support novice and expert level challenges to practice.

Research Focus features current research linking theory to practice. Information is presented in an abstract format appropriate for a research project.

Perspectives at the beginning of each of the eight units set the tone for the chapters within the unit. This feature may be insight from the perspective of a client or practitioner. It may also take the form of "food for thought" before beginning the chapter content.

Making the Connection at the beginning of each chapter helps the student and instructor link the information across the holistic care continuum and tie new content to previously learned content within the text.

Think About it boxes aim to develop sensitivity to and awareness of ethical and moral issues, providing an opportunity to think critically and develop problem-solving skills in clinical situations.

Clinical Alert boxes alert the learner to those situations that require immediate attention to ensure client health and safety.

Ask Yourself boxes use ethical and social issues to encourage self-reflection and examination of values. This feature also helps to evaluate how a person's values will affect nursing care.

Nursing Tips contain hints to assist with a more practical and efficient approach to on-the-job nursing practice. The variety of tips and strategies presented can help toward professional advancement.

Care Plans are framed in a case study format and then proceed through the nursing process to establish, administer, and evaluate a specific plan of care. These are also helpful in strengthening critical thinking skills.

Resources located at the end of each chapter provide Internet addresses to enhance research and technology skills.

Support Materials

The Clinical Companion for Assessment of the Older Adult (authored by Cora D. Zembrzuski, RN, MSN, CS) is a convenient pocket-size quick reference for the student or practitioner. It utilizes a systems approach to nursing care, with numerous easy-to-reference tables and figures. Special features such as Nursing Tips, Nursing Alerts, Nursing Checklists, and Tips from the Experts are tailored to the care of the older adult. Appendices include laboratory parameters specific to older adults, developmental tasks of later maturity, and pressure ulcer assessment guides for care, management, and nutrition. The companion has been specially designed for easy access of information in a clinical environment.

Mildred Hogstel, editor of this book, has been involved in gerontological nursing in the United States since the 1960s when she first taught nursing students in a nursing facility. She edited one of the early textbooks in gerontological nursing in the United States, which was first published in 1981. She received a diploma in nursing from Providence Hospital School of Nursing and a bachelor of science in nursing education from Baylor University in Waco, Texas; a master of science in nursing from the University of Texas in Austin, Texas; and a doctor of philosophy in higher education from the University of North Texas in Denton, Texas. She also studied health care at the University of Oslo in Norway. She has worked as a nurse in surgery, an emergency department, general medical-surgical units in hospitals, and in home health care. She has been continuously certified as a gerontological nurse generalist by the American Nurses Credentialing Center from 1985–2004. She taught nursing at Baylor University School of Nursing in Dallas, Texas and Harris School of Nursing at Texas Christian University in Fort Worth, Texas, where she currently is a Professor Emeritus and occasional faculty.

Besides her professional nursing credentials and experience, she also cared for her parents in their later years in her home for almost twenty-five years. Her primary professional goals have always been and continue to be providing, teaching, and advocating for quality health care and quality of life for older people. She is currently a gerontological nursing consultant in Fort Worth, Texas, where she consults with a variety of agencies and organizations working with older adults.

ACKNOWLEDGMENTS

Sincere appreciation is expressed to the publisher, Delmar, for its interest in gerontological nursing and patience in completing this book. I also want to thank all of the contributing authors, who have a variety of educational backgrounds, experience, and expertise in geriatric care, for their hard work and ultimate successful outcome. Most of all, I want to thank my typist, Susan Moore, for her excellent organization and work. She has the ability to make rough drafts look and read well. She is definitely a miracle worker. By now she knows exactly how to revise format, and sometimes the use of words for consistency, without my noting it in writing. Thank you, Susan.

The holistic care of older adults and their family members who have a variety of complex needs is the most challenging and rewarding area of nursing I have ever experienced. I hope that many readers of this book will experience that same joy.

Mildred O. Hogstel

CONTRIBUTORS

Margaret C. Basiliadis, DO
Director Family Geriatrics
Fort Worth, Texas

Carolyn Spence Cagle, PhD, RN, C
Texas Christian University
Harris School of Nursing
Associate Professor
Fort Worth, Texas

Beth L. Cameron, MS, RN, FNP
Trinity College of Nursing
Assistant Professor, Community Health
Moline, Illinois

Dianne M. Chiu, RD, LD
University of Texas Southwestern Medical Center at Dallas
Consultant Dietitian in Long-Term Care, Renal Dialysis,
    and Nutrition Support
Fort Worth, Texas

Perle Slavik Cowen, PhD, RN
The University of Iowa
College of Nursing
Associate Professor
Iowa City, Iowa

Marsha Cox, PhD, RN, CS, GNP, ANP
Baylor Senior Health Network
Dallas, Texas

Linda Cox Curry, PhD, RN
Texas Christian University
Harris School of Nursing
Professor of Nursing
Fort Worth, Texas

Gail C. Davis, RN, EdD
Texas Woman's University
College of Nursing
Professor
Denton, Texas

M. Nelia Davis, RN, MSN
Clinical Nurse Specialist, Gerontology
The University of Texas Medical Branch at Galveston
Galveston, Texas

Susan Brown Eve, PhD
University of North Texas
Department of Applied Gerontology
Denton, Texas

Janis M. Fleming, PhD, RN
The University of Akron
College of Nursing
Associate Professor
Akron, Ohio

Deborah K. Fultner, PhDc, MS, RN, CS
The Methodist Hospital
Advanced Practice Nurse
Houston, Texas

Mary S. Harper, PhD, RN, FAAN
The University of Alabama
Geropsychiatric Research Consultant and
    Distinguished Adjunct Professor
Tuscaloosa, Alabama

Barbara Harty, RN, MSN, CS
University of North Texas
Health Science Center
Fort Worth, Texas

Bert Hayslip, Jr., PhD
University of North Texas
Regents Professor of Psychology
Denton, Texas

Janice A. Knebl, DO, CMD, FACP
University of North Texas
Health Science Center
Chief, Division of Geriatrics/Department of Medicine
Associate Professor of Medicine
Fort Worth, Texas

Susan Margolis, PhD, RN, CNS—P/MH
Director of Geriatric Services
Psychiatric Center of North Texas
DeSoto, Texas

Libby High Poston, NP, PhDc, MS, RN
Preceptor, University of Texas at Arlington
School of Nursing
Arlington, Texas
and
Nurse Practitioner
Senior Med Services
Dallas, Texas

Sharon Beth Prentice, RN, MS
University of North Texas
Fort Worth, Texas

Charlie D. Pruett, Jr., MS
Abilene Christian University
Director of the Gerontology Center
Abilene, Texas

Barbara M. Raudonis, PhD, RN, CS
The University of Texas at Arlington
School of Nursing
Assistant Professor
Arlington, Texas

Katy Scherger, RN, MSN, CS
Gerontological Nurse Practioner/Clinical Nurse Specialist
Evercare
Tucson, Arizona

Carol A. Stephenson, EdD, RN, C, CRNH
Texas Christian University
Harris School of Nursing
Associate Professor
Fort Worth, Texas

Jacqueline M. Stolley, PhD, RN, CS
Trinity College of Nursing
Professor
Moline, Illinois

Laura Talbot, RN, CS, EdD, PhD
Johns Hopkins University
Program Director for Geriatric Nursing
Assistant Professor
School of Nursing
Baltimore, Maryland

Debra Schutkowski, LMSW, CCM, MS
Director of Senior Services
Osteopathic Health Systems of Texas
Fort Worth, Texas

Diana J. Torrez, PhD
University of New Mexico
Albuquerque, New Mexico

Jan W. Weaver, PhD, RN
Director of Services and Education
Alzheimer's Association, Greater Dallas Chapter
Dallas, Texas

JoAnn Wedig, RN, MA
Trinity College of Nursing
Associate Professor
Moline, Illinois

Kay Weiler, RN, MA, JD
CompleWare Corporation
Vice President
Iowa City, IA

REVIEWERS

Mary Bliesmer, DNSc, GNP
Professor, School of Nursing
Minnesota State University, Mankato
Mankato, Minnesota

Ada Romaine Davis, PhD, RN, CANP
Johns Hopkins University
Baltimore, Maryland

Annette R. Gibson, RN, MEd, MSN
Professor, School of Nursing
Miami-Dade Community College
Medical Center Campus
Miami, Florida
Joan K. Stout, RN Endowed Teaching Chair Recipient
    1999–2002

Brenda Morris, BSN, MS, EdD
Clinical Associate Professor of Nursing
Arizona State University, College of Nursing
Tempe, Arizona

Jayne F. Moore, PhD, RN, CNS
Assistant Professor
Orvis School of Nursing
University of Nevada, Reno
Reno, Nevada

Max B. Rothman, JD
Executive Director
Southeast Florida Center on Aging
North Miami, Florida

Maureen Straight, RN, MSED
Regents College
Albany, New York

Marilyn J. Vontz, PhD, RN, MSN, MA, BS
Professor
Bryan Hospital School of Nursing
Lincoln, Nebraska

Cora D. Zembrzuski RN, MSN, CS, PhDc
New York University
New York, New York
and
The Connecticut Visiting Nurses Association

HOW TO USE THIS BOOK

▲ Key Terms

Review this list before reading the chapter to familiarize yourself with new terms and revisit those terms you already know to link them with the content of the new chapter.

COMPETENCIES

After completing this chapter, the reader should be able to:

- Describe structural lag theory.
- Review data on race and ethnic differences in aging.
- Identify the different social roles commonly associated with older adults.
- Describe how the role of grandparenthood has evolved into parenthood the second time around.
- Discuss how the role of retirement has changed in recent years.
- Compare and contrast the differences experienced in widowhood by gender.
- Examine special issues of spirituality as it relates to the aging process.

▲ Competencies

Read the chapter competencies before reading the chapter content to set the stage for learning. Return to the competencies when the chapter study is completed to see which entries you can respond to with "yes, I can do that."

MAKING THE CONNECTION

Refer to the following chapters to increase your understanding of the successful aspects of aging:

- **Chapter 6** Psychological Aspects of Aging
- **Chapter 9** Geriatric Nutrition
- **Chapter 10** Informal Support Systems
- **Chapter 24** Community Organizations and Services

▲ Making the Connection

Read these boxes before beginning a chapter to link material across the holistic care continuum and to tie new content to material you have already encountered.

CLINICAL ALERT

Absolute contraindications for physical activity include such conditions as severe coronary heart disease, decompensated congestive heart failure, uncontrolled arrhythmia, valvular disease, uncontrolled hypertension, acute myocarditis or infectious illness, recent pulmonary embolism, and deep vein thrombosis.

▲ Clinical Alert

Certain situations require immediate action to ensure client health and safety. Pay careful attention to this feature as it will assist effective and efficient responses to critical situations.

Ask Yourself

You are seeing a client from a culture that does not believe in traditional Western medicine. This client has a condition that would respond to antibiotics; however, the client refuses and informs you she has been using her culture's traditional herbs and roots. She is only seeing you because of her employer's insistence. She has missed work days because of her condition. How would you respond to her situation?

▲ Ask Yourself

Deals with self-reflection and opinions on various ethical and social issues. It may be useful to keep a journal to record responses. After completing each chapter, reviewing journal entries will help evaluate how a person's values will affect nursing care.

Nursing Tip

It is important for health care providers to remain alert to situations that require ethical decision-making skills (Robbins, 1996). Ethics in health care often involve choosing between two equally good or equally bad alternatives. Health care providers often are faced with dilemmas about deciding to do what is best for someone versus allowing individual autonomy. Health care providers must use their communication skills and listen to individual needs before determining the best course of action.

▲ Nursing Tip

Presents helpful hints that assist with more efficient job performance. The wide variety of tips, hints, and strategies presented will help with professional advancement. This feature provides the opportunity for discussion and idea sharing.

Think About It

How would you begin to assess how satisfied an older adult is with his or her intimate relationships?

▲ Think About It

Helps develop sensitivity to ethical and moral issues, providing an opportunity to think critically in clinical situations and be active in problem solving. Issues can be explored before reading the chapter content or as the chapter progresses.

Research Focus

Citation:
Kelley, S. J., Yorker, B. C., & Whitley, D. (1997). To grandmother's house we go . . . and stay: Children raised in intergenerational families. *Journal of Gerontological Nursing, 23*(9), 13–20.

Purpose:
An estimated 1.1 million children in foster care have been placed with relatives, especially grandparents, where neither biological parent is present in the home. This study focused on the issues older adults experience when parenting the second time around.

Methods:
Review of U.S. Census Bureau statistics, personal interviews of grandparents with children in prisons, and studies of low-income and minority neighborhoods.

Findings:
There is a severe increase in recent years of grandparents formally and informally becoming the primary caregivers of grandchildren.

Implications:
Health care providers need to be alert to the fact that the most vulnerable grandparents tend to be the ones forced into full-time caregiving. This group needs extensive support with child caregiving responsibilities and monitoring of personal health care.

▲ Research Focus

Emphasizes the importance of clinical research in nursing by linking theory to practice. This useful learning tool focuses attention on current issues and trends in nursing, as well as illustrating the correct way to write an abstract for a research project.

CARE PLAN

Case Study

Mr. and Mrs. O'Connor are in their early seventies. They met at law school in their college years and have had long, successful careers as lawyers. Although over the years they admit to "making some bad financial decisions," they are thankful for their good health. They live modestly in a condominium in the northeast.

Both have remained very active over the years. Mrs. O. loves the water. She swims at the pool on a daily basis in good weather. In the winter, she goes to the town's indoor pool. In addition, as a child she enjoyed horseback riding, something she misses. Mr. O. enjoyed a very active childhood full of competitive sports. His favorite sports were basketball and wrestling, both of which he learned to appreciate from his mother. Over the past 20 years, he has played golf and even won a few trophies.

Mr. O. has a family history of prostate cancer and MI (myocardial infarction). His only brother died of a heart attack at the age of 62. His father had "hardening of the arteries" and died at 73. Mrs. O. has a history of cystic breasts and severe endometriosis. Her 90-year-old mother (still alive) was hospitalized for PID (pelvic inflammatory disease). All deliveries of the four children were "agonizing and long," according to Mrs. O.'s mother. One of Mrs. O.'s sisters died of uterine cancer, the other two are alive and living on the West Coast. Mrs. O. misses them.

As part of their overall philosophy of health and wellness, the O'Connors embrace traditional medicine supplemented by alternative medicine. Both are informed on some of the conflicting issues with alternative medicine. They are aware that the use of herbal therapies can enhance or detract from medication effectiveness, even causing life-threatening interactions. Mrs. O. takes ginkgo biloba for memory stimulation, plus a vitamin prescribed by her physician-nutritionist. Mr. O. takes Kavatrol (kava kava) for relaxation, along with specifically prescribed vitamins from the same physician-nutritionist.

Mr. and Mrs. O'Connor want to improve upon their good health and have sought your expertise.

Assessment

These are two healthy older adults who enjoy a fulfilling life. They are active and well informed. They take their health seriously—as a lifetime job—and cope with shortcomings in a productive manner. Reflect on how their health history affects their health outcome. What other steps could they take to stay at optimal health? Each has a family history of concern to the clinician. The following care plan reflects some preventive measures aimed at health screening and disease prevention.

NURSING DIAGNOSIS

Health-seeking behaviors related to desire for enhanced health, movement toward a higher level of health, and disease prevention.

Outcomes:

Mr. O. will:
- *Control and screen for risk factors of cardiac and prostate disease.*
- *Learn anxiety-reducing exercises and possibly using biofeedback.*

Mrs. O. will:
- *Control and screen for uterine, breast, and other reproductive-related disorders.*
- *Enhance social well-being by visiting her sister.*

▲ Care Plan

Walks through the process of assessment, diagnosis, planning care, performing interventions, and evaluating the success of the course of care. These are helpful in strengthening the understanding of the nursing process through a case study approach and in exercising critical thinking skills.

Review Questions and Activities

1. What are the major components of successful aging?

2. Discuss ways to promote successful aging in an older adult population.

3. How are nutritional needs different for older adults?

4. What are the effects of a regular exercise program?

5. What effect does a support system or significant other have on successful aging?

6. What are two major factors that determine whether an older adult will want to be employed?

7. What role does formal and informal education have in the life of an older adult?

8. What kinds of group activities are helpful to older adults?

9. Describe the roles health care providers can assume in relation to nutrition, social support systems, activities, and exercise.

10. Develop an exercise program for an older adult using the principles of adult learning and taking into consideration their unique physiological changes.

▲ Review Questions and Activities

At the end of each chapter, exercises assist in the learning process and assimilation of the information presented in the chapter.

Resources

American Dietetic Association: **www.eatright.org**

Extended Care: **www.elderconnect.com**

▲ Resources

Found at the end of each chapter, Internet addresses provide the opportunity to enhance research and technology skills.

UNIT 1

An Overview of Aging Issues

PERSPECTIVE...

Mrs. O'Dwyer, an 85-year-old widow, lived alone in a home where she and her husband and children had lived for many years. Her two sons and their families lived in another state. When walking down her back steps late one afternoon, Mrs. O'Dwyer fell down the steps to the sidewalk. Although she often spoke to her next-door neighbors, the family on one side was out of town and the neighbor on the other side was in the hospital.

After she fell, Mrs. O'Dwyer felt severe pain in her left hip and could not get up to walk or even crawl up the stairs to get to a phone. She lay on the sidewalk all night because she knew that no one would hear her if she called for help. Fortunately, it was summer so it was not cold weather, but she was in pain and was thirsty and hungry by morning. About noon she heard someone in her driveway. It was a telephone repairman checking on her telephone line because one of her sons had gotten no response when he called several times the night before. An ambulance was called and Mrs. O'Dwyer was taken to the hospital where her family was notified about her condition.

She had hip replacement surgery for a fractured hip the next afternoon after one of her sons had flown in to be with her. She recovered from the surgery well and needed a period of rehabilitation. A gerontological clinical nurse specialist (GCNS) met with her several times and made arrangements for Mrs. O'Dwyer's care.

These arrangements included physical therapy on the rehab unit for a couple of weeks, the purchase of a walker, transfer to a skilled nursing facility for a month, and then home with home health care, including attendants and homemakers, for several weeks. The hospital GCNS arranged for an emergency response system in case of another emergency and called Mrs. O'Dwyer frequently for several months.

The case of Mrs. O'Dwyer illustrates many of the issues of aging. Comprehensive, coordinated, holistic, quality care is the goal of gerontological nursing. Mrs. O'Dwyer was able to return to her own home in a realistic period of time and her family felt assured that she was getting the care and help she needed even though they could only be there for short visits.

CHAPTER 1

Aging Yesterday, Today, and Tomorrow

Mildred O. Hogstel, PhD, RN, C

COMPETENCIES

After completing this chapter, the reader should be able to:

- *Differentiate life expectancy, life span, and longevity.*
- *Identify the most common chronic diseases in older adults.*
- *Describe the reasons for most accidental injuries in the older population.*
- *List common myths related to the aging process.*
- *Discuss three major needs of older adults.*
- *Explore housing options for older people.*
- *Identify sources of income for older people.*
- *Summarize the Aging Network.*
- *Describe the primary functions and services of the Older Americans Act and the American Association of Retired Persons.*

MAKING THE CONNECTION

Refer to the following chapters to increase your understanding of aging yesterday, today, and tomorrow:

Demographics

The new century brings to our society a host of formative issues important to health care: rapid advancements in computer technology, the reality of cloning, the changing concepts of health care treatments (such as alternative therapies), and questions about continuing economic growth. A rapidly expanding aging population is one of the factors that will impact the entire world and especially health care in this century. The rapid increase in the number of older people in the United States is shown in Table 1-1. In 1998, 8% of adults age 65 and older were African Americans, 5.1% were of Hispanic origin, and 2.1% were Asian or Pacific Islander. There were 143 women for every 100 men (American Association of Retired Persons & Administration on Aging, 1999).

In 1997 the fastest growing age group in terms of percentage of total population was those age 85 and over (Figure 1-1). In 2000 the fastest growing age group was those age 95 and older (Atchley, 1997). The states with the greatest percentage of people age 65 and older are listed in Table 1-2.

Definitions

Most aging statistics are based on age 65 and older because full Social Security and **Medicare** benefits become available at that age; however, there is no one age that classifies people as older adults. There is no mandatory retirement age except in certain occupations such as airline pilot. Some people retire from a full-time position at age 50 and some never retire. Aging is a developmental process that begins at conception and ends at death. Because everyone ages at a different rate and body systems and organs age at different rates in different individuals, it is impossible to categorize

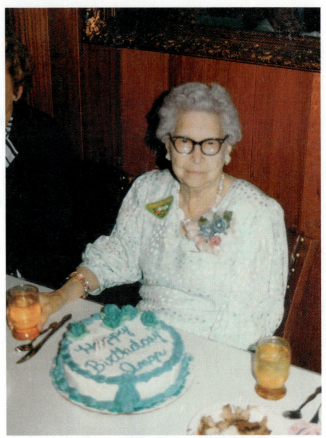

FIGURE 1-1 A 90th birthday party.

people based on chronological age alone. However, age groups have been classified using the model shown in Table 1-3.

There are several basic terms related to aging that need to be explored. These are listed and defined in Box 1-1. "A child born in 1997 could expect to live 76.5

TABLE 1-1   Number and Percentage of People in the United States Age 65 and Older from 1900 to 2030

	Number	Percentage
1900	3.1 million	4.1
1998	34.4 million	12.7
2000	34.7 million	13
2030	69.4 million	20

From A Profile of Older Americans: 1999 *(pp. 1–2), 1999, Washington, DC: American Association of Retired Persons and the Administration on Aging, U.S. Department of Health and Human Services.*

TABLE 1-2   States with the Greatest Percentage of People Age 65 and Older in 1998

	Number	Percentage
1. Florida	2,734,145	18.3
2. Pennsylvania	1,904,312	15.9
3. Rhode Island	154,327	15.6
4. West Virginia	274,689	15.2
5. Iowa	431,018	15.1

From A Profile of Older Americans: 1999 *(p. 8), 1999, Washington, DC: American Association of Retired Persons, and the Administration on Aging, U.S. Department of Health and Human Services.*

TABLE 1-3 Chronological Classification of Age Groups	
Age	**Classification**
65–74	Young-old
75–84	Old
85–94	Old-old
95 and older	**Elite-old/chronologically gifted**

From National Institute on Aging, August 30, 1994.

BOX 1-1 Gerontology Definitions

- **Centenarian**—a person who has lived to be 100 years of age
- **Gerontology**—the study of the aging process
- **Geriatrician**—a physician who has special, formal postgraduate education in geriatric medicine
- **Geriatrics**—the specialty of geriatric medicine
- **Life expectancy**—the number of years one can be expected to live based on a specific age or year of birth according to statistical probability
- **Life span**—the total number of years that a human is likely to live or has lived
- **Longevity**—living a long time

years," but a person who was age 65 in 1997 had an average life expectancy of 82.6 (AARP & AOA, 1999, p. 1). Those who were age 65 in 1997 had survived childhood and young adult diseases and accidents, thus increasing their life expectancy. Table 1-4 shows statistical projections of life expectancy.

Ask Yourself

Think of your definition of *quality of life*. Can there be quality of life at age 100?

Morbidity and Mortality

Although normal aging does not imply disease, the incidence of chronic diseases increases with increasing age. The most common chronic diseases that occur in the older age group are listed in Table 1-5. Chronic diseases are more common than acute illnesses in the older age group. Chronic diseases refer to those illnesses that last three to six months or more and are usually treatable—but not curable—such as arthritis.

Another major problem in this age group is the prevalence of comorbidity, or the presence of several chronic diseases in one person, which makes treatment and quality of care and life more difficult. Health care services for chronic illnesses are expensive because they are long-term, often needed for months, if not years. For example, rehabilitation after a cerebrovascular accident (CVA) may require physical therapy and speech pathology as well as skilled and custodial nursing care for a year or more. Nurses can have a major role in coordinating comprehensive long-term care. Most older people with chronic conditions are able to function well with relatively minor adaptations and assistance.

The major causes of death in people age 65 and older are not much different from those of other adults, as shown in Table 1-6. The most common types of accidents and injuries resulting in death in older people differ from those of younger adults, however. Younger adults are more likely to die from motor vehicle accidents (MVAs) and work-related injuries, while older people die more often as a result of complications following accidental falls.

TABLE 1-4 Projections of Life Expectancy, 1995 to 2010

	White		Black		Other	
Year	**Male**	**Female**	**Male**	**Female**	**Male**	**Female**
1995	73.6	80.1	64.8	74.5	68.2	76.8
2000	74.2	80.5	64.6	74.7	68.3	77.5
2005	74.7	81.0	64.5	75.0	69.1	78.1
2010	75.5	81.6	65.1	75.5	69.9	78.7

Adapted from Table No. 118, Statistical Abstract of the United States, 1996, Washington, DC: U.S. Government Printing Office.

TABLE 1-5   Most Common Chronic Illnesses in the Older Age Group (1994–1995)

Disease	Percentage of Older Population
• Arthritis	49
• Hypertension	40
• Heart disease	31
• Hearing impairments	28
• Orthopedic impairments	18
• Cataracts	16
• Sinusitis	15
• Diabetes mellitus	13

From A Profile of Older Americans: 1999 *(p. 13), 1999, Washington, DC: American Association of Retired Persons, and the Administration on Aging, U.S. Department of Health and Human Services.*

Other differences in **mortality** relate to heart disease. Whereas younger adults (those less than age 65) have higher rates of myocardial infarctions (MI), older people have more decompensated heart problems such as congestive heart failure (CHF). Some studies have shown that adverse effects of medications complicate 2.43% of hospital admissions (Classen et al., 1997). Considering the fact that older people take more medications than younger adults, this could be a factor in their **morbidity.**

People are living longer as health and medical technology successfully treat the chronic diseases that begin to develop and as there is more emphasis on promotion

TABLE 1-6   Major Causes of Death in Adults Age 65 and Older

Cause	Percent
• Cardiovascular	47
• Cancer	20
• Cerebrovascular accident (CVA)/ stroke	11
• Lung disease	6
• Accident and/or a fall	2

From "Primary and Secondary Prevention Strategies in the Older Adult," by L. Z. Rubenstein & R. Nahas, 1998, Geriatric Nursing, *19(1), pp. 11–18.*

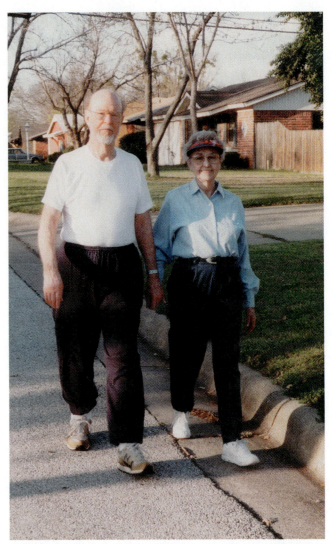

FIGURE 1-2 Today many older adults enjoy healthy, active lifestyles.

of health and wellness such as good nutrition and exercise (Figures 1-2 and 1-3).

Issues and Problems

The major issues and problems that affect the quality of health and life for older people are listed in Table 1-7.

Think About It

What do you think will be the major issues and problems of the baby boomers when they reach age 65 in 2011?

Ageism: Myths and Facts

Unfortunately, there is much misinformation and a lack of accurate facts about the aging process and older

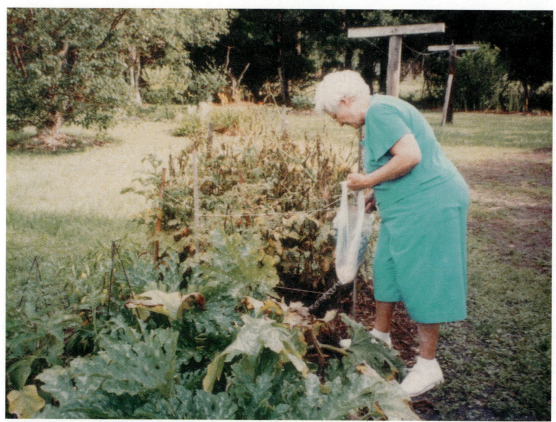

FIGURE 1-3 An active gardener.

people, both in society as a whole and among health care providers (Box 1-2). Ageism in health care can be noted in the following examples:

- A 93-year-old man was told by an orthopedic surgeon that he was too old to have knee replacement surgery for severe osteoarthritis that limited his mobility and usual preferred activities. He eventually had both knees replaced so he could dance and play golf again.

- A 75-year-old woman was told by her physician during her annual physical examination that she did not need a pelvic exam or Pap smear because she had had a hysterectomy. With encouragement she changed physicians.

- An 85-year-old woman was told by her physician that she did not need an annual mammogram. However, the nurse in her senior center encouraged her to get one.

- A physician stated that a 95-year-old woman living independently needed to be in a nursing home after she was raped by a homeless man in her private home. A community group paid for and erected a high fence around her house and the police started to patrol her street more frequently.

Think About It

What kind of examples of ageism have you seen?
How did the older person react?
If you encounter ageism in the future, what will you do about it?

TABLE 1-7   Major Issues and Problems Affecting Older People

- Transportation, both in urban and rural areas
- Safe, adequate, and comfortable housing
- Crime, abuse, and financial exploitation
- Prevalence of **ageism** in society and among health care providers
- Inadequate access to quality health care and long-term care
- Multiple chronic illnesses (comorbidity)
- Inadequate financial resources
- Limited family or friend support (outlive family and friends)
- Isolation, loneliness, and depression

Despite the many statements reflecting ageism, there are greater individual differences among older people than among any other age category. They are not only more mature but also more independent and often more assertive in expressing their thoughts and ideas because they are not subject to peer pressure or employment status. *Senile* is a word that should never be used. Although the term simply means aging, it has come to mean the normal mental deterioration in old age. However, there is no normal mental deterioration in old age.

Myths persist for various reasons. Children and young people growing up today often do not have personal contact with an older family member such as a grandparent. They therefore may feel uncomfortable around older people. Health care providers routinely see only older people who are acutely and/or chronically ill, such as in a hospital or nursing facility. Therefore, if they have not had much direct contact with healthy, happy, active older adults, they may perceive that all older people are like their clients. Also, medical and nursing care of chronic, long-term illnesses may not seem as exciting or as rewarding (especially when the client is not likely to have a rapid recovery) as surgery, delivery, or the newborn nursery. The more one learns about some type of health problem and care, the more one realizes that there is much more to learn. Geriatric health care and education are still somewhat new, even after decades of struggle.

BOX 1-2   Myths about Older Adults

Older people:

- cannot change
- like to live in the past
- cannot learn new information
- are grouchy all the time
- are childish, have a second childhood
- are all cute
- live in nursing homes
- lose interest in life
- are sick most of the time
- become children to their adult children
- have hypertension, arthritis, presbycusis, and urinary incontinence
- are sick, senile, senseless, and sexless

Major Needs of Older Adults

Needs are individualized at all ages based on personal preferences and current physical and mental status. The basic needs of older adults discussed in this chapter include: health care and long-term care, housing, nutrition, safety, transportation, education, employment, finances, and social support.

Health Care and Long-Term Care

The need for comprehensive health care for older adults, including health promotion, wellness strategies, and long-term care, is the major focus of this book.

Housing

When chronic illnesses and/or disabilities occur, independent living may not be possible. There are many more choices now than in previous years when the nursing facility was considered the only alternative to independent living.

The continuum of care and places for that care are illustrated in Table 1-8 and Figure 1-4. Many older people

---

TABLE 1-8   Housing Alternatives for Older Adults

- Private home or apartment (alone or with a family member)
- Mobile home parks (perhaps designed for older people)
- Subsidized low-rent apartment housing (for those with minimal income)
- Share a house (with a friend or family member)
- Retirement center (independent living with some services provided)
- Single room occupancy (SRO) hotel (room and meals)
- Echo home (home or apartment close to an adult child's home)
- Board and care homes (some assistance provided)
- Adult foster care home (live with a nonrelative family or person)
- Assisted living facility (ALF) (in between independent living and institutional care)
- Continuing care retirement community (CCRC) (independent living to skilled care)
- Institutional living (need of skilled nursing care and/or custodial care on a 24-hour basis)

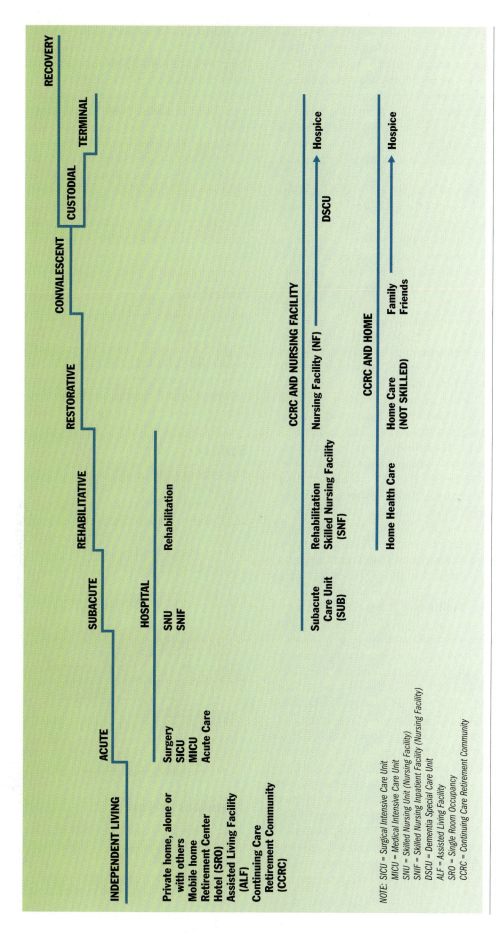

FIGURE 1-4 Continuum of living arrangements and care.

are fortunate to have paid for a home over many years. However, sometimes these homes are in areas of cities where the living environment has changed (perhaps more crime) and/or the home needs repair and upkeep that older residents cannot afford. They may want to move to a different area but not have the financial resources to relocate. Some older couples who like to travel sell their home and plan to spend all of their time in a recreational vehicle (RV), often visiting children and grandchildren throughout the country.

Subsidized low-rent housing in an apartment complex may be the best option for those who qualify for local or federal assistance because of minimal income. If they qualify financially, they pay 30% of their gross income in rent. An increasing number of older people are sharing private homes with nonrelatives for financial and companionship reasons. Retirement centers offer independent living in a protected environment where residents may have the option to pay for specific services such as yard work, housecleaning, and meals. Most such housing arrangements also have a 24-hour emergency alert system that provides a sense of security for residents and their family members.

Another option is a single-room occupancy (SRO) hotel that provides room and meals on a monthly basis, usually for a relatively low fee depending on location and type of hotel. An **echo home** is a small apartment, duplex, or other type of housing that is on the same property as the family home. The older family member lives independently but is still within a short distance of others when needed. Board and care homes provide housing, meals, and other needs such as housekeeping and laundry. Adult foster care homes are used by some older people who need temporary living arrangements. Foster home owners are paid to provide shelter, meals, and other support.

Assisted living facilities (ALFs) are the most recent and fastest expanding type of housing for older adults. ALFs provide personal care such as assistance with bathing, eating, toileting, and supervision of medication self-administration. Such facilities are ideal for older adults in their late 80s, 90s, and 100s who cannot manage at home alone but who do not need to be in a nursing facility. Additional regulation and licensing of these homes are being studied because as people age in place and develop multiple health problems, they often require more physical care than the facility is capable of providing or allowed to provide legally. However, as these facilities need to provide as much independence as possible within a safe and secure environment, there is a question about how much regulation is appropriate. Some people prefer to take a risk to remain independent if they have the mental capacity to make that choice, but "the line between autonomy and need for protection is difficult to draw" (Moncrief, 1998, p. 15).

Continuing care retirement communities (CCRCs) are unique and ideal for those who can afford them (Figure 1-5). These programs provide lifetime care—from independent living to skilled nursing and hospice care, if needed. The person buys into this arrangement with a somewhat high entry fee (for example, $100,000) and then pays a monthly fee for utilities and other services. When home health care or skilled nursing care is needed, that care is available on site, often for an additional fee. Contracts differ among CCRCs.

The last type of housing is institutional living, as may take place first in a **skilled nursing facility (SNF)** and later a **nursing facility (NF)** where custodial care is provided for as long as needed.

Nutrition

One of the most important needs of older adults is adequate, available, and nutritious food based on their age, physical condition, and possible health problems. Lack of adequate nutrition can cause major health problems, prevent recovery from acute illnesses, and cause major decline in many chronic health conditions. For a variety of reasons, older adults are at risk for poor nutrition.

Safety

The importance of safety is relevant when remembering that the fifth leading cause of death among older adults is accidents and/or falls. Decreasing vision, poor balance, dizziness from low blood pressure and/or medications, and environmental factors such as inadequately marked steps, broken furniture, loose rugs, and poorly equipped bath areas are the most common causes. Older people should be helped to function safely in their homes and other places they visit.

> ### *Nursing Tip*
>
> Teach older clients how to prevent falls.
> - Stand up slowly.
> - Wear comfortable, well-fitting shoes.
> - Keep a night light on.
> - Eliminate loose rugs in the house.
> - Have grab bars installed in the tub and by the commode in the bathroom.

Transportation

When asking older adults in the community about their major needs, one of the first ones listed is transportation, both in urban and rural areas. Some older people may not have the financial resources to purchase and/or maintain a personal car or they may have vision and/or hear-

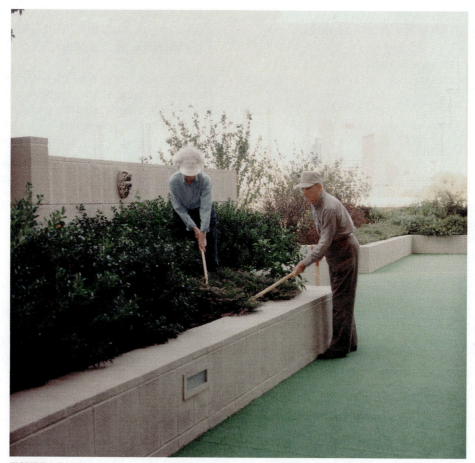

FIGURE 1-5 Active residents in a Continuing Care Retirement Community (CCRC).

ing deficits that make driving hazardous. Rural area residents may have to depend on neighbors, family, or friends for transportation for essential needs, such as visits to the physician and shopping for food. Many urban areas also have inadequate public transportation routes to the suburbs. Some grocery stores and pharmacies deliver, but this service is usually limited to certain geographical areas. One of the advantages of retirement centers, ALFs, and some nursing facilities is that they usually provide transportation for medical appointments and shopping. Some small businesses and individuals provide transportation for older adults for a monthly membership charge and per-use service fee. Transportation is an area for increased community awareness, development, and allocation of municipal and state funds.

Education

Older people continue to want to learn, both formally and informally. Many colleges and universities offer short courses and/or reduced tuition for regular credit courses as well as specially designed courses often taught by older instructors. A program called **Elderhostel** arranges for older people to live on a university or college campus

and take selected courses, usually during the summer. These programs have been offered throughout the country and in Europe so that participants can travel to an area, live on the campus, and attend classes. Local communities also offer workshops and seminars on topics of interest to older people (Boxes 1-3 and 1-4). Many older people can and do want to continue to learn. The simple saying "use it or lose it" refers to the brain as well as to the muscles. An active mind can decrease depression, enhance memory, and give meaning and purpose to existence.

Employment

Some older people prefer and need (for personal and financial reasons) to continue employment, either full- or part-time, beyond the common retirement ages of 62 or 65. Sometimes they continue in work similar to what they had done for years. In other instances, they try something new that they have always wanted to do. Continuing employment in the latter years fills many needs (Box 1-5).

In 2000, Congress eliminated the Social Security penalty for people age 65 to 69 who continue to work.

BOX 1-3   Educational Program about Social Security Benefits

What you need to know:

- How Social Security works

- Understanding SSI and Medicare

- Future of Social Security

Date: Thursday
Time: 3:00–4:30 PM
Place: First United Methodist Church
Cost: Free
Presenter: Field Representative, Social Security
               Administration

Please share this information with anyone who might be interested. Thank you for your assistance in sharing this educational opportunity.

BOX 1-4   A Seminar for Older Adults on Spirituality and Aging

Join us for a seminar—*"At Last, God's Best!"*—to learn more about spiritual gifts in later life and ways to develop a deep and personal relationship with God. A *gerontologist* will lead the seminar on spirituality and aging.

In this seminar, the speaker will explore with us ways to answer questions about spiritual gifts:

- Are you aware of the gifts you have received over the course of your lifetime?

- Do you realize also that you are a gift and a source of new gifts to others?

- Do you recognize the ways in which the gifts you have received and the gifts that you have given have shaped your life?

Bring your questions to the seminar to share as we discover more about ourselves, our spiritual gifts, and our relationship with God.

As of January 1, 2000, Social Security recipients age 65 through 69 can earn as much as they wish and still receive their full Social Security benefits. Before that legislation was passed, workers age 65 through 69 had $1.00 deducted from their Social Security benefit for every $3.00 they made over a set amount. This legislation encourages more older adults to continue working after age 65.

Finances

Adequate finances to meet needs and provide a comfortable lifestyle are essential, especially to provide adequate housing, nutrition, and health care. Sources of income after retirement from full-time work come from the following: employer pension, Social Security, full-time or part-time employment, savings, and investments. Unfortunately, for many older people Social Security is the primary source, if not the only source of income. The Social Security system has been under much scrutiny in recent years. The goal is for it to continue to be available to future generations, especially the **baby boomers** (those born between 1946 and 1964) who will become eligible for Social Security benefits beginning in 2011.

Social Support

One of the most important needs of older adults is the need for social support from others such as family, friends, neighbors, church members, and other individuals in the person's life. A person needs to have contact with others to call for help when needs arise. One of the most important factors in successful aging is a strong support system. It is helpful when older people develop

friendships with younger people because as one reaches the oldest age group (85 and older), peers such as one's spouse, friends, and even children may die first (Hogstel, Smith, & Reckling, 2000).

The Aging Network

Community resources available for older adults have been expanding over many years. The **Older Americans Act (OAA)** of 1965, as amended, has guided and governed many of the nation's efforts to respond to the problems of and enhance the opportunities for a rapidly growing population of older Americans. The OAA, through the federal **Administration on Aging (AOA)** and a network of state, area, and local agencies, promotes economic and personal independence for older persons (Figure 1-6).

Although many people point to the first White House Conference on Aging in 1961 as the catalyst that brought together the necessary congressional forces to enact the OAA, the struggle began before then. For a number of years prior to 1961, educators, social scientists, human service providers, and special interest groups representing the older population had been stressing the need for a focal point for older adults' concerns at the national level. This national concern, plus the favorable climate for social legislative action during the Great Society years of Lyndon B. Johnson's presidency, led to the passage into law of the OAA of 1965.

BOX 1-5 **Advantages of Continued Employment in Later Years**

- Additional income
- Health insurance coverage (e.g., benefits not covered by Medicare)
- Mental stimulation
- Physical activity
- Personal satisfaction
- Contact with peers, colleagues
- Sense of purpose
- New interests, friends, activities

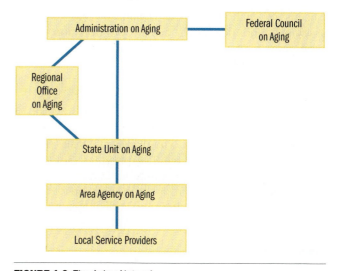

FIGURE 1-6 The Aging Network.

The OAA made major strides towards organizing and establishing programs and services for many older people across the country. It designated a special office—the Administration on Aging, within what is now the federal Department of Health and Human Services—to be the agency through which concerns of older Americans were to be addressed.

Some older people had problems that could not be solved solely by increases in Social Society benefits and payments for health care. Some of them needed safe, reliable transportation to the grocery store or medical facilities; some needed more nutritious diets; some had lost their friends and family and needed companions and advisors; and some older people needed information and motivation to maintain active, healthy lifestyles. Through the Aging Network, gerontologists, social service providers, planners, and others interested in older people have taken action to alleviate these and similar problems. The OAA programs offer services that can be of specific use to older people in a variety of settings.

 OAA programs are not based on income and, therefore, are not welfare programs. Under Title III of the OAA, programs are available to persons age 60 or older without regard to income. Individuals cannot be refused service based on their inability or unwillingness to pay a fee but are encouraged to contribute toward the cost of services. Depending on the service, some services, such as fitness classes, may request voluntary contributions, while others, such as home health care services, may rely on a sliding contribution scale to encourage appropriate levels of participant cost-sharing.

The OAA is reauthorized periodically. With each amendment comes new areas of emphasis. The act was amended in 1991, but Congress did not develop an amendment that could pass both the House and the Senate. Therefore, it was 1992 before the amendment was finalized. Reauthorization issues that continue to be debated include the need for additional levels of funding, outreach efforts to minority and dependent older people, the need for more local flexibility to meet local needs, more appropriate funding formulas, and the role of area agencies on aging in providing direct services such as information and referral.

The uniqueness of the Aging Network is that it provides for a nationwide network of locally administered and coordinated aging services. Although the specific services may vary, the generic services—information and referral, **case management,** senior centers, nutrition services including congregate and home-delivered meals, home health care services, legal services, and nursing home ombudsmen programs—should be available in most regions throughout the country. To nurses and social workers one value of this network is in being able to refer families and those caring for older relatives to similar services in other areas of the country.

Nursing Tip

Find out about the Aging Network in your community. Find out what services are available and lacking. Find out where to call to find needed resources and services for your clients.

Structure

The AOA is the heart of the federal government's attempt to formulate policy and influence and coordinate the delivery of services to older people across the country. The early programs of services to the older citizens of each state were organized with technical assistance and depended heavily on donations from local sources to meet the needs that have outstripped federal funding increases.

The needs of those older people requiring special diets have not been overlooked. Nutrition sites are required to provide low-cholesterol meals, low-salt or salt-free meals, soft diets, and the like, both at the congregate site and in the home-delivered meals service. From the inception of the nutrition program, participants have been given the opportunity to contribute to the cost of the meals. Funds from participants must go back into the program to provide for additional meals.

Services

Services for older adults provided for by the OAA cover many of the needs previously identified in this chapter through the local **Area Agency on Aging (AAA).** The most important services are:

- Nutrition at congregate sites (senior centers, for example) and home-delivered meals

- Transportation of older adults to senior centers and to medical or social service appointments

- Information and assistance related to services available in the community

- Case management to assess, plan, and meet the need for in-home services

- In-home services such as homemaker, home health aide, and chore services; programs not usually covered by Medicare

- Benefits counseling and education regarding assistance with financial and other issues such as Medicare, **Medicaid,** and **managed care**

- Long-term care ombudsman programs that provide staff and volunteer advocates for residents in nursing facilities and assisted living facilities

- Prevention of elder abuse, neglect, and exploitation

- Preventive health services

- Family caregiving education and support programs

National Institute on Aging (NIA)

The **National Institute on Aging (NIA)** was established in 1974. It conducts research on biomedical, social, and behavioral aspects of aging at its Gerontology Research Center. It also supports research by others at universities and laboratories across the United States. It has a limited publications program but does not engage in support of service delivery.

Veterans Affairs

The Department of Veterans Affairs (VA) is responsible for meeting the health, human services, and income maintenance needs of eligible veterans. The VA's health care system includes acute medical, surgical, and psychiatric inpatient and outpatient care; extended hospital, nursing home, and custodial care; noninstitutional extended care; and a range of special programs and professional services for older veterans in both inpatient and outpatient settings. Disability and survivor benefits, such as pension, compensation, and dependency, administered by the Department of Veterans Affairs provide all or part of the income for certain persons age 65 or older.

National Organizations

There are nongovernmental groups that are also excellent sources of education and support for aging issues. Two of these are the American Association of Retired Persons (AARP) and the National Council on the Aging (NCOA).

American Association of Retired Persons (AARP)

The **American Association of Retired Persons (AARP)** is the nation's leading and most powerful organization for people aged 50 and older. The name is somewhat misleading because many people who are employed full time or part time are members. The annual membership dues are very nominal, so it is available to almost anyone in that age group who has an interest in aging activities. It is a nonprofit, nonpartisan membership organization whose primary goal is to help older people live with independence, dignity, and purpose. In support of that goal, AARP offers a wide range of services, programs, volunteer opportunities, and benefits to its members. Millions of people are helped each year through its free or low-cost programs such as Tax-Aide (tax counseling) and the "55 Alive" driver's training program. The association publishes and gives away millions of informational publications on health, consumer, and financial issues.

AARP has about 32 million members, which represents about half of all Americans age 50 and older. One-third of the members work full time or part time. The membership includes about 300,000 active volunteers. Many members are active in local chapters.

AARP's motto is: "To serve, not to be served," and its vision statement is: "AARP excels as a dynamic presence in every community, shaping and enriching the experience of aging for each member and for society."

AARP's legislative advocacy grows out of the membership's desire to help create an economically strong and healthy nation. The legislative agenda, policies, and activities are determined by the volunteers who serve on its National Legislative Council and Board of Directors. The Council bases its policy positions on suggestions from AARP members across the country. Advocacy is carried out on the state level by the State Legislative Committee and in each congressional district by AARP/VOTE volunteers.

The members of AARP have a deep interest in many of the issues facing the country. Foremost is the commitment to improve the nation's health care system—especially Medicare—and to maintain strong, effective Social Security, retirement, and pension programs. These programs assist older Americans to live independently and with dignity. The more that older people are able to live independently, the less they need financial support from their children and grandchildren. This is important because in most cases, the caregivers for dependent older people are their adult children. The financial and emotional toll of caregiving on those adult children directly affects their ability to provide for themselves and their own retirement as well as their own children.

AARP is concerned about the future of young people and families. The members are committed to building a more secure, purposeful, independent life for the young people today who will be the older people of tomorrow. AARP understands the deep economic and social interdependence of the generations. Ensuring access to health care, containing medical costs, and making long-term care affordable for the chronically ill all serve to help people, regardless of age. The members are sensitive to the needs of other generations and work in support of children's funding priorities such as eliminating child poverty and improving education.

The members of AARP come from different political parties and the association is totally nonpartisan. AARP neither supports nor opposes candidates for public office, nor does it contribute financial aid to any candidate or party at any level of government. It does not target candidates for defeat.

AARP volunteers and employees are committed to attracting, developing, and maintaining a volunteer force that reflects diversity in the areas of governance, management, and service. AARP regards volunteer diversity as including, but not limited to, differences of age, gender, race, sexual orientation, national and ethnic origins, religion, economic status, and physical and mental ability.

Other programs and services include educational opportunities, a monthly newspaper and magazine, chapters for participation at the local level, mail-order pharmacy services, and various products of companies (such as health, life, and auto insurance) that are evaluated for quality and marketed through AARP membership. They provide research and special project grants through the Andrus Foundation and are very active in advocating for national and state legislation that will improve the health and life of older people (for example, Medicare, Social Security, and nursing facility care). According to Mary Scott, a member of the National Legislative Council of the AARP, "The AARP is very influential in legislation because of the large number of active voters they represent" (personal communication, March, 1998).

The National Council on the Aging (NCOA)

The **National Council on the Aging (NCOA)** is a nonprofit, membership-driven organization for professionals and volunteers. It is a national resource for information, technical assistance, training, and research in the field of aging. Some of their activities and services include:

- maintaining a national information center related to the field of aging

- planning conferences on aging issues

- conducting research on the aging process

- supporting demonstration programs related to aging

- providing a library of materials related to the psychological, economic, and social aspects of aging

(NIA, 1993, pp. 148–149)

Summary

Nurses caring for older people in all settings need to have a broad view of aging, a basic understanding of the total process of aging, the special needs and problems of older people, and the national and community resources available to meet their needs. Older people have different needs and problems than other age groups. A 50-year-old person usually has much different needs than a 100-year-old. With an increasing population of people age 85 and older, the needs of this group will increase tremendously in this century. Will their needs be different? Will the current local, state, and national resources be able to meet those needs? All health care providers, including nurses, need to look to the future and begin to determine how those needs can best be met.

Review Questions and Activities

1. What was the percentage of the population age 65 and older in 2000?

2. Which state has the greatest percentage of people age 65 and older?

3. What is the most common chronic disease in older people?

4. What is the most common type of accidental injury in older people?

5. In what type of housing do most people age 65 and older live?

6. Why is transportation a problem for older people?

7. What are some advantages of continued employment in the later years?

8. What is the most common source of income for older people who are retired from full-time employment?

9. What are major functions of the American Association of Retired Persons and the National Council on Aging?

10. What kinds of programs and services are funded by the Older Americans Act?

References

American Association of Retired Persons (AARP) & the Administration on Aging (AOA). (1999). *A profile of older Americans: 1999.* Washington, DC: U.S. Dept. of Health and Human Services.

Atchley, R. C. (1997). *Social forces and aging* (8th ed.). Belmont, CA: Wadsworth.

Classen, D. C., Pestotnik, S. L., Evans, R. S., et al. (1997). Adverse drug events in hospitalized patients. *Journal of the American Medical Association, 277* (4), 301–306.

Hogstel, M. O., Smith, H. N., & Reckling, D. (2000). *Eldercare/Faith in action program* (5th ed.). Fort Worth, TX: Tarrant Area Community of Churches.

McIver, D. (1998). Senior housing—The next millennium. *Texas Journal on Aging, 1*(1): 18–22.

Moncrief, M. (1998). Regulatory issues with assisted living. *Texas Journal on Aging, 1*(1): 14–17.

National Institute on Aging (NIA). (1993). *Resource directory for older people.* Bethesda, MD: U.S. Dept. of Health and Human Services.

Rubenstein, L. Z., & Nahas, R. (1998). Primary and secondary prevention strategies in the older adult. *Geriatric Nursing, 19*(1): 11–18.

Resources

Administration on Aging: `http://www.aoa.dhhs.gov`

American Association of Retired Persons: `http://www.aarp.org`

White River Area Agency on Aging: `http://www.wraaa.com`

CHAPTER 2

Gerontological Nursing

Mary S. Harper, PhD, RN, FAAN
Mildred O. Hogstel, PhD, RN, C

COMPETENCIES

After completing this chapter, the reader should be able to:

- *Provide an overview of the history of gerontological nursing.*
- *Discuss the processes, procedures, standards, and activities of gerontological nurses.*
- *Discuss some of the principles and techniques of gerontological nursing that are useful to all nurses caring for older adults whether in an institution or community-based program.*
- *Analyze the roles of the nurse or other health care provider in enhancing the quality of life for older adults by teaching informal family caregivers.*
- *Discuss the interrelatedness of behavioral and physical care when caring for older adults.*
- *Evaluate the impact of illiteracy, poverty, and other demographic variables on successful aging.*
- *Analyze information that may serve as a reference for researchers and health care providers who provide culturally sensitive care to older adults.*
- *Identify information essential for health care providers to become active members of the interdisciplinary team.*

MAKING THE CONNECTION

Refer to the following chapters to increase your understanding of gerontological nursing:

Historical Development

Gerontological nursing is slowly gaining momentum in the profession of nursing (Figure 2-1). It has had more than its share of challenges and barriers, as manifested by the absence of gerontological content in nursing education programs and the lack of nurse faculty with advanced education in gerontological nursing. This status is difficult to accept when one thinks that over half of the adults in the health care system are over 50 years of age. As early as 1904, the *American Journal of Nursing* published an article on old age and disease. However, it was not until 1966 that the **American Nurses Association (ANA)** formed a Division of Geriatric Nursing and established the appropriate gerontological nursing advisory committee. In 1976, ANA's Gerontological Nursing Division first developed and published Standards for Gerontological Nursing Practice.

In the nursing literature, the terms *geriatric nursing, gerontological nursing,* and *gerontic nursing* are used interchangeably; however, **geriatric nursing** relates more to the treatment of older people with health problems, **gerontological nursing** is a broader term that includes health promotion, education, and disease prevention, and **gerontic nursing** is a combination term from *geriatric* and *gerontological* that encompasses both the health problems and holistic aspects of older adult nursing care.

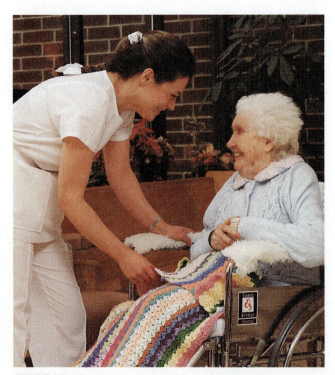

FIGURE 2-1   Care of the older adult is gaining momentum in the nursing profession.

Educational Programs

In the mid 1970s, postbaccalaureate programs were developed in gerontological nursing when graduate and certificate programs were offered by such universities as Cornell (PRIME Geriatric Nursing training program), the University of Colorado, the State University of New York, and Duke University (graduate geriatric nurse practitioner program). The Division of Nursing of the United States Public Health Service (USPHS) funded most of these programs. In fact, 141 advanced nurse education programs were funded at the cost of $17 million under Title VIII of the United States Public Health Service Act (PHSA). In 1993 there were nearly 50,000 nurse practitioners. More than half of these were certified but only 1,572 were certified as **gerontological nurse practitioners (GNPs).** Although there were 58,000 clinical nurse specialists (CNSs), only 493 of them were certified as **gerontological clinical nurse specialists (GCNSs)** (USDHHS, 1993).

In 1998, 3,469 nurses became certified as gerontological nurses, 55 became certified as gerontological clinical nurse specialists, and 332 became certified as gerontological nurse practitioners. ("Passing Scores and Rates," 1999, p. 5.). Requirements for **certification** vary depending on the specialty. A national examination in the area of specialty is required for initial certification (personal communication, ANCC, June 23, 2000). Recertification by the **American Nurses Credentialing Center (ANCC)** requires 1,500 clinical hours of nursing practice in gerontological nursing over the previous five-year period and satisfactory completion of a national examination or five options of continuing education requirements in that specialty (Figure 2-2) (ANCC, 1999). Gerontological nurses can be certified as generalists, clinical nurse specialists, or nurse practitioners. The first **geropsychiatric nursing** program was offered at the Frances Payne Bolton School of Nursing at Case Western Reserve University through a special grant from the **National Institute of Mental Health (NIMH).**

Specialty Roles

Gerontological nursing has made substantial progress in the 34 years since ANA formally recognized it as a specialty with the need for special knowledge and practices in the care of older Americans. In 1987, the ANA designated two categories for gerontological nursing practice: generalist or specialist. The specialist requires a minimum of a master's degree in gerontological nursing (ANA, 1987). The generalist functions in a variety of settings (institutional and community) and utilizes the resources and experience of the specialist. Gerontological nurses function as health care providers, supervi-

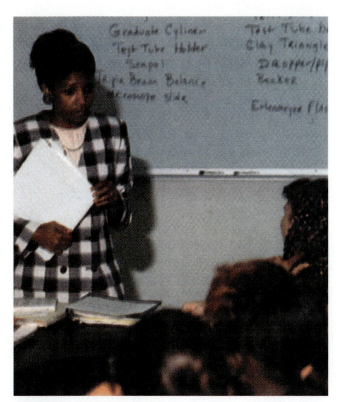

FIGURE 2-2 Nursing students.

in the home and community-based programs as well as in institutions. Roles of the NP include: teaching, conducting/participating in clinical research, private practice, practice with physician groups, and functioning as director of nursing in a skilled nursing facility. The nurse may function as a clinician. There are over 31 nurse-managed community clinics supported by the Division of Nursing in the United States Public Health Service. The NP performs physicals, takes histories for all residents in long-term care facilities or clinics, and prescribes specific types of medications if allowed by state law. A 1986 **Office of Technology Assessment (OTA)** study determined that nurse practitioners provided quality care equivalent to that provided by physicians. In the areas of communication and preventive care, NPs were judged more adept than physicians (Knopp, 1998). Another study found that nursing facility administrators and medical directors have positive attitudes toward nurse practitioners in that they provide timely access to medical services and continual monitoring of the clients and care plans (Knopp, 1998).

The Primary Care Health Practitioner Incentive Act, part of the Balanced Budget Act (BBA) of 1997, enabled direct payment by the Medicare program for services provided by nurse practitioners (NPs) and clinical nurse specialists (CNSs) in all practice settings (Figure 2-3).

sors, client/family educators, health promoters, and in disease management and prevention. They also provide guidance in self-care, participate in policy making and implementation, as well as collaborate in research.

Although the USPHS Division of Nursing has spent $67 million on professional traineeships for gerontological nurse practitioners (GNPs) and baccalaureate nursing graduates since 1989, many hospitals do not employ gerontological nursing specialists. There are 17,000 Medicare and Medicaid certified nursing facilities in the United States, but fewer than 70 certified nurse practitioners and/or specialists are employed in these facilities (HRSA, 1991). Twenty years ago, Senator Daniel K. Inouye recommended that every nursing facility with over 100 beds should employ a geriatric nurse practitioner (Institute of Medicine, 1983). Few hospitals have a gerontological clinical nurse specialist and/or gerontological nurse practitioner on their staffs. Gerontology specialists are beginning to be employed in Primary Health Care Centers, sometimes owned by hospital systems, in the community.

Nurse Practitioners (NPs)

To receive national certification today, clinical nurse specialists and nurse practitioners must have baccalaureate and master's degrees in nursing. There are now nearly 50,000 nurse practitioners. With this number of NPs, older people should have greater access to health care

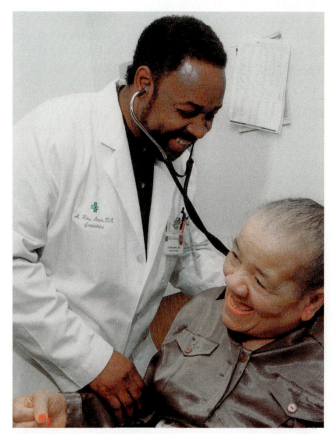

FIGURE 2-3 GNP in clinical setting.

TABLE 2-1 Barriers to Utilizing Nurse Practitioners

- *Legal.* State law may impose restrictions on the scope of practice and prescription of medications, especially controlled substances.
- *Financial.* Public and private third-party payers may not reimburse services performed by NPs (for example, commercial health maintenance organizations).
- *Professional.* NPs may be prohibited from working in hospitals and managed care organizations or may be unable to purchase malpractice insurance. Barriers may arise when physicians' competition restricts NP practice.

Prior to this legislation, NPs could only be reimbursed for services provided in rural areas. This historical policy change gives high visibility to nurses and provides more access to health services for older adults (Buerhaus, 1998; Grzeczkowski & Knapp, 1998). Some of the barriers to utilizing the NP are listed in Table 2-1.

Organizations

There are several national nursing organizations specifically for gerontological nurses. The **National Gerontological Nursing Association (NGNA)** was founded in 1984 and has 1,676 active members (NGNA, personal communication, August 24, 1999). The NGNA is open to all registered nurses that are interested in nursing care of older adults. It meets annually at various sites and offers educational programs as well as provides nurses an opportunity to share their research with others. Members receive a bimonthly newsletter. Call 1-800-723-0560 for more information.

The **National Conference of the Gerontological Nurse Practitioners (NCGNP)** was founded in 1981 and is specifically for gerontological nurse practitioners. They also have an annual conference with presentation of research and other educational programs as well as a quarterly newsletter. A goal is to be active in legislative efforts that affect their practice and the health care of older people. Call 1-800-268-9678 for more details about this organization.

Standards

Nursing

The American Nurses Association first published the standards for gerontological nursing in 1976 with revi-

TABLE 2-2 Standards of Clinical Gerontological Nursing Care

- Standard I: *Assessment.* The gerontological nurse collects client health data.
- Standard II: *Diagnosis.* The gerontological nurse analyzes the assessment data in determining diagnosis.
- Standard III: *Outcome Identification.* The gerontological nurse identifies expected outcomes individualized to the client.
- Standard IV: *Planning.* The gerontological nurse develops a plan of care that prescribes interventions to attain expected outcomes.
- Standard V: *Implementation.* The gerontological nurse implements the interventions identified in the care plan.
- Standard VI: *Evaluation.* The gerontological nurse evaluates the aging person's progress toward attainment of expected outcomes.

From Scope and Standards of Gerontological Nursing Practice *(pp. 11–18), by American Nurses Association, 1995, Washington, DC: Author. Copyright 1995 by American Nurses Publishing, American Nurses Foundation/American Nurses' Association. Reprinted with permission.*

sions in 1987 and 1995. See Tables 2-2 and 2-3 for a list of the most recent (1995) categories of standards.

Unfortunately, some of the prevailing standards and practices of health care for older people in the United States are based on an inadequate understanding of the normal aging process and the care needs of older adults. Problems regarding high-quality health care for this age group are apparent in acute care, community-based, and long-term care settings. The U.S. health care system is currently focused on institutional acute care, reimbursement, length of stay, and financial savings. However, enhancement of the quality of life, health and wellness, maintenance of independence, and a sense of worth and usefulness, especially for older people, are beginning to be more highly valued.

Federal Programs

There are federal and state regulations governing the qualifications and continuing education for licensed nurses and nurse aides in nursing facilities (NFs). The staff and care in nursing facilities are guided by the **Omnibus Budget Reconciliation Act of 1987 (OBRA).** OBRA 1987 was federal legislation that mandated changes that improved the quality of care in nursing facilities.

TABLE 2-3 Standards of Professional Gerontological Nursing Performance

- Standard I: *Quality of Care.* The gerontological nurse systematically evaluates the quality of care and effectiveness of nursing practice.
- Standard II: *Performance Appraisal.* The gerontological nurse evaluates his or her own nursing practice in relation to professional standards and relevant statutes and regulations.
- Standard III: *Education.* The gerontological nurse acquires and maintains current knowledge in nursing practice.
- Standard IV: *Collegiality.* The gerontological nurse contributes to the professional development of peers, colleagues, and others.
- Standard V: *Ethics.* The gerontological nurse's decisions and actions on behalf of clients are determined in an ethical manner.
- Standard VI: *Collaboration.* The gerontological nurse collaborates with the aging person, significant others, and health care providers in providing client care.
- Standard VII: *Research.* The gerontological nurse uses research findings in practice.
- Standard VIII: *Resource Utilization.* The gerontological nurse considers factors related to safety, effectiveness, and cost in planning and delivering client care.

From *Scope and Standards of Gerontological Nursing Practice (pp. 19–26)*, by American Nurses Association, 1995, Washington, DC: Author. Copyright 1995 by American Nurses Publishing, American Nurses Foundation/American Nurses' Association. Reprinted with permission.

TABLE 2-4 Sections of the Older Americans Act (OAA)

Title I. Declaration of Objectives: Definitions
Title II. Administration on Aging
Title III. Grants for State and Community Programs on Aging
Title IV. Training, Research, and Discretionary Projects and Programs
Title V. Community Service Employment for Older Americans
Title VI. Grants for Native Americans
Title VII. Elder Rights (Ombudsman)

The **Older Americans Act (OAA)** was first passed in 1965 and subsequently has been amended during reauthorization. In its current version, the act includes the sections found in Table 2-4. Medicare and Medicaid, which began as part of the OAA of 1965, are federal programs that help to finance and regulate health care and social services of older adults.

Case Management and Teaching

The gerontological nurse has a major and sometimes difficult role in helping older clients and their families to negotiate through the current health care delivery system in the United States. The older client may require specialized care in a variety of settings over months and perhaps years. Whether a clinical nurse specialist or nurse practitioner, the gerontological nurse—frequently functioning as a **case manager** who understands the physical and psychosocial needs involved as well as the best community resources to meet those needs—can be of enormous value to the client and family. Family members still provide most of the **long-term care (LTC)** needed by older relatives. The caregiver may be a long-distance caregiver or a primary day-to-day caregiver. There are 22 million such caregivers in the United States, which means that one in four adults are caregivers.

The typical caregiver is a woman between the ages of 50 and 78 who is married, has a high school education, and is employed full-time ("Who's Taking Care," 1997). The caregiver may have two parents and probably has abandoned many of her social roles with her immediate family. Decreased self-esteem, high stress levels, and other multiple roles of the primary caregiver are major concerns (Penning, 1998). In a study of sons as caregivers, more help was needed in planning and organizing the household chores and care (Harris, 1998). The sons' ages ranged from 24 to 46. The results showed that the sons accepted the caregiver role as a duty and struggled to cope. In a study of minority caregivers, the black caregiver spent 20.6 hours per week caregiving and was older—50 to 80 years old—than the typical Caucasian caregiver ("Who's Taking Care," 1998).

Older clients have a short length of stay in the hospital and are discharged sicker and quicker. In one study, it was revealed that less than half of the 264 clients in the study received any discharge planning or were offered any personal assistance in care after discharge (Bowman, Rose, & Kresevic, 1998).

In counseling and conferencing with the caregiver as part of discharge planning, the nurse should be aware of earlier parental issues. There may be times when the older adult was not a responsible and supportive parent. There are caregivers that do not accept their roles in

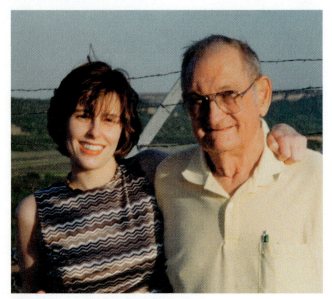

FIGURE 2-4   Older adult with daughter.

Mental and Behavioral Health Care

Mental health disorders are a particular challenge to gerontological nurses. The most common problem is depression, which is often not diagnosed. Studies of residents in nursing facilities have found that 30% to 45% of that population probably have some degree of depression (Parmelee, 1992; Kelsey, 1998).

The Mental Health Statistics Improvement Program (MHSIP) has developed minimum data set elements in three categories that should be collected on older adults (Manderscheid & Henderson, 1995). There is a co-occurrence of depression with heart disease. In coronary heart disease clients with a history of myocardial infarction (heart attack), the prevalence of various forms of depression is estimated from 40 to 65% (NIMH, 1997).

Older people frequently present their illness in nonspecific or altered presentation. Frequent presentation of illness includes failure to eat or drink, despair/depression, weight loss, and/or disturbance of gait. Some will have pneumonia without an elevated temperature or white blood cell count and will appear confused (Ham & Sloan, 1997). A common symptom of dehydration is confusion (Harper, 1991). Diagnosis, therefore, is often difficult and some conditions, especially mental illness, go untreated (Kelsey, 1998). Without adequate education, some health care providers wrongly assume that the presenting symptoms are a part of the normal aging process (Colenda, Banazak, & Mickus, 1998).

care of a person who was an irresponsible and nonsupportive parent. Therefore, earlier parental transfer of emotions must be considered (Henretta, Hill, Li, Saldo, & Wolf, 1997). It is the responsibility of the gerontological nurse to plan a series of conferences with the client and significant members of the family to prepare the older person for the best setting and highest quality of care at an affordable cost. The nurse should work closely with a variety of other health care providers in an interdisciplinary manner to provide the specific types of services needed for that client and family (Figure 2-4).

Special Issues

Rationing of Health Care

Another societal problem regarding health care for the older population concerns the possibility of rationing certain services and resources through definitions, legislation, policies, copayments, limitations on the number of days or visits, length of stay in the hospital, and determination of medical necessity. For example, is there or should there be an age limit for dialysis; heart, liver, and kidney transplants (as there is in some countries); or even hip or knee replacements?

CLINICAL ALERT

A thorough and complete assessment should be performed when there is *any* change in a client's physical or mental condition, recognizing that the typical signs and symptoms for many problems such as an infection may not be present.

Minority Older Adults

There is a higher incidence of mortality among minorities than among Caucasians. "Blacks get sick, stay sick, and die sooner than whites" (Meckler, 1998, G-13). In many instances the disease has more to do with lifestyle and/or sociodemographics than with pathology. Diabetes preva-

Research Focus

Citation:

Schoenbaum, M., & Waidmann, T. (1997). Race, socioeconomic status, and health: Accounting for race differences in health. *The Journals of Gerontology,* 52B, 61–73.

Purpose:

To study differences in the chronic conditions and functional limitations between black and Caucasian adults age 70 and older.

Methods:

Self-reports of health and socioeconomic status (SES) of nonHispanic whites and nonHispanic black subjects age 70 and older. Data from the Asset and Health Dynamics Among the Oldest Old (AHEAD) study were used.

Findings:

Socioeconomic factors affect many of the differences in health status, but not all. Low SES and being black do not alone cause poor health.

Implications:

Further research and public policy should focus on lack or degree of wealth, education, and other SES measures that could affect health status.

Think About It

What are some of the issues and problems specific to the nursing care of older minority groups that need to be studied? What difficulties do you anticipate, if any, in conducting research with minority groups?

lence is 70% higher in black and Hispanic individuals than in Caucasians. The death rate of heart disease in blacks is 40% higher than it is in Caucasians, blacks die of strokes 50% more than Caucasians, and blacks die of cancer 35% more than whites. Vietnamese women have more cervical cancer and American Indians have more diabetes than whites (Meckler, 1998, G-13). The fastest growing groups in the United States are minorities, and they are aging also. This phenomenon must be considered in planning sites and types of care. Also, more research on health status and care of these groups is needed, especially identification of the differences among these groups. Are these differences caused by lifestyle, diet, type or lack of adequate health care, economic status, educational levels, or biological differences?

Future Projections and Visions

By 2030, the projected need for full-time gerontological nurses in all settings is expected to reach 1.1 million. A 1989 study conducted by the American Academy of Nurse Practitioners revealed that 79% of the family nurse practi-

tioners (FNPs), 78% of adult nurse practitioners (ANPs), 99% of gerontological nurse practitioners (GNPs), and 42% of women's health nurse practitioners (WHNPs) cared for clients 65 years of age and older (Select Committee, 1993). These and other data (Klein, 1995) clearly point to the need for increasing the number of nurses with the knowledge and skills needed to provide quality primary health and chronic health care for older adults.

Presently most of the direct nursing care in long-term care settings is provided by nurse aides or technicians of various types and licensed vocational/practical nurses with minimal supervision. Clients in a Medicare-certified skilled nursing facility (SNF) receive 254.73 minutes of nursing care per day (68.63 minutes from an RN; 43.59 minutes from an LPN, and 142.52 minutes from nursing aides) (Mohler, 1998). Therefore, gerontological nurses have a major responsibility to supervise and monitor those personnel to ensure that all older clients receive quality care.

The field of gerontology has been preoccupied with loss; with studies of disability, chronic disease, nursing facility admission, long-term care, and medication use. There has been neglect of the positive aspects of aging and the factors that permit older people to continue to function well despite the changes of aging. The most exciting, most optimistic, and most challenging role for nurses is to teach older adults about things that are modifiable. It is never too late to change behaviors (for example, smoking and diet) and to improve health status and quality of life for the older population. That is the role of the gerontological nurse.

Gerontological nurses also must become partners in outcomes research. Health outcomes research is research that studies the end results of the structure and processes of health care on the health and well-being of the client population. Health outcomes in gerontological nursing include specific measures that focus on:

- clinical signs or symptoms (physiological, biological, psychological),
- well-being or mental functioning,
- physical, cognitive, and social functioning,
- satisfaction with care,
- health related quality of life,
- cost and appropriate use of resources, and
- impact of ethnicity, culture, race, and poverty (Feasley, 1998).

BOX 2-1   Suggestions for In-Service Education for Staff

- Safety factors in ambulating and transferring clients using walkers, canes, and wheelchairs

- Communication techniques, including appropriate terminology to use

- The normal aging process

- Common physical and psychological changes with related nursing interventions (for example, skin and musculoskeletal system)

- Ethical and legal issues

- Signs of physical and psychological abuse and neglect and how to report such findings

The Advocacy Role

All nurses who care for older adults in any setting need to be knowledgeable about the specific differences in the diagnosis, treatment, and care of older clients. It is hoped that more and more nurses will seek additional formal education in this specialty and share that knowl-

Nursing Tip

Suggest and encourage your employer to provide regular inservice education on topics that are important in providing quality nursing care to older patients in your institution.

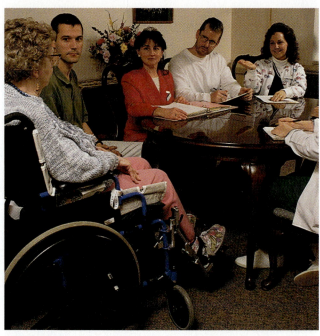

FIGURE 2-5   Nurses need to advocate for their older clients.

edge with other staff in the work setting. If additional formal education is not possible, there are many topics for possible in-service education for staff (Box 2-1).

Nurses need to advocate for quality care for their clients with other professional and technical staff who may not be aware of some of the complexities of geriatric care. Nurses also should become aware of the broad range of community agencies and services that their older clients and their families might need after discharge, especially when leaving an acute care facility (Figures 2-5 and 2-6).

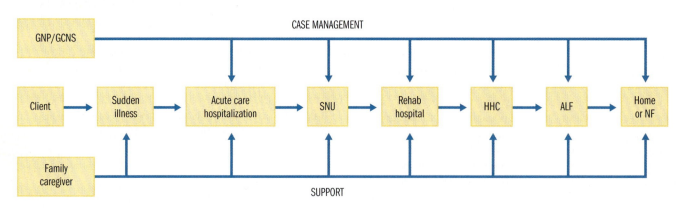

Note:

ALF	Assisted living facility
GCNS	Gerontological clinical nurse specialist
GNP	Gerontological nurse practitioner
HHC	Home health care
NF	Nursing facility (home)
SNU	Skilled nursing unit (in the hospital)

FIGURE 2-6   The gerontological nurse case manager helps the client and family negotiate the continuum of care.

Summary

Gerontological nursing has made progress in the past 30 years. It is essential that all nursing education programs at all levels of preparation of nurses and other health care providers include curricula content in the care of older adults in institutional and noninstitutional settings. Because most of the care provided to older adults is given by informal/family caregivers in the community, it is essential that nurses provide education, support, guidance, and supervision to clients as well as to their informal caregivers. As the health care delivery system in the United States moves to focus on quality of health care through outcomes research, gerontological nurses need to be actively involved in the interdisciplinary care of older adults in all settings.

Review Questions and Activities

1. Why has gerontological nursing as a specialized field of study been slow to develop?

2. Name three types of national certification in the field of gerontological nursing.

3. What are the purposes of national nursing standards for gerontological nurses?

4. What are some of the programs covered in the Older Americans Act (OAA)?

5. Where are gerontological nurse practitioners (GNPs) especially needed?

6. How effective are gerontological nurse practitioners (GNPs)?

7. How do the health care needs of minority older adults differ from those of Caucasians?

8. What are two major areas that gerontological nurses need to focus on in the future?

References

American Nurses Association (ANA). (1987). *Standards and scope of gerontological nursing practice,* Kansas City, MO: Author.

American Nurses Association (ANA). (1995). *Standards and scope of gerontological nursing practice.* Washington, DC: Author.

American Nurses Credentialing Center (ANCC). (1999). *Recertification catalog.* Washington, DC: Author.

Bowman, K. F., Rose, J. H., & Kresevic, D. (1998). Family caregiving of hospitalized patients. *Gerontological Nursing, 24*(8–9), 16.

Buerhaus, P. I. (1998). Medicare payment for advanced practice nurses: What are the research questions: *Nursing Outlook, 46*(4), 151–153.

Colenda, C. C., Banazak, D., & Mickus, M. (1998). Mental health services in managed care: Quality questions remain. *Geriatrics, 53*(8): 49–64.

Feasley, J. C. (1998). *Health outcomes for older people: Questions for the coming decade.* Washington, DC: National Academy Press 1996 (Institute of Medicine).

Greczkowski, A. M., & Knapp, M. (1998). The gerontological nurse practitioner as director of nursing in the long-term care facility. *Nursing Management, 19*(2), 19–22.

Ham, R. A., & Sloan, P. D. (1997). *Primary care geriatrics: A care-based approach* (3rd ed.). St. Louis: Mosby.

Harper, M. S. (1991). *Management and care of the elderly.* Newbury Park, CA: Sage.

Harris, P. B. (1998). Listening to caregiver sons: Misunderstood realities. *The Gerontologist, 38*(3), 342–352.

Health Resources and Services Administration (HRSA). (1991). *National employment estimates of selected health care personnel in home health care agencies, hospices, nursing homes, board and care (residential homes).* Washington, DC: Author.

Henretta, J. C., Hill, M. S., Li, W., Saldo, B. J., & Wolf, D. A. (1997). *Selection of children to provide care, the effect of earlier parental transfers,* 52B:S.I., 110–119.

Institute of Medicine. (1983). *Nursing and nursing education: Public policies and private actions.* Washington, DC: National Academy Press.

Kelsey, J. E. (1998a). Introduction. *Geriatrics, 53*(suppl. 4), 53.

Kelsey, J. E. (1998b). The use of antidepressants in long-term care and the geriatric patient: Primary care issues. *Geriatrics, 53*(Suppl. 4), 512–521.

Klein, S. (1995). *A national agenda for geriatric education: white papers.* Washington, DC: HRSA, Administrative Document.

Knopp, M. (1998, March 14). Nurse practitioner: Expanded role in long-term care. *The Brown University Long-Term Care Quality Letter, 6,* 5. Providence, RI: Brown University.

Manderscheid R.W., & Henderson, M. J. (1995). *Speaking with a common language: The past, present, and future for managed behavioral healthcare.* Rockville, MD: Center for Mental Health Services.

Meckler, L. (1998, November 29). Health inequalities. *Fort Worth Star-Telegram,* p. G-13.

Mohler, M. M. (1998). Commentary from the capital: R.U.G.s, the director. *Official Publication National Association of Directors of Nursing Administration in Long-Term Care, 6*(1), 25–31.

NIMH/D/ART Program. (1997). *Co-Occurrence of depression with heart disease.* Rockville, MD: Author.

Parmelee, P. A., Katz, I. R., & Lawton, M. P. (1992). Incidence of depression in long-term care settings. *Journal of Gerontology, 47*(6), M189–M196.

Passing scores and rates, 1998 ANCC certification examinations. (1999). *Credentialing News, 2*(1), 5.

Penning, M. J. (1998). In the middle: Parental caregiving in the context of other roles. *Journal of Gerontology, 53B*(1–5), 188–197.

Schoenbaum, M., & Waidmann, T. (1997). Race, socioeconomic status, and health: Accounting for race differences in health. *The Journals of Gerontology, 52B,* 61–73.

Select committee on aging: Shortage of health care professionals caring for the elderly: Recommendations for change. (1993). Washington, DC: U.S. Government Printing Office (Comm. Pub. No. 102-915).

USDHHS, Public Health Services, Bureau of Health Professions (1993). *An agenda for health professions reform.* Rockville, MD: Author.

Who's taking care of older people? (1997). *Global Aging Report. 2*(3), 3.

Who takes care of the sick? (1998, October 10). *Washington Post: Cutting Edge,* p. 21.

Resources

American Nurses Association: `http://www.nursingworld.org`

American Nurses Credentialing Center: `http://www.nursingworld.org/ancc`

National Conference of Gerontological Nurse Practitioners, Inc.: `http://www.ncgnp.org`

CHAPTER 3

Changes in the Health Care Delivery System Affecting Older Adults

Mildred O. Hogstel PhD, RN, C

COMPETENCIES

After completing this chapter, the reader should be able to:

- List the major problems older people have in accessing adequate quality health care.
- Compare the primary methods older people use to pay for health care.
- Differentiate the primary purposes and benefits of Medicare and Medicaid.
- Discuss the advantages and disadvantages of managed care organizations for older people.
- Evaluate the need for long-term care insurance.
- Describe the health care benefits for military veterans.
- Critique the effect of the Medicare prospective payment system on the care of older adults.
- Describe how health care is changing for older adults, including the use of alternative therapies.
- Discuss the function and role of the geriatric care coordinator (case manager).
- Explore reasons for the lack of geriatric health care providers.

MAKING THE CONNECTION

Refer to the following chapters to increase your understanding of changes in the health care delivery system affecting older adults:

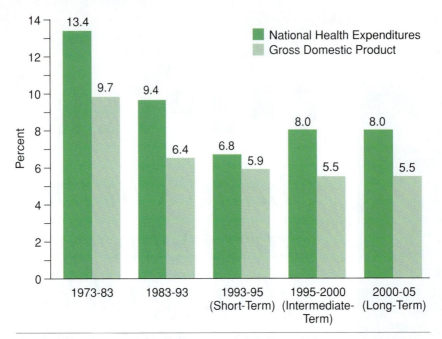

FIGURE 3-1   Average annual growth in national health expenditures and gross domestic product for selected periods: 1973–2005.
[Reprinted from Healthcare Financing Review, *16(4), p. 224, 1995, Health Care Finance Administration.]*

There have been major changes in the health care delivery system in the United States in the last 10 years. Changes and improvements in health care treatments have been dramatic and continuous for decades (for example, transplants, new medications, and other technology). However, changes in the methods of delivering health care have been more recent. The primary driving force causing these changes has been the increasing cost of health care. Health care costs increased 12%–14% per year in the 1970s and began to decrease slightly in the 1980s. The increase was approximately 10% per year in the late 1990s (Kadlec, 2000). Payment mechanisms were affected through changes in health insurance such as managed health care plans and federal legislation related to **Medicare** such as the way hospitals were paid. See Figure 3-1 for a comparison of national health expenditures and **gross national product (GNP)** from 1973 to 2005. These changes have affected and will continue to affect the way older people receive health care as well as the quality and quantity of their care.

Problems Related to Geriatric Health Care

The primary problems older adults have in receiving an adequate quantity and quality of health care are shown in Box 3-1. Most outpatient prescription medications are expensive and not covered by Medicare, although federal legislation has been proposed to provide assis-

tance with the purchase of medications. Transportation to physicians' offices, clinics, and other health care providers is a major problem for those who can no longer drive or afford to maintain a car. Many physicians, nurses, and other health care providers are not aware of the specialized care older adults may need. Only recently have medical schools and nursing schools

BOX 3-1   Problems in Geriatric Health Care

- High cost (even with Medicare)

- Transportation to receive health care (hospital, physician's office, pharmacy)

- Lack of health care providers (physicians, nurses, social workers, and others), with special educational preparation, experience, and interest in geriatric health care

- Comorbidity (multiple chronic illnesses)

- Long-term cultural belief that the "doctor knows best" and physicians or other health care providers should not be questioned

- Changing and confusing choices of paying for health care

- Limited funding available for long-term care

started to require specific courses in geriatrics although these students care for many older clients in many clinical settings. Older adults often do not feel comfortable asking questions and being more assertive with their health care providers. When an older person has several chronic health problems, many medications may be prescribed by multiple providers of care that cause adverse and interactive side effects. Paying for health care not covered by Medicare and using all of Medicare choices available may be confusing or not known to the older adult.

Financing Health Care

To help understand how the multiple changes have affected health care for older adults, it is necessary to discuss how that care is financed because that affects the delivery of care. Health care for older people is primarily paid for by the following methods:

- Medicare
- **Medigap** supplemental insurance
- **Managed care organizations (MCOs)**
- **Medicaid**
- **Long-term care insurance**
- Veterans' Affairs (VA)
- Private pay

> ### *Nursing Tip*
>
> Nurses need to be familiar with the methods of paying for health care so that they can clarify questions their clients and family members have. Nurses also need to be advocates for their clients so needed care is not limited because of health care provider and/or insurance company policies regarding medically necessary care. The nurse can assist the client and/or family in the appeals process if services are denied.

Medicare

The large majority of people age 65 and older are enrolled in Medicare if they contributed to Social Security and Medicare during their working years. People younger than 65 years of age also are eligible for Medicare if they had contributed to Social Security and became too disabled to be employed. People younger than 65 with **end-stage renal disease (ESRD),** including those on dialysis, are also eligible for Medicare benefits if they have participated in the Social Security program during their working years.

Medicare is a federal government program that was enacted into law in 1965 during the period known as "The Great Society." There were several programs started that were aimed to assist the poor, the disabled, and older people to have a better quality of health care and life. At that time people age 65 and older often had difficulty purchasing private health insurance because they were considered a poor risk based on their age and a belief that they would soon require costly health care. Some groups, including the American Medical Association (AMA), opposed the Medicare legislation because they believed it was a step toward socialized medicine. However, socialized medicine means that health care is paid for, controlled, and delivered by the government. Medicare is paid for by the government and therefore involves some regulation, but health care under Medicare is delivered by the private sector (physicians, hospitals, and laboratories). Physicians decide whether or not to

Research Focus

Citation:
Hoerger, T. J., Downs, K. E., Lakshmanan, M. C., Lindrooth, R. C., Plouffe, L., Wendling, B., West, B., West, S. L., & Ohsfeldt, R. L. (1999). Healthcare use among U.S. women aged 45 and older: Total costs and costs for selected postmenopausal health risks. *Journal of Women's Health and Gender Based Medicine, 8*(8), 1077–1089.

Study problem/purpose:
To identify the costs and resource utilization of postmenopausal women relative to specific diseases

Methods:
National discharge data were used for women age 45 and older in identifying diseases and associated resources. Costs based on Medicare reimbursement were estimated.

Findings:
Costs indicated the following: $186 billion was spent in 1997; $16 billion for cardiovascular diseases; $13 billion for osteoporosis; $5 billion for breast and gynecological diseases.

Implications:
The resource and cost estimates are substantial for health care for the population of postmenopausal women. A logical conclusion suggests that monies spent in preventive care of cardiovascular disease, osteoporosis prevention, and reproductive health are worthwhile and cost-saving interventions.

BOX 3-2   Medicare Key Points

History: 1965 Amendment to the Social Security Act—Title XVIII, Medicare implemented July 1, 1966

Eligibility: 65 and older, less than 65 if disabled on Social Security or chronic ESRD

Number on Medicare: 39 million (4 million <65)— 78% with incomes <$25,000

Major Benefits

- Part A—inpatient hospital, skilled nursing facility, home health care following hospitalization, hospice care (includes a deductible that changes annually)

- Part B—outpatient, physician, durable medical equipment, supplies, ambulance, advanced practice nurses, home health care not following hospitalization and after 100 visits (includes an annual deductible)

Source of Funding

- Part A—Medicare Trust Fund (1.45% payroll tax employee and employer each)

- Part B—participants' premiums (pays about 25% of costs) and general federal revenues (people who

did not apply for Part B at the same time that Part A became available to them have to pay higher premiums for Part B)

Major Problems

- Costs are increasing 10% a year.

- Medicare trustees predicted a shortfall in the Trust Fund by 2001.

- Number of Medicare recipients are increasing yearly (approximately 5,500 become 65 every day); 76 million baby boomers become eligible in 2011.

- Health technology and costs continue to increase.

- Minimal preventive care is covered.

- Prescription medications out of a clinical setting are not covered.

- Fraud (duplicate and other payments to providers for services not provided).

- Dental care, hearing devices, and eye glasses are not covered (unless related to a covered surgical benefit).

accept Medicare clients. If they do, they receive 80% of the **usual customary and reasonable (UCR)** fee for services provided if they accept **assignment.** They do not have to accept assignment but may legally charge no more than 115% of the Medicare allowed amount. The client then pays 20% of the UCR and any other amount up to 115%. Medicare has undoubtedly had an impact on the increasing life expectancy and quality of health care and life of older adults in the United States since 1965.

A summary of the key points for Medicare is presented in Box 3-2.

Medigap Supplemental Insurance

Medigap is the name given to private nongovernmental health insurance that Medicare recipients may purchase to help pay for what Medicare does not cover, especially Parts A and B **copays, deductibles,** health care out of the United States, and assistance with the purchase of medications. The federal government has set regulations for these plans in that there are 10 standard plans that must cover some of the essentials such as coverage of

Medicare deductibles (2000 Guide, 2000). However, each insurance plan can have additional benefits and set its own premiums. Many Medicare recipients purchase a Medicare supplement policy, but some, of course, cannot afford the additional monthly premium. A brief description of the ten standard plans is shown in Figure 3-2.

Managed Care Organizations

One of the most prevalent and controversial influences on the delivery of health care in the last decade has been managed health care (see Box 3-3). This concept originated in Oklahoma in the 1920s, and some plans started in the Washington, D.C., area and California in the 1930s and 1940s. Even though federal legislation in 1973 allowed the further development of for-profit managed health care companies (Sultz & Young, 1999), they did not expand throughout the country until the 1990s (Kongstvedt, 1995). They became available to Medicare recipients in 1982.

The primary purpose of an MCO is to deliver quality health care at a competitive price by focusing

The 10 Standard Medicare Supplement Plans

Every company must have plan A

Basic Benefits *(Included in All 10 Plans)*
- **Hospitalization:** Part A coinsurance plus coverage for 365 additional days after Medicare benefits end.
- **Medical Expenses:** Part B coinsurance (20 percent of Medicare-approved expenses).
- **Blood:** First three pints of blood each year.

Plan A	Plan B	Plan C	Plan D	Plan E	Plan F*	Plan G	Plan H	Plan I	Plan J*
Basic Benefits	Basic Benefits	Basic Benefits	Basic Benefits	Basic Benefits	Basic Benefits	Basic Benefits	Basic Benefits	Basic Benefits	Basic Benefits
		Skilled Nursing Coinsurance	Skilled Nursing Coinsurance	Skilled Nursing Coinsurance	Skilled Nursing Coinsurance	Skilled Nursing Coinsurance	Skilled Nursing Coinsurance	Skilled Nursing Coinsurance	Skilled Nursing Coinsurance
	Part A Deductible	Part A Deductible	Part A Deductible	Part A Deductible	Part A Deductible	Part A Deductible	Part A Deductible	Part A Deductible	Part A Deductible
		Part B Deductible			Part B Deductible				Part B Deductible
					Part B Excess (100%)	Part B Excess (80%)		Part B Excess (100%)	Part B Excess (100%)
		Foreign Travel Emergency	Foreign Travel Emergency	Foreign Travel Emergency	Foreign Travel Emergency	Foreign Travel Emergency	Foreign Travel Emergency	Foreign Travel Emergency	Foreign Travel Emergency
			At Home Recovery			At Home Recovery		At Home Recovery	At Home Recovery
							Basic Drugs ($1250 Limit)	Basic Drugs ($1250 Limit)	Extended Drugs ($3000 Limit)
				Preventive Care					Preventive Care

*Plans F and J also have a high deductible option for a lower cost.
NOTE: This chart does not apply in Massachusetts, Minnesota, or Wisconsin.
Call the State Insurance Department for details.
A chart like this must be included in the sales material of every company.

FIGURE 3-2 Ten standard Medicare supplement plans. [*Adapted from* 2000 Guide to Health Insurance for People with Medicare *(p. 10), 2000, Baltimore, MD: National Association of Insurance Commissioners and the Health Care Financing Administration of the U.S. Department of Health and Human Services.*]

BOX 3-3   Types of Managed Care Organizations

- **Health maintenance organization (HMO).** All health care must be provided or arranged by a **primary care physician (PCP),** often called a **gatekeeper,** who agrees to provide **medically necessary** care at a discount of the fee—for service rate or a set monthly rate (called capitation) for each member, thus assuming some financial risk. It is the most common type and has the most limited choices.
  - Staff model—the physicians who care for the clients in the HMO are employed by the HMO.
  - Group model—the HMO makes contracts with groups of physicians to provide medical care to the customers of the HMO. They are in independent practice and are not employed by the HMO. They may have contracts with several HMOs as well as care for clients not in HMOs.

- **Medicare risk HMO.** An HMO specifically for persons on Medicare.
  - Low or no monthly fee other than the Part B premium taken out of the Social Security payment, small copayments for physician office visits (e.g., $5.00–$7.00).
  - The **Health Care Financing Administration (HCFA)** pays the HMO monthly (e.g., $200–$800 depending on geographic region) for each member in the plan whether or not any care is given.

  - The HMO then is obligated to provide the same type of benefits as Medicare regardless of cost, so the HMO takes the risk, although the extent of the benefits may be less.
  - The member must receive all care through the HMO (if the member goes outside the HMO network, neither the HMO nor Medicare Parts A and B will pay anything).
  - **HMO with a point-of-service (POS) option.** The patient can use the network of providers approved by the HMO or go to another provider of choice and pay more.
  - **Preferred provider organizations (PPOs).** Similar to an HMO but with more choice of provider. There is a list of approved physicians, but patients can go outside the network of approved physicians for an extra charge.
  - **Provider-sponsored organizations (PSOs).** Physicians and/or hospitals form their own health plans (similar to HMOs). Owned and operated by health care providers rather than insurance companies. May be helpful in rural areas where there are fewer HMOs.

Note: There are various combinations of all these plans. Very few insurance plans offer the POS, PPO, or PSO option for Medicare clients.

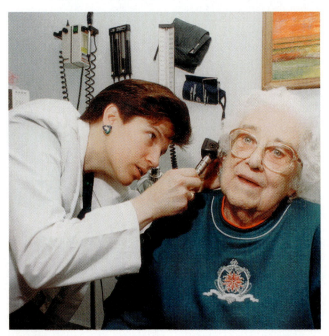

FIGURE 3-3   MCOs focus on preventive health care at all stages of life.

on wellness and *preventive* health care, thus decreasing more costly care later (Figure 3-3). Managed care organizations expanded rapidly in the mid-1990s, primarily as a result of employers attempting to reduce the cost of health insurance coverage for their employees. In 1998 almost 85% of insured employees and 15% of Medicare recipients were enrolled in some type of MCO. Physicians and sometimes hospitals are paid by **capitation,** which means that they receive a designated amount of money either per month **[per member per month (PMPM)]** or per year, regardless of whether or not any care has been provided during that period of time.

However, in the late 1990s consumers' complaints about access to choice and quality health care gained momentum and federal and state legislation to protect clients was enacted. Also, because of expanding competition among MCOs in some metropolitan areas, they had kept premiums as low as possible and soon found that they were losing money as health care expenses continued to rise and federal and state legislation mandated more patient protection (Ornstein,

BOX 3-4 Advantages and Disadvantages of HMOs for Medicare Recipients

Advantages

- Less expensive than Medigap supplemental health insurance

- All care coordinated by one physician so less likelihood of unneeded duplication (for example, same or similar medicines prescribed by two or more physicians)

- Must accept *all* Medicare patients regardless of medical condition (except kidney failure)

- Monitors quality of hospitals and physicians (e.g., licensure, certification, experience)

- May cover benefits not included in original Medicare (e.g., prescription medications, eye care, dental care, hearing devices) for minimal or no cost

- Good coverage of acute-care short-term illnesses

Disadvantages

- There is limited choice of physicians, hospitals, laboratories, and other health care providers.

- Services are provided in a limited geographic area (e.g., one county and/or surrounding counties); only emergency and urgent care covered out of the service area; coverage may be canceled if out of area more than 90 consecutive days.

- It may take weeks or months to get an appointment with a PCP who has a heavy load of patients as required in his or her contract with the HMO.

- It requires HMO preauthorization/precertification for specific diagnostic tests, medications, and surgery, thus possibly delaying treatment.

- Primary care physicians may schedule 40 patients or more a day, thus limiting time available to one patient.

- Access to diagnostic tests and specialists may be limited if the PCP must pay for these services out of his or her capitated payments.

- Physicians must use laboratories and prescription medicines approved by the HMO (if medicines are covered in the plan), even though a different medicine may be preferred by the physician and be more effective for a particular patient.

- The HMO and/or physician may delay or deny care to meet financial goals (save money).

- Primary care physicians may treat conditions or do procedures for which they are not trained (e.g., a gynecologist doing a sigmoidoscopy) instead of referring to a specialist.

- There is questionable coverage of chronic long-term health problems, a major concern for patients on Medicare.

1998). Managed care organizations started to merge in an increasingly competitive market to decrease administrative costs and reduce losses (Fuquay, 1998). In 2000, many insurance plans nationwide dropped their Medicare HMOs because of financial losses. Clients had to choose between returning to original Medicare or looking for another HMO. See Box 3-4 for some of the advantages and disadvantages of MCOs.

Over the years of development, variations of the first type of MCO, the **health maintenance organization (HMO),** evolved to meet consumers' needs for more freedom of choice and quality of care. Questions to be evaluated when considering a managed care plan are in Box 3-5; what to do if one has concerns or complaints about a managed health care plan is discussed in Box 3-6.

Medicaid

Medicaid is also a governmental health care program enacted by the same legislation as Medicare. The primary difference is that Medicaid is a state-administered *welfare* program of health care for all ages that meet the eligibility requirements related to income. Older people who have minimum financial resources and who qualify for income assistance through a federal program called Supplemental Security Income (SSI) also become eligible for Medicaid health care benefits. A person age 65 and older may have Medicare benefits and also qualify for Medicaid. Medicaid covers more than Medicare, such as some prescription medications, dental care, and eye care that Medicare does not cover. The most extensive Medicaid program for older adults is the coverage of long-term custodial care in nursing facilities that Medicare does not cover (Figure 3-4). The essential key points for Medicaid are listed in Box 3-7.

Long-Term Care Insurance

Long-term care insurance is relatively new and has been developed by insurance companies to help customers

BOX 3-5   Questions to Ask When Considering a Managed Care Plan

What is covered by the plan? What is not?

- Does the plan cover dental, podiatry, mental health, or other specific care needs I have?

- Are prescriptions covered and, if so, what are the copayments and maximum out-of-pocket expenses per year?

- What pharmacies can I use and are they convenient to me?

- Does the plan have a list of covered prescriptions (formulary) and, if so, does it cover the drugs I use?

- What preventive care screenings are covered and how often can I have them?

- Does the plan cover hearing aids, eye exams, eyeglasses, or contacts?

What are the costs and financial arrangements of the plan?

- What are the monthly premiums, any copayments, or any deductibles?

- Are physicians paid a salary or on a per-person basis? Do they receive bonuses for fewer referrals? Will the plan let me see a copy of any physician incentive programs?

What physicians and hospitals are available to me through the plan?

- What are the rules on the PCP and can I change PCPs?

- How many PCPs have left the plan in the past three years?

- What can I do if a PCP will not refer me to a specialist I feel I need to see?

- Are physicians/specialists I currently see on the approved provider list and, if so, can I continue to see them? How will I feel if they are later dropped from the provider list?

- Are the physicians and hospitals convenient to me?

- How long does it take to get an appointment with a physician or specialist?

- What type of quality reviews are conducted on the physicians and other providers? Are the hospitals accredited? Are the physicians board certified?

- Will the plan cover an out-of-network specialist?

What do other enrollees think of the health plan?

- Does the plan have any customer satisfaction survey results I may see?

- How many people have disenrolled from the plan in the past three years?

Is the HMO accredited by the National Committee on Quality Assurance?

BOX 3-6   What to Do If One Has Concerns or Problems About an MCO

- Ask for copies of claim forms filed by the physician to determine exact treatment and costs.

- Ask the physician why he or she will not order certain tests or make referrals to a specialist. Ask for the denial in writing and call the MCO to see if it is a covered service.

- Get a second opinion and send copies to the physician and the MCO.

- Appeal the denial of treatment to the MCO by registered mail with a threat to go to court. Seek the assistance of a lawyer if needed.

- If this process is likely to take too long a time, pay for the needed treatment and try to obtain reimbursement from the MCO later.

- Write an official complaint to your state's Department of Insurance.

- Call your state's Peer Review Organization to report complaints related to Medicare clients.

- If the MCO has not provided what they advertised or promised, call an investigator in the office of the State Attorney General.

- Be *assertive* as needed to ensure that quality health care is available.

- Change physicians, if necessary.

- Change health insurance plans, if possible.

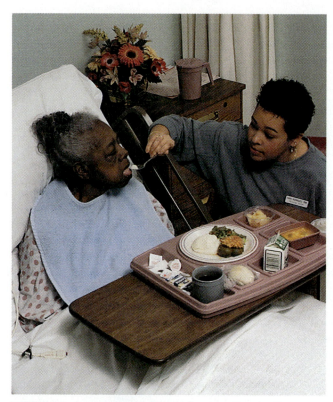

FIGURE 3-4 Long-term custodial care is a benefit under the Medicaid health care program.

pay for long-term health care services when multiple chronic health problems occur that require custodial care not covered by Medicare or other insurance. This type of insurance provides a daily payment (e.g., $50–$250) for approved care in nursing facilities, care in the home by health care providers, care at adult day centers, and care in assisted-living facilities. Monthly

premiums vary depending on age at the time of purchase, the length of desired coverage (e.g., <2–6 years), waiting period (e.g., qualify after 6 months of care), and amount of daily payments. See Box 3-8 for summary.

Long-term care insurance may be appropriate for middle-income individuals and couples who have too many financial assets to qualify for Medicaid and not enough assets to pay for long-term care for years for one or two people (e.g., $35,000–$80,000 per person per year). However, the premiums are relatively high, although comparison shopping will help to identify the lowest cost for the most complete coverage. There may also be a monetary policy limit. The younger a person is when purchased, the lower the premiums. However, a 50- or 60-year-old could pay premiums for 30–40 years and never need the insurance. Some would argue that using that money for a wise investment would probably provide sufficient funds if and when it is needed for long-term care.

Some people buy this type of insurance for two primary reasons: It gives them a sense of security about the future for their own long-term care if needed, and it saves their assets for their heirs, who many feel strongly about it. The decision to spend their money for long-term care insurance will depend upon individual assets, needs, and choices. Information and guidance should be sought from an objective person, not from an insurance salesperson who would benefit from selling the insurance. See Figure 3-5.

Veterans' Benefits

Veterans age 65 and older can choose to use their veterans' health care benefits or Medicare if they have it by qualifying for Social Security. There are veterans' hospitals and outpatient clinics throughout the country,

---

BOX 3-7 Medicaid Key Points

History: 1965 Amendment to the Social Security Act—Title XIX

Eligibility: Needy poor of all ages based on income and other resources

Number: 34 million

Major Benefits: Assistance with all health care needs including nursing home care (50%–70% of residents' nursing home cost paid for by Medicaid)

Source of Funding: General revenues from federal and state budgets based on a ratio (60% federal and 40% state)

Major Problems
- Increasing costs, especially for long-term custodial nursing facility costs as the population ages

- 44 million U.S. citizens with no health insurance (Kadlec, 2000)

Possible Changes
- Block grant all federal funds to states based on a formula yet to be determined

- Trials in some states to place Medicaid recipients who enter nursing homes in MCOs

BOX 3-8   Long-Term Care Insurance

Purpose: Helps pay for long-term care (e.g., 6 months or longer) in a variety of situations:

- Home health care
- Respite care
- Adult day services
- Assisted-living facilities
- Nursing facilities

Benefit Eligibility: Eligible for services after a waiting period (e.g., 6 months). Qualify if have functional impairment or impairment of cognitive ability requiring continual supervision. For example, the person cannot perform two of six basic activities of daily living (ADL) such as bathing, eating, toileting, transferring, walking, and dressing.

Daily Benefit: About $50–$250 (annual cost of nursing home care can range from $35,000 to $80,000 or more).

Length of Benefit: Twelve months to 5 years. Average length of stay in a nursing facility is about $2\frac{1}{2}$ years.

Premium Costs: Increases with increasing age. Some plans will not sell a policy to anyone over a specific age (e.g., 80–85). Higher cost if select an inflation rider, shorter waiting period for eligibility, higher daily benefit, and longer benefit period. Examples of premiums based on age:

Age (years)	Monthly Premium
60	About $ 90
65	About $125
70	About $185

Advantages

1. Gives peace of mind about future need and cost of long-term care

2. Part of premium cost tax deductible depending on total health care costs (currently if health care expenses exceed $2\frac{1}{2}$% of adjusted gross income)

3. Wish to save assets for heirs instead of using on personal long-term care

Disadvantages

1. Expensive premiums

2. May pay premiums for many years and never use the benefits

3. May be policy payment limits (e.g., $150,000) and/or years of coverage limit

4. May not cover inflation costs

5. Could invest premium amounts and possibly make enough to pay for years of care

Note: All policies will differ on benefits and costs. Need to compare benefits and costs of competing policies.

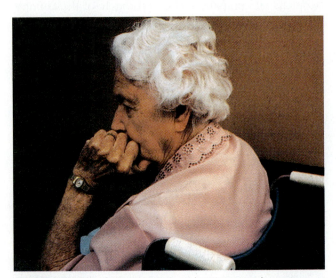

FIGURE 3-5 The decision to purchase long-term care insurance may not be feasible for some older adults.

but mostly in urban areas, so not all veterans have easy access to these sources. There are only a few separate veterans' nursing facilities, although most general veterans' hospitals also have a skilled nursing unit.

Outpatient clinics provide physician services, diagnostic testing including laboratory tests, minor surgery, and other needed benefits, such as prescription medications, for a nominal fee (e.g., $2) for non–service connected patients. This service is available even if the prescription was written by a physician other than at the VA clinic. For example, the service-connected veteran could see a physician under the Medicare program, receive a prescription for a medication, and obtain the medication at the VA clinic. Veterans with service-connected health problems are usually given priority status, but because all veterans can receive health care at these clinics, waiting times for appointments and services may be long. See Box 3-9 for a benefit summary.

Private Pay

Older people pay privately for health care services not covered by Medicare, Medicaid, or other government or insurance sources. Some of the types of care not usually covered by any of the above sources are:

- Cosmetic and/or experimental surgery
- Private duty nurses
- Convenience items
- Homemaker, companion, and chore services in the home (unless they also qualify for other skilled services)

Effects of Health Care Delivery System Changes on Older Adults

The dramatic changes in the health care delivery system in the last 10–15 years have had an effect on the delivery of health care to older people. Decreased Medicare and HMO payments to hospitals, home health agencies, and nursing facilities and decreased coverage of outpatient

and rehabilitation services have caused reductions in numbers of staff and closure of some of these programs.

Hospital-Based Care

Because of the increasing costs of health care in the 1970s to the 1980s, federal legislation in 1983 changed how hospitals were paid for the care of Medicare patients. Prior to that time, hospitals were paid on a cost basis. That is, hospitals provided the care and then billed Medicare for the cost of the care. In 1983, a **prospective payment system (PPS)** was initiated that involved a set payment amount before care based on the diagnosis of the patient. This prospective payment system was based on defined **diagnostic-related groups (DRGs)** (Sultz & Young, 1999). This system did not set a limit on days in the hospital, as some clients are told, but set a limit on

---

Nursing Tip

If a Medicare client and/or family member believe that the client is being asked to leave the hospital too soon, suggest that they speak to the physician about the problem and/or remind them that they can call the state **Peer Review Organization (PRO)** telephone number, which they should have received in their admission papers. The purpose of the PRO is to ensure quality of care for Medicare patients.

BOX 3-9   Veterans' Benefits

Eligibility for VA Care
- Honorable discharge from one of the armed services
- Active duty service (at least 2 years if service after 1980)
- Service-connected injuries/illnesses given priority (incurred or activated by military service)
- Spouses not covered

Types of Care
- Veterans' Affairs outpatient clinics provide full diagnostic and treatment services such as physician care, laboratory tests, and prescription medications for a nominal fee (e.g., $2.00).
- Veterans' Affairs hospital care provides a full range of services, but the veteran may not live close to one.

- Nursing facilities:
  - VA hospital nursing facility for short-term rehabilitation care (e.g., 6 months to 1 year), wound care, hospice care, and interim placement (3–6 months)
  - VA or private nursing facility for long-term custodial care as long as needed if a service-connected diagnosis and/or disability

Coverage
- Veterans age 65 and older may choose to use their veteran's health care benefits or Medicare if they have it by qualifying for Social Security.
- Veterans who do not have a service-connected disease or disability would benefit from both Parts A and B Medicare.

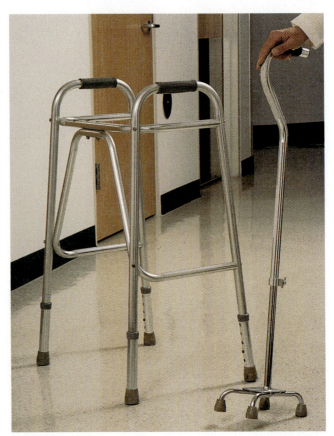

FIGURE 3-6 DME is a covered benefit under Medicare guidelines for home health care.

the amount of money paid by Medicare to the hospital. See Box 3-10 for an example of how a PPS works.

As a result of this change in payment mechanisms, clients on Medicare were discharged quicker and sicker, thus requiring rehabilitative care in their home or a skilled nursing facility (SNF). Previous to this change, older clients who had a fractured hip often were hospitalized for 10–14 days with more time to adapt to their condition and receive skilled rehabilitation services. Because of the DRGs, more clients were transferred to nursing facilities than to their home and never completely recovered enough to live independently again.

The MCO expansion in the 1990s also greatly affected hospital care. As hospitals were paid less by Medicare and by MCOs, their staffing patterns changed from fewer professional nursing staff to more unskilled, unlicensed, minimally trained nursing technicians called **unlicensed assistive personnel (UAP).** Changes in hospital staffing and lack of an adequate quantity and quality of staff prepared in gerontology raised serious questions about the quality of care of older hospital clients with acute illnesses who also had coexisting multiple chronic diseases.

Because of both the PPS and MCOs, more surgery and other treatments were on an outpatient basis for all patients, causing multiple problems for many older adults who did not have the ability or support to care for themselves at home in the immediate postoperative period.

Think About It

Can an 85-year-old woman who has just had a simple mastectomy at 7 AM be expected to be discharged at 3 PM to her home, where she lives alone with no close supportive assistance? What could you do as a nurse advocate to assist this client?

Home Health Care

The need for more extensive home health care became obvious when considering the shorter hospital stays and patients' wishes to be at home if at all possible. Home health care was one of the fastest growing areas of health care in the mid- and late 1990s. Although home health care is available for all ages, approximately 90%–95% of the patients receiving care are those age 65 and over and thus are eligible for Medicare benefits. While home health care was expanding rapidly, there was an increasing amount of fraud and abuse of Medicare by unscrupulous home health care and **durable medical equipment (DME)** providers. See examples of DME in Figure 3-6. Fraud in Medicare home health care has been reduced by half by changes made in federal legislation in 1997 and better surveillance of requests for payments from Medicare. Some of the typical Medicare home health abuses are listed in Box 3-11.

However, as health care costs and the aging population both continued to increase, there was a need to decrease the growth of Medicare expenses to maintain the program for the future. There was a federal moratorium on the opening of new home health agencies under Medicare for a period of time in late 1997. The

BOX 3-11 Fraud in Home Health Care

- Care was provided to clients who did not qualify because they were not confined to the home (a requirement for Medicare reimbursement).

- Medicare was billed for specific supplies that were never provided to the clients.

- Medicare was billed for care to clients that were never seen.

- Medicare was billed for a 3-hr visit when the aide might have been there only 5 or 10 min.

- New home health agencies opened that did not have the financial resources, staff, or knowledge to provide quality care for older adults in the home. There were minimal criteria for obtaining state licensure and Medicare reimbursement.

Balanced Budget Act of 1997 (Public Law 105-33) made specific changes in the way home health care agencies operated. The new law made several major changes as presented in Box 3-12.

These changes caused some home health agencies to have to close or merge with others and, unfortunately, forced some older clients into nursing facilities because, for one reason or another, they could no longer receive home health care services. Either they could not qualify or, more likely, the home health agency could no longer continue to provide the needed care because of their

BOX 3-12 Effects of the Balanced Budget Act of 1997 on Home Health Care Agencies

- Payment mechanisms moved from cost-based to an interim system based on previous costs to a PPS similar to that required since 1983 for hospital payments.

- Medicare would no longer pay for a blood draw (for monitoring medication levels in the blood) if that was the only need.

- Home health care not following a hospitalization or after 100 visits was moved from Part A to Part B.

decreased payments from Medicare. Payments under a PPS are not enough to care for chronically ill clients who need extensive care for long periods of time.

Nursing Facility Care

As noted earlier, Medicare pays for very little nursing facility care, primarily short-term skilled rehabilitation following an acute illness or surgery such as a fractured hip. Most of the long-term custodial care in nursing facilities is paid for by Medicaid, a welfare program that is funded by both the federal and state governments. Pilot projects to place Medicaid clients who need long-term custodial care in an MCO have been tried and the progress and results need to be evaluated.

Think About It

How will client care in nursing facilities be affected by the fiscal policies of Medicaid managed care?

Nursing facilities are licensed and regulated by state governmental agencies, so each state has different criteria. The American Association of Retired Persons (AARP) has been very active in getting state legislation passed to improve the quality of life and care in nursing facilities in recent years (Figure 3-7). Some of these regulations relate to:

- Residents' Bill of Rights

- Higher monetary penalties when complaints and deficiencies are substantiated

- Public awareness of facilities' state survey reports

The issue of nursing facility occupancy, federal regulation, state licensure, nurse staffing, and payment mechanisms will continue to be of concern.

Think About It

Will nursing facilities as we know them today be available in the year 2020? Where will the dependent sick older adults be cared for in the future?

Mental Health Care

Mental health care for older adults has not received much emphasis in the past, especially in home health care or nursing facilities. Because of expense and insurance fraud, most mental health care for all ages moved from a

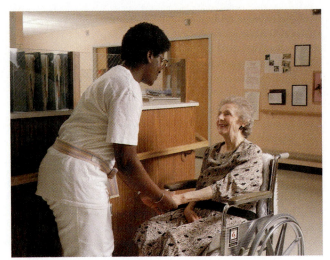

FIGURE 3-7 Nursing facilities are licensed and regulated by each state.

month-long inpatient care setting to an outpatient and/or partial hospitalization program to decrease costs. The diagnosis and treatment of mental disorders in nursing facilities needs to be studied. Some hospitals that had been providing behavioral health care in the Medicare partial hospitalization program have been discontinuing these services because of decreasing payments.

Alternative Therapies

Alternative types of health care increased tremendously in the 1990s. As individual responsibility for wellness and health promotion became more prevalent, more people sought options that could be used without consulting a physician. According to Greenwald (1998), "more and more Americans are supplementing and replacing prescription medicines with a profusion of pills and potions that contain various herbs, vitamins, and minerals" (p. 59). Some of these therapies are "herbology, homeopathy, nutrition, Chinese medicine, body work and Ayurvedic medicine" (Levin, 1998, p. 1). Traditional medicine also became more accepting of alternative therapies and began to suggest some choices as an option (Gorman, 1998). It is especially important that older adults consult their physicians when deciding to try a new alternative substance. Because many of them are also taking several prescription medications, there may be a **synergistic** or **antagonistic reaction** that could be harmful and cause severe adverse effects. For example, if a person is taking an antidepressant, it could be dangerous to take St. John's wort, an herb that is used to treat mild or moderate depression. Drug-herb interactions can be potentially serious (Gorman, 1998). Even high doses of some vitamins can be toxic.

Although research has been increasing on the safety and effectiveness of many of these herbal products, "herbs and other supplements have been all but exempt from federal oversight" since the Federal Dietary Supplement Health and Education Act was passed in 1994, thus expanding the market for the herbal industry (Greenwald, 1998, p. 63). People believe that herbs are *safe* because they come from *natural* sources. However, herbs also contain chemicals, just like prescription medications do (Greenwald, 1998). Sample alternative substances are listed in Table 3-1 and other alternative therapies may be found in Table 3-2 and Figure 3-8.

CLINICAL ALERT

Be sure to ask clients about their use of specific alternative substances and include information about those substances and/or therapies in their health history and assessment because of the risk of changing the effects of prescription medications being taken.

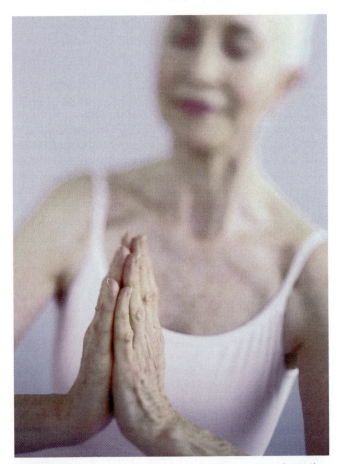

FIGURE 3-8 Alternative therapies have become an attractive option to traditional medicine.

TABLE 3-1 Alternative Therapy Substances

Substance	Possible Action/Use/Precautions
Green tea (polyphenols)	Antioxidant/anticancer, hypertension/high cholesterol
Ginkgo biloba (flavonoid glycosides and ginkolides)	Increases cerebral blood flow/Alzheimer's disease (inhibits platelet-activating factors and can interact with warfarin)
Coenzyme Q10 (ubiquinone)	Various types of heart disease, weight reduction
Kava-Kava	Treats anxiety and reduces fatigue
St. John's wort	Depression, treatment of wounds
Alfalfa	Laxative, diuretic, urinary infections
Bilberry	Improves vision, treats thrombosis and angina
Devil's claw root	Relief of pain
Glucosamine sulfate	Osteoarthritis
Cayenne pepper	Relief of pain
Chondroitin	Joint pain and mobility
Aloe vera	Skin conditions (acne, burns)
Dehydropiandrosterone (DHEA) steroid	Transformed into androgens or estrogens in tissues
Echinacea purpurea	Treats and prevents colds and flu (increases immune system action)
Vitamins, especially	
A	Antioxidant/eyes, skin
B_3 niacin	Nervous and digestive systems
C	Antioxidant, hair, skin, gums
D	Bones, teeth
E	Antioxidant, circulation, skin, hair, prostate
Minerals, especially	
Boron	Arthritis
Calcium	Bones
Magnesium	Migraine headache
Selenium	Skin, male fertility, anticancer
Zinc	Prostate, skin
Onions	Heart, circulation, lowers cholesterol
Garlic	Infections, decreases blood cholesterol, lowers blood pressure, anticancer effects
Ginger root	Relieves pain in arthritis and migraine headaches
Melatonin	Antioxidant/sleep
Ganqulipid	Decreases fats and cholesterol
Cat's claw	Anticancer effects, acquired immunodeficiency syndrome (AIDS)
Lecithin	Lowers low-density lipoprotein (LDL) cholesterol, less likely to form gallstones
Hawthorne	Increases blood to heart, lowers blood pressure
Cabbage juice	Stomach ulcers
Primrose oil	Cancer, menopausal symptoms
Garcinia cambogia	Weight loss
Milk thistle	Hepatitis C, liver
Dimethylsulfoxide (DMSO)	Relieves pain, tinnitus, arthritis (anti-inflammatory)
Psyllium	Cholesterol, constipation
Ginseng	Improves memory and ability to learn, increases energy, antioxidant, anticancer, lowers blood pressure and cholesterol
Saw palmetto	Anti-inflammatory, treats benign prostatic hyperplasia
Monosodium glutamate (MSG)	
Feverfew herb *(Tanacetum parthenium)*	Migraine headache

Adapted from Gorman, C. (1998, November 23). Is it good medicine? Time, *69. Greenwald, J. (1998, November 23). Herbal healing.* Time, *58–67. The healthy cell news. (1998, Summer). Young, AZ: ALV Publishers. Williams, D. (1997) The real miracle of natural healing.* Alternatives. *Ingram, TX: Mountain Home Publishing. Williamson, J. S., & Wyandt, C. M. (1997, August 4). Herbal therapies: The facts and the fiction.* Drug Topics, *78–88. Williamson, J. S., & Wyandt, C. M. (1998, June 1). An herbal update.* Drug Topics, *60–80.*

Note: None of these substances have been approved by the U.S. Food and Drug Administration (FDA) for the prevention or treatment of disease.

TABLE 3-2 Other Alternative Therapies

Therapy	Action/Use
Acupressure, acupuncture	Relieve pain and nausea
Aromatherapy	
Basil	Promotes peace and happiness
Broom, catnip	Calm nerves
Carnation, cardamom	Increase sexual desire
Lavender	Relaxes
Marigold	Cheers the soul
Cedar	Increases spirituality
Sage	Relieves depression
Rosemary	Enhances memory
Violet	Eases headaches
Lily, rose	Promotes love and tranquility
Guided imagery	Depression, anxiety
Music therapy	Relaxation
Light therapy	Mood enhancer, osteoarthritis, skin problems
Aerobic exercise	Energy, relaxation, enhances mood
Massage therapy	Relaxation
Magnet therapy	Relieves pain
Pet therapy	Improves social interaction and cardiovascular health, decreases depression, decreases blood pressure
Color therapy	
Purple	Asthma
Indigo	Burns
Lemon	Angina
Orange	Digestive problems

Adapted from Mindell, E. (1995). Flower power makes scents. Joy of Health, 3(6), 3. Douglas, W. C. (ND). The incredible healing power of color and light. Second opinion. Atlanta, GA: Author. Rosenfeld, I. (1998, August 16). Acupuncture goes mainstream (almost). Parade Magazine, 10–11. Jorgenson, J. (1997). Therapeutic use of companion animals in health care. Image: Journal of Nursing Scholarship, 29(3), 249–254.

Interdisciplinary Approach to Geriatric Health Care

The major history, problems, and issues related to the delivery of health care to older adults have been presented. This section will focus more on trends and suggestions for continued progress and improvement. Gerontology is interdisciplinary by nature and involves psychology, sociology, economics, religion, ethics, medicine, nursing, social work, and all other major health care providers. See Figure 3-10. Gerontology involves the total person, physically, psychologically, socially, emotionally, intellectually, and spiritually. Therefore, an interdisciplinary team is essential to identify, predict, and meet the total needs of older adults. It is an ideal setting when individuals from all of the disciplines mentioned can work together to improve the lives of older adults in any setting. Some rehabilitation and **hospice** organizations come close to this goal, but many other health care agencies, including hospitals, clinics, and MCOs, lack the interest, communication skills, information, education, insight, or resources to use such an approach.

Primary and Long-Term Care

The health care delivery system of the United States has clearly been a sick system (focusing on illness once it is present) and *not* a well system, where the focus is primary care including prevention and early diagnosis and treatment of illnesses. There needs to be more focus on primary care, including all elements to keep people well and to identify health problems early to prevent later client complications and decline at a higher cost. Sultz and Young (1999) noted that "medicine and medical education . . . have a history of being incredibly inept in establishing health promotion and disease prevention as a high priority in the U.S. health care system" (p. 157). However, prevention and primary care costs money, and traditionally neither health insurance nor Medicare has covered the prevention components of primary care. Although most people age 65 and older are fortunate to have Medicare for essential treatment and care, it is estimated that there are approximately 44 million U.S. citizens without any kind of health insurance. A number of these uninsured fall in the 55–64 age group, and in 1998 the federal government proposed to allow these people to purchase Medicare early at a higher cost (e.g., $300–$400 a month). It was estimated that about 300,000 people would take advantage of this opportunity (Bedlin, 1998, p. 2). They have often lost their employer's health insurance because of termination, mergers, or retirement and cannot purchase private insurance independently because of age, preexisting health care conditions, or excessive cost.

Providing and paying for long-term care, whether in the home, assisted-living facility, or nursing facility are probably the most critical problems facing the U.S. health care delivery system in the future.

Think About It

How will the baby boomer generation receive long-term care in 2030?

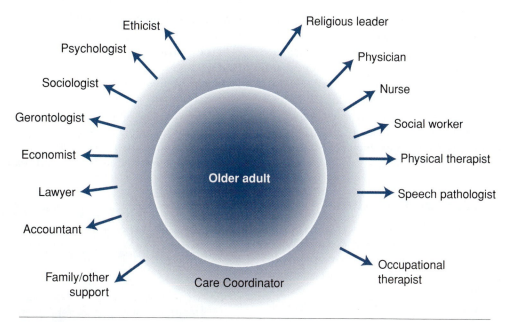

FIGURE 3-9 An interdisciplinarian approach to geriatric health care.

When presented with these problems, some national policy makers state that the family, church, and community will have to give that care. However, society has changed since the early 1900s, when health care costs were less and family members, usually a wife or daughter, were at home to care for older parents and grandparents. The role of the church/synagogue in health care is increasing, however, with the expanding role of elder care programs and parish nurses.

Care Coordination (Case Management)

An emerging and very important role in health care delivery in the future is that of **care coordination** (more commonly called case management). Care coordination is considered a more compassionate and caring term than managing a case. This role is especially important in the field of gerontology and a growing field of study and practice in nursing, social work, and other related health care fields. There is a national organization of private geriatric case managers and more nurses are entering this field. A geriatric care coordinator assesses the total needs of an older adult and provides and/or enables the person to receive the right care from the right person or agency at the right time (see Figure 3-9). The care coordinator works with the family or takes on the role of the family when there is no family in close proximity (Figure 3-10). This need is especially important for the older adult (age 85 and older) who is

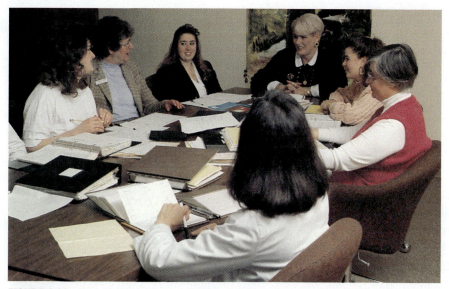

FIGURE 3-10 The care coordinator facilitates appropriate care for each client.

living alone in the community and who has lost spouse, siblings, and perhaps children by death.

The care coordinator has to know how to get a wheelchair ramp built on a porch; where to obtain safe, comfortable, inexpensive transportation for someone who cannot drive; as well as how to assist older adults in selecting a physician right for them. This role can be very rewarding because of the independence of practice and the rewards of seeing a person receive the right assistance when it is needed.

Geriatric Health Care Providers

A major problem in the health care of older adults is the lack of health care providers with specific educational preparation in geriatrics. Some physicians have postresidency fellowships in geriatric medicine. Physicians can become board certified in geriatric medicine as a subspecialty of internal medicine (American Board of Medical Specialties, personal communication, June 2, 1999). It is estimated that there are only about 9,500 certified geriatricians in the United States when at least 20,000 are needed (Neergaard, 2000). In one county in one southwestern state, there are only four fellowship-trained geriatricians out of about 2,200 licensed physicians.

Nurses with special education and experience in the care of older adults may receive national certification by the American Nurses Credentialing Center as a generalist, clinical specialist, or nurse practitioner. Although the number of certified gerontological nurses has increased tremendously in recent years, there is still a great need for more geriatric prepared nurses in all areas where older people receive health care. There is no degree or certification in geriatrics for most of the other professional health care fields, although social workers are initiating such action in some states.

Legislation Affecting Health Care Delivery

Because of many of the changes discussed in this chapter, health care has become a national issue for discussion and debate since 1994. Medicare is a major part of that debate because it is a significant portion of the federal budget.

Federal

The Family Medical Leave Act of 1994 allowed employees to receive up to 12 weeks of leave without pay to care for the health care needs of a family member. For example, an adult child can take off from work for a period of time to care for and be with an older family member after a serious illness or surgery or while waiting for a pending death.

The Balanced Budget Act of 1997 made major changes in Medicare as previously mentioned. The key elements of this legislation are listed in Box 3-13. A National Bipartisan Commission on the Future of Medicare also was appointed in 1997 to make recommendations to Congress for legislation related to the Medicare program. However, they were unable to agree on a specific proposal in 1999 and disbanded.

BOX 3-13   Major Changes in Medicare as a Result of the Balanced Budget Act of 1997 (Public Law 105-33)

- Increased choices for participants
  - Original Medicare fee-for-service
  - Health maintenance organization (HMO)
  - HMO with a point-of-service (POS)
  - Preferred provider organization (PPO)
  - Provider-sponsored organization (PSO)
  - Religious Fraternal Benefit Plan
  - Private fee-for-service
  - Medical saving's account (MSA)
  - Private physician contracting

- Increased preventive health care services
  - Mammogram and Pap smear
  - Colorectal cancer screening
  - Prostate cancer screening
  - Bone density measurement
  - Outpatient diabetes self-management

- Cost savings
  - Prospective payment system (PPS) for home health care, skilled nursing facilities (SNF), rehabilitation facilities, hospital outpatient care, and ambulance services
  - Greater penalties for fraud and abuse
  - Decreased payments to some Medicare HMOs

- Added consumer protection
  - Care must be provided 24 hr a day 7 days a week
  - Prohibits gag rule (limiting advice to clients for care not covered by the HMO)
  - Prudent lay person definition of an emergency
  - Confidentiality of client records
  - No physician incentives to limit care

Adapted from O'Sullivan, J., Franco, C., Fuchs, B., Lyke B., Price, R., & Swendiman, K. (August 18, 1997). Medicare provisions in the Balanced Budget Act of 1997 (BBA 97, Public Law 105-33). Washington, DC: CRS Report for Congress.

More legislation related to health care was proposed in 1998 such as allowing certain people age 55–64 to buy into Medicare, as previously discussed, and consumer protection for people in MCOs. Many other possible changes have been discussed to provide more benefits and to save Medicare for the future. See the range of possibilities in Table 3-3.

State

The most common type of state legislation passed in recent years related to health care has been regulations regarding consumer protection in MCOs. Some states have passed legislation that allows consumers to sue HMOs when delay or denial of treatment causes harm. Prior to that legislation physicians could be

---

TABLE 3-3 Possible Future Medicare Changes

Changes	Issues and Questions
• Raise eligibility age from 65 to 67 or even 70 over the next 25 years (eligibility age for Social Security has already been increased gradually to 67 for those born in 1960 and later).	People are living longer and healthier. Could they buy private health insurance at 65 or 66?
• Implement premium support (voucher) in which Medicare would provide so much money for recipients to purchase some type of private health insurance if they wished.	Would there be guaranteed benefits? Would there be limits on premiums? Would the insurance companies have to accept anyone who applied? Government-run insurance could still be an option, but it would have more financial problems if the sickest, poorest, and oldest stayed in that program.
• Require affluent recipients to pay more for Part B premiums (2000, $45.50).	Should Medicare involve means testing? How would it be done? How much would that cost?
• Increase the deductibles (2000, Part A, $776; Part B, $100) and copays (2000, Part B, 20% of Medicare-allowed amount).	Increase how much?
• Allow people age 62–64 to buy into Medicare (about $300/month) and 55–61 (about $400/month) if they lose their job and employer paid health insurance. Would have to pay more per month for Medicare monthly premiums once they became eligible for Medicare at age 65 or 67.	Could they afford it? Would it cause more financial problems for Medicare?
• Add a prescription medication benefit to Medicare.	How much? A high-cost benefit. How to pay for benefit? Many federal bills were introduced in 1999 and 2000 to meet this need. These proposals became a major issue in the 2000 presidential campaign.
• Increase payroll taxes by 1/4%. Saves Medicare until 2035.	Baby boomers begin to reach 65 in 2011.
• Set aside 15% of the federal budget surplus for future Medicare costs.	Not approved by Congress. Where is the surplus going?
• Encourage more people into MCOs and other similar private plans such as medical savings accounts (MSAs).	Will patients receive needed quality care?
• Add coverage for assisted-living facilities, adult day services, and respite care for family caregivers.	Caregiving is a major problem for many families.
• Reduce premiums for healthy lifestyles (e.g., proof of exercise and weight control).	How could this be monitored?
• Integrate a case management system into fee-for-service Medicare to focus on getting the right care at the best site early.	Improves quality of care and saves money.

BOX 3-14   Examples of State Legislation Related to Health Care

- Require insurance to pay for 48 hr of hospital stay after a mastectomy and postmastectomy breast reconstruction.

- All women can self-refer to a gynecologist (not permitted in some HMOs).

- Must cover a prostate-specific antigen (PSA) blood test to screen for prostate cancer.

- Allow pharmacists to give immunizations and vaccinations under a physician's written protocol.

- Insurance must pay for diabetes supplies if the insurance pays for diabetes treatment.

- More mental health coverage by the insurance plan.

Adapted from Summary of Health Care Legislation (July 1997). Austin, TX: Texas Department of Insurance.

sued, even if they were following the MCO guidelines, but not the MCO.

Other state legislation relates to health care for immigrants, Medicaid eligibility (it differs from state to state), and physician-assisted suicide. See Box 3-14 for other examples of recent state legislation related to health care.

Summary

The health care delivery system in the United States has been in the process of change for the last decade. These changes are affecting the health care of older adults. The cost of care has initiated many of these changes, including how and where older adults receive health care. Shorter hospital stays, outpatient surgery and treatment, and decreased home health care services have caused problems for older clients. The major methods older people use to pay for health care are Medicare, Medigap supplemental health insurance, managed care organizations (MCOs), Medicaid, long-term care insurance, veterans' benefits, and private pay.

The fastest growing area of health care in the mid-1990s was home health care, but more recently that has changed to assisted-living facilities as they expand. The greatest problem for the future is the provision of long-term custodial care for the chronically ill very old as the oldest age group increases in numbers. There is a severe shortage of all kinds of health care providers who have the education and interest to specialize in the care of older adults.

The ever-changing health care delivery system in the United States is likely to be open to public debate and discussion as well as possible legislation for many years to come. Two of those changes are the increasing use of alternative therapies and changes in the methods of paying for health care. Advocates for older adults, including nurses, need to be sure that they are involved in this public debate and policy formation for the future. Nurses also need to understand the various payment mechanisms used by their older clients, so they can answer questions and be a strong advocate for quality care when needed.

Review Questions and Activities

1. How do older people pay for their health care?

2. What is the difference between Medicare and Medicaid?

3. What are the major benefits of Medicare Parts A and B?

4. What are the primary goals of managed care organizations (MCOs)?

5. Discuss pro's and con's of buying long-term care insurance.

6. Visit a Medicare risk MCO sales presentation, VA outpatient clinic, or a partial hospitalization program for the treatment of mental health in older adults. Describe what you think is the perspective or agenda and purpose of each.

7. What is a prospective payment system (PPS)? What kind of care does it affect?

8. Is there too much federal and state legislation regarding MCOs? Explain your answer.

9. Can physicians obtain national specialization board certification in geriatric medicine? Do you think credentialing is necessary? Explain and support your answer.

10. Why is there a shortage of health care professionals in gerontology?

References

Bedlin, H. (February, 1998). Congress expected to tackle seniors' issues. *Networks,* National Council on the Aging, p. 2.

Douglas, W. C. (ND). The incredible healing power of color and light. *Second opinion*. Atlanta, GA: Author.

Fuquay, J. (March 3, 1998). Dwindling HMOs. *Fort Worth Star Telegram,* pp. C-1, 12.

Gorman, C. (1998, November 23). Is it good medicine? *Time,* p. 69

Greenwald, J. (1998, November 23). Herbal healing. *Time,* pp. 58–67.

The healthy cell news. (1998, Summer). Young, AZ: ALV Publishers.

Jorgenson, J. (1997). Therapeutic use of companion animals in health care. *Image: Journal of Nursing Scholarship, 29*(3), 249–254.

Kadlec, D. (2000, July 17). Focus on prohibitive health care costs. *Time,* B13.

Kongstvedt, P. R. (1995). *Essentials of managed care.* Gaithersburg, MD: Aspen.

Levin, J. (1998, Spring). Alternative health care. *The NCGNP Newsletter, 59,* 1–2.

Mindell, E. (1995). Flower power makes scents. *Joy of Health, 3*(6), 3.

2000 guide to health insurance for people with Medicare. (2000). Bethesda, MD: National Association of Insurance Commissioners and the Health Care Financing Administration of the U. S. Department of Health and Human Services.

Neergaard, L. (2000, July). Too few doctors trained as geriatricians. *Senior News, 13*(7), 10.

Ornstein, C. (March 13, 1998). Area's HMOs report massive losses in '97. *The Dallas Morning News,* pp. A-1, 24.

O'Sullivan, J., Franco, C., Fuchs, B., Lyke, B., Price, R., & Swendiman, K. (August 18, 1997). Medicare provisions in the Balanced Budget Act of 1997 (BBA 97, Public Law 105-33). Washington, DC: CRS Report for Congress.

Rosenfeld, I. (1998, August 16). Acupuncture goes mainstream (almost). *Parade Magazine,* pp. 10–11.

Sultz, H. A., & Young, K. M. (1999). *Health care USA* (2nd ed.). Gaithersburg, MD: Aspen.

Summary of health care legislation. (July 1997). Austin, TX: Texas Department of Insurance.

Williams, D. (1997). The real miracle of natural healing. *Alternatives.* Ingram, TX: Mountain Home Publishing.

Williamson, J. S., & Wyandt, C. M. (1997, August 4). Herbal therapies: The facts and the fiction. *Drug Topics,* pp. 78–88.

Williamson, J. S., & Wyandt, C. M. (1998, June 1). An herbal update. *Drug Topics,* pp. 60–80.

Resources

American Association of Retired Persons Medicare and Social Security: **www.aarp.org**

Congress: **www.house.gov or www.senate.gov**

Health Care Financing Administration (HCFA): **http://www.hcfa.gov**

Medicare: **www.medicare.gov**

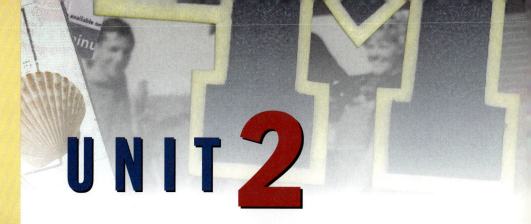

UNIT 2

The Process of Aging

PERSPECTIVE...

Retirement is a time of change. For many older adults the transition is made easy by pre-retirement planning, which includes not only the financial aspects but the psychosocial adaptations that accompany retirement from full-time employment.

Mr. Edwards is a 75-year-old Caucasian male who is an excellent example of a smooth transition from full-time career employment to full-time retiree. This change for him reflects the same personality characteristics that have allowed him to age successfully. He demonstrates ego strength, social integration, and personal control.

Mr. Edwards is an optimist whose ego identity exists well beyond the boundaries of his employment. He is the one who can always find the way to make a difficult situation better. He visits those who are sick, plans surprises to make someone's day special, and does not forget those less fortunate than he. At Christmas he is Santa Claus. At Halloween he dresses in costume and works at the church carnival. Now that he is retired he has become more active in his neighborhood association, he volunteers in the neighborhood citizen patrol, he has expanded his work within the church, he spends more time entertaining his young grandchildren, and he continues to reach out to help others when he is needed. He wonders now how he ever had time to work.

Good health is fundamental to enjoying a high quality of life. Mr. Edwards is the youngest of eight siblings who have enjoyed good physical health, but he is very health conscious. He has joined a health club and works out regularly. He eagerly does his own yard work and frequently helps others who are unable to do the physical labor around their home. He sees this as an opportunity to stay active and help others.

Mr. Edwards is an example of a person who has always possessed a strong ego identity and sense of self-worth, which are not confined to his concept of self within the employment arena. He has always been a person who valued strong social ties and led an active life. He sees life as challenging, enjoys participating in new activities, freely gives of himself to others, seeks new learning opportunities of interest to him, has a strong value system, exhibits good health practices, plans for the future, and manages his financial resources well. Successful aging for Mr. Edwards has allowed him to see retirement as just another chapter in his book of life. For him, life is full and pleasurable.

CHAPTER 4

Developmental Aspects of Aging

Linda Cox Curry PhD, RN

COMPETENCIES

After completing this chapter, the reader should be able to:

- List the developmental tasks for later maturity.
- Compare and contrast the developmental tasks projected for later maturity by several different authors.
- Identify the role of developmental tasks in later maturity to promote healthy aging.
- Discuss selected theoretical views that explain psychosocial development during later maturity: Erikson, Maslow, Havighurst, Peck, Fowler, and Atchley.
- State common life events during later maturity where adaptation is made easier by healthy resolution of earlier developmental tasks.
- Describe how one can plan ahead to contribute to retirement adjustment and satisfaction.
- Discuss the faith process as proposed by James Fowler.
- Discuss how the focus of continuity theory differs from that of Erikson.
- Describe psychosocial characteristics of healthy aging adults.
- Develop an understanding of theories of human development within the context that each person is unique.

MAKING THE CONNECTION

Refer to the following chapters to increase your understanding of the developmental aspects of aging:

Developmental Tasks

Life is constantly evolving within a changing environment. Enjoyment of life is no longer seen as only a right of youth (Figure 4-1). Humans adapt and develop with new experiences throughout life. The changes of the older adult's life may be more subtle, but they are equal in importance to those of the younger years when development is more rapid and dramatic.

A theory is an organized set of ideas, not fact, that attempts to explain interrelationships. Psychosocial theories of development help to understand human behavior. There are many theories of psychosocial development, with no one theory being complete in itself to explain the variety and complexity of human behavior. By examining different theories, it is possible to develop a more holistic concept of the dynamics of development. The theoretical approaches of Erikson, Peck, Maslow, Havighurst, and Fowler will be presented in this chapter to give a broad view of the psychosocial dynamics for adults age 60 and older (Neugarten & Havighurst, 1979).

Developmental tasks are an integral part of many developmental theories. How an adult has met earlier developmental tasks determines behavior during **later maturity.** A developmental task is a growth responsibility that occurs at a particular time in life (Havighurst, 1974). The tasks vary by stage of development and each stage builds on previous stages. The tasks for later maturity fall into three broad categories: (1) adjusting to physical and physiological changes, (2) adjusting to changes in the family life cycle and relationships with friends, and (3) changes in lifestyle (e.g., retirement, income changes, and changes in living accommodations).

Successful completion of developmental tasks leads to satisfaction and forms the foundation for a healthy adjustment during the later years. If a task is not met at the time when the task is usually met, achievement can occur but it may be more difficult, and there may be difficulty with other developmental tasks. The tasks focus on meet-

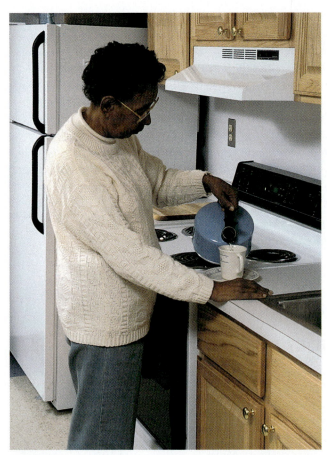

FIGURE 4-1   Most mature adults continue to live in their own homes. Many communities have services that assist them to continue living at home when help is needed with activities like food preparation or transportation.

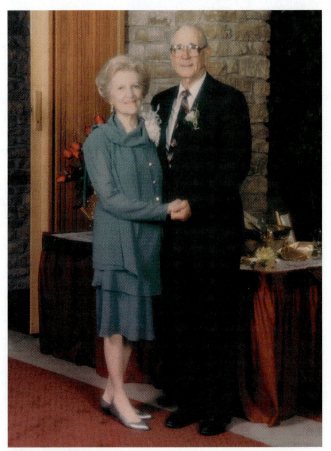

FIGURE 4-2   Long-lasting marital relationships can form the basis for gratifying companionship and promote extended social relationships.

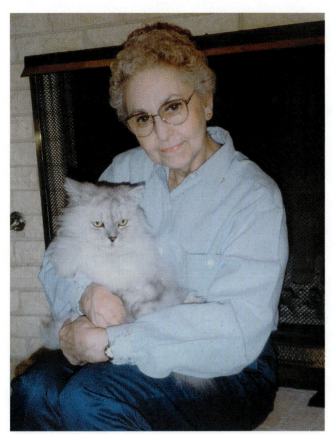

FIGURE 4-3 When developmental tasks are met, older adults experience a high degree of personal satisfaction, feeling that life has been and continues to be rewarding.

ing basic needs in all areas of development—cognitive, physical, psychosocial, and spiritual (Figures 4-2 and 4-3). When the tasks go unmet, individuals may experience anxiety, unhappiness, or maladjustment (Havighurst, 1974). Table 4-1 summarizes these developmental tasks.

> ### *Nursing Tip*
>
> How an adult has met earlier developmental tasks determines behavior during later maturity. Abrupt behavioral changes may indicate an illness or stressor.

Traits necessary for **successful aging** include **ego strength, social integration,** and personal control. Box 4-1 summarizes the key points of the theories being discussed.

Think About It

How can you utilize the developmental tasks for later maturity in your nursing practice?

BOX 4-1   Traits for Successful Aging

1. Ego strength
   - Feels satisfaction with life accomplishments
   - Goals identified and met, and new goals set
   - Positive feelings about past and future
   - Sees life as stimulating; optimistic
   - Demonstrates sense of self-worth
   - Accepting of self and others
   - Remembers good things from the past
   - Adapts to changing physical abilities
   - Experiences pleasure in life
   - Accurate self-concept
   - Adjusts to death of loved ones
   - Adjusts to changes with retirement
   - Value system is clear and guides behavior
2. Social integration
   - Learns new social roles
   - Involved with family and friends
   - Able to receive and give emotionally
   - Willing to accept help when needed
   - Continues to seek new experiences
   - Enjoys learning new things
   - Enjoys company of others
3. Personal control
   - Independent within realistic constraints
   - Able to make decisions based on current life status
   - Exhibits good health practices
   - Manages financial resources well
   - Makes plans for future
   - Adjusts to reduced income accompanying retirement
   - Utilizes needed community resources
   - Adjusts to changes in living accommodations

TABLE 4-1 Developmental Tasks of Later Maturity

Author	Identified Tasks
1. Erikson (1950)	• **Ego integrity versus despair**
2. Peck (1968)	• **Ego differentiation versus work-role preoccupation** • **Body transcendence versus body preoccupation** • **Ego transcendence versus ego preoccupation**
3. (Duvall (1977) (Duvall & Miller, 1985)	*Individual:* • Make satisfying living arrangements • Adjust to retirement • Establish comfortable routines • Maintain physical and mental health • Maintain love, sex, and marital relations • Remain in touch with other family members • Keep active • Find the meaning in life *Family:* • Aging family stage—retirement to death of both spouses • Cope with bereavement • Adapt home for aging • Adjust to retirement • Adjust to living alone
4. Brown (1978)	*Young old* (approximately 65–85): • Prepare for and adjust to retirement • Adjust to lower and fixed income of retirement • Establish physical living arrangements • Adjust to new relationships with adult children and their offspring • Manage leisure time • Adjust to slower physical and intellectual responses • Deal with death of parents, spouses, and friends *Old-old* (over 85): • Learn to combine new dependency needs with continued need for independence • Adapt to living alone • Accept and adjust to possible institutional living • Establish affiliation with age group • Adjust to increased vulnerability to physical and emotional stress • Adjust to loss of physical strength, illness, and approach of one's own death • Adjust to losses of spouse, home, and friends
5. Havighurst (1974)	• Adjust to decreasing physical strength and health • Adjust to retirement and reduced income • Adjust to death of spouse • Establish an explicit affiliation with one's age group • Adjust and adapt social roles in a flexible way • Establish satisfactory physical living arrangements
6. Fowler (1981)	• Internalize a frame of meaning for life • Deal with personal paradoxes offered by a personal openness to the viewpoint of others • Develop an openness to new social, political, economic, and ideological concepts • See past as a way to the future
7. Atchley (1997)	• Use information from life experiences to select developmental goals and life activities • Establish coping patterns and adapt to change • Develop a consistent view of self and personality

Theories

Eric Erikson

Eric Erikson (1902–1993), a student of Sigmund Freud's daughter, Anna Freud, believed the ego to be the center of personality. Ego functioning is influenced by social, biological, and environmental forces that create inner conflicts as a part of normal maturation. Throughout life, the person's energy is directed at maintaining balance. He defined eight specific developmental states organized by broad age ranges that build upon each other and lead to maturation throughout life. He does not identify cognitive or moral development. Each state is expressed as two opposing forces, or nuclear conflicts. Successful resolution of each conflict moves the person to the next stage, all contributing to one's developing ego identity (Erikson, 1950, 1980).

The eighth stage, **ego integrity versus despair**, is one of maturity, where one strives to reach acceptance of self. Erikson describes this stage, which is applicable to the years of later maturity, where one reaches **self-acceptance** (Erikson, 1950, 1968, 1980; Erikson, Erikson, & Kivnick, 1986). Integrity represents the aging person's struggle to integrate the strength and purpose necessary to maintain wholeness despite declining physical abilities. It suggests the need to make the experiences of one's life form a meaningful whole. This stage begins in retirement, punctuated with reflection on the past, reviewing ups and downs, and integrating memories and experiences into a meaningful set of beliefs not only about oneself but about the world. To achieve positive resolution one must have successfully achieved earlier developmental tasks throughout the previous seven stages; if, upon review, the previous stages form a meaningful whole, the person is left with a feeling of satisfaction and self-worth. There is an acceptance of both the failures and the successes in one's life. The person feels in control of one's life and accepts self and others. With resolution comes wisdom, which allows the person to approach death with less fear. Individuals who are able to accept responsibility for their behavior throughout life, feel pleasure and appreciation (Figures 4-4 and 4-5) with life experiences, and accept death as a part of life are most likely to reach this final stage of development (Hamachek, 1990).

Negative resolution is represented by a feeling of despair and regret, accompanied by a feeling of self contempt. The person may feel incomplete, be disappointed, feel that time is short, there is no chance to do things over, and fear death (Erikson, 1950, 1968, 1980; Erikson et al., 1986). People experiencing despair may have difficulty accepting responsibility for their lives, blame others for personal failures or difficulties, be pessimistic, and feel dissatisfied with their lives (Hamachek, 1990). Life is not acceptable to the person in despair. Those who feel a lack of control, feel they have little to be thankful for, have poor self acceptance, and wish others were different are more prone to experience despair. One's inner contempt of self may be directed at others or society in general. Such feelings may precede ego integrity as individuals work through their **life review** and thoughtfully evaluate their life. Refer to Table 4-2.

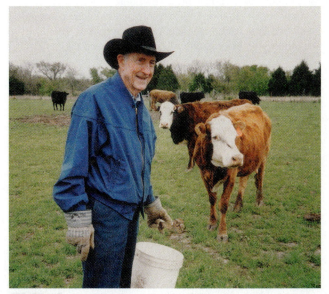

FIGURE 4-4 Ego integrity is evident when older adults appreciate life and experience pleasure in meaningful activities.

FIGURE 4-5 Ego integrity is maintained when older adults continue to use their time in satisfying ways that reaffirm their self-worth. This man and his wife continue to maintain their own home and he tends a small herd of cattle.

TABLE 4-2 Signs of Ego Integrity and Despair

Signs of Ego Integrity	Signs of Despair
Talks of past without pessimism, accepting mistakes	Easily discouraged or frustrated
Expresses satisfaction with life accomplishments	Has difficulty accepting status/lifestyle
Optimistic outlook about life	Sees little in life to be thankful for
Reminiscent but able to focus on present/future	Expresses feelings of hopelessness
Involved with family and community activities	Focuses on unresolved problems in the past
Accepting of self and others	Wishes others were different
Shares self and talents with others	Wishes to live one's life again
Able to see continued purpose in life and set meaningful, realistic goals	Emphasizes failures more than successes
Accepting of declining physical capabilities	Unable to forgive oneself for mistakes
Able to experience pleasure in life	Blames others for one's mistakes
Takes personal responsibility for self within realistic limits	Critical of self/others/society
Able to resolve feelings related to death of others	Feels they have nothing to offer others
Talks of death without overwhelming fear	Pessimistic about everyday life events
Periods of despair self-limiting and lead to self-understanding/acceptance of event	Unwilling to take control of own activities
	Withdraws from other
	Obsessive fear of death
	Unable to adjust/cope with death of others

Adapted from Erikson, E. H. (1980). Identity and the life cycle. *New York: Norton.*

Think About It

Recognizing signs of ego integrity or signs of despair can help the nurse to intervene appropriately to support the older adult's psychosocial needs. What nursing interventions would be appropriate to promote ego integrity when signs of despair are evident?

Robert Peck

Robert Peck (1968) expanded Erikson's concepts. Peck believed more emphasis should be placed on the stages of development for middle and later adulthood. His work is an effort to more specifically define stages for this period of life. He defines three psychological developmental tasks of old age: (1) **ego differentiation versus work-role preoccupation,** (2) **body transcendence versus body preoccupation,** and (3) **ego transcendence versus ego preoccupation.**

The stage of ego differentiation versus work-role preoccupation is concerned with the value a person places on job and, to a certain extent, family. A person needs to prevent feelings of uselessness and loss of ego identity that can occur with retirement. If ego integrity is chiefly obtained through one's job, retirement may disrupt ego functioning. Activities other than work that result in a sense of continued value to self and society are increasingly important with retirement. For the person whose life has centered around childrearing activities, activities need to be identified that provide a continued sense of value and ego identity. Peck has suggested that a person needs to develop valued alternatives before retirement and old age to use leisure time in a satisfying way that reaffirms self-worth. Family, friends, and the community are important avenues for ego differentiation (Figure 4-6).

Think About It

How can a person achieve ego differentiation after retirement or after all the children have left home?

Body transcendence versus body preoccupation is the second dimension according to Peck. The person who exhibits body transcendence is able to enjoy life to its fullest extent despite minor physical discomforts. The person who is preoccupied with physical discomforts will have problems enjoying life. Decrease in physical health and recuperative powers should not dominate a

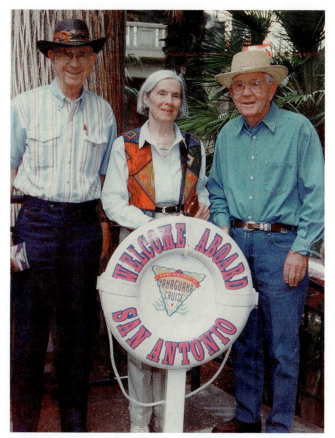

FIGURE 4-6 Traveling with family members and friends is a common activity after retirement.

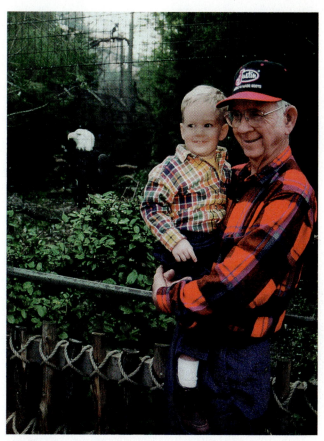

FIGURE 4-7 Grandparenting can be one of the most satisfying social relationships for the older adult. Devoting energy to the welfare of future generations helps a person achieve ego transcendence.

person's life. This stage should find the older adult sharing with others in a satisfying manner or using the creative abilities developed earlier in life. Body transcendence can occur as people emphasize their cognitive and social skills to compensate for the physical limitations that become a part of their everyday lives. To do this, they must see beyond the aging of the physical body and recognize the satisfaction other areas of life have to offer.

Think About It

What kinds of activities can a person choose to maintain a sense of purpose and self-worth during later maturity, when physical limitations are present?

People who are preoccupied with physical discomforts will be unable to see the joy and rewards other spheres of their life have to offer. Such self-focus frequently alienates others, further decreasing the opportunity for achieving happiness as social support is withdrawn. Their world becomes smaller, entrapping them physically and psychologically within their own bodies.

Ego transcendence versus ego preoccupation is the third and final dimension according to Peck. The older adult should be able to devote energies to the welfare of future generations and avoid becoming overly concerned with his or her own death. A person exhibiting ego transcendence has usually lived a generous and unselfish life. One's philosophy of life includes a healthy acceptance of death, realizing that death is an inevitable end of living. People experiencing ego preoccupation are overly concerned about their own death. The ego-transcending person is active, working to make the world a better place in which to live for familial and cultural descendants. By assuming an active role, the person leaves a legacy to be admired and emulated by others (Figure 4-7).

The person exhibiting ego preoccupation approaches and lives through this stage of life in a selfish and despondent manner. Because of a preoccupation with personal needs and death, the person is unable to care about and give of himself to the younger generations in a meaningful and satisfying manner. The older adult may be

BOX 4-2   Peck's Theory

- Ego differentiation is achieved by developing valued alternatives to work before retirement and old age to use leisure time in a satisfying way that reaffirms self-worth.

- Ego transcendence is achieved by being active, working to make the world a better place in which to live for familial and cultural descendants.

- Body transcendence occurs as one emphasizes cognitive and social skills to compensate for the physical limitations that become part of everyday living.

lonely, as a negative and self-centered attitude will cause others to avoid him.

Older adults who successfully meet the three tasks identified by Peck have successfully made a life beyond that of their life's occupation and their physical bodies (see Box 4-2). In addition, they have a vision beyond themselves that influences future generations in a positive way. Internally, they feel a sense of satisfaction that allows them to be a positive role model for youth.

Abraham Maslow

The humanist Abraham Maslow (1908–1970) proposed that psychosocial maturation and maintenance of a healthy personality occurred by meeting a **hierarchy of needs** (1954). He emphasized health, wellness, and the capacity to grow and change as basic needs are met. The individual is unique, constantly evolving, and changing for the positive as the person journeys through life. The hierarchy is not age specific but provides a framework for understanding the level of functioning at any given time and the motivations guiding behavior.

Think About It

Imagine yourself at age 80. Describe the psychosocial aspects of your life. What actions can you take now to achieve healthy psychosocial aging?

A person must meet the lower levels of the hierarchy, the strongest, in order to reach peak functioning. Like Erikson's theory, successful completion of one stage prepares one for reaching potential in the next stage, but gratification does not necessarily progress in a fixed order. Maslow proposed that although one level of needs predominates at any given time, complete resolution of a stage is not necessary to focus on another level. Some people may be satisfied functioning below their full potential. For others, once they have reached full potential, they must continually reassess and alter goals to maintain a peak level of functioning. The ability to meet potential is influenced by many constraints, both personal and environmental. Poverty, emotional deprivation, and cultural constraints are but a few environmental factors influencing a person's ability to meet inherent potential. A supportive social network and healthy view of self are other mediating factors (Figure 4-8).

The first and most basic level of needs within the hierarchy is physiological needs. This type of need includes the need for food, oxygen, water, and temperature regulation. The physical needs must be met before an individual may move to fulfilling the second level, the safety needs. These needs include having a safe non-threatening environment and an orderly nonchaotic life. The third level, the need for love and belonging, means being an accepted part of a group, being loved, and receiving affection. The fourth level, **esteem,** includes the need to be viewed by oneself and others in a positive fashion (e.g., to have self-esteem and to be held in esteem by others). People feel satisfied with themselves, their relationships, and accomplishments. The fifth and highest level of personal growth is defined as the level of **self-actualization.**

Self-actualized individuals are very content with themselves. They are open, autonomous, creative, and accepting of themselves and others. Because their needs

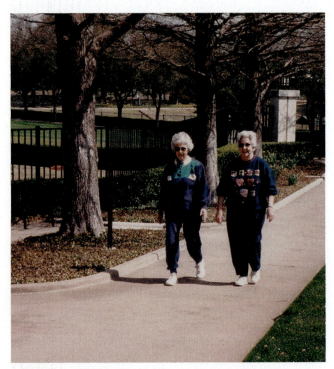

FIGURE 4-8   More people are living longer and enjoying life.

are fulfilled, they are able to look beyond themselves to help others. When self-actualization is combined with the need to know and understand and the need for art and beauty, a person has met the highest level of potential. Maslow believed that only a small percentage of the population achieve this highest level of development. Unemployment, crime, and illness are but a few factors that can block the full maturational development of many individuals, even though each individual possesses the internal characteristics to become self-actualized. When growth potential is thwarted, psychosocial problems can develop, such as feelings of despair or depression.

Think About It

Do you agree or disagree with Maslow's belief that only a small percentage of people reach their highest level of potential?

Robert Havighurst

Robert Havighurst (1974) described socially defined tasks for six developmental periods during life, the last being later maturity. He identified six tasks he believed crucial for healthy development during the last period of life. See Table 4-1.

Adjusting to decreasing physical strength and health is the first identified task. Biological aging is the result of a decrease in the functioning of cells and cellular systems. If cells are unable to rid themselves of noxious substances, cellular nutrition is impaired, and there is a decrease in the cell's ability to repair itself. Impairment of one system affects another. For instance, cardiac disease can lead to immobility and affect one's emotional well-being. In the absence of disease, there is an adjustment to the body's common changes with aging. One must adjust to the reduced immune response, longer rehabilitation time, observable physical signs of aging, and need to alter exercise habits to reduce chance of injury. People can no longer ignore the body's changing needs with age no matter how young-at-heart they feel.

Adjusting to retirement and reduced income is the second developmental task. This task is directly related to the degree of importance a job has held for the individual. People never stop working; they simply retire from positions of employment (Atchley, 1997). If retirees achieved a sense of worthiness mainly through an occupation, they are likely to suffer ego disintegration after retirement. One-half of U.S. heads of households retire before age 60 (Atchley, 1997), which is particularly hard for the person whose identity is formed mainly through work. Others look forward to retirement, having more time to spend on various areas of interest. Volunteerism,

spending time with grandchildren, hobbies, and travel are but a few activities for older adults to focus on once retired (Figure 4-9). The individual usually does not abandon the former job-related identity but adds the identity of a retired person (Atchley, 1997).

Reduced income is a serious problem. Seventy percent of male retirees receive a retirement pension, with 57% adding to the income working 20 hours or less a week (Atchley, 1997). They may not be able to maintain memberships in clubs and organizations that have been central to their social lives. Travel and lifestyle may be severely restricted. Such changes can affect emotional well-being. The degree to which people will have problems from reduced income depends on the activities they are forced to eliminate and how important these activities are to them. Planning leads to better retirement adjustment and satisfaction, yet most middle-agers do not plan ahead effectively (Atchley, 1997). Those who have made long-range retirement plans find a comfortable style of living postretirement, especially in the absence of devastating health problems.

Think About It

Is life different for single persons compared to couples when they reach later maturity?

Adjusting to death of a spouse is the third task. Women are more affected by the death of a spouse than men, partly because they are less likely to remarry and will live [alone] longer. The loss of one's spouse is a major psychological adjustment as one experiences the grieving process. Such a change can alter finances, lead

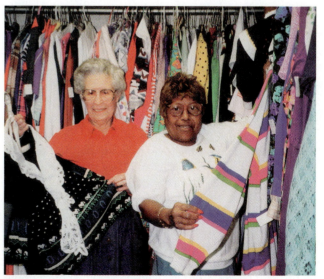

FIGURE 4-9 Following retirement, there is more time for hobbies, community service, or other activities. These women volunteer at a ministry that provides clothing for needy families.

to a change in residence, expose one to vulnerabilities by living alone, and eventually lead to the awkwardness of dating and seeking a new mate. How much a person will experience difficulty from the death of a spouse depends on the emotional ties between the two, the availability of supportive family members and friends, and how dependent the person was on the spouse for solving the problems of everyday living. Some older women are totally dependent on the husband in business matters and household repairs. Men tend to be more dependent on their wives for cooking and housekeeping chores. The need to acquire a new skill or perform a new task because of the loss of a spouse comes at a time when learning new skills and ways of coping are the hardest.

Think About It

Death of a spouse is one of the most difficult adjustments for the older adult. What nursing assessment would be appropriate to determine how well a person is making a satisfactory adaptation?

Establishing an explicit affiliation with one's age group is the fourth development task identified by Havighurst. An affiliation with one's own age group is biologically, psychologically, and sociologically determined to a certain extent.

Biological aging causes older people to slow down, making it more difficult to keep up with the activities of younger groups. From a psychological perspective one is forced to look at the concept of rewards and punishments. Sometimes older adults are rewarded internally and externally for continuing the activities of their middle adulthood (Figure 4-10). Conversely, older adults may be punished internally and externally if they are no longer able to keep up with those same activities. Internal rewards result when the older adult experiences a sense of achievement for being able to continue to participate in activities of middle age. External rewards result when they are accepted by the younger group. The reverse is true for punishment. Older adults may be unable to perform the activities of middle age not only because of biological slowing down but because of reduced income or other factors. They may be shunned by the middle-aged group because they are not able to keep up.

It can be psychologically rewarding for people to associate with their own age group or cohort. There is less need for competition, companionship is less difficult to find, and one can find prestige in organizations closed to the middle-aged group. Unfortunately, some people may feel a sense of failure or punishment when they are more or less forced to associate with their own age group. This is particularly true of those people who have

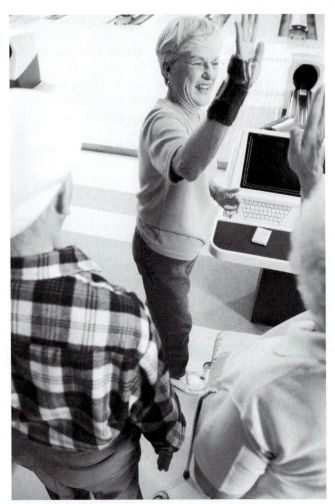

FIGURE 4-10   Older adults high-fiving at a bowling alley.

a negative view of aging and are unable to appreciate its positive aspects.

Think About It

Is it realistic to expect healthy people to be accepting and less fearful of death?

Adjusting and adapting social roles in a flexible way is the fifth of Havighurst's tasks for later maturity. Most older people receive great satisfaction and happiness once they compensate for the loss of middle-age roles. Satisfactory patterns of living are usually met by expanding family roles, being involved in the community (Figure 4-11), cultivating new activities, and maintaining a balanced slowdown of activity.

Establishing satisfactory physical living arrangements is the sixth and last of the tasks identified by Havighurst. The biological, psychological, and sociological changes associated with aging often necessitate a change in living arrangements.

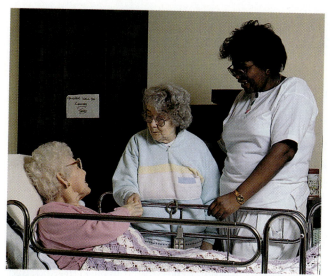

FIGURE 4-11 Volunteer work such as visiting those who are ill can be very rewarding.

Think About It

Why do the biological, psychological, and sociological changes associated with aging often necessitate a change in living arrangements?

Biological limitations caused by the presence of disease or physical changes can lead to a change in residence. For instance, a person may no longer be able to live in an upstairs apartment where there is no elevator.

Psychological needs are important. Housing areas change over the years. What was once a quiet, safe neighborhood can come to be a center of crime activity or populated by much younger families than the older person. Or they may no longer be near family. The main psychological values important to older adults in their place of residence are quietness, privacy, independence of action, nearness to relatives and friends, cost, and closeness to transportation lines and communal institutional libraries, shops, movies, and churches.

Ask Yourself

How would you feel as an older adult having to change your living accommodations because of physical limitations?

Sociological needs tend to remain similar to those of the middle-aged years. Older adults tend to continue to live as couples and maintain homes in much the same manner as in their middle adult years. If they are unable to do so, women tend to move in with their children more often than do men because women usually take care of an older husband at home until he dies. Some older adults tend to seek living arrangements in warmer climates. For example, Florida has the highest percentage of people age 65 and older, which was 18.3% in 1998 (*A profile of older Americans,* 1999, p. 8). Others prefer not to move far away from family or friends. A small number seek housing communities that consist mostly of people their own age. As the needs of the older adult become better understood, more varied choices of living accommodations will become available.

Think About It

Will there be new developmental tasks for the older adult 30 or 40 years from now?

James Fowler

James Fowler (1981) proposed that faith develops as we age, based on one's cognitive and moral development. He used the theories of Jean Piaget (1973) and Lawrence Kohlberg (1964) to explain ones' readiness for faith development. Fowler defined faith as one's basic value system, but not necessarily religious. Faith gives meaning to our lives, involving both self and others. Development of faith is a dynamic, lifelong process, based on the trust, courage, hope, and love experienced during infancy. The first three stages of faith development usually occur during childhood: (a) intuitive-projective faith—behavior is imitative and mixed with fantasy; (b) mythic-literal faith—beginning to internalize beliefs; and (c) synthetic-conventional faith—becoming more group oriented with life experiences beyond the family. The last three phases are based on adult cognitive abilities and developmental needs. Rarely is the last stage achieved. The last three stages are **individuative-reflective faith, conjunctive faith,** and **universalizing faith** and are summarized in Table 4-3.

Robert C. Atchley

Continuity theory (Atchley, 1971, 1989, 1995) focused on the process of development and proposed that adults evolve through the use of information about effectiveness of life structure, self-concept, and personality. The individual is responsible for shaping personal development and goals for developmental direction. At the core of development is the ability to adapt. Hence development occurs when adults use life experiences to select personal aspects to develop and to select activities in which to engage (Atchley, 1997).

With aging, continuity is stronger than discontinuity in both the self and personality and stability develops. Such stability is seen as a natural consequence of adult development. Information for development is continuously provided by the duration and multiplicity of relationships and environments. Individuals develop a consistent view of

TABLE 4-3   Fowler: Cognitive—Faith Theory—Adult Stages

Stage	Task
Individuative-reflective faith	Turn inward development of moral and spiritual orientation; faith and value conflicts arise
Conjunctive faith	Resolution of faith and value conflicts, reaching an improved self-understanding; openness to the views of others
Universalizing faith	Freedom to see future without constraints of past; absolute love and justice; commit oneself and life to making values a living reality (rarely achieved)

their personality and self, which includes a customary strategy for coping with the demands and opportunities of life (Atchley, 1997). Assumptions inherent in continuity theory are presented in Table 4-4.

Summary

There are many theories of development. This chapter has presented those most pertinent to later maturity. Erikson proposed eight nuclear conflicts within a socialization focus. The last, ego integrity versus despair, described the healthy older adult as content and satisfied with life. Peck extended the work of Erikson and emphasized the psychosocial development of middle

TABLE 4-4   Assumptions of Continuity Theory

- Development is continuous.
- Adults actively construct patterns of thinking in order to adapt, change, and seek individual goals.
- Adults have goals for developmental direction.
- Developing, maintaining, and preserving **adaptation** capacity are the core of adult development.
- People constantly learn about themselves and their world and use information to increase, maintain, or retain adaptive capacity.

and later adulthood. He described three specific tasks for this time of life that focused on ego differentiation, body transcendence, and ego transcendence for the adult to successfully make the transition to old age. Maslow proposed that healthy people matured within a hierarchy of basic needs. As those needs were met, they were able to achieve healthy functioning, with self-actualization representing the highest level. Havighurst identified six developmental tasks for healthy development during the last period of life. These centered around physiological changes, retirement/income changes, role changes, relationships with others, and changes in living arrangements.

Fowler proposed that cognitive and moral development forms the foundation for the development of faith, one's basic value system, and discussed six stages of development. Atchley discussed the process of development, contending that adults evolve through the use of information gained with life experiences. Adaptation through use of coping mechanisms directs the adult's development as the person chooses what aspects of self and personality to develop and what activities in which he will invest his time. With aging, continuity develops as a natural consequence of continuous development.

All theorists stress that the healthy older adults are able to successfully adapt in meeting their own needs with changing life events and the realities of physiological aging. They are content with their own life and are able to share themselves and their talents with others. New experiences and accomplishments continue to enrich their lives. Aging brings new challenges, new relationships, new discoveries, and new personal rewards.

Review Questions and Activities

1. Identify common themes among the developmental tasks identified by various authors for older adults.

2. How are Maslow's achievement of self-actualization, Erikson's attainment of ego integrity, and Peck's three stages of adaptation similar?

3. Describe characteristics of someone you know who exemplifies Erikson's older adult who projects ego integrity and someone who projects despair.

4. Identify factors in one's history that may interrupt meeting developmental tasks important for healthy aging.

5. Describe how resolution of developmental tasks throughout life promote the development of faith.

6. What major life events common to later maturity cause major transitions psychosocially?

7. What is the impact of physiological changes common to aging on psychosocial functioning?

8. According to Peck and Havighurst, adjustment to retirement is a major developmental task. What factors assist the transition to retirement?

9. How does psychosocial maturity help prepare a person for death?

References

A profile of older Americans: 1999. (1999). American Association of Retired Persons and the Administration on Aging, U.S. Department of Health and Human Services.

Atchley, R. C. (1971). Retirement and leisure participation: Continuity or crisis? *The Gerontologist, 11*(1, part 1), 13–17.

Atchley, R. C. (1989). A continuity theory of normal aging. *The Gerontologist, 29,* 183–190.

Atchley, R. C. (1995). Continuity theory. In G. L. Maddox et al. (Eds.), *Encyclopedia of aging* (2nd ed., pp. 227–230). New York: Springer.

Atchley, R. C. (1997). *Social forces and aging: An introduction to social gerontology* (8th ed.). New York: Wadsworth.

Brown, M. (1978). *Readings in gerontology.* St. Louis: Mosby.

Duvall, E. M. (1977). *Marriage and family development* (5th ed.). New York: Lippincott.

Duvall, E. M., & Miller, B. C. (1985). *Marriage and family development* (6th ed.). New York: Harper & Row.

Erikson, E. H. (1950). *Childhood and society.* New York: Norton

Erikson, E. H. (1968). Generativity and ego-integrity. In B. Neugarten (Ed.), *Middle age and aging,* (pp. 85–87). Chicago: University of Chicago Press.

Erikson, E. H. (1980). *Identity and the life cycle.* New York: Norton

Erikson, E. H., Erikson, J., & Kivnick, H. (1986). *Vital involvement in old age.* New York: Norton.

Fowler, J. W. (1981). *Stages of faith: The psychology of human development and the quest for meaning.* San Fancisco: Harper & Row.

Hamachek, D. (1990). Evaluating self-concept and ego status in Erikson's last three psychosocial stages. *Journal of Counseling and Developing, 68,* 677–683.

Havighurst, R. J. (1974). *Development tasks and education* (3rd ed.). New York: David McKay.

Kohlberg, L. (1964). Development of moral character and moral ideology. In M. L. Hoffman & L. W. Hoffman (Eds.), *Review of child research* (Vol 1). New York: Russell Sage Foundation.

Maslow, A. (1954). *Motivation and personality.* New York: Harper & Row.

Neugarten. B. L., & Havighurst, R. J. (1979). Aging and the future. In J. Hendricks & C. D. Hendricks (Eds.), *Dimensions of aging: Readings.* Cambridge, MA: Winthrop.

Peck, R. (1968). Psychological development in the second half of life. In B. L. Neugarten (Ed.), *Middle age and aging.* Chicago: University Press of Chicago.

Piaget, J. (1973). *The moral judgment of the child.* New York: Free Press.

Resources

University of Michigan Health and Retirement Study: **www.umich.edu/~hrswww**

Social Security Administration: **www.ssa.gov**

CHAPTER 5

Biological and Physiological Aging

Laura Talbot RN, CS, EdD, PhD
Mildred O. Hogstel PhD, RN, C

COMPETENCIES

After completing this chapter, the reader should be able to:

- *Discuss the concept of reserve functional capacity.*
- *State the two major theoretical categories of biological aging.*
- *Discuss age-related changes associated with the integumentary system*
- *Describe methods that the older adult can use to compensate for the age-related sensory-neurological changes that occur.*
- *Explain the relationship between nutrition and muscle/bone integrity in the older adult.*
- *Identify the single factor that retards the loss of lung function in the aging adult.*
- *Describe aging changes in the gastrointestinal system.*
- *Discuss the hormonal changes seen in the older adult.*
- *Describe the physical changes that affect sexual activities.*
- *Relate nursing implications to changes in each organ system.*

MAKING THE CONNECTION

Refer to the following chapters to increase your understanding of biological and physiological aging:

- **Chapter 17** *Management of Medications*
- **Chapter 21** *Hospice and Palliative Care*

Theories of Biological Aging

Because more people are living to old age than ever before and more is being learned about changes in body functioning with aging, chronological age is not a reliable indicator of organ system functioning. There is great variability in the rate of physiological aging among people and among the organ systems of any one person.

Rapidity of aging depends on a person's heredity, lifelong dietary patterns, the amount of habitual exercise, past illnesses, the presence of one or more chronic illnesses, and the stresses experienced throughout life. Some generalizations can be made regarding changes attributed specifically to aging. These generalized changes include:

- A decrease in the rate of **mitosis** in tissue composed of cells that regenerate, for example, epithelial tissue

- A deterioration of more specialized nondividing cells, particularly neurons and skeletal muscle cells, leading to a decreased functional capacity

- Changes in connective tissue leading to increased rigidity and loss of elasticity, producing change in organ systems

Aside from individual differences, there is a general loss of **reserve functional capacity** in all organ systems with increasing age. Body systems ordinarily maintain homeostasis, but when they are under stress, a longer time is required to adjust and return the body to a state of homeostasis.

Many theories have been proposed to determine why people age. None has been able to explain satisfactorily all aging processes or why people age at different rates. Aging theories can be grouped into two categories: those that assert a preexisting biological clock and those citing random occurrences (Hayflick, 1994). A list of generally accepted theories of physiological aging follows (Davies, 1992; Luggen, 1996; Miller, 1994).

1. Biological clock theories:

   (a) Finite doubling potential theory states the control for aging is found in the nucleus of the cells. Cells are postulated to be able to reproduce themselves a limited number of times. This limited ability to divide has been shown to occur in the laboratory, but whether the same is true within the living body is not yet known.

   (b) The neuroendocrine theory—the endocrine gland secretes hormones that regulate many body functions, such as metabolism, reproduction, and immune function.

Hormones can accelerate as well as slow the aging process, such as the role of hormones in reproductivity. The hypothalamus is thought to be one of the biological clocks associated with aging.

   (c) The immunologic theory—the immune system produces fewer antibodies with age and, as a person ages, more instances of autoimmune problems occur. Atrophy of the thymus gland occurs before the decrease in the immune system (Kay, 1979).

2. Random-chance theories:

   (a) Free-radical theory—free radicals are unpaired electrons that are by-products of oxygen metabolism. The free radicals then react with lipids, proteins, and other substances and disrupt normal chemical bonds or membranes (Harmon, 1956). Antioxidants such as vitamins E and C inhibit the formation of free radicals and may possibly retard aging.

   (b) Cross-linking theory—changes in aging occur when macromolecules are linked by a hydrogen bond or by other means. DNA may be damaged and result in cell death. In the 1950s, cross-linking in collagen was thought to decrease elasticity and permeability (Verzar, 1956). It is speculated that the cross-linkages in the strands of DNA also relate to this theory (Bjorksten, 1974).

   (c) **Lipofuscin** accumulation—lipofuscin is thought to result from the breakdown of mitochondria or lyposomes. It increases as a person ages but has not clearly been linked to changes in normal cell function (Nagy, 1988).

None of the preceding theories is accepted widely, and it is still thought that the primary reason why aging occurs has not yet been determined. It is apparent from the list of theories of aging that although scientists are not in agreement about the basic cause of aging, much is known concerning the effects of aging on different organ systems. Nurses should be aware of this information so they can provide quality care to aging clients.

Changes in Organ Systems

It is important to remember that no two people age at the same rate and that different organ systems show great variations in aging in each individual (Kain et al, 1990). Because the rate of aging is so individual, nurses should evaluate older clients carefully to identify their individual capabilities and needs when planning nursing care or helping clients meet their own needs for health maintenance.

Changes in Integument

Several changes occur in the skin and its appendages—hair and nails—with aging. Well-known changes are the graying of hair and wrinkling of the skin that lead to feelings of loss of self-esteem in many people in American society because these changes are so obvious to others and not respected in our culture (Balin, 1990).

Skin

Wrinkling is caused by the loss of subcutaneous fat and water in epidermal layers and exposure to the sun over many years. Highly pigmented skin is less prone to wrinkling and sun damage causing thinning, although cyanosis may be more difficult to detect. There are also fewer elastic fibers, resulting in reduced skin turgor, so that pinching the skin is no longer a valid indication of the state of hydration in an older person. The condition of the tongue may be a better indicator of dehydration than the skin. Sebaceous glands produce less sebum in the aging adult, so the skin may feel dry and scaly and itch. This condition can be partially overcome by using tepid rather than hot water when bathing, using less soap or an oily soap, and by eliminating the use of powder. An emollient lotion can be applied after the bath. With the thinning of the epidermis, the skin is easily injured and healing is slow if the blood flow to the dermis is impaired, as it frequently is. Because of the changes in the skin, prolonged bed rest can cause major problems such as pressure ulcers. Special beds, mattresses, and lotions can help to prevent skin breakdown (Figure 5-1).

Nails

The nails of older clients may be thick and easily split (Jarvis, 1996). It is imperative that nails be soaked in warm water before being cut or shaped to prevent splintering and to avoid possible trauma leading to infection. The condition of an older client's toenails may help to indicate whether the person is capable of living alone and caring for personal hygienic needs. An older client should be encouraged to seek professional care for the feet from a podiatrist at periodic intervals to prevent trauma, especially if the client has a severe visual deficit, vascular problems, and diabetes or if the client's body is no longer flexible enough to allow him or her to care for the feet.

Benign Changes

Older adults develop brown, pigmented areas called lentigo senilis on the dorsum of the hands, arms, and

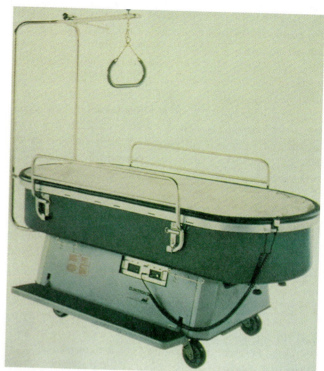

FIGURE 5-1 Clinitron® Air Fluidized Therapy Unit Model CII. *(Courtesy of Support Systems International, Inc., Charleston, SC)*

face. Lay people sometimes refer to these areas as liver spots, although they have no relationship to the liver, or age spots (Figure 5-2). These areas are harmless but may result in a feeling of self-consciousness on the part of the person who develops them.

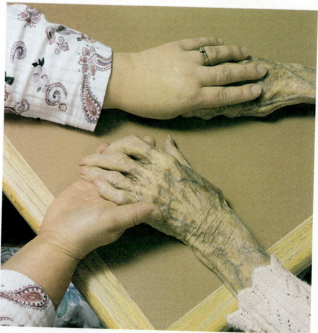

FIGURE 5-2 Pigmented areas on the hands are a normal part of the aging process.

Keratoses frequently occur on the exposed skin of the older person. Actinic keratoses are identified by raised areas that appear scaly and may bleed at the edges. There may be an area of inflammation around the border of the lesion. The lesions are unsightly and may become malignant, so they should be seen by a physician, particularly if any change in character of a keratosis is noted. Seborrheic keratoses are yellowish-to-brownish wartlike areas and are usually covered with an oily scale (Eaglstein et al., 1994). These lesions are more common in persons with oily skin and do not usually become malignant.

Cancer

Older adults exposed to the sun or other irritants for long intervals are susceptible to the development of skin cancer on the exposed surfaces of the skin. Cancer of the skin can be of either the basal cell or squamous cell type (Seidel et al., 1995). Basal cell tumors grow slowly and rarely metastasize, but they are locally invasive (Figure 5-3). Early medical treatment is essential. Squamous cell carcinoma may begin as a lesion with central ulceration or with increased keratinization (Figure 5-4). Squamous cell carcinoma will metastasize to regional lymph nodes if not treated early. Since many skin lesions in older adults appear similar early in their occurrence, medical advice should be obtained soon after a lesion is noted (Balin, 1990). Complete skin assessments should be obtained each year to assess hard-to-see areas.

CLINICAL ALERT

It is important to be very careful in turning or lifting the thin oldest old adult to prevent shearing forces from causing a tear in the skin or a fracture of the ribs, hip, or spine. Use the palms of the hands and not the fingers to lift or move an arm or a leg and roll as a log from one side to the other carefully.

Neurological Changes

There is much discussion among biologists concerning the neurological changes that occur with the normal aging process. Most research has been conducted with animals and may or may not apply to human beings.

The brain has great reserve capacity. However, in very old people there is a decrease in the size and weight of the brain, with some decrease in the number of functioning neurons, especially in the substantia nigra, striatum, and dorsal nucleus of the vagus nerve (Lukacs, 1996). It should be noted that no real correlation has been drawn between brain size and functioning (Poirier & Finch, 1990). Nurses should evaluate each client's ability to respond to the environment when deciding whether there are several pathological conditions or none. It is generally conceded that nerve transmission is slower in older adults. Nerve conduction velocity is reduced, so that by the age of 70 there is somewhat slower voluntary movement, slower decision making, and a slowed startle response.

Think About It

Why do you think some older adults have memory loss and decreased cognitive functioning when others do not?

Thought processes, reasoning, learning, and memory are retained in normal aging. Nurses need to treat older adults as intelligent people, who are capable of comprehending events unless they have a pathological condition superimposed upon the aging process. However, response time will vary for each individual.

There seems to be a consensus among biologists that the number of neurons decreases with age (Lewis, 1992). There is a depletion of dopamine and some of the enzymes in the brain of aging adults (Poirier & Finch,

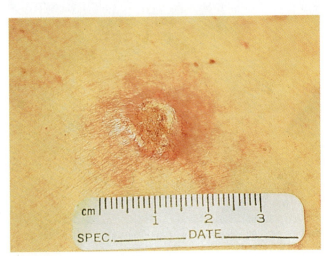

FIGURE 5-3 Basal cell carcinoma.

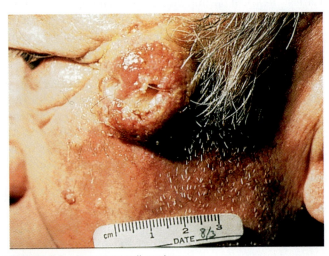

FIGURE 5-4 Squamous cell carcinoma.

1990). Older adults who appear to have reduced response to environmental stimuli increase their ability to respond spontaneously and appropriately when in an environment of consistent stimulation. There appears to be a consistent increase in the amount of the pigment lipofuscin in the cytoplasm of neurons in older adults, but there is no consensus whether this pigment is harmful to neuronal activity.

Although older adults need about the same amount of sleep as other adults (7–8 hr a night), the total amount of time spent in stages III and IV and **rapid eye movement (REM) sleep** declines with age (Gorbien, 1993). As a result the older adult may not only have more difficulty going to sleep but also awaken with a feeling of inadequate sleep (Figure 5-5). Many people resort to hypnotic drugs as they get older. A nap during the day may interfere with an older adult's sleep at night. The nurse should identify the part of the night during which the person sleeps best and help to direct the time of retiring to suit individual sleep patterns. Some older adults find that spending more time sleeping will compensate for changing sleep patterns. For some older adults a later bedtime, a change from a light to a heavier evening meal, or both will enhance sleep and the person will sleep longer in the morning. However, the majority of fluids should be taken early in the day rather than after 5:00 PM to reduce waking up to go to the bathroom during the night. A light snack at 5:00 PM with no bedtime snack may cause older people to awaken early because of hunger. Increasing physical and mental exercise during the day may also improve the ability to go to sleep at bedtime.

Because of physiological and behavioral changes, older adults have increased susceptibility to either heatstroke or hypothermia, depending on the environmental temperature (Macey & Schneider, 1993). Very old people who develop hypothermia do not shiver to increase body heat; vasoconstriction of peripheral vessels does not occur as in a young person. So the person who feels cold may have skin that is pink rather than blue or pale (Abrass, 1990). Because of the reduction in the functioning of the sweat glands and skin capillaries, the very old person cannot dissipate heat from the body and is predisposed to heatstroke if subjected to high environmental temperatures. Using this knowledge, nurses should educate older adults about the necessity of protecting themselves from direct exposure to the sun and severe heat during periods of very hot weather. Conversely, during periods of very cold weather, older adults need to be protected from developing hypothermia. Because of the loss of subcutaneous fat, the reduction in vasoconstriction, and the inability to increase body metabolism enough to increase heat production, older adults are more susceptible than the young to exposure to cold. Older adults should be encouraged to wear more layers of clothing and to wear materials that prevent loss of body heat, particularly wool garments or newer synthetics that trap body heat. Adequate covering for the feet and legs is especially important because there is less heat near the floor. Older adults should be encouraged to participate in activities that increase the body's heat production and to maintain adequate nutrition for body metabolism to provide heat.

Sensory Changes

Some sensory changes begin in early middle age. They are progressive and are apt to cause limitation of activity in later years. All the sensory organs show some degree of altered function by the age of 70 and older. In general, the changes in sensory function with aging include a higher sensory threshold and a decrease in sensory acuity. Sensory impairment in older adults can lead to malnutrition, food poisoning, and impaired immunocompetence (Schiffman, 1997). See Table 5-1 for a summary of the major sensory changes with age and suggested interventions.

The sensation of pain varies considerably in older adults. It may be more difficult to evaluate acute pain because of poor localization of pain. Pain may be referred from the site of origin. The autonomic response to pain may not occur in older adults so that rapid pulse, elevated blood pressure, pallor, and nausea may be absent (Payne & Pasternak, 1990). However, every person exhibits learned behaviors in response to pain, and older adults may have experienced chronic discomfort for such a long time that they fail to respond to a new stimulus. Also, with the oldest-old, the inflammatory response is often reduced or delayed, resulting in a

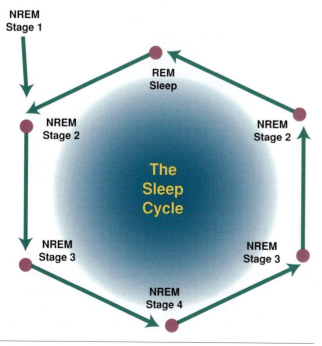

FIGURE 5-5 The sleep cycle.

TABLE 5-1   Sensory Changes and Nursing Interventions

Sensory Changes with Age	Interventions
Vision	
• Decreased visual acuity; presbyopia	Assessment of eyes and vision Eyeglasses with corrective lenses Optical devices: high-powered spectacles, hand-held magnifying glasses, telescopic devices Nonglare environmental lighting Nonoptical devices: large-print reading material, audio books (see Box 5-1).
• Delayed glare recovery	Sunglasses and antireflective coatings for corrective lenses; avoid high-gloss reading material
• Decreased light/dark adaptation with impaired night vision	Night light; decreased driving at night; pause until vision improves when transitioning from light to dark
• Decreased color discrimination and depth perception	Blue-green and blue-violet colors difficult to differentiate, use warm colors (orange, red, and yellow) to contrast backgrounds; establish well-lighted areas, especially stairs
Hearing	
• Presbycusis, reduced ability to hear high-pitched sounds	Examine for excess cerumen in the ear Use facial expressions and gestures; lower pitch of voice; install flashing lights for smoke detectors, telephones, and all safety devices; amplify volume of telephone, hearing aid; picture board (client points to needs) (Figure 5-6)
Taste	
• Decreased taste acuity with decreased saliva flow	Decreased ability to taste sweet and salty, then sour and bitter; reduced ability to detect spoiled food; check stored food for spoilage using dates; contrast food with hot and cold temperatures; use spices, herbs, lemon juice, and vinegar for seasoning; good oral hygiene. Do not increase sodium intake indiscriminately.
Smell	
• Diminished ability to smell and taste	Ensure that smoke detector is functioning; date stored food; visually check pilot light for gas appliances

decreased stimulus for pain. The pain associated with myocardial infarction described by most older adults is different in location and intensity from the pain experienced by young adults with the same condition. Such pain may not be intense because the older adult has developed collateral circulation, and the amount of **necrosis** is actually less in the aging heart. The distention of the colon associated with progressive cancer may be significant before an older adult complains of discomfort. The nurse must use a combination of assessment skills to detect the presence of pain, because the usual signs and symptoms are often not present. It is essential to differentiate acute from chronic pain because the cause and treatment may be quite different (Young, 1999).

Tactile Sensation

Because the sense of touch may be decreased in an older adult, a firmer touch may be needed to elicit a response. Many older clients respond to touch, perhaps it indicates a special sense of caring by another person. Nurses should think about this fact and use a hand on the shoulder or a hand-clasp to establish contact and provide support.

BOX 5-1   Sample Large-Print Reading Material

Prayer for Courage

Lord, it is so easy to blend in and to be like everyone else. I know I am to let my light shine, but hiding it takes less effort. Lord, help me to realize that You have not given me a spirit of timidity but a spirit of power and love and self-control. Help me to make the good confession as Jesus did before Pilate. Strengthen me through my Baptism and Your Holy Supper that I may speak Your Word with boldness. Help me to be watchful, to stand firm in the faith, to be courageous and strong, and to do all that I do in love, for Jesus' sake. Amen.

Source: Portals of prayer. *(July-September, 1998). St. Louis, MO: Concordia Publishing House. Used with permission.*

The sense of balance is precarious in many very old people, particularly when they try to hurry. The coordination of muscular activity for bodily movement may require a longer interval for processing than in younger adults. Older adults should be reminded to sit up slowly, stand firmly, and be sure of their balance before walking (Figure 5-7).

Vestibular and Kinesthetic Senses

The response to both vestibular and kinesthetic stimuli is reduced in very old people. Vestibular sense receptors are located in muscles and tendons and relay signals to the central nervous system concerning joint motion and body position in space. Because both these senses help maintain equilibrium, coordination, and body position, a diminution in their effectiveness produces a general unsteadiness, a lack of coordination in movements, and an increase in the amount of body sway in the older adult. Because a longer time is required for stimuli to reach the central nervous system and be interpreted and for messages then to be sent to the periphery, there is a great need for very old people to move slowly, have a wide stance, and perhaps use a cane for support when walking. When balance is precarious in older adults,

they should be encouraged to walk slowly, refrain from rapid body or head turning to maintain balance and prevent falls, and walk with a wider stance than in youth. Older people should be instructed not to make rapid changes in direction because such movements may cause loss of balance.

Visual Changes

A decrease in visual accommodation begins in the thirties and progresses with aging, so that **presbyopia,** or an inability to change the shape of the lens for near vision, affects most people 45–50 years old, making glasses necessary for reading fine print. The size of the pupil decreases with aging, necessitating a brighter light for vision. Sensitivity to glare also increases with age because of changes in the opacity of the lens (Castor & Carter, 1995); therefore, for reading, older adults should have a bright but diffused light (Figure 5-8). Color discrimination decreases with the yellowing of the lens in the aging process (Kee, 1990). The blue-greens and violet are difficult to see because the yellow lens screens out these colors. The yellow, orange, and red hues remain more clearly visible. Sharp contrasts in color, such as pairing yellow and black, provide an effective

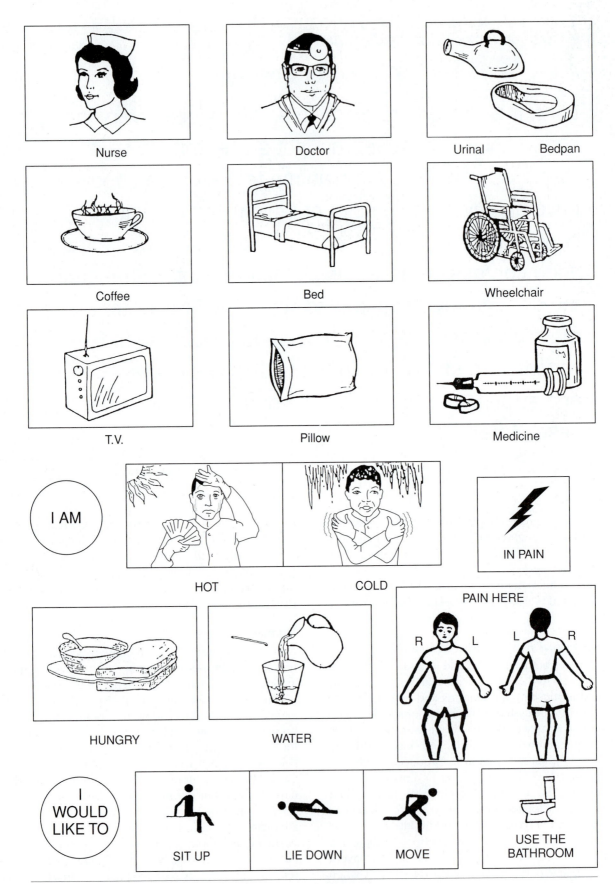

FIGURE 5-6 The picture communication board. *(Courtesy of the Seratoma Club of Fort Worth)*

medium for visual discrimination. The colors mentioned above are a valuable medium for orientation to a setting. These different colors can be used to provide highly visible landmarks for older clients in hospitals and nursing facilities. Because of the reduced color discrimination, some older adults may wear clashing colors and need guidance in selecting clothing. As vision decreases, depth perception is altered. Because of these changes, some method of determining where the steps of a staircase begin and end and the edge of each step becomes important. A narrow strip of red or yellow at the edge of each step will help an older person avoid a misstep and be aware of where the steps end.

Older people need a longer time to focus on near objects. The inability to focus quickly and the lessened ability to adapt to light-dark changes contribute to accidents that happen when an older adult moves from a lighted area to a dark area, especially if there are stairs to be negotiated. Older adults should be encouraged to allow time for their vision to adapt before they begin to move in a dark area. Hand rails are necessary on stairs to prevent falls from poor vision as well as poor balance (Figure 5-9).

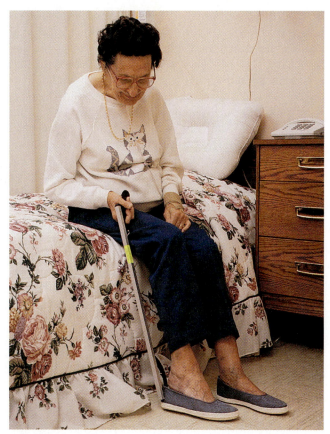

FIGURE 5-7   Older adults should be instructed to take their time when sitting, standing, and walking.

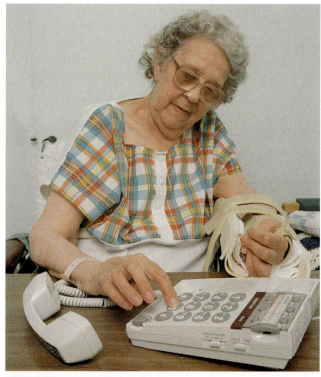

FIGURE 5-8   Good lighting and a large button phone helps improve vision.

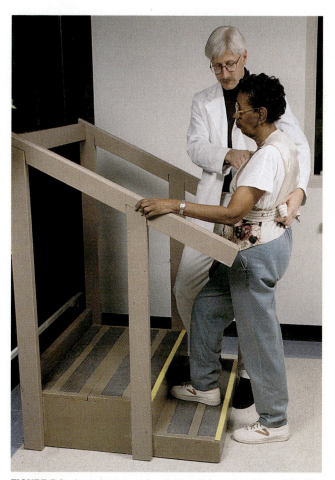

FIGURE 5-9   Learning to use handrails will help the older adult with poor balance or vision.

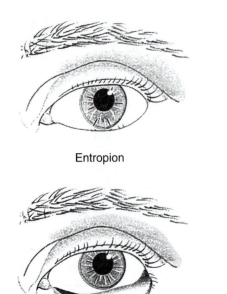

Entropion

Ectropion

FIGURE 5-10   Entropion and ectropion of the eyelids.

Another change in the eyes that accompanies aging is **arcus senilis,** or the accumulation of a lipid substance in the outer rim of the cornea. This appears as a grayish or white circle at the edge of the cornea. Such a change usually does not affect vision, although its appearance may be disturbing to the client. **Flashes** and **floaters** also increase in the eyes as one ages. They are usually harmless but may affect vision. Large flashes of light could indicate a more serious problem such as **retinal detachment,** which needs to be treated quickly.

The lacrimal glands produce fewer tears, resulting in a dry, irritated cornea that can be relieved by eye drops of the methylcellulose variety. The oldest old adult may have **entropion** (lower eyelid turning in) or **ectropion** (lower eyelid turning outward) of the eyelids, leading to more dryness or chronic irritation caused by the lashes rubbing the cornea or sclera (Figure 5-10). Minor surgical correction of entropion or ectropion will relieve this discomfort. Glasses must be free of scratches to prevent distortion of vision.

Hearing

Presbycusis, the progressive loss of hearing and sound discrimination with age, is related to changes in the organ of Corti, or the loss of nerve cells in the eighth cranial nerve, accompanied by the loss of perception of high tones. Presbycusis is more common in men than in women. Exposure to loud noises over a long period of time, such as loud music at concerts, the use of earphones with radios played at exaggerated volumes, and increased noise levels in the workplace, community, or in homes, increases hearing losses, so that in middle and

old age the deficits may be severe. Impacted cerumen also is a common occurrence in older adults and may lead to the assumption that the person has a hearing loss. This cerumen may need to be removed by the physician or nurse. Drops may be recommended to soften the wax before removal. The ability to discriminate among higher frequencies is often impaired by the age of 50 and markedly declines for most individuals after the age of 65. Most people who are described as *hard of hearing* have a selective high-frequency loss rather than a generalized decrease in hearing acuity. Thus voices, horns, telephones, and doorbells are more easily heard by older adults if they have a low tone and high intensity. Because men usually have low-tone voices, they can be heard better than women. Their decreased ability to identify high-frequency tones causes older adults difficulty in discerning the subtle tones and pitches in human speech. The older adult has increased difficulty in discriminating among sounds, particularly the consonants, *s, f, t,* and *g.* Further, pitch discrimination and threshold may decrease, so that older adults have difficulty hearing accurately because of an impairment in their ability to filter words from interfering background noise.

Hearing loss progresses slowly and unevenly. Such loss may first be noticed when the older adult complains that everyone seems to be mumbling. The increase in a person's threshold of hearing can be especially troublesome. The older adult may have to increase the volume of sounds to a point that is intolerable to anyone with normal hearing who happens to be close by. Although an older adult may hear little of a conversation held at a normal voice level, increasing the volume does little to help. The older adult hears the higher level of sound as shouting, because of the impairment in hearing at the upper frequencies.

Ask Yourself

What do you think are some of the concerns of an older adult who cannot see or hear well? What behaviors might you notice in such individuals?

Taste Buds

It is believed by some that the number of taste buds decreases with age, but such a decrease has not been shown. There seems to be decreased taste sensation, which leads to a change in the type of foods preferred. Older adults seem to like more spices, highly seasoned foods, or simply more sugar or salt in food so it can be tasted (Figure 5-11). Among healthy older adults only minimal changes occur with aging; however, prescription medications increase the frequency of complaints associated with taste (Baum & Ship, 1994). Among institutionalized older adults sometimes an elevated taste

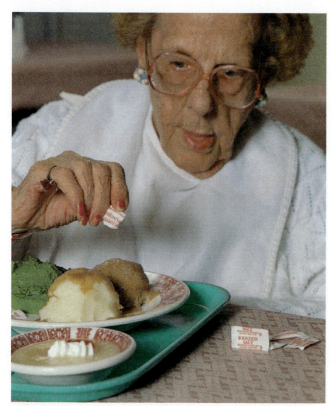

FIGURE 5-11 Adding salt to food is common due to a decreased sense of taste.

There is a concomitant loss of elastic fibers in muscle tissue, leading to reduced flexibility and increased stiffness. People who remain physically active show less muscle atrophy and stiffness. Proper nutrition is essential to help reduce muscle atrophy. Many older adults do not have enough protein, vitamins, and minerals in their diets to maintain muscle and bone integrity. Older adults are subject to loss of both muscle and bone structure over time. Any teeth that can be retained should be, and partial plates should be fitted around the intact teeth. The presence of teeth helps prevent bone resorption in the jaw. Old people who have been edentulous for a long time may not be able to tolerate dentures. Poor dental health or lack of all teeth interferes with mastication, swallowing, and good nutrition.

CLINICAL ALERT

Take special precautions while turning, lifting, and helping to ambulate older adults who are at high risk for falling. Know and follow fall precaution and restraint policies in the institution where you work.

threshold exists, possibly associated with increased use of prescription medications. Changes in taste sensation should be considered by people who prepare food for older clients. Many of the oldest old continue to taste sweets, and because high-carbohydrate foods are easier to chew, they tend to consume large amounts of sweets and neglect other types of foods.

Olfactory Nerves

The olfactory nerves are also thought to have fewer cells functioning in older adults. Because the odor of foods stimulates salivation and hunger, a diminished sense of smell often contributes to a decreased appetite. A decreased sense of smell also leads to the inability to smell danger in the environment, such as leaking gas, stove burners that are not completely turned off, and spoiled food. The oldest old person living alone should develop the habits of checking all burners after use to be certain they are turned completely off and marking the date food is placed in the refrigerator to prevent eating spoiled food.

Musculoskeletal System

With advancing years there is a gradual loss of muscular strength and endurance because the muscle cells atrophy and because of the loss of lean muscle mass.

Osteoporosis is a common manifestation of bone abnormality in older adults and occurs more frequently and at an earlier age in women than in men. Both trabecular and cortical bones are affected by osteoporosis, but trabecular bone is more severely involved. In older adults, resorption exceeds accretion of bone, resulting in a thinning of the vertebrae, long bones, and pelvic bones. Bone thinning increases the possibility of fracture resulting from weight bearing or stress. Vertebral osteoporosis leads to fracture and skeletal deformities of aging (kyphosis and scoliosis) as well as severe back pain or pressure on the spinal nerves (Kessenich & Rosen, 1996). Vertebrae are particularly vulnerable to osteoporosis because of their high proportion of trabecular bone. New effective treatment regimens use alendronate (Fosamax), calcitonin (Miacalcin), and raloxifene (Evista) in addition to calcium, vitamin D, and estrogen to prevent and treat osteoporosis (Miller, 1996; Taxel, 1998). Women age 65 years and older should consume dairy products to provide 1500 mg calcium daily or take calcium fortified with vitamin D (Johnson et al., 1995).

Nursing Tip

Good sources of calcium are skim milk, low fat yogurt, cheddar cheese, sardines, salmon, broccoli, and turnip greens. If a calcium supplement is also needed, calcium citrate and calcium gluconate are more easily absorbed in the stomach than calcium carbonate because of decreased gastric acid in many older people.

Many chronic illnesses of older people, such as intestinal malabsorption, diabetes mellitus, and uremia, increase the rapidity with which osteoporosis occurs. **Osteomalacia,** the adult equivalent of rickets, is an

Research Focus

Citation:

Schilke, J. M., Johnson, G. O., Housh, T. J., & O'Dell, J. R. (1996). Effects of muscle-strength training on the functional status of patients with osteoarthritis of the knee joint. *Nursing Research, 45*(2), 68–72.

Purpose:

The purpose of the study was to determine if 8 weeks of isokinetic strength training would improve functional health status and muscle strength in patients with osteoarthritis (OA) of the knee joint.

Methods:

Twenty patients ranging in age from 59 to 85 who were attending a rheumatology clinic were randomly assigned into either an experimental ($n = 10$) or a control ($n = 10$) group. Both groups were pre- and posttested for muscle strength, walk time, and range of motion. In addition, the Arthritis Impact Measurement Scales and Osteoarthritis Screening Index were used to measure physical health status, psychological status, pain, joint stiffness, joint mobility, and energy level. Training sessions for the experimental group included a 5-min warm-up on a stationary bike with no resistance applied, followed by a progressive protocol of muscle-strengthening exercises performed three times each week for 8 weeks. The control group received a pretest and posttest session.

Findings:

For the experimental group, there was a significant decrease in pain and stiffness with a significant increase in mobility. In addition, the experimental group also increased in all strength measures. Strength training had no effect on walk time.

Implications:

With OA of the knee, painful knee joints can lead to weakened leg muscles causing an increased workload on the affected joints. Muscle-strengthening exercises can increase mobility and decrease pain. Additional research is needed to validate these findings and examine the long-term effects of isokinetic muscle-strength training on OA of the knee.

abnormality of increased resorption of bone resulting from reduced absorption of calcium from the small intestines. Resorption occurs to maintain blood serum calcium levels, but there is concomitantly less formation of new bone.

Active exercise and a nutritionally adequate diet are now thought to decrease the rapidity with which muscle mass and bone density decrease, so the older adult should be encouraged to be as active as he or she is physically capable. Walking is a good exercise for older adults, as is swimming, if neither is carried to excess. Walking has the added advantage of providing a change of environment and sensory stimuli. But the pace must be slow enough for safety and the person should stop and rest when tired. The older adult should be reminded to stand as erect as possible while walking to help retain balance. Well-fitting supportive shoes should be worn.

Cardiovascular Changes

As with other muscles, the cardiac muscle has increased amounts of collagen and fat with increasing age. There is much discussion concerning the specific causes of the declining functioning capacity of the heart with aging, but it is generally agreed that cardiac output in response to stress declines with age (Rich, 1997). Cardiac output may be adequate for normal activity, but when undergoing vigorous exercise, stress, or illness, the heart of an older adult cannot meet the additional demands placed on it. This is thought to be a factor in the rapidity with which older adults tire. In aging, a greater percentage of the total cardiac output of blood is sent to the brain and coronary arteries, with the result that the skeletal muscles and viscera may receive inadequate blood supplies when there is increased demand for blood flow. Consistent exercise throughout one's lifetime is felt to be the best and safest way to maintain an adequate cardiac output throughout old age. With vigorous exercise the maximum heart rate of the older adult is consistently less than the maximum heart rate attained by a young person and requires a longer time to return to its usual rate (Wenger, 1990). The valves of the older adult's heart become more rigid and may compromise cardiac function, and preexisting valvular heart disease tends to become more pronounced with age, further compromising cardiac output.

The vascular system of older Americans typically shows some degree of atherosclerosis affecting the aorta, coronary arteries, and carotid arteries. The changes associated with atherosclerosis reduce the distensibility and elasticity of the large arteries and limit, to the degree of the pathological condition, the ability to increase the amount of blood available to vital organs. The effect is greatest when tissue demands increase because the diseased arteries make the work load of the heart greater. Neither the heart nor the arteries can respond to the increased need to the degree possible in young people. Therefore anything that greatly increases the need for blood, for example, fever, vasodilation, strenuous exercise, or any stress, can produce angina or syncope because the heart or brain becomes hypoxic. The aged heart can exhibit arrhythmia, which can also reduce the amount of blood flow available to tissues and cause further cardiac or cerebral problems.

Respiratory Changes

The changes in the respiratory systems of older adults are similar to those in other systems. There is generally a decreased functional reserve capacity. Medications often produce a significant negative effect on respiration so that breathing is very slow and shallow. Hypoventilation is ineffective for maximal gas exchange. Pulmonary tissue in the older adult has an altered level of function because of loss of elasticity, leading to some degree of hyperinflation of the lung. Bony changes in the thorax and vertebrae further reduce the ability of the lungs to distend. Therefore, if any circumstance occurs that demands greater oxygen consumption, the lungs are not able to respond appropriately. The poor response is also partly because of impaired cardiac function. During the aging process there is a larger portion of dead air space in the respiratory tree, so that even if the respiratory rate increases with need, the ventilation/perfusion ratio is decreased, resulting in less gas exchange. Lung vital capacity is reduced with aging, so that the amount of air that can be forcibly exhaled decreases. With the gradual decline in respiratory muscle structure and function, there is a corresponding decrease in strength for breathing and/or coughing. In older adults the vital capacity is reduced primarily because of the increase in the residual volume of air. Residual volume is the amount of air remaining in the lung at the end of a forced exhalation. The exchange of oxygen and carbon dioxide in the alveoli and capillaries decreases with the aging process. Older people who exercise consistently have less decrease in lung function. The major decrease in lung function occurs when the older adult requires maximal breathing for a period of time.

The respiratory system usually is able to meet the needs of a normal older adult, but when illness or stress precipitates a need for increased respiratory function, the reserve capacity may be inadequate to meet the need. For most people the reserve capacity is greater if they have remained active throughout life.

Gastrointestinal Changes

The salivary glands secrete less ptyalin and amylase as age advances, the saliva becomes more alkaline, and the bony structure of the mouth begins to shrink. Many older adults have missing or decayed teeth, making eating difficult and less pleasurable than in younger years. Because of changes in the smooth muscle of the digestive tract and reduced stimuli to the autonomic nervous system, peristalsis is slowed from the esophagus to the colon in the oldest old, resulting in **dysphagia.** There is delayed emptying of the esophagus and the stomach, causing a feeling of fullness. With the shrinking of the gastric mucosa, there is a decrease in the stomach secretions pepsinogen and hydrochloric acid, delaying digestion. In addition, many older adults show a decrease in the intrinsic factor, leading to pernicious anemia.

There is also a slight decrease in the amount of pancreatic enzymes with aging, which further decreases digestion and the absorption of nutrients. Bile tends to be thicker and the gallbladder empties slowly. Thus digestion is slowed but remains fairly adequate until an advanced age. Slowed peristalsis, reduced abdominal muscular strength, inadequate exercise, and reduced food and fluid intake are responsible for a high prevalence of constipation. Some older adults may have problems related to relaxation of the anal sphincter because of cold environments, anal ulcers, or hemorrhoids that lead to constipation.

Endocrine Changes

There seems to be no major decrease in hormone secretions with aging with the exception of estrogen and testosterone. It appears that there is a lack of response to some hormones and even an increase in the secretion of some hormones, notably antidiuretic hormone. Although growth hormones continue to be secreted, less of the hormone is secreted in older adults than in younger people in response to a stimulus such as a low blood sugar level.

There is some evidence that the hormones cortisol and thyroxin are not degraded as rapidly in older adults as in the young, so that the negative-feedback mechanisms cause a decline in secretions. There are two theories that attempt to explain the increasing incidence of diabetes mellitus with aging. One states that there are specific cell membrane receptors for insulin on tissue cells and that the number or sensitivity of these receptors declines with age. According to the other theory, the aging body produces antibodies against insulin. Regardless of what future research reveals, older adults generally show fairly normal fasting blood sugar levels but cannot respond to a glucose load. A glucose tolerance test will reveal glucose levels that are high and remain so longer than in younger adult nondiabetic subjects. Because older adults exhibit delayed responses in other areas of homeostasis control, it is not surprising that the complex mechanism for maintaining their blood glucose levels and glucose metabolism is slowed or inadequate.

In women, after **menopause** and the resulting decrease in estrogen levels, there are changes in breast tissue that result in less glandular tissue, reduced elasticity, and more connective tissue and fat. These changes lead to the sagging seen in older women's breast tissue, but the size of the breast may not change, because the glandular tissue is replaced by fat. Cancer of the breast may increase and there is also an increased incidence of hypothyroidism in postmenopausal women.

In men, a gradual decline in the secretion of testosterone from young adulthood to old age is assumed to occur, although there is no abrupt decline in hormone secretion or in spermatogenesis. With aging there is an increased incidence of **benign prostatic hyperplasia (BPH)** and consequent difficulty starting the voiding stream. The incidence of cancer of the prostate increases with age, so any indication of prostate enlargement should be referred for medical diagnosis and treatment.

Genitourinary Changes

The number of nephron units of the kidney decreases during the aging process, but this decrease does not account for the primary age-related changes of renal function unless the person is severely stressed. There is also a gradual degenerative change in the remaining nephron units. The renal blood flow gradually decreases—about 6% per decade after the age of 30—and is accompanied by a proportional decrease in glomerular filtration. By the age of 70 or 80 the filtration rate is approximately one-half of the rate at age 30.

Because of decreased filtration, there is a decrease in the clearance of substances normally excreted in the urine. Some of the substances that show an increase with advanced age are blood urea nitrogen, creatinine, and uric acid. Also, with decreased glomerular filtration, drugs previously excreted in the urine may remain in the bloodstream and produce toxic levels. The tubule cells decline in their reabsorption and selective secretion abilities, which can lead to loss of water and electrolytes. Steroids such as glucocorticoids and sex hormones that were formerly excreted in the urine are also retained. The function of the kidneys is usually adequate until some event occurs that demands a rapid change, for example, an event that precipitates acidosis, alkalosis, dehydration, or electrolyte imbalance.

Because of a reduced response to antidiuretic hormones in older adults, there is a decreased ability to concentrate urine. The total quantity of extracellular fluid remains fairly constant, but the intracellular fluid compartment decreases. The composition of body fluids remains relatively normal. In the aging adult the renal system is inefficient in its ability to regain normal fluid

and electrolyte balance after a rapid loss of fluids. The renal tubules of older adults are not as responsive to an increased acid or base load as those of a younger person. The tubules are not as active in secreting ammonia to be converted to ammonium chloride that aids in the removal of excess hydrogen ions from body fluids. Therefore acidosis is not corrected as quickly as in a young person. The mechanism for correcting alkalosis is also less effective and requires a much longer time than in the young person. The kidney also requires a longer time to correct electrolyte disturbances (O'Donnell, 1995).

During the aging process the ureters and bladder tend to lose muscle tone and the bladder loses enough tone to result in incomplete emptying that leads to accumulation of residual urine, increasing the risk of retention and cystitis (Sale, 1995). Usually bladder capacity decreases with age, and because the kidneys no longer concentrate urine well, frequent urination and nocturia result. Many older women, particularly those who are multiparous, experience **incontinence** because of the relaxation of the pelvic muscles with or without the presence of a cystocele. Incontinence is embarrassing in our society. Older women should be reminded that the external urethral sphincter is controlled by the pelvic muscles and should be taught to contract these muscles **(Kegel exercises)** several times throughout the day to strengthen their external urethral control.

Older men may experience frequency of urination because of hyperplasia of the prostate and decreased bladder capacity. Both men and women may avoid shopping trips or social interactions because of frequent or urgent urination or the fear of incontinence. Frequent rest stops during a trip and an understanding that the older adult may hesitate to state the need for relief should be anticipated by family, associates, and nurses.

Many older adults also restrict their fluid intake to prevent frequent micturition. They need clear, concise explanations of the hazards of dehydration that can result from this restriction and should be encouraged to take at least 2,000 mL of liquids in 24 hr unless contraindicated because of other medical conditions.

Urinary incontinence is not a normal part of the aging process. It is a symptom with an underlying cause. Still, age-related changes to the genitourinary system can predispose the older adult to incontinent episodes. Pharmacological and pathological insults to the older adult can trigger transient incontinent episodes, which, if left unchecked, can lead to the misconception that incontinence is part of the aging process and untreatable.

Treatment of incontinence focuses on finding the underlying pathology through urodynamic testing and a complete history and physical examination. Once the cause is identified, the goal of the practitioner is to restore continence. If incontinence persists, the focus will be directed toward assisting the individual to modify the environment and utilize available resources so that activities of daily living can be carried out with minimal disruption. For example, an older adult who has a stroke may have irreparable damage to the neurological system that innervates the urinary system. Incontinence may be a result. Because a cure may not be possible, managing incontinence through modifying the environment would be the management approach, such as bedside commodes and night lights for safety.

Many older adults who develop an acute illness and are in bed for a period of time will develop a problem related to continence. The person who is aware of the problem may feel a loss of self-worth. Efforts should be directed toward establishing urinary control as the person recovers from the illness. Environmental factors can also play a vital part in achieving continence. Functional incontinence may occur if the older client's request for assistance to the bathroom is not met when needed. Older adults may not have the ability to hold their urine for an extended period of time. When the sensation of urinary urgency occurs, action needs to be taken immediately. Nursing care should be focused on finding a means of restoring continence, because success can mean the difference between home care and institutionalization for the older adult.

Sexual Changes

Physical changes occur after menopause (cessation of menses) and **andropause** (midlife changes in the male) that may affect sexuality and sexual activity. Of concern to many men and women are the changes that are noticed in the sexual response cycle. In the female, the ovaries cease to produce ova (eggs) and have less estrogen hormone that may cause physiological symptoms in some women. The uterus becomes smaller and in old age is about one-half the size of the uterus of the young adult woman. The fallopian tubes also decrease in size and, with the decline in estrogen levels, become less motile. The vulva and external genitalia shrink with aging because of a loss of subcutaneous fat. The vagina loses elasticity and may decrease in breadth and depth, especially if the woman has had a hysterectomy. There is also less vaginal lubrication and penetration is more difficult. These physical changes may cause **dyspareunia.** Treatments include **hormone replacement therapy (HRT)** (somewhat controversial because of the possible adverse effects) and vaginal hormone creams and lubricants. Once the couple understands why it takes longer for vaginal lubrication to occur in the woman past the age of menopause and the need for extended foreplay, the problem may be resolved. Older women should be informed that water-soluble lubricants may relieve the pain and discomfort and allow sexual activity to continue. Without the nurse's intervention the conditions that cause the pain might continue, so that the woman may lose interest in sexual activity and avoid it whenever possible. This avoidance of sexual intimacy can have a negative effect on the relationship. Stereotypical attitudes of family members and health professionals may dictate the sexual expression of older couples more than the couple's own wishes.

In the male the penis may decrease in size and conditions/surgery of the prostate gland may affect the ability to have an erection. **Erectile dysfunction (ED)** (also known as impotence) is the consistent inability of the male to achieve and/or maintain an erection that is sufficient for intercourse and affects some 30 million men of all ages (Rosenfeld, 1998). Erection may take longer to achieve, not last as long, and require a longer interval between erections. New medications developed in recent years (e.g., Viagra) have helped older men with this condition that is often caused by other physical diagnoses or problems. These newer medications are simpler and easier to use than previous treatments such as penile implants or injections. However, as with all medications, Viagra can cause adverse effects, especially for those with cardiovascular conditions. The development and wide publicity about the newer treatments have made the issue of erectile dysfunction more open so that men have felt more comfortable talking about the problem and seeking treatment (Rosenfeld, 1998). Sexual activity is normal and possible in the older age group if there are no major health problems. Couples can learn to enjoy experimenting with new and different techniques, such as variations in foreplay, positions, and roles that make adjustments for physical conditions such as arthritis. Older couples may also find increased pleasure in other types of intimacy, such as holding hands, hugging, and sharing personal thoughts and feelings (Figure 5-12).

Sexual activity also occurs in retirement centers, assisted-living facilities, and nursing facilities. Facility staff should be accepting of such behavior and ensure

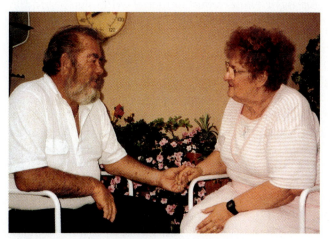

FIGURE 5-12   Older adults still need companionship and intimacy.

privacy if the activity is between cognitive consenting adults and no harm occurs. Family members, however, may disagree and protest. Even on a dementia unit, a resident may enjoy and find support in spending time talking with and holding hands with a member of the opposite sex. Sometimes these types of activities decrease agitation and anxiety of the residents.

Nurses should discuss the topic of sexuality with clients when the need is identified. Older adults should be reminded about the dangers of sexually transmitted diseases and the related precautions because these might not have been major problems when they were younger. The nurse can also teach the client and his or her partner about the effects of drugs on sexual desire. Some drugs, such as tranquilizers and antihypertensive agents, will decrease libido. Some men and women refrain from taking antihypertensive drugs because they fear a loss of their sexual potency, because the risk of having a stroke may be less anxiety producing for them than being unable to perform sexually in a satisfactory manner. The nurse who understands these factors can be more understanding of and helpful to clients who have problems with sexuality.

Immunological System Changes

Research is being pursued to learn more about the immune system in humans. Two views are held concerning changes in this system as people age. One theory that is widely accepted is that the very old have a delayed or inadequate response of the immune system to infectious agents, so that infections in the very old, as in children, are more likely to be fatal than they are in younger adulthood.

The second theory that seems to be recognized by the scientific community holds that as people age, there is an increase in the production of antibodies that fail to recognize the person's own tissue and cause an increasing incidence of autoimmune diseases. Shock (1984) stated that the T lymphocytes are decreased in number and in their ability to function as efficiently as in young individuals. This is thought to be due to the involution of the thymus gland.

In addition to having a delayed immune response to infections, older adults have a delayed or inadequate response to the stress of an infection, so there is a real hazard for the older adult who develops conditions such as pneumonia or cholecystitis. The altered inflammatory response leads to altered signs and symptoms, such as little or no fever, less pain sensation, and minimal leukocytosis, that, unaltered, would alert both a younger adult and the physician or other health care provider to a medical problem. Nurses should have a high index of suspicion when early warning signs of illness are present in older people. More research is needed concerning the differences in the responses of older adults

to social as well as physiological stress. Nurses must be particularly alert in assessing early changes in homeostasis maintenance mechanisms in older adults and should refer the person for medical attention when stressful situations occur.

In the older adult the total blood volume is about the same as in a young person of comparable size and sex. However, the older adult may not be able to redistribute blood volume when anemia, blood loss, or congestive heart failure is present. The veins in the feet and legs may be enlarged and have loss of elasticity (Lipschitz, 1990). Hemoglobin values vary greatly in individuals of the same age and sex with aging, but this is thought to be caused by disease rather than aging alone. However, Lee and Walsh (1990) stated that bone marrow studies show a decrease in erythropoietic function in the older adult. There is a decrease in the formation of leukocytes as one ages, so the ability to respond effectively to infection is decreased. Iron deficiency anemia is common because of poor nutrition or blood loss.

Nursing Implications

Nurses should divest themselves of the stereotypes they hold of older adults and consider each client as an individual with unique capabilities and needs. Nursing actions to meet the needs of older adults should be based on a knowledge of common physical changes and a specific data base for each individual.

Some generalizations about care can be made, however. Older adults should be encouraged to remain as active and independent as their physical condition allows so as to maintain their current level of functional capacity. The speed of activities should be well paced. Rest should be encouraged before fatigue occurs. Explanations or instructions should be clear and given in a relaxed manner. Enough time should be allowed for a response. If detailed explanations are needed, reinforcement is helpful. Nurses should encourage an adequate fluid intake, because the sensation of thirst may be reduced and the ability to concentrate urine may be decreased. Nurses should always be aware that older clients often show minimal signs and symptoms of serious physical problems. Careful attention should be given to early changes in behavior and other aspects of the physical and psychosocial assessment and such changes should be promptly reported to the physician or other appropriate health care provider.

Summary

Chronological age is not a good indicator of physiological age or of organ system functioning. The rate of age change varies among people and among organ systems in each person. As a general rule the client who is 85 years or older is expected to show the greatest accumulation of age-related change.

There is a decrease in the reserve capacity in all organ systems with aging. Body systems have greater difficulty maintaining homeostasis when they undergo illness or social or psychological stresses. The organ systems require a longer time to respond to the stress and return to a state of equilibrium. In the oldest old client the reserve capacity may not be great enough to restore equilibrium, and death may result from a situation that would be a lesser problem in a young adult, for example, diarrhea with severe fluid and electrolyte loss.

In addition to physiological changes in most organ systems, older clients are apt to experience multiple chronic illnesses that require several drugs for treatment, thereby increasing the risks of adverse effects of drug interactions. Symptoms of illness in older adults are often nonspecific and easily ignored because of the general belief that the symptoms result from the normal aging process. Age alters the response to disease by causing a slower and lower level of response; for example, there is often little if any temperature rise with infection. Pain perception is usually decreased and therefore its protective function is lost.

Review Questions and Activities

1. Explain the difference between normal and pathological physical changes of aging.

2. Why is proper toenail care so important in older adults?

3. What is the major characteristic of keratoses?

4. What is a major difference between basal cell and squamous cell carcinoma?

5. What is the effect of changes in REM sleep in older people?

6. What colors can older adults see best? Why?

7. What are the consequences of decreased sensitivity of taste buds?

8. What are the major changes in the cardiac and respiratory function of older adults?

9. Explain the physiological changes of both women and men that affect sexual functioning in old age. Discuss how ageism affects attitudes about sexuality in older adults.

10. Describe at least one nursing intervention related to physical changes in each of the major systems.

References

Abrass, I. (1990). Disorders of temperature regulation. In W. R. Hazzard, R. Anders, E. Bierman, & J. Blass (Eds.), *Principles of geriatric medicine and gerontology* (2nd ed.). New York: McGraw-Hill.

Balin, A. (1990). Aging of human skin. In W. R. Hazzard, R. Anders, E. Bierman, & J. Blass (Eds.), *Principles of geriatric medicine and gerontology* (2nd ed.). New York: McGraw-Hill.

Baum, B. J., & Ship, J. A. (1994). The oral cavity. In W. R. Hazzard, E. Bierman, J. Blass, W. H. Ettinger, Jr., & J. B. Halter (Eds.), *Principles of geriatric medicine and gerontology* (3rd ed.). New York: McGraw-Hill.

Bjorksten, J. (1974). Crosslinkage and the aging process. In M. Rockstein (Ed.), *Theoretical aspects of aging*. New York: Academic Press.

Castor, T. D., & Carter, T. L. (1995). Low vision: Physician screening helps to improve patient function. *Geriatrics, 50*(12), 51–58.

Davies, I. (1992). Theories and general principles of aging. In J. C. Brocklehurst, R. C. Tallis, & H. M. Fillit (Eds.), *Textbook of geriatric medicine and gerontology* (4th ed.). Edinburgh: Churchill Livingston.

Eaglstein, W. H., McKay, M., & Pariser, D. M. (1994, April 15). The problems that plague aging skin. *Patient Care*, pp. 89–107.

Gorbien, J. J. (1993). When your older patient can't sleep: How to put insomnia to rest. *Geriatrics, 48*(9), 65–75.

Harmon, D. (1956). Aging: A theory based on free radical and radiation chemistry. *Journal of Gerontology, 11*, 298.

Hayflick, L. (1994). *How and why we age*. New York: Ballantine Books.

Jarvis, C. (1996). *Physical examination and health assessment*. Philadelphia: Saunders.

Johnson, R. M., Kaiser, F. E., Kerstetter, J. E., & Reuben, D. B. (1995). Calcium and other help for your bones. *Patient Care, 29*(18), 68–77.

Kain, C., Reilly, N., & Schultz, E. (1990). The older adult: A comparative assessment. *Nursing Clinics of North America, 25*(4), 833–848.

Kay, M. B. (1979). The thymus: Clock for immunological aging? *Journal of Investigative Dermatology, 73*(1), 29.

Kee, C. (1990). Sensory impairment: Factor X in providing nursing care to the older adult. *Journal of Community Health Nursing, 7*(1), 45–52.

Kessenich, C. R., & Rosen, C. J. (1996). Osteoporosis: Implications for elderly men. *Geriatric Nursing, 17*(4), 171–174.

Lee, M., & Walsh, J. (1990). Hematology. In C. Cassel, D. Riensenberg, L. Sorensen, & J. Walsh (Eds.), *Geriatric medicine* (2nd ed.). New York: Springer-Verglag.

Lewis, P. D. (1992). The neuropathology of old age. In J. C. Brocklehurst, R. C. Tallis, & H. M. Fillit (Eds.), *Textbook of geriatric medicine and gerontology* (4th ed.). Edinburgh: Churchill Livingston.

Lipschitz, D. (1990). Anemia in the elderly. In W. R. Hazzard, R. Anders, E. Bierman, & J. Blass (Eds.), *Principles of geriatric medicine and gerontology* (2nd ed.). New York: McGraw-Hill.

Luggen, A. S. (1996). Theories of aging. In A. S. Schmidt (Ed.), *Core curriculum for gerontological nursing.* St. Louis: Mosby.

Lukacs, K. (1996). Neurological/Alzheimer's disease. In A. S. Schmidt (Ed.), *Core curriculum for gerontological nursing.* St. Louis: Mosby.

Macey, S. M., & Schneider, D. F. (1993). Deaths from excessive heat and excessive cold among elderly. *The Gerontologist, 33*(4), 497–500.

Miller, M. M. (1996). Endocrine disorders: New technology allows quick, accurate diagnosis. *Geriatrics, 51*(1), 52–58.

Miller, R. A. (1994). The biology of aging and longevity. In W. R. Hazzard, E. L. Bierman, J. P. Blass, W. H. Ettinger, Jr., & J. B. Halter (Eds.), *Principles of geriatric medicine and gerontology* (3rd ed.). New York: McGraw-Hill.

Nagy, I. Zs. (Ed.). (1988). Lipofusin—1987 state of the art. *Excerpta Medica,* International Congress Series 782.

O'Donnell, M. (1995). Assessing fluid and electrolyte balance in elders. *American Journal of Nursing, 95*(11), 41–46.

Payne, R., & Pasternak, G. (1990). Pain and pain management. In C. Cassel, D. Riensenberg, L. Sorensen, & J. Walsh (Eds.), *Geriatric medicine* (2nd ed.). New York: Springer-Verlag.

Poirier, J., & Finch, C. (1990). Neurochemistry of the aging human brain. In W. R. Hazzard, R. Anders, E. Bierman, & J. Blass (Eds.), *Principles of geriatric medicine and gerontology* (2nd ed.). New York: McGraw-Hill.

Rich, M. W. (1997). Epidemiology, pathophysiology, and etiology of congestive heart failure in older adults. *Journal of the American Geriatrics Society, 45,* 968–974.

Rosenfeld, I. (1998, July 19). When impotence is curable. *Parade Magazine,* pp. 14–16.

Sale, P. G. (1995). Genitourinary infection in older women. *Journal of Obstetric, Gynecologic Neonatal Nursing, 24*(8), 769–775.

Schiffman, S. S. (1997). Taste and smell losses in normal aging and disease. *Journal of the American Medical Association, 278,* 1357–1362.

Seidel, H. M., Ball, J. W., Dains, J. E., & Benedict, G. W. (1995). *Mosby's guide to physical examination,* St. Louis: Mosby.

Shock, N. W. (1984). Energy metabolism, caloric intake and physical activity of the aging. In N. Shock (Ed.), *Normal human aging: The Baltimore longitudinal study of aging.* Washington, DC: NIH Publication.

Taxel, P. (1998). Osteoporosis: Detection, prevention, and treatment in primary care. *Geriatrics, 53*(8), 22–40.

Verzar, F. (1956). Aging of collagen fibres. In *Experimental research on aging. Experientia,* supplement 4:35. Basel: Birkauser Verlag.

Wenger, N. (1990). Cardiovascular disease. In C. Cassel, D. Riesenberg, L. Sorensen, & J. Walsh (Eds.), *Geriatric medicine* (2nd ed.). New York: Springer-Verlag.

Young, D. M. (1999). Acute pain management protocol. *Journal of Gerontological Nursing, 25*(6), 10–21.

Resources

Advanstar Communications: **geriatrics@advanstar.com**

Geriatrics: **www.geri.com**

CHAPTER 6

Psychological Aspects of Aging

Bert Hayslip, Jr., PhD

COMPETENCIES

After completing this chapter, the reader should be able to:

- *Discuss the characteristics of aging from a life span perspective.*
- *Understand aspects of perceptual functioning that do and do not decline with age.*
- *Compare the distinction between learning and memory in later life.*
- *Distinguish between memory structures and memory processes.*
- *Discuss the influences on memory performance of older adults.*
- *Define the conditions under which intelligence does and does not decline with age.*
- *Discuss the major theoretical views on personality and aging.*
- *Answer the questions "Does personality change with age?" and "How do different older adults cope with the aging process?"*
- *Discuss ways older adults might improve their memory and intellectual functioning.*
- *Discuss therapeutic options for psychological interventions.*

MAKING THE CONNECTION

Refer to the following chapters to increase your understanding of the psychological aspects of aging:

The Life Span Developmental Approach to Aging

As it becomes necessary for many to care for aging parents or other older family members, aging is likely to be perceived as either a problem or something to be looked forward to, valued, and treasured. Changes in how the body functions or appears may demonstrate how people are treated as they age (Karp, 1988). People with positive self-images will interpret such events positively (though perhaps inaccurately), while those with fragile, negative self-views will likely adopt a negative view of aging (Atchley, 1982, 1997).

This chapter provides a view of psychological aging that reflects the immense diversity among older adults, stressing the larger developmental framework in which aging occurs. Also discussed will be many of the aging-related changes in psychological functioning that research conducted over the last 20 years has revealed, stressing their role in the everyday lives of older adults. These changes are of importance to not only those who conduct aging research but also to those professionals and laypersons who care for older adults.

A model that examines psychological aging in light of the complexity of both describing and explaining the aging process is the **life span developmental approach** (Baltes, 1987, 1997; Baltes, Reese, & Nesslroade, 1986; Lerner, 1996; Riegel, 1976). The life span approach views the process of aging as being affected by many mediating or moderating factors. Consequently, older adults are best understood in the context of these factors and their relationship to one another. These include *inner-biological* factors (health or illness), the *physical* or *cultural* aspects of the environment (outer-physical and cultural-sociological factors), and *individual-psychological* influences. The nature of how people experience aging as well as both the quantity and quality of their lives varies in terms of the extent to which these factors are working together, or at cross-purposes with one another (Riegel, 1976). All older adults, as do all adults, go through smooth and bumpy periods in their lives, where they are more or less in synchrony with others as well as with physical or social changes in their everyday lives. For example, after the death of a spouse, one may wish to remarry but not find a suitable mate, illness may interfere with one's plans after retirement, or one may be forced to retire prematurely because of poor health or other factors.

The life span developmental model views development and aging as multidimensional and multidirectional. **Multidimensionality** refers to the fact that it is necessary to both describe and explain aging in terms of many different dimensions or aspects of development.

For example, intelligence and sensory abilities are very distinct and independent processes, and each is likely to be caused by different sets of underlying factors. Aging and development are also multidirectional, which suggests that change can take on many forms or directions. For example, some abilities will decrease with age, others will increase with age, and still others will be age irrelevant; that is, they do not change with age.

Causes of Change in Adulthood

Development and aging are universal characteristics of all living organisms and thus entail and imply change. The life span perspective suggests that to adequately understand changes in the context of adulthood and aging, one must consider three types of influences: (a) **age-normative,** (b) **history-normative,** and (c) **nonnormative influences** (Baltes, 1987, 1997).

Age-normative influences are general to the process of development and are highly related to chronological age. Although the timing in terms of onset may vary for different persons, these influences generally affect people of a specific age in a particular manner. Age-normative influences can be the result of either bio-physiological processes, such as the onset of puberty or menopause, or social-environmental factors, such as mandating a specific age for marriage, getting a driver's license, or retirement. History-normative influences are events that occur at a specific point in time (day, month, or year) and theoretically affect everyone in a given society or culture. Within a given historical context or cohort these influences, nevertheless, can have different effects on individuals as a function of age. For example, the Great Depression of the 1930s, or being a member of the baby-boom generation are each factors that differentiate people by cohort membership. The personal values, expectations about family or career, access to health care, or level of education of people who are members of a particular birth cohort are shaped by the historical context in which they are born, raised, grow into adulthood, age, and die. Nonnormative influences are factors that are not related to age or historical change but whose effects are unique to specific individuals. For example, having an accident, becoming seriously ill, winning the lottery, or being fired from a job are all examples of nonnormative events.

Each of these influences is considered ongoing and interactive in terms of its effect across the life span, and each affects individuals differently as a function of age. Because age-normative influences are maturational and often under genetic control, they have the most pronounced effects during childhood and old age. History-normative influences are most pronounced among adolescents and young adults, and nonnormative events increase in significance with increasing age (Baltes et al., 1986; Danish, 1981).

Several core ideas about psychological aging can be derived from the life span approach: (a) the person-environment interaction, (b) pluralism, (c) decrement with compensation, and (d) plasticity.

Think About It

What are important factors in the environment that affect how people adapt to aging changes?

Person-Environment Interaction

The concept of person-environment interaction suggests that behavior and performance are the result of the interactions or transactions between older individuals and their environments (Panek, 1997). Thus, to age successfully, people must continually and selectively match their skills to the environment, which is also changing (Baltes, 1997). This concept is illustrated by the transactional model of Lawton and Nahemow (1973). The components of the transactional model are presented in

Table 6-1. According to this model, psychological aging is viewed in terms of the demands and pressures from the external environment as well as the changes in physical and cognitive functioning that take place. Consequently, for most older adults, to deal effectively and competently with the environment, they must engage in tasks and activities that match their ability levels.

Pluralism and Psychological Aging

As noted above, aging is a complex phenomenon. It is perhaps best described as pluralistic in nature, reflecting diversity rather than sameness among older adults (Baltes, 1987; Hoyer, 1974). This diversity expresses itself most directly in the life experiences of older adults, and the parameters along which such differential experiences can be understood are in many ways as diverse as older adults themselves. Childhood experiences with parents and gains and losses of significant relationships with others through geographic mobility or death exemplify factors that differentiate one person from another. One's experiences with marriage, parenting, divorce, or illness, expected and unexpected turns in one's career, or role changes (that is, grandparenting, widowhood,

TABLE 6-1 Components of the Transactional Model

Component	Description and Example
Degree of individual competence	The diverse collection of abilities and skills the person possesses, for example, sensory processes or intelligence. Each of these abilities or skill levels is unique to the person and varies over time between minimum and maximum limits that are specific to each person.
Environmental press	The demands from the environment impinging upon and affecting the individual, for example, demands or requirements of the task, job, or situation.
Adaptive behavior	The outer manifestation of individual competence. For example, in the work environment, adaptive behavior can be considered the observable (measurable) performance on the job.
Affective responses	The inner, unobservable aspects of the individual-environmental transaction, including the person's evaluation and emotional reaction to the environment. For example, if the person is critical of his or her performance, the person may respond by becoming angry or depressed.
Adaptation level	The point or level where the person is functioning at a comfortable level relative to the external demands. Beyond this comfort zone, positive affect decreases and becomes negative as demands push the person past an adaptation level. For example, if the person's adaptation level is driving 55 mph, 60 might be challenging, and attempting or being required to drive 65 mph would cause the person discomfort and may result in an accident.

Adapted from Lawton and Nahemow (1973) and Panek (1997).

institutionalization) are also examples of factors that differentiate people along biological, interpersonal, intrapersonal, or cultural lines.

The point to be made most strongly is that the differences among older adults are of sufficient magnitude to preclude general statements about aging-related changes in sensory, perceptual, cognitive, personality, or interpersonal aspects of functioning. While it is tempting to draw general, all-encompassing conclusions about older adults or the aging process, the fact is that individual differences among older adults are indeed great (Nelson & Dannefer, 1992). This variability among older adults in personalities, interests, attitudes, and capabilities should be recognized and encouraged.

Ask Yourself

Do you believe older adults tend to think, feel, and act alike as they age? If not, why do younger people sometimes refer to them as a group?

Pluralism is consistent with multidimensionality and **multidirectionality,** that is, strength versus speed of response, short-term versus long-term memory, and verbal versus performance aspects of intelligence. Each changes in diverse ways with age. Pluralism also embraces different theoretical models or explanations to account for changes with aging. A broader, more flexible theoretical stance can be adopted that encompasses a variety of viewpoints regarding why persons age in the ways they do.

Decrement with Compensation

If one assumes that losses in functional skills with age are necessarily and causally related to biological/physiological changes associated with the aging process, that person is using an irreversible decrement philosophy of aging (Schaie & Gribbin, 1975). There are some decrements that accompany aging, for example, cardiac output, nerve conduction velocity, vital capacity, and cortical size and composition clearly decline with age (Fries & Crapo, 1981; Hayflick, 1994). Declines with age in memory function, certain dimensions of intelligence, and the efficiency of information processing and **reaction time** can easily be documented (Hayslip & Panek, 1999; Kausler, 1991; Salthouse, 1991). While it would be easy to conclude that such declines are biologically based (maturational), such conclusions would be unjustified for a number of reasons: (1) in many cases, such data are cross-sectional in nature, and age effects are confounded with **cohort effects** in such comparisons; (b) such declines are in many cases products of disease, the disuse of skills, or artifacts of what have been termed

ability-extraneous influences (for example, depressed affect, task-specific influences, sensory loss, speededness, fatigue, or response bias) (Hayslip & Kennelly, 1985; Kausler, 1990). Ability-extraneous influences either exacerbate what would otherwise be mild decline or mask genuine positive change. The irreversible decrement model of psychological aging is also undermined by (1) the wide individual differences in rates of decline and/or levels of function late in life and (2) the pluralistic nature of such changes.

While some older adults show declines in their cognitive skills, upon closer examination they discover that they lack confidence in themselves for various reasons. Older adults who believe they cannot continue to acquire new cognitive skills with age decrease their efforts at new learning; such individuals lack what Bandura terms self-efficacy (Bandura, 1989). Disuse of once proficient skills, related to social isolation, disease, or lack of support by significant others, can lead to apparent declines in proficiency, reflecting the popular notion of "use it or lose it" (Hayslip et al., 1995).

Think About It

How would you apply the concept of use it or lose it to your nursing care of older adults?

Laypersons and professionals alike often fail to distinguish between aging and disease and are willing to attribute declines in functioning to aging. For example, declines in memory function thought to be causally related to aging are often found to be consequences of pathology (for example, Alzheimer's disease) (Butler et al., 1991; Heston & White, 1991). This problem reflects the importance of the distinction between **normal, optimal** or **healthy,** and **pathological aging** (Abeles, 1997). Normal aging involves changes in functioning and behavior that are inevitable. They occur as the natural result of maturation or the passage of time and affect all persons. Optimal or healthy aging refers to the aging of individuals who have no identified physical illness, while typical aging describes the aging of individuals who have one or more medical conditions that become prevalent in later life. Pathological aging refers to changes with age that are the result of abnormal conditions or disease processes, rather than to age per se.

Rather than accept an irreversible decrement model of aging, most professionals now endorse a *decrement-with-compensation* model of the aging process. In this case, by virtue of changes older adults themselves make or via environments that supplement and enrich older adults' lives, declines in function can be minimized or even reversed. For example, simply taking care of one's own health, developing effective strategies for coping with threats to one's well-being and self-esteem (Atchley, 1997), seeking out others for support and advice (Foster & Gallagher, 1986), or involving oneself in new and challenging activities or opportunities are all ways in which older adults can forestall declines in health, well-being, or cognitive skills that may vary with but not be causally related to growing older. Such strategies may also allow older adults to compensate for declines in their cognitive or physical skills (Baltes, 1993).

Perhaps most important is to foster in all the view that aging need not be a time in our lives when loss and decline are seen as inevitable. Where declines are present, drawing upon experience and the acquired wisdom of years of solving everyday problems (Sternberg, 1991) can lead to positive growth and change even into very advanced old age. Seeing aging-related declines in functioning as multicausal (causally related to both maturational and experiential factors) is also consistent with pluralism and contextual embeddedness.

Plasticity

Baltes (1987, 1997) uses the term *selective optimization with compensation* to refer to the fact that human change is adaptive. Because aging consists of gains and losses in (intellectual) function, adaptive functioning is characterized by the tendency to selectively optimize one's skills. While one's information processing, memory, or intellectual skills can selectively decline, individuals can take steps to compensate for such declines by purposefully developing those skills that depend upon experience or new learning. Individuals, when they reach their biological limits, can choose to channel their resources or energies into those domains in which high levels of proficiency are still possible while seeking to maintain their problem-solving, intellectual, or memory skills to the fullest extent. These actions can be beneficial despite the fact that the limits of such skills are to a certain extent dictated by maturation, heredity, or the effects of illness/ disease.

The literature in the area of aging clearly substantiates the plasticity of intellectual and physical functioning through deliberate intervention and skill training, changes in one's lifestyle, or focusing on individuals' beliefs and feelings regarding their continued ability to function adaptively (Baltes, 1987; Fries & Crapo, 1981; Elias, Elias, & Elias, 1990; Hayslip, 1989). Thus, relative to levels of function prior to training, older adults can improve their skills significantly. Recent interest in creativity, expertise, and wisdom as well as an emphasis on the motivational and psychosocial determinants of cognitive performance in late adulthood reflect the inherently plastic nature of human change (Kausler, 1990; Schooler, 1987; Simonton, 1990). Thus, while some older adults do experience declines, such losses are not uni-

versal and are subject to the demands of the everyday context in which humans function. Human growth and change are not only desirable but also quite realistic and attainable. Enhancing the quality of later life has become the focus of study rather than the documentation of decline.

Having discussed life span development in which psychological aging is best viewed, it is important to examine what is not known about a variety of domains of psychological aging: reaction time, learning and memory, intelligence, personality, and psychological interventions with older adults. In each case, several questions will be addressed: (a) To what extent are changes in late adulthood to be expected? (b) What factors explain such changes? and (c) To what extent are such changes amenable to training or intervention? For most laypersons and professionals, the answers to such questions will have a major influence on their interactions with older adults, be they clients, friends, or family members.

Perception

Perceptional changes with age have major implications for the everyday functioning of older adults (Kline & Scialfa, 1997). Several of the most important perceptual processes for everyday functioning are **vigilance, selective attention,** and reaction time.

Vigilance

Vigilance is the ability to maintain attention on a task for a sustained period. It is very important on tasks such as driving, assembly-line work, air-traffic control, computer programming, and other activities where the person must maintain attention for a fairly long period of time (Panek, 1997; Panek et al., 1977). Performance on vigilance tasks decreases with age; young-old differences on vigilance tasks do not seem to be changed with practice (Parasuraman & Giambra, 1991). Age differences in vigilance vary as a function of the nature of the task, the sensory modality studied, the length of time one is expected to be vigilant, the time one has to respond, memory, the number of items to be monitored, and fatigue (Belmont, Epperson, & Anderson, 1989; Kausler, 1991). Kausler (1991) suggested that vigilance is most impaired in older adults when a task is rapidly paced or lengthy or when individuals must hold information in memory.

Perceptual/Cognitive Style

Perceptual or cognitive style has been developed to help explain individual differences in perception (Rogers, 1997). One's perceptual style more or less sets the stage for those aspects of the environment to which one attends. How attention is divided, as well as what information one chooses to process, is likely to be influenced by a general perceptual orientation to the environment. One aspect of cognitive style is field dependence/independence. People who are field dependent make judgments that are heavily influenced by the immediate environment, while the judgment of field-independent people is not. Extensive cross-sectional data suggest that there is a shift from field dependence to independence during adolescence, continuity during adulthood, and a return to field dependence during old age (Panek, Barrett, Sterns, & Alexander, 1978; Rogers, 1997).

Selective Attention

Selective attention is an essential aspect of perception, information processing, and everyday behavior. In many situations, people engage in divided attention, or the allocation of attentional resources to two simultaneous sources of stimulation (reading this text and watching the television). On divided-attention tasks, the performance of both young and old individuals declines as the tasks increase in difficulty. However, the decline is generally greater and more rapid for older adults (Wright, 1981). When the attentional demands of the task decrease, the performance of older adults improves (Lorsbach & Simpson, 1988).

Overall, research indicates that as people get older they are less able to concentrate on two simultaneous tasks (Kausler, 1991). Explanations include a diminished ability to divide attention, short-term memory impairment, left hemispheric dominance, and complexity (Kline & Scialfa, 1997; McDowd & Craik 1988). Research suggests that older adults, when confronted with difficult or complex tasks, often respond anxiously (Hayslip, 1989). Anxiety can interfere with attentional resources in situations where mental effort is expected, as can depression and fatigue (Hayslip, Kennelly, & Maloy, 1990).

> ### Nursing Tip
>
> Do not rush ill older clients on admission to a clinical facility. Take time to explain carefully what you want them to do, such as changing into a gown or going to the bathroom to obtain a urine specimen. It may take just a little longer for them to process those requests and complete the task.

Reaction Time

One of the most documented age-related changes is a slowdown in behavior and performance (Panek, 1997; Vercruyssen, 1997). From age 40 onward, accuracy ap-

pears to be emphasized at the expense of speed in performing a psychomotor task (Welford, 1977), which is referred to as the **speed versus accuracy trade-off.** By age 60, the maximum speed of movement may decline by as much as 90% and often continues to slow at an increasing rate as one gets older (Vercruyssen, 1997).

This slowdown in behavior has often been studied with reaction time tasks. In a reaction time task, the person must (a) perceive that an event has occurred, (b) decide what to do about it, and (c) carry out the decided-upon action (Welford, 1977). Thus, poor performance can often be attributed to one or more of these other factors rather than to just the speed of motor performance. When studying perceptual-motor reaction time, researchers derive two components: (a) **premotor time,** which is the time from the onset of a stimulus to initiating the response, and (b) **motor time,** or the time from initiating the response to completing the response. Although there are consistent age-related differences on each of these components, the most pronounced age differences are in the **decision or premotor time** component (Kausler, 1991; Panek, Barrett, Sterns, & Alexander, 1978; Vercruyssen, 1997). That is, it takes older adults a longer time to initiate the response (decision time) than those who are younger. Although age-related slowing is well documented, it is still largely unexplained (Salthouse, 1993). The many explanations for the slowing of behavior with age can, however, be classified into either the neurobiological (hardware) or the psychological (software) perspective (Vercruyssen, 1997). Explanations in the former category suggest that the slowdown in behavior and performance can be attributed to some change in the central nervous system, that is, a generalized slowing of central nervous system function. Aging also disrupts decision-making processes and higher cortical functions (Fozard et al., 1994); these decision-making processes and higher cortical functions are the basis of the software perspective.

> ### Think About It
>
> How would you apply the perceptual processes of vigilance, selective attention, and reaction time to the discharge plan of an older newly-diagnosed insulin-dependent client who is going home to live alone?

Learning and Memory

All people have memory lapses or have difficulty in **learning** new information from time to time. Unfortunately, when people reach their fifties and sixties, even temporary slips of memory or difficulty in learning new ideas is interpreted as a sign that they must be getting old, or worse still, that they might have Alzheimer's disease, and thus is cause for alarm, anxiety, or depression. Such memory failures might even cause a son or a daughter to consider institutionalizing a parent. Learning difficulties or memory loss with increased age may become a self-fulfilling prophecy for some middle-aged and older adults (Figure 6-1).

In thinking about memory and aging, it is important to distinguish between normal, maturational changes in our memory skills that are independent of disease, which have been termed **age-associated memory impairments** (Crook et al., 1986), and pathological changes in memory, which are caused by the effects of disease or injury, for example, Alzheimer's disease or vascular dementia (Cherry & Smith, 1998). While age differences in memory depend on the nature of the memory system and associated processes, what it is that one is trying to remember and how one accesses memory (Cherry & Smith, 1998) show that there are great differences among adults in the nature of their memory skills (Powell, 1994).

Learning can be understood in terms of the acquisition of *stimulus-response (S-R) associations* (Kausler, 1991), while forgetting is caused by a weakening or breakdown of these associations. The stimuli (S) evoking a response (R) that may lie in the environment (a sound causes one to turn his head), must first evoke an internal connection that may be a particular thought or image, (for example, the sound just heard means class is over). This internal connection mediates (links) the observable, external response (R), such as putting one's notes away and leaving the classroom. In contrast to a stimulus-response perspective, the *information-processing approach* stresses that learning and memory are best understood in terms of **registration, encoding, storage,** and **retrieval**—the adult learner is an *active processor of information* (Schwartz & Reisberg, 1991). For example, one might organize or categorize information and store for later retrieval or recall, as people often do when trying to remember grocery items to be purchased or learning and recalling names at a party.

Though learning and memory are often treated as separate, in reality they are related to one another. When one's ability to learn a list of words is assessed, for example, it is often only through the *recall* of that list that conclusions about how many words one has learned can be reached. Because both learning and memory cannot be observed directly, they must be *inferred* from performance.

One can distinguish between memory for general rules or basic meanings, termed **generic** or **semantic memory,** and memory for specific events, termed **episodic memory** (Kausler, 1994; Smith, 1996). Memory may be intentional or explicit, or it may exist without an awareness for remembering, in which case it is termed implicit (Hultsch & Dixon, 1990). Relative to explicit memory, implicit memory performance is relatively stable with increased age (Hultsch & Dixon, 1990). This is true for recall for the occurrence of specific bits of information (items) known to the learner as well as memory for associations between unrelated items.

Memory Structures

Memory in adulthood can also be understood by studying memory structures and **memory processes,** as illustrated in Table 6.2. With the former approach there are distinct structures or hypothetical entities defining memory. Typically, differences between sensory, primary, secondary, and **tertiary memory** stores are expressed in terms of the time elapsing from exposure to recall of information.

Each memory store serves a different function within the multistore memory system. **Sensory memory** is preattentive or precategorical—what exists is in the form of unprocessed image. Material in sensory memory decays very rapidly (within ⅓ to 1 sec). There are few clear age differences/age changes favoring young adults regarding sensory memory (Kausler, 1994), especially

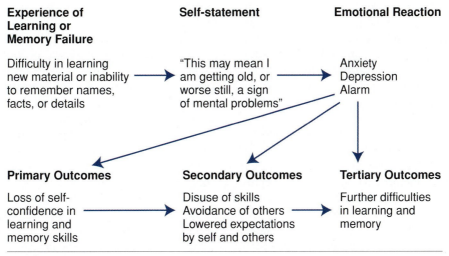

FIGURE 6-1 Learning and the cycle of memory loss.

TABLE 6-2   Memory Structures and Aging

Memory Structure	Defining Characteristics
Sensory memory	Rapid decay of memory (e.g., ½ sec) preattentive in nature, little aging decline, depends on sensory integrity
Primary memory	Limited to what one can consciously retain at present. Reliable but modest age declines in both active and passive aspects.
Secondary memory	Less limited capacity. Age deficits are common and reflect the nature of how material is actively processed, stored, and retrieved.
Tertiary memory	Almost unlimited capacity. Age effects depend upon the date of the material and extent of rehearsal.

both **iconic** (visual) and **echoic** (auditory) sensory memory. It may be difficult to demonstrate that sensory memory even exists for older adults who may be experiencing serious sensory or attentional deficits.

Primary memory contains items that are within one's conscious awareness; such information decays if it is not processed further. While its capacity is small, primary memory plays an important role in the control and assimilation of information (Poon, 1985), serving more as a temporary holding and organizing reservoir and less as a formal storehouse of information. In general, there seems to be at best a moderate age decrement in primary memory (Hultsch & Dixon, 1990; Kausler, 1994; Smith, 1996), using, for example, a *digit span* task, where digits of varying span lengths (two to seven digits) are read to the individual, who repeats this span in the same order. When digits are repeated in reverse order, however, age differences favoring younger people are stronger, largely because of deficits in primary memory (Hultsch & Dixon, 1990; Dobbs & Rule, 1990).

When material to be remembered exceeds primary memory, it enters the **secondary memory** store, whose capacity is less limited (five to seven items). When age deficits in secondary memory occur, they generally reflect its lessened capacity by primary memory deficits (Kausler, 1991). Older adults may be slower or less efficient in searching the content of the secondary store, and they may organize information to be stored less efficiently (Kausler, 1991). Older adults rehearse to-be-

remembered items less actively and search for such items less efficiently. This problem contributes to both primary and secondary short-term memory deficits (Kausler, 1994). Age deficits are also found in an aspect of secondary memory—working memory—the simultaneous processing of two tasks, one of which must be stored while the other is being actively processed (for example, having to remember a guest's name at a party while being introduced to someone else).

Tertiary, or long-term, memory, whose storehouse is in theory limitless and permanent, refers to recall of remote events or extended recall for recent events. Researchers studying remote or tertiary memory typically use questionnaires to gather their data. While age differences in tertiary memory do exist, they tend to favor older adults (Perlmutter & Mitchell, 1982). However, deficits with age in tertiary memory are difficult to demonstrate, given the confounding of the age of the individual and the date of that which is to be recalled (Botwinick, 1984). Because it is not known exactly what persons knew at the time the memory was *originally* encoded and stored, it is difficult to know who has the better long-term memory, younger persons whose store is less extensive and for whom searching its contents is less cumbersome or older persons who have accumulated more knowledge and who have perhaps rehearsed more often that which is personally important (Kausler, 1994). The latter suggests cohort differences to influence tertiary memory performance (Storandt, Grant, & Gordon, 1978).

Memory Processes

As opposed to memory structures, a newer approach to memory emphasizes *processes* that explain *how* material is transferred from one memory store to another (Craik, 1977; Poon, 1985). Figure 6-2 illustrates how each of these stores can be linked together via memory processes. These processes are referred to as registration, encoding, storage, and retrieval, and they build upon and interact with one another.

Registration refers to whether the material is literally heard or seen, that is, its size or loudness exceeds one's sensory threshold—this is a prerequisite for further processing such information. If, for example, an older adult has some sensory loss (e.g., poor eyesight), it is unlikely that what has been presented visually will be adequately registered. Encoding refers to the process of giving meaning to information after it has been registered and has entered the sensory store. Creating a visual or verbal mediator (a rhyme or an image) to help one learn and recall a list of words reflects encoding. Encoding information requires that one attend to and rehearse (actively process) information that has been registered. The ease with which material stays in the system is determined by the efficiency of the learner's encoding system. Storage

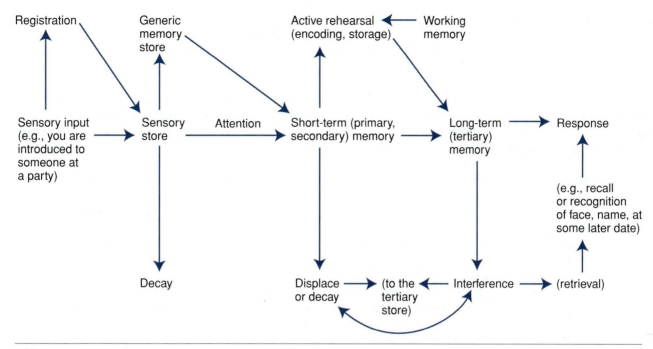

FIGURE 6-2 Links between memory stores via memory processes.

suggests that information, having been encoded in some form, is then organized in a hierarchic (general-to-specific) pattern, where general categories are first created, within which more specific categories are developed.

It appears that older adults are less likely spontaneously to organize or to use mediators, and they store information less efficiently (Kausler, 1994). A good way of expressing the distinction between encoding and storage is that encoding involves establishing a memory trace, whereas in storage, this trace is maintained (rehearsed) until it can be retrieved (Kausler, 1994). Retrieval is, quite simply, getting out information that presumably has been registered, encoded, and stored. Typically, recognition formats show fewer age differences than do recall tasks (Poon, 1985), highlighting retrieval as a critical skill that is essential to both secondary and tertiary memory (Craik, 1977; Poon, 1985).

Influences on Learning and Memory in Later Life

As a general rule, whether a given older adult is a superior learner or has a good memory is relative to (a) the nature of the information to be learned; (b) the needs, abilities, and motives of the individual; and (c) the requirements of the situation in which one uses learning and memory skills (Cockburn & Smith, 1991; Hultsch & Dixon, 1990; Willis, 1985). For this reason, those interventions used to help other adults improve their learning and memory skills must be flexible.

When various aspects of the task, such as the amount of time given to originally learn an item or to

search one's memory for a correct response, are paced, age deficits in secondary memory are increased. In paced tasks, the time per item or between items is restricted. For example, a paced task would require that one learn and recall material at a fixed rate of presentation (e.g., one item per minute). However, proceeding through each item at one's own speed would be learning in an unpaced situation. Older adults recall the fewest correct words when they are not given sufficient time to respond. Increasing the time available to search and retrieve a correct response seems to be more important in lessening age differences in learning and memory (Monge & Hultsch, 1971).

Much research has suggested that the extent to which encoding is supported or impaired may determine secondary memory deficits among adults. For example, encouraging and training adults in the use of **verbal mediators** (a verbal association involving the words to be learned) or **visual mediators** (a mental picture involving the words to be linked) seem to help matters greatly (Rowe & Schnore, 1971).

Robertson-Tchabo, Hausman, and Arenberg (1976) and Anschultz et al. (1985) have had great success with the **method of loci,** by which the learner is asked to imagine a walk through his or her home, picking out several stopping points during the journey. The learning and memory of words were greatly helped by instructions to associate each of the familiar loci with each word. Closely related to the method of loci is the keyword method, where the learner forms a word *(whale)* that sounds like the word to be remembered (the name *Whalen*), which also elicits a clear image (a whale swimming). This too was found to be helpful for both younger and older learners. Unfortunately, in the long term (3 years after training), older learners frequently abandon the method of loci even though it had been effective (Anschultz et al., 1987). Likewise, specific instructions to *organize* the material, for example, using the alphabet, creating categories (Schmidt, Murphy, & Sanders, 1981), have been shown to enhance learning/memory.

Helping older adults learn to manage their anxiety about failure is also very important (Kooken & Hayslip, 1984). The debilitating effect of the inappropriate use of attention is also observed in older adults when the task requires a great deal of cognitive effort or concentration. This issue is based on a fixed-resources view of older adults' attentional capacity (Smith, 1996). When older adults must *divide their attention* when they are anxious or when they are confronted with a complex task such as learning to give their own insulin or a simple task requiring a complex response, their attentional resources are further compromised by having to devote effort to how their attention is used (Perlmutter, 1983; Plude & Hoyer, 1981). This situation leaves them few resources with which to deal with the task itself and respond appropriately (Smith, 1996). A clinical example of such a situation might be learning how to give the insulin injection while still in a busy hospital setting.

One's personality as a noncognitive factor (something that influences one's performance) also has an important influence on learning and memory in later life (Kausler, 1990). Personal beliefs about whether it is even important to maintain one's skills or not can and do influence learning and memory skills (Kausler, 1990, 1991).

Recent discussions of how to best improve learning and memory in adulthood reflect a sensitivity to a variety of these influences on learning and memory performance (Cherry & Smith, 1998; West, 1989). Enhancement techniques involve (a) assessing the learning and memory demands one faces, (b) identifying helpful strategies that individuals are capable of and are willing to use in improving their skills (e.g., organization, mnemonic aids, overlearning, verbal elaboration), and (c) ensuring that such gains can be maintained and that they are generalizable (West, 1989).

Practical Memory in Late Adulthood

Practical memory refers to the use of learning and memory skills to cope with the everyday demands that are made on us in real life. The use of our memory skills depends upon our beliefs about and estimates of our memory skills, termed **metamemory** (Dixon, 1989). Related to metamemory is (a) **memory self-efficacy**—the confidence one has in his or her memory skills; (b) **memory management**—the strategies and techniques one

uses to make best use of one's memory; (c) **memory remediation**—the efforts we make to improve our memories; and (d) **memory fears**—concerns about memory loss that affect people personally (Reese, Cherry, & Norris, 1998). Reese et al. (1998) found that older adults could remember important dates (birthdays, anniversaries) but not names, used external memory aids most often, wanted to improve their memory for names and for verbal information, and linked the loss of their independence to memory failures. These findings suggest much potential for enhancing everyday memory performance among middle-aged and older adults. This might be achieved by providing (a) skills for memory improvement, (b) skills to best use one's existing memory skills, and (c) techniques to cope with fears over memory failures. An interest in how adults use their memory and learning skills is important because it helps us to understand how cognitive processes can be used and improved to enhance the quality of life and everyday functioning for adults of all ages.

> ### Nursing Tip
>
> A newly admitted older client in the hospital may not remember your name after one introduction; repeat your name every time you enter the client's room. Giving the client your name, title (e.g., registered nurse or nursing student), and the reason for being in the room each time you enter will facilitate future communication and the client's trust in you and your care.

Intelligence

What is known about intelligence in later life is nearly as complex as that for learning and memory. Primary mental abilities and fluid and crystallized abilities are discussed to illustrate this varied picture of intellectual aging.

Primary Mental Abilities

The primary mental abilities (PMA) approach has served as the framework within which K. W. Schaie has conducted perhaps the most extensive studies of adult intellectual development to date (Schaie, 1979), beginning with a series of cross-sectional and longitudinal studies that began in 1956. Data from the first cross-sectional study conducted in 1956 suggested that different types of abilities demonstrated diverse age-related peaks of functioning. Schaie found PMA reasoning (predicting a letter having seen a string of letters preceding it, e.g., *abcd_*) to peak most early, versus Space (thinking about objects in two or three dimensions), Verbal Meaning (vocabulary), Word Fluency (naming as many words as possible that begin with the letter *B* in 30 sec), and Number (arithmetic), which all peaked later. Younger adults had strengths in different areas than did those who were older. The 1963 data found evidence for a **time of measurement effect,** where those tested in 1963 at comparable ages were superior to those tested in 1956. Longitudinal (1956–1963) findings suggested that age-related changes in intelligence were minimal until people reached their sixties. Schaie's data suggested that cohort differences were more important in explaining the cross-sectional or longitudinal age effects found for many abilities than was chronological age (Schaie & Willis, 1996). Further, analyses suggested positive cohort effects, that is, more favorable performance for successively younger cohorts for Verbal Meaning, Space, and Reasoning. For Number, cohort effects were minimal, while for Word Fluency, cohort effects were slightly negative, where young cohorts scored more poorly. Thus, the extent to which age decrements in intelligence vary with (a) the type of ability examined and (b) cohort membership (Schaie, 1996). Schaie's 21-year study of adult intelligence clearly indicates that the notion of irreversible, biologically based decline with age in abilities is clearly unfounded. In most cases, depending upon the interaction of the sociocultural environment (whether it is stimulating or not) and aging, the age decrement in intelligence may be reduced or intensified—different cohorts age intellectually in unique ways. Thus, there is no such thing as universal, true decline (Baltes & Schaie, 1976). Schaie's data also indicate that declines in ability are largely restricted to those 70 or over.

Crystallized and Fluid Intelligence

The distinction between **crystallized (Gc) intelligence** and **fluid (Gf) intelligence** abilities is especially suited to adult development in that both are defined in such a way that predictions about developmental change are possible. What is perhaps most distinctive about fluid ability is that it can be measured by tasks in which relatively little advantage comes from intensive or extended education and acculturation (Horn, 1978). Crystallized skills come about as a function of more organized, systematic, acculturated learning. Gf is *fluid,* or fluctuates with the demands made in novel situations. On the other hand, Gc *crystallizes* or takes on a definite form or character with experience—early learned skills are the basis for those acquired later on in life. In some cases, where the problem or situation demands a novel response to it, Gf will come into play, whereas when previously learned skills are required, Gc will be called upon. Fluid intelligence is thought to increase and then decline over the life span, whereas Gc should generally increase or remain stable over the adult years (Horn &

Cattell, 1967; Horn, 1978). The distinction between Gf and Gc (Horn, 1978, 1982) suggested that in adulthood a more complex picture of intelligence is necessary (Figure 6-3). Thus, a global measure of intelligence (IQ) fails to separate crystallized and fluid intelligences. As is true for PMA measures of intelligence, considerable variation can also be observed both within and across individuals in Gf and Gc functioning. For example, some adults may make more effort to sharpen their skills than do others (Horn, 1978). Some people are more prone to fatigue, anxiety, or attentional lapses than are others (Horn, 1978; Kennelly, Hayslip, & Richardson, 1985). These factors should be considered when caring for ill clients in any clinical setting.

Research Focus

Citation:
Hayslip, B. (1988). Personality-ability relationships in aged adults. *Journal of Gerontology: Psychological Sciences, 43,* 74–84.

Purpose:
To investigate relationships between crystallized and fluid abilities and dimensions of personality in older adults.

Methods:
One-hundred and two community-residing older adults were administered measures of crystallized (e.g., vocabulary) and fluid (e.g., letter series) abilities as well as the Holtzman inkblot technique, a projective (inkblot) measure of personality. Five dimensions of personality, based on previous work, were derived from the Holtzman inkblot technique.

Findings:
Statistical analysis (factor analysis) of ability and personality data indicated that crystallized ability correlated with a personality dimension labeled Anxiety over Ideational Sufficiency and that fluid ability correlated with a personality dimension labeled Intellectual Resources to deal with Reality.

Implications:
These findings indicate that intellectual functioning in later life may be influenced by personality dynamics. More specifically, it may be that some older adults accumulate information to protect them from feelings of intellectual decline while at the same time develop intellectual skills that reflect the everyday requirements of problem solving and decision making.

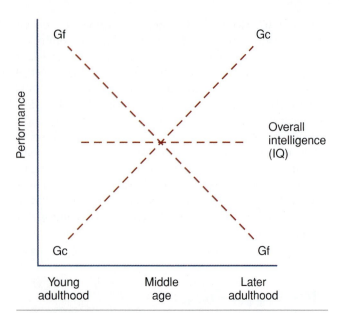

FIGURE 6-3   Age curves for Gf and Gc versus an overall measure of intelligence.

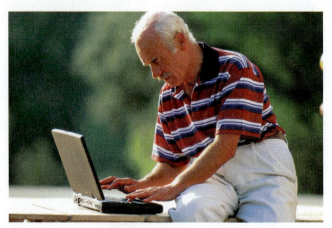

FIGURE 6-4   Activities that are enjoyable provide diversion and help to stimulate mental functioning.

Factors Influencing Intelligence in Later Life

While cohort effects may modify the aging of intelligence, a number of other factors influence declines in intelligence with age. For example, sensory deficits in hearing and vision may put many older adults at a disadvantage (Sands & Meredith, 1989). Persons who are in poor physical and mental health tend to perform more poorly on a measure of fluid ability (Perlmutter & Nyquist, 1990), while Hertzog et al. (1978) found that persons diagnosed with hypertension perform more poorly over time. Another factor found to influence intelligence is education. On the average, those who are more highly educated tend to age less, intellectually speaking. For those who are initially more able, declines may be more rapid because they have more to lose, while those who are less able appear to gain somewhat (Adler et al., 1990). An additional influence on intelligence is speed, where an emphasis on speed unfairly penalizes those adults who respond slowly in timed tests (Kausler, 1991). Also slower performance could result from lessened ability to process information quickly (Hertzog, 1989; Kausler, 1991, Schaie & Willis, 1996). There may also be a relationship between personality factors and intellectual performance, but the reasons for this relationship remain unclear (Schaie & Willis, 1996). It may be that persons who have adaptive personalities age better intellectually or intelligence may permit more flexibility in adulthood. In one study, the relationship between personality and Gf and Gc was examined (Hayslip, 1988), wherein Gf and Gc were found to be

linked to distinct personality attributes. As with learning and memory, **self-efficacy** may be especially relevant to intelligence in adulthood. Lachman and Leff (1989) reported that over a 5-year period, control beliefs about one's skills did not predict changes in Gf functioning. However, changes in intellectual control beliefs were predicted by fluid intelligence. Decrements in perceived changes in one's ability over time may also contribute to declines in intelligence (Schaie, Willis, & O'Hanlon, 1994). Schooler (1987) and Schaie and Willis (1996) have emphasized the impact that the complexity of our everyday (work) environment may have on cognitive performance. Individuals in optimally complex environments who are reinforced for using their brains may develop higher cognitive skills (Figure 6-4).

Optimizing Intelligence in Later Life

Many investigators have developed training programs to help older adults enhance their intellectual skills by comparing those who received such training with those who received no training or with those who simply practiced (without benefit of any training). Baltes and Willis (1982) were able to enhance the fluid intellectual skills of older adults. These effects were specific to fluid abilities and were maintained over time. For those who had simply been allowed to practice, no specific pattern of improvement was found. Schaie and Willis (1986) have demonstrated that training can apparently reverse 14-year declines in PMA performance. Over a 7-year interval, intellectual performance still exceeded original levels 7 years earlier. Improvements in fluid ability performance can be achieved by other means as well. For example, Hayslip (1989) found that providing older adults with anxiety-reduction techniques, such as substituting success self-statements for failure self-statements (Meichenbaum, 1989) and relaxation, was almost as effective as direct specific rule-based training and superior to persons who were not trained at all. Practice seemed to help all persons.

Personality

Two questions about personality in adulthood can be asked: Does aging affect personality (do people change with increased age) and does personality affect aging (does one's personality influence adaptation to the aging process)? The answer to each is a qualified yes: (a) people do change in some ways as they age and (b) different types of persons do cope with aging in unique ways. The answer(s) to each question are a function of (a) one's definition of stability or change, (b) one's theoretical biases, (c) the particular design (e.g., cross-sectional versus longitudinal) used to gather our facts about personality, (d) the level of personality that one studies, and (e) how one assesses personality. Depending upon these factors, personality can be stable and yet change throughout adulthood.

Erikson's Psychosocial Approach

Erikson's (1959) psychosocial crisis theory is an age-graded approach to ego development. While Erikson suggested that individuals deal with each crisis in a cumulative manner, difficulties in resolving earlier crises can seriously interfere with but do not completely prevent adults from resolving later crises. Each psychosocial crisis, regardless of its resolution, comes to help redefine later crises. These crises are **epigenetic,** that is, they arise out of a maturational ground plan and eventually come together to form the whole individual. Integrity versus despair characterizes old age. Integrity implies a sense of completeness, of having come full circle. Persons who have integrity have, through the process of introspection (looking inward and examining what one finds), been able to integrate a lifetime full of successes and failures to reach a point where they have a sense of the life cycle. Despairing individuals fear death as a premature end to a life (good or bad) that they have not been able to take personal responsibility for, while those who have a sense of integrity accept death as the inevitable end of having lived. **Life review** and **reminiscence** (Butler, 1963) refer to a similar process of evaluating and reevaluating one's life by focusing on the past and its relationship to the present.

Whitbourne's Identity Styles

Whitbourne's (1986, 1987) approach to personality emphasizes the concept of **identity style,** which is one's manner of representing and responding to life experiences, based on the accumulated self-representations of experiences that date back to one's childhood. These identity styles can be assimilative, accommodative, or balanced. In identity assimilation, new experiences are fit into the existing identity of the individual, while in identity accommodation, one's identity is changed to fit a new experience. As people have new experiences or interactions with others, they attempt to fit these into how they see themselves along those dimensions that are important to them. For example, if it is important to be a loving grandparent, the experiences with one's children will be processed in a way that reinforces the perception of oneself as a loving father or mother (Whitbourne, 1987). In other words, these new experiences are assimilated into one's existing identity. Likewise, if being productive is an important aspect of the self, then retiring will be processed in a way that complements one's view about oneself as productive.

Successful adaptation occurs when there is a balance between identity assimilation and identity accommodation. Persons with balanced styles are more consistent, yet flexible enough to deal with experiences that contradict their self-views. As aging involves adaptation to physical change and to new roles, this approach suggests that persons with each identity style will cope with stress and change differently, and each style has its advantages and disadvantages (Table 6-3). For example, becoming defensive, withdrawing, denial, or acting out, which are all emotion-focused coping styles, may be helpful in an emergency. In contrast, seeking advice and information, or problem solving, both cognitive coping styles, are more advantageous when making an important new purchase (e.g., a car or a house) (Pearlin & Skaff, 1995; Roth & Cohen, 1986).

Trait Approaches to Personality and Aging

Using a trait approach, different individuals can be located along a continuum, in that people can be described as possessing a certain degree of one trait, which is bipolar in nature, that is, it has a negative and a positive pole (aggressive versus passive, dominant versus submissive). Lerner (1996) suggested that by using traits one can understand whether, through development, people sort themselves out (are differentiated) along a number of bipolar trait dimensions: for example, as they age, some people become more aggressive than do others.

Perhaps the most impressive evidence for personality stability comes from a series of investigations emphasizing psychological traits (Costa, et al., 1983; McCrae, 1991; McCrae & Costa, 1990). Costa et al. (1983) found stability in what they term the *N* (Neuroticism)–*E* (Extro-

TABLE 6-3   Benefits and Costs of Identity Styles in Later Life

Identity Style	Benefits	Costs	Manifestations
Assimilative	Optimism toward present situation	Use of projection as defensive strategy, leading to social isolation	Unwillingness to change one's identity
	Self-perception of good health	Depletion of psychological energy required to maintain denial of age changes	Attributing negative identity attributes to others rather than oneself
	Positive evaluation of life accomplishments	Alienation from real, aging, self	Unwillingness to recognize that a negative identity attribute exists
Accommodative	Secure basis of self-definition in identity of aging person	Overreaction to physical symptoms of aging and disease that blocks effective remediation	Accepting into one's identity positive or negative identity attributes, considering a neutral identity attribute
Balanced	High motivation to take advantage of preventive as well as therapeutic health practices, favorable adjustment to aging integrating	Frustration and a sense of helplessness in the face of age changes and events beyond one's personal control, direct confrontation with loss and mortality	
	Favorable adjustment to aging that integrates age changes into a consistent sense of the self	Direct confrontation of issues related to loss and mortality	

Adapted from Whitbourne, S. K. (1987). Personality development in adulthood and old age. Annual Review of Gerontology and Geriatrics, 7, 201. Used by permission of Springer Publishing Company.

version)–O (Openness to Experience) trait model of personality. Somewhat later (Costa & McCrae, 1989), two other factors (Agreeableness and Conscientiousness) were added to form a five-factor model of personality.

Costa and McCrae (1980) also have found that the structure of personality itself remains basically the same across age, regardless of time of measurement and/or cohort effects. This means that the cluster of traits defining the five-factor model of personality is itself stable over time. There are also cohort effects in some personality traits (e.g., superego strength, ascendance, flexibility, restraint, social adjustment), as well as some indication of time of measurement effects (e.g., thoughtfulness, tolerance of others, friendliness) (Schaie & Willis 1991; Woodruff & Birren, 1972). More recently, Field and Milsap (1991) studied 51 women and 21 men from the Berkeley study who were aged 69 in 1969 and 83 in 1983 using a five-factor approach similar to that of Costa and McCrae (1980). They found that satisfaction (an absence of Neuroticism) showed the greatest absolute stability

(stability of averages) and relative stability (stability of individual differences). Three other aspects of personality (extroversion, agreeableness, intellect) all showed high relative stability over 14 years. In terms of absolute stability, satisfaction and agreeableness were highest, while energy, intellect, and extroversion showed declines. These findings for the most part confirm our picture of personality and stability and extend it to very late in life, where absolute stability is less often observed. It is very important to understand, however, that while socialization and peer pressure may foster stability, life events such as divorce, serious illness, or death of a child or spouse can change people forever (Field, 1991).

State-Dependent Aspects of Personality

Recent interest has emerged in what are termed state-dependent aspects of personality, which fluctuate from day to day or from week to week, because of hormonal, biological, or social factors (Nesselroade, 1988). Such variations in our personalities affect our relationships with parents, children, care providers, or spouses. Fatigue, anxiety, feelings of control, mood states (feeling good or bad), and hostility are aspects of our personalities that show short-term fluctuations over days or weeks (Nesselroade, 1988). Because these changes influence and are often influenced by the everyday context, they are termed contextual (Kogan, 1990).

Stress and Coping in Later Life

When older adults are confronted with a life change, they engage in a series of cognitive appraisals that lead to behaviors that may or may not be successful in helping them adapt to change. Primary appraisals allow persons to evaluate the event in terms of its being positive, neutral, or stressful and negative (Lazarus & Delongis, 1983). Secondary appraisal allows the individual to decide what options are available to cope with the event, if a chosen course of action is possible, and if the behaviors chosen will produce positive or negative outcomes. Tertiary appraisal or reappraisal allows one to incorporate new information into the situation. At this point, one might evaluate whether the course of action taken was effective; in other words, "Did things actually work out as I planned? Are there outcomes that I did not anticipate?" (Figure 6-5).

An emphasis on stress and coping processes also highlights the individual's beliefs about personal control over events or personal commitments to a set of values and ideals as influences on how people assess and respond to change over the life span (Lazarus and Delongis,

1983; Pearlin & Skaff, 1995). Lazarus and Delongis (1983), for example, suggested that with increased age, individuals may pull away from commitments they have made earlier in their lives because of poor health (they can no longer work, which has been very important to them) or nonreward (they are passed over for a promotion, or demoted, even though their work may be of high quality). Such changes are adaptive—they allow the individual to cope with stress. Such beliefs are central to the compensation and optimization of personal functioning (Baltes, 1997).

For example, as people age, they divest themselves of relationships that are not crucial to the maintenance of their convoy of social support (Kahn & Antonucci, 1980) in favor of those that are more meaningful, valuable, and satisfying, termed socioemotional selectivity (Carstensen, 1992). Similarly, as they age, individuals may decide that they lack primary control over events in their lives and consequently exert secondary control over such events by reinterpreting what these events mean to them personally (Schulz & Heckhausen, 1996). Primary control is directed to the external world, while secondary control is directed at the self. Individuals may also redefine what goals they see as important to reach (Brandstadter, Krampen, & Grieve, 1987). Through such processes, people can maintain their self-esteem, establish satisfying relationships with others, and develop new interests and skills (Figure 6-6).

Self-Concept

A positive self-concept is pivotal in defining the experience of growing older (Atchley, 1982, 1997). Those with

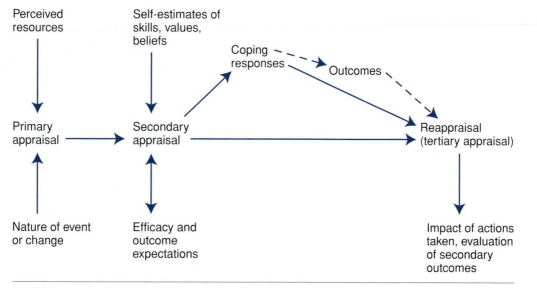

FIGURE 6-5 Stress and coping in later adulthood.

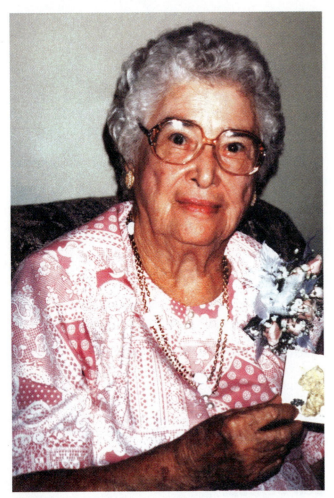

FIGURE 6-6   A positive self-concept is important at all ages.

positive self-concepts experience greater life satisfaction, less anxiety, and more control over events in their lives (George, 1981; Lawton, 1983). They also have a more positive view of their own development and aging (Brubaker & Powers, 1976). Markus and Herzog (1991) and Wells and Stryker (1988) noted that the self-concept is dynamic—our self-concept influences what we know about ourselves: our goals, hopes, preferences, values, and relationships. It is also social in nature—influenced by the many interpersonal and societal factors that we all encounter. The self-concept is composed of many domain-specific self-schemas (areas of the self such as family or work) that include past, current, and future selves (Cross & Markus, 1991). With age, self-schemas are bolstered and strengthened, and these same schemas are influenced by how successful people are in carrying out these roles (Markus & Herzog, 1991). If these roles confirm our self-knowledge, then self-schemas are strengthened. If they do not, our self-schemas may need to be redefined.

Locus of Control

The preceding discussion of personal control highlights what is termed **locus of control,** which is domain specific—it has intellectual and health dimensions (Lachman et al., 1982; Lachman, 1986a; Lefcourt, 1981). Each dimension is distinct from generalized locus of control, where distinctions between internal (I perceive control over my life) and external (other people or events control my life) locus of control are generally made (Levenson, 1972). While generalized locus of control seems to show adequate differential stability (Gatz et al., 1986; Lachman, 1986b), some studies suggest that with age, individuals generally become less internal and more external, while other studies do not (Lachman, 1983, 1985). The change toward more externality with age is stronger for domain-specific locus of control (Lachman, 1986a).

Psychological Interventions with Older Persons

Fortunately, a great deal of research stemming from the life span tradition has demonstrated that older adults are equally amenable to change (Baltes, 1987; Knight, 1992). Ideally, this should provide additional impetus for professionals to actively treat older clients by focusing on their potential for change in the context of the relationship with a counselor or therapist (Steenbarger, 1991). However, research does not show age to be a predictor of therapeutic success (Garfield, 1986; Knight, 1992). These results may relate to the small numbers of older adults studied.

Specific goals in therapy with adults and older adults are (a) insight into one's behavior, (b) symptom relief, (c) enhancing coping skills in light of one's life situation, (d) improving the ability to make independent decisions, (e) facilitating activity and independence, (f) becoming more self-accepting, and (g) improving interpersonal relationships. In addition to generalized approaches to helping older adults (e.g., individual psychoanalytic therapy, behavioral approaches), more specific techniques geared to the older person's capabilities and environment have also become popular in recent years. Reality orientation and life review are examples of these more specialized techniques. While it is tempting to focus solely upon these narrower approaches, serious consideration must be given to the therapeutic options open to the older adult in distress. Unfortunately, because the field of clinical psychogerontology is relatively new, interest in these specific treatment modalities with the older adults has, in most cases, preceded an evaluation of their effectiveness. An array of counseling and inter-

TABLE 6-4	Counseling and Therapy Strategies with Older People			
Approach	**Examples**	**Domains of Use**	**Advantages**	**Disadvantages**
Psychoanalytic	Time-limited therapy, classical psychoanalysis	Emotional and behavior difficulties	Helpful in some cases, especially if goals are short term in nature	Difficult to document objectively, treatment can be very long, only certain older people can benefit
Cognitive	Alter thinking strategies and problem-solving/coping skills	Adjustment to life change, stress reduction, cognitive change	Easily used by most older adults	Real-life environment may not support new thinking skills, not all older people can benefit
Behavioral	Define undesirable and desirable behavior in behavioral terms; reinforce desired behavior; withdraw reinforcers from undesired behavior	All types of general behavioral problems	Easily learned; outcomes timely if used correctly	Does not address itself to the social context that influences behaviors, ethical concerns
Family	Alter patterns of communication and behavior within the family	All types of family dysfunction	Can be used with a variety of family-related problems (marital, caregiving)	Difficult to document
Group	Small-group dynamics are used to help individuals profit from feedback from others facing similar difficulties	Help people deal with emotional, behavioral, and interpersonal difficulties in the context of a group setting	Building on the older adult's dependency needs, creates sense of safety, can be issue oriented	Benefits difficult to document; only certain older people can benefit

vention approaches used with older adults is presented in Table 6-4.

Psychoanalysis

Some advocate brief psychoanalytic therapy with older adults, where more realistic goals of reducing anxiety and restoring the person to a more functional state can be achieved (Silberschatz & Curtis, 1991). Silberschatz and Curtis (1991) term this variation on classical **psychoanalysis** time-limited psychodynamic therapy. Rather than spend years in therapy, clients spend 3–4 months. Pathogenic (abnormal, destructive) beliefs about oneself rooted in childhood can be dealt with through therapy by clearly defining goals with the client. As older clients may believe that they are too old to change, or simply unworthy of help, they may test the therapist by being hostile, late for appointments, argumentative, or passive. All of these maneuvers are designed to find out if the painfully destructive beliefs about oneself formed in

childhood need to be maintained or whether they can be challenged. Silberschatz and Curtis (1991) emphasized that these tests be understood as an outgrowth of painful experiences early in life (Semel, 1996). They should not be interpreted as evidence for the adult's rigidity or resistance to therapy. Reports of classical psychoanalysis are rare with older clients (see Newton, Brauer, Gutmann, & Grunes, 1986; Semel, 1996), and they are often poorly designed and documented. However, recent well-designed studies indicate that psychoanalytic therapy can be quite helpful, leading to less anxiety, less depression, greater self-esteem, and more functional behavior (Lazarus et al., 1987). Good candidates for psychoanalysis should have some insight into their own unconscious motives, be committed to changing, be able to tolerate very strong emotions, and have had some success in relating to others (Myers, 1991).

An extension of psychoanalytic thought is to be found in life review therapy (see Knight, 1996). As Butler et al. (1991) point out, life review therapy is more extensive than a simple recall of the past, although reminiscence is important in this approach. Obtaining an extensive autobiography from the older adult is important, allowing the elder the opportunity to put his or her life in order. Resolving internal conflict, improving relationships with one's family, making decisions about success and failure, resolving guilt, clarifying one's own values, and simply expressing one's feelings about painful past experiences are all benefits of the life review (Knight, 1996; Newton et al., 1986).

Group Therapy

The distinguishing feature of **group therapy** with older adults is that dependency needs can be used to their best advantage (Spayd & Smyer, 1996). As many older adults are isolated, group therapy may be especially suited to them (Finkel, 1991). It may also be quite helpful for adult caregivers, who often must shoulder the burden of caring for an ill or dying family member (Smyer et al., 1990; Waters, 1995). In many cases, simply being with others may make one feel safer. Problems, fears, and hidden emotions can be shared with others. These may range from relationship difficulties to illness, retirement, or simply feeling alone or less worthy. Face-to-face contact, touching another person, and sharing experiences are quite important to many older adults (Finkel, 1991). Group therapy can take many forms, ranging from issue-oriented (life event) discussion groups to groups designed to stimulate interaction among group members (Finkel, 1991; Smyer et al., 1990; Waters, 1984). Groups can also be designed to promote independence and a positive sense of self. Common themes often include social losses, independence, illness, sensory loss, death, or loneliness (Finkel, 1991; Spayd & Smyer, 1996). Groups are typically short term (when used within the institution) and informal in nature. They may be self-help, educational in nature, or more formally therapeutic. Both self-help and educational groups may not carry the stigma of being in therapy. Group therapy is often used in a variety of settings in combination with art therapy, dance therapy, or music therapy for older adults and is especially appropriate for older adults living in long-term care environments (Spayd & Smyer, 1996).

Family Therapy

Family therapy is another attractive alternative in treating older adults whose difficulties are communicative in nature (Qualls, 1996). Family therapy can aid in adjustment to roles such as retirement or grandparenthood and help resolve problems accompanying caring for an ill spouse, institutionalizing one's parent(s) or spouse, or conflicts arising when an older parent is being cared for

at home by a middle-aged child. Each family member can be involved in setting up clear expectations for behavior, improving communication, lessening distrust and guilt, or dealing with hostility and anxiety.

Family therapy can also help older couples reestablish intimacy, learn to enjoy life without being preoccupied with illness, enable them to nurture and let go of children, and help them grieve over losses of loved ones. For some couples dealing with their sexuality, education and instruction in sexual techniques can be helpful in reestablishing sexual intimacy and lessening marital tension (Kaplan, 1991; Knight, 1996; O'Donohue, 1987; Whitlatch & Zarit, 1989). Family therapy is appropriate in dealing with parent-child conflicts centering around remarriage, struggles for power within the home, or restrictions on the older adult brought about by ill health or by the divorce of an adult child. Family therapy can also help children cope with the terminal illness of an older family member or help them care for a parent who is chronically ill. For example, Zarit (1996) suggested that giving information, active problem solving, support, and one-on-one counseling can help families make decisions about caring for a family member.

Behavior Therapy

Behavior therapy is most often used in an institutional, inpatient setting, where control over reinforcers (rewards) and those behaviors one wants to change is more likely. According to this approach, application of a behavioral strategy requires that three primary tasks be carried out (a) definition and assessment prior to intervention of the desired target behavior; (b) identifying a reinforcer defined as a stimulus whose impact makes the desired behavior more frequent or of longer duration, a reinforcer that may be self-administered or administered by the therapist; and (c) establishment of specific behavior-reinforcer contingencies. Of all the forms of intervention with older adults, behavior therapy is perhaps easiest to document and there is ample, well-designed research to support its efficacy in dealing with a variety of behavior problems (Smyer et al., 1990; Zeiss & Steffen, 1996). For example, overly dependent interactions with other older adults as well as with nursing home staff, incontinence, assertive behavior, withdrawal, inappropriate sexual behavior, wandering, anxiety, and self-care can all be treated behaviorally (Smyer et al., 1990). Many of these behaviors are a consequence of being institutionalized and have been termed excess disabilities (Kahn & Miller, 1978).

Cognitive Therapy

Closely related to behavioral approaches is **cognitive behavior therapy** (Ellis & Velten, 1998; Meichenbaum,

1977; Beck, 1976). In general, cognitive behavior therapists believe that the way a person thinks largely determines the way he or she feels. In other words, thought causes emotional response. Older adults, perhaps lacking realistic comments about themselves from others, often make thinking errors that are not realistic (Hayslip & Caraway, 1989). For example, irrational assumptions about one's age or about the loss of skills once had, may lead to feelings of self-depreciation in many older people. These feelings can lead to anger, guilt, and depression. Cognitive techniques are available to instruct the older adult to substitute more rational thoughts for these irrational ones (Hayslip & Caraway, 1989). Specific techniques are available for this purpose and have been discussed in detail by Thompson et al. (1991) and by Zeiss and Steffen (1996). Regarding older adults (Thompson et al., 1991; Zeiss & Steffen, 1996), the therapist must be more flexible, special attention should be given to cohort differences in education, background and interests, an assessment of one's physical history must be made, and a conference with the client's physician and family should be arranged. In addition, the therapist may have to be more active with older clients, keeping them focused on the issue at hand, and should expect the pace of therapy to be slower, because of fatigue or resistance in giving up long-held assumptions about oneself or others (Hayslip & Caraway, 1989; Thompson et al., 1991). Cognitive-behavioral approaches to therapy have been successfully utilized to treat a variety of cognitive and emotional problems such as depression, memory loss, test anxiety, performance on intellectual tasks, and response slowness (Zeiss & Steffen, 1996).

Summary

In light of the complexity of the aging process, this chapter examined psychological aging within the context of a life span development approach. The life span approach makes several assumptions about aging that are critical to the adequate description and explanation of change in late adulthood: (1) that aging is inherently complex in terms of both the multidimensional and multidirectional nature of change, (b) that the determinants of psychological aging are many rather than few, (c) that the diversity of older adults requires an attention to how and why older adults are different from one another, (d) that the psychological functioning of older adults is best understood in light of the relationship between the older adult and the demands of the environmental context in which one finds himself or herself, and (e) that aging persons are capable of a great deal of plasticity, which enables one to reject an irreversible decrement model of the aging process.

A number of dimensions of psychological aging were discussed that are of importance to understanding the everyday functioning of older adults: perception, learning and memory, intelligence, personality, and psychological interventions with older adults. In each case, the picture of age-related change is a complex one, dependent on the particular dimensions of change one examines. In most cases, it is best to understand psychological aging in relative terms, wherein the particular patterns of change with aging depend upon the interaction of many factors that reside within the individual as well as those in the environment as they bear on the cognitive and personality functioning of older adults. Consistent with a decrement-with-compensation model of psychological aging, many interventions are available that have proven to be effective in enhancing the cognitive functioning of older adults, as well as being able to effectively treat those who are experiencing a variety of functional psychological disorders. A sensitivity to the distinction between normal, pathological, and optimal aging is essential if the quality of life for older adults is to be improved.

Review Questions and Activities

1. What are the characteristics of psychological aging viewed from a life span perspective?

2. What is vigilance, and why is it important to the everyday functioning of older adults?

3. What aspects of reaction time do and do not change with age? What factors might explain this?

4. What is the distinction between learning and memory?

5. What is the difference between a memory structure and a memory process approach to memory and learning? How do memory structures and memory processes change with age?

6. What is practical memory?

7. What aspects of intelligence change with age? Why?

8. How might older adults improve their cognitive skills?

9. What approaches to personality and aging are relevant to the question of whether personality changes with age?

10. What are personality types? Why are they relevant to how people cope with aging?

11. What psychological intervention techniques have proven most effective with older adults?

References

Abeles, N. (1997). *What practitioners should know about working with older adults.* Washington, DC: American Psychological Association.

Adler, A. G., Adam, J., & Arenberg, D. (1990). Individual differences assessment of the relationship between change and initial level of adult cognitive functioning. *Psychology and Aging, 5,* 560–568.

Anschultz, L., Camp, C. J., Markley, R. P., & Kramer, J. J. (1985). Maintenance and generalization of mnemonic for grocery shopping by older adults. *Experimental Aging Research, 11,* 157–160.

Anschultz, L., Camp, C. J., Markley, R. P., & Kramer, J. J. (1987). A three-year follow-up on the effects of mnemonic training in elderly adults. *Experimental Aging Research, 13,* 141–143.

Atchley, R. C. (1982). The aging self. *Psychotherapy: Theory, Research, and Practice, 19,* 388–396.

Atchley, R. (1997). *Social forces and aging* (8th ed.). Belmont, CA: Wadsworth.

Baltes, P. B. (1987). Theoretical propositions of life-span developmental psychology: On the dynamics between growth and decline. *Developmental Psychology, 23,* 611–626.

Baltes, P. (1993). The aging mind: Potential and limits. *The Gerontologist, 33,* 580–594.

Baltes, P. (1997). On the incomplete architecture of human ontogeny: Selection, optimization, and compensation as a foundation of developmental theory. *American Psychologist, 52,* 366–380.

Baltes, P. B., & Schaie, K. W. (1976). On the plasticity of intelligence in adulthood and old age: Where Horn and Donaldson fail. *American Psychologist, 31,* 720–725.

Baltes, P. B., & Willis, S. L. (1982). Plasticity and enhancement of intellectual functioning in old age: Penn State's Adult Development and Enrichment Program (ADEPT). In F. I. M. Craik & S. E. Trehub (Eds.), *Aging and cognitive process* (pp. 353–389). New York: Plenum.

Baltes, P. B., Reese, H., & Nesselroade, J. R. (1986). *Life-span developmental psychology: Introduction to research methods.* Hillsdale, NJ: Erlbaum.

Bandura, A. (1989). Regulation of cognitive processes through self-efficacy. *Developmental Psychology, 25,* 729–735.

Beck, A. (1976). *Cognitive therapy and the emotional disorders.* New York: International Universities Press.

Belmont, J., Epperson, J., & Anderson, N. (1989, November). *Simple reaction time as problem-solving: Relations to fluid and crystallized intelligence.* Paper presented at the annual meeting of the Gerontological Society, Minneapolis, MN.

Botwinick, J. (1984). *Aging and behavior.* New York: Springer.

Braudstadter, J., Krampen, G., & Grieve, W. (1987). Personal control over development: Effects on the perception and emotional evaluation of personal development in adulthood. *International Journal of Behavioral Development, 10,* 99–120.

Brubaker, T. H., & Powers, E. A. (1976). The stereotype of "old": A review and alternative approach. *Journal of Gerontology, 31,* 441–447.

Butler, R. N. (1963). The life review: An interpretation of reminiscence in the aged. *Psychiatry, 26,* 65–76.

Butler, R. N., Lewis, M., & Sunderland, A. (1991). *Aging and mental health: Positive psychosocial and biomedical approaches.* New York: Springer.

Carstensen, L. L. (1992). Social and emotional patterns in adulthood: Support for socioemotional selectivity theory. *Psychology and Aging, 7,* 331–338.

Cherry, K., & Smith, A. (1998). Normal memory aging. In M. Herson & V. VanHasselt (Eds.), *Handbook of clinical geropsychology.* New York: Plenum.

Cockburn, J., & Smith, P. T. (1991). The relative influence of intelligence and age on everyday memory. *Journal of Gerontology: Psychological Sciences, 46,* 31–36.

Costa, P. T., Jr., & McCrae, R. (1980). Still stable after all these years: Personality as a key to some issues in adulthood and old age. In P. Baltes & O. Brim (Eds.), *Life-span development and behavior* (pp. 66–103). New York: Academic Press.

Costa, P. T., & McCrae, R. R. (1989). Personality continuity and the changes of adult life. In M. Storandt & G. VandenBos (Eds.), *The adult years: Continuity and change* (pp. 45–77). Washington, DC: American Psychological Association.

Costa, P. T., Jr., McCrae, R., & Arenberg, D. (1983). Recent longitudinal research on personality and aging. In K. W. Schaie (Ed.), *Longitudinal studies of adult psychological development* (pp. 222–265). New York: Guilford Press.

Craik, F. I. M. (1977). Age difference in human memory. In J. E. Birren & K. W. Schaie (Eds.), *Handbook of the psychology of aging* (pp. 384–429). New York: Van Nostrand Reinhold.

Crook, T. H., Bartus, R. T., Ferris, S. H., Whitehouse, P., Cohen, G. D., & Gershon, S. (1986). Age-associated memory impairment: Proposed diagnostic criteria and measures of clinical change (report of an NIMH work group). *Developmental Neuropsychology, 2,* 261–276.

Cross, S., & Markus, H. (1991). Possible selves across the life course. *Human Development, 34,* 230–255.

Danish, S. (1981). Life-span development and intervention: A necessary link. *Counseling Psychologist, 9,* 40–43.

Dixon, R. (1989). Questionnaire research on metamemory and aging: Issues of structure and function. In L. Poon, D. Rubin, & B. Wilson (Eds.), *Everyday cognition in adulthood and late life* (pp. 394–415). New York: Cambridge.

Dobbs, A. R., & Rule, B. G. (1990). Adult age differences in working memory. *Psychology and Aging, 4,* 500–503.

Elias, M., Elias, J., & Elias, P. (1990). Biological and health influences on behavior. In J. Birren & K. Schaie (Eds.), *Handbook of the psychology of aging* (pp. 80–102). New York: Academic Press.

Ellis, A., & Velten, E. (1998). *Optimal aging: Getting over getting older.* New York: Open Court.

Erikson, E. H. (1959). Identity and the life cycle. *Psychological Issues, 1.*

Field, D. (1991). Continuity and change in personality in old age: Evidence from five longitudinal studies. *Journal of Gerontology: Psychological Sciences, 46,* 271–274.

Field, D., & Milsap, R. E. (1991). Personality in advanced old age: Continuity or change. *Journal of Gerontology: Psychological Sciences, 46,* 299–308.

Finkel, S. I. (1991). Group psychotherapy in later life. In W. A. Myers (Ed.), *New techniques in psychotherapy of older patients* (pp. 223–244). Washington, DC: American Psychiatric Press.

Foster, J., & Gallagher, D. (1986). An exploratory study comparing depressed and nondepressed elders' coping strategies. *Journal of Gerontology, 41,* 91–93.

Fozard, J. E., Vercruyssen, M., Reynolds, S. L., Hancock, P. A., & Quilter, R. E. (1994). Age differences and changes in reaction time: The Baltimore longitudinal study of aging. *Journal of Gerontology: Psychological Sciences, 49,* 179–189.

Fries, J. F., & Crapo, L. M. (1981). *Vitality and aging.* San Francisco: Freeman.

Garfield, S. L. (1986). Research on client variables in psychotherapy. In S. L. Garfield & A. E. Bergin (Eds.), *Handbook of psychotherapy and behavior change* (pp. 271–298). New York: Wiley.

Gatz, M., Siegler, I., George, L. K., & Tyler, F. B. (1986). Attributional components of locus of control: Longitudinal, retrospective, and contemporaneous analyses. In M. M. Baltes & P. B. Baltes (Eds.), *The psychology of control and aging* (pp. 237–263). Hillsdale, NJ: Erlbaum.

George, L. K. (1981). *Role transitions in later life.* Monterey, CA: Wadsworth.

Hayflick, L. (1994). *How and why we age.* New York: Ballantine.

Hayslip, B. (1988). Personality-ability relationships in aged adults. *Journal of Gerontology: Psychological Sciences, 43,* 74–84.

Hayslip, B. (1989). Alternative mechanisms for improvements in fluid-ability performance in aged persons. *Psychology and Aging, 4,* 122–124.

Hayslip, B., & Caraway, M. (1989). Cognitive therapy with aged persons: Implications of research design for its implementation and evaluation. *Journal of Cognitive Psychotherapy, 3,* 255–271.

Hayslip, B., & Kennelly, K. (1985). Cognitive and non-cognitive factors affecting learning among older adults. In B. Lundsden (Ed.), *The older adult as learner* (pp. 73–98). Washington, DC: Hemisphere.

Hayslip, B., & Panek, P. (1999). *Adult development and aging.* Melbourne, FL: Krieger.

Hayslip, B., Kennelly, K., & Maloy, R. (1990). Fatigue, depression, and cognitive performance among aged persons. *Experimental Aging Research, 16,* 111–115.

Hayslip, B., Maloy, R. M., & Kohl, R. (1995). Long term efficacy of fluid ability interventions with older adults. *Journal of Gerontology: Psychological Sciences, 50B,* 141–149.

Hertzog, C. (1989). The influence of cognitive slowing on age differences in intelligence. *Developmental Psychology, 25,* 636–651.

Hertzog, C., Schaie, K. W., & Gribbin, N. (1978). Cardiovascular disease and changes in intellectual function from middle to old age. *Journal of Gerontology, 33,* 872–883.

Heston, L. L., & White, J. A. (1991). *The vanishing mind.* New York: Freeman.

Horn, J. L. (1978). Human ability systems. In P. Baltes (Ed.), *Life-span development and behavior* (Vol. 1, pp. 211–256). New York: Academic Press.

Horn, J. L. (1982). The aging of human abilities. In B. B. Wolman (Ed.), *Handbook of intelligence: Theories, measurements, and applications* (pp. 267–300). New York: Wiley Interscience.

Horn, J. L., & Cattell, R. B. (1967). Age differences in fluid and crystallized intelligence. *Acta Psychologica, 26,* 107–129.

Hoyer, W. J. (1974). Aging and intraindividual change. *Developmental Psychology, 10,* 821–826.

Hultsch, D. F., & Dixon, R. A. (1990). Learning and memory in aging. In J. E. Birren & K. W. Schaie (Eds.), *Handbook of the psychology of aging* (pp. 258–274). New York: Academic Press.

Kahn, R., & Antonucci, T. (1980). Convoys over the life course: Attachment, roles, and social support. In P. B. Baltes, & O. G. Brim, Jr., (Eds.), *Life-Span Development and Behavior* (pp. 254–286). New York: Academic Press.

Kahn, R., & Miller, N. (1978). Assessment of altered brain function in the aged. In M. Storandt, I. Siegler, & M. Elias (Eds.), *The clinical psychology of aging* (pp. 43–69). New York: Plenum.

Kaplan, H. S. (1991). Sex therapy with older patients. In W. Myers (Ed.), *New techniques in psychotherapy with older patients* (pp. 21–38). Washington, DC: American Psychiatric Press.

Karp, D. A. (1988). A decade of reminders: Changing age consciousness between fifty and sixty years old. *Gerontologist, 28,* 727–738.

Kausler, D. (1990). Motivation, human aging, and cognitive performance. In J. E. Birren & K. W. Schaie (Eds.), *Handbook of the psychology of aging* (pp. 172–183). New York: Academic Press.

Kausler, D. (1991). *Experimental psychology and human aging* (2nd ed.). New York: Springer-Verlag.

Kausler, D. (1994). *Learning and memory in normal aging.* San Diego: Academic Press.

Kennelly, K., Hayslip, B., & Richardson, S. (1985). Depression and helplessness-induced cognitive deficits in the aged. *Experimental Aging Research, 8,* 169–173.

Kline, D. W., & Scialfa, C. T. (1997). Sensory and perceptual functioning: Basic research and human factors implications. In A. D. Fisk & W. A. Rogers (Eds.), *Handbook of human factors and the older adult* (pp. 27–54). New York: Academic Press.

Knight, B. (1992). *Older adults in psychotherapy.* Newbury Park, CA: Sage.

Knight, B. (1996). *Psychotherapy with older adults.* Thousand Oaks, CA: Sage

Kogan, N. (1990). Personality and aging. In J. E. Birren & K. W. Schaie (Eds.), *Handbook of the psychology of aging* (pp. 330–346). New York: Academic Press.

Kooken, R. A., & Hayslip, B. (1984). The use of stress inoculation in the treatment of text anxiety in older students. *Educational Gerontology, 11,* 39–58.

Lachman, M. E. (1983). Perceptions of intellectual aging: Antecedent or consequences of intellectual functioning? *Developmental Psychology, 19,* 482–498.

Lachman, M. E. (1985). Personal efficacy in middle and old age: Differential and normative patterns of change. In G. Elder, Jr. (Ed.), *Life-course dynamics: Trajectories and transitions, 1968–1980* (pp. 188–213). Ithaca, NY: Cornell University Press.

Lachman, M. E. (1986a). Locus of control in aging research: A case for multidimensional and domain-specific assessment. *Psychology and Aging, 1,* 34–40.

Lachman, M. E. (1986b). The role of personality and social factors in intellectual aging. *Educational Gerontology, 12,* 399–444.

Lachman, M. E., & Leff, L. (1989). Perceived control and intellectual functioning: A five-year longitudinal study. *Developmental Psychology, 25,* 722–728.

Lachman, M. E., Baltes, P. B., Nesselroade, J. R., & Willis, S. L. (1982). Examination of personality-ability relationships in the elderly: The role of contextual (interface) assessment mode. *Journal of Research in Personality, 16,* 485–501.

Lawton, M. P. (1983). Environment and other determinants of well-being in older people. *Gerontologist, 23,* 349–357.

Lawton, M. P., & Nahemow, L. (1973). Ecology and the aging process. In C. Eisdorfer & M. P. Lawton (Eds.), *The Psychology of Adult Development and Aging* (pp. 619–674). Washington, DC: American Psychological Association.

Lazarus, L. W., Groves, L., Guttmann, D., Ripkyjin, A., Frankel, R., Newton, N., Gruner, J., & Havasy-Galloway, S. (1987). Brief psychotherapy with the elderly: A study of process and outcome. In J. Sadavoy & M. Leszca (Eds.), *Treating the elderly with psychotherapy* (pp. 5–22). Madison, CT: International University Press.

Lazarus, R. S., & Delongis, A. (1983). Psychological stress and coping in aging. *American Psychologist, 38,* 245–254.

Lefcourt, H. M. (1981). *Research with the locus-of-control construct: Assessment methods* (Vol. 1). New York: Academic Press.

Lerner, R. M. (1996). *Concepts and theories of human development*. New York: Random House.

Levenson, H. (1972). *Distinctions within the concept of internal-external control: Development of a new scale*. Proceedings of the 80th Annual Convention of the American Psychological Association, pp. 261–262. Washington, DC: American Psychological Association.

Lorsbach, T. C., & Simpson, G. B. (1988). Dual-task performance as a function of adult age and task complexity. *Psychology and Aging, 3,* 210–212.

Markus, H. R., & Herzog, A. R. (1991). The role of self-concept in aging. In K. W. Schaie & M. P. Lawton (Eds.), *Annual review of gerontology and geriatrics* (pp. 110–143). New York: Springer.

McCrae, R. R. (1991). The five-factor model and its assessment in clinical settings. *Journal of Personality Assessment, 57,* 399–414.

McCrae, R. R., & Costa, P. T. (1990). *Personality in adulthood*. New York: Guilford Press.

McDowd, J. E., & Craig, F. (1988). Effects of aging and task difficulty on divided attention performance. *Journal of Experimental Psychology: Human Perception and Performance, 14,* 267–280.

Meichenbaum, D. (1977). *Cognitive behavior modification*. New York: Plenum.

Meichenbaum, D. (1989). *Cognitive behavior modification: An integrative approach*. New York: Plenum.

Monge, R. H., & Hultsch, D. (1971). Paired-associate learning as a function of adult age and the length of the anticipation and inspection intervals. *Journal of Gerontology, 26,* 157–162.

Myers, W. A. (1991). *New techniques in the psychotherapy of older patients*. Washington, DC: American Psychiatric Press.

Nelson, E. A., & Daneffer, D. (1992). Aged heterogeneity: Fact or fiction? The fate of diversity in gerontological research. *Gerontologist, 32,* 17–23.

Nesselroade, J.R. (1988). Some implications of the state-trait distinction for the study of development over the life-span: The case of personality. In P. Baltes & O. Brim (Eds.), *Life-span development and behavior* (Vol. 8, pp. 163–191). Hillsdale, NJ: Erlbaum.

Newton, N. A., Brauer, D., Gutman, D., & Grunes, J. (1986). Psychodynamic therapy with the aged: A review. In T. L. Brink (Ed.), *Clinical gerontology* (pp. 205–230). New York: Haworth Press.

O'Donohue, W. T. (1987). The sexual behavior and problems of the elderly. In L. Carstensen & B. Edelstein (Eds.), *Handbook of clinical gerontology* (pp. 66–75). New York: Pergamon.

Panek, P. (1997). The older worker. In A. D. Fisk & W. A. Rogers (Eds.), *Handbook of human factors and the older adult* (pp. 61–96). San Diego, CA: Academic Press.

Panek, P. E., Barrett, G. V., Sterns, H. L., & Alexander, R. A. (1977). A review of age changes in perceptual information processing ability with regard to driving. *Experimental Aging Research, 3,* 387–449.

Panek, P. E., Barrett, G. V., Sterns, H. L., & Alexander, R. A. (1978). Age differences in perceptual style, selective attention, and perceptual-motor reaction time. *Experimental Aging Research, 4,* 377–387.

Parasuraman, R., & Giambra, L. (1991). Skill development in vigilance: Effects of event rate and age. *Psychology and Aging, 6,* 155–169.

Pearlin, L., & Skaff, M. (1995). Stressors and adaptation in later life. In M. Gatz (Ed.), *Emerging issues in mental health and aging* (pp. 97–123). Washington, DC: American Psychological Association.

Perlmutter, M. (1983). Learning and memory through adulthood. In M. W. Riley, B. B. Hess, & K. Bond (Eds.), *Aging in society* (pp. 219–242). Hillsdale, NJ: Erlbaum.

Perlmutter, M., & Mitchell, D. (1982). The appearance and disappearance of age differences in adult memory. In F. Craik & S. Trehub (Eds.), *Aging and cognitive processes* (pp. 127–142). New York: Plenum.

Perlmutter, M., & Nyquist, L. (1990). Relationships between self-reported physical and mental health and intelligence performance across adulthood. *Journal of Gerontology: Psychological Sciences, 45,* 145–155.

Plude, D. J., & Hoyer, W. J. (1981). Adult age differences in visual search as a function of stimulus-mapping and processing load. *Journal of Gerontology, 36,* 596–604.

Poon, L. (1985). Differences in human memory with aging. In J. E. Birren & K. W. Schaie (Eds.), *Handbook of the psychology of aging* (pp. 427–462). New York: Van Nostrand Reinhold.

Powell, D. (1994). *Profiles in cognitive aging.* Cambridge, MA: Harvard University Press.

Qualls, S. (1996). Family therapy with aging families. In S. Zarit & B. Knight (Eds.), *A guide to psychotherapy and aging* (pp. 121–138). Washington, DC: American Psychological Association.

Reese, C., Cherry, K., & Norris, L. (1998). *Practical memory concerns of older adults.* Unpublished manuscript.

Riegel, K. F. (1976). The dialectics of human development. *American Psychologist, 31,* 689–700.

Robertson-Tchabo, E. A., Hausman, C., & Arenberg, D. (1976). A classical mnemonic for older learners: A trip that works. *Educational Gerontology, 1,* 215–226.

Rogers, W. A. (1997). Individual differences, aging, and human factors: An overview. In A. D. Fisk & W. A. Rogers (Eds.), *Handbook of human factors and the older adult* (pp. 151–170). New York: Academic Press.

Roth, S., & Cohen, J. L. (1986). Approach-avoidance and coping with stress. *American Psychologist, 41,* 813–819.

Rowe, E. J., & Schnore, M. M. (1971). Item concreteness and reported strategies in paired-associate learning as a function of old age. *Journal of Gerontology, 26,* 470–475.

Salthouse, T. A. (1991). *Theoretical perspectives on cognitive aging.* Hillsdale, NJ: Erlbaum.

Salthouse, T. A. (1993). Attentional blocks are not responsible for age-related slowing. *Journal of Gerontology: Psychological Sciences, 48,* 263–270.

Sands, L. P., & Meredith, W. (1989). Effects of sensory and motor functioning on adult intellectual performance. *Journal of Gerontology: Psychological Sciences, 44,* P56–P58.

Schaie, K. W. (1996). Intellectual development in adulthood. In J. Birren & K. W. Schaie (Eds.), *Handbook of the Psychology of Aging* (pp. 266–286). San Diego, CA: Academic Press.

Schaie, K. W. (1979). The primary mental abilities in adulthood: An exploration in the development of psychometric intelligence. In P. Baltes & O. Brim (Eds.), *Life-span development and behavior* (Vol. 2, pp. 68–115). New York: Academic Press.

Schaie, K. W., & Gribbin, K. (1975). Adult development and aging. *Annual Review of Psychology, 26,* 65–96.

Schaie, K. W., & Willis, S. L. (1986). Can decline in adult intellectual functioning be reversed? *Developmental Psychology, 22,* 223–232.

Schaie, K. W., & Willis, S. L. (1991). Adult personality and psychomotor performance: Cross-sectional and longitudinal analyses. *Journal of Gerontology: Psychological Sciences, 46,* 275–284.

Schaie, K. W., & Willis, S. L. (1996). Psychometric intelligence and aging. In F. Blandchard-Fields & T. Hess (Eds.), *Perspectives on cognitive change in adulthood and aging* (pp. 293–322). New York: McGraw-Hill.

Schaie, K. W., Willis, S. L., & O'Hanlon, A. (1994). Perceived intellectual change over several years. *Journal of Gerontology: Psychological Sciences, 19,* 108–119.

Schmidt, F., Murphy, M., & Sanders, R. E. (1981). Training older adults free-recall rehearsal strategies. *Journal of Gerontology, 36,* 329–337.

Schooler, C. (1987). Effects of complex environments during the life-span: A review and theory. In C. Schooler & K. W. Schaie (Eds.), *Cognitive functioning and social structure over the life course* (pp. 24–29). Norwood, NJ: Ablex.

Schulz, R., & Heckhausen, D. (1996). A life span model of successful aging. *American Psychologist, 51,* 702–714.

Schwartz, B., & Reisberg, D. (1991). *Learning and memory.* New York: Norton.

Semel, V. (1996). Modern psychoanalytic treatment of the older patient. In S. Zarit & B. Knight (Eds.), *A guide to psychotherapy and aging* (pp. 102–120). Washington, DC: American Psychological Association.

Silberschatz, G., & Curtis, J. T. (1991). Time-limited psychodynamic therapy with older adults. In W. Myers (Ed.), *New techniques in the psychotherapy of older clients* (pp. 95–110). Washington, DC: American Psychiatric Press.

Simonton, D. K. (1990). Creativity and wisdom in aging. In J. E. Birren & K. W. Schaie (Eds.), *Handbook of the psychology of aging* (pp. 320–329). New York: Academic Press.

Smith, A. (1996). Memory. In J. E. Birren & K. W. Schaie (Eds.), *Handbook of the psychology of aging* (pp. 236–250). San Diego: Academic Press.

Smyer, M. A., Zarit, S. H., & Qualls, S. H. (1990). Psychological intervention with the aged individual. In J. E. Birren & K. W. Schaie (Eds.), *Handbook of the psychology of aging* (pp. 375–404). New York: Academic Press.

Spayd, C., & Smyer, M. (1996). Psychological interventions in nursing homes. In S. Zarit & B. Knight (Eds.), *A guide to psychotherapy and aging* (pp. 241–268). Washington, DC: American Psychological Association.

Steenbarger, B. N. (1991). All the world is not a stage: Emerging contextualist themes in counseling and development. *Journal of Counseling and Development, 70,* 288–296.

Sternberg, R. J. (1991). Theory-based testing of intellectual abilities: Rationale for the triarchic abilities test. In H. Row (Ed.), *Intelligence: Reconceptualization and measurement* (pp. 183–202). Hillsdale, NJ: Erlbaum.

Storandt, M., Grant, E. A., & Gordon, B. C. (1978). Remote memory as a function of age and sex. *Experimental Aging Research, 4,* 365–375.

Storandt, M., & VandenBos, G. (1994). *Neuropsychological assessment of dementia and depression in older adults: A clinician's guide.* Washington, DC: American Psychological Association.

Thompson, L. W., Gantz, F., Florsheim, M., DelMaestro, S., Rodman, J., Gallagher-Thompson, D., & Bryan, S. (1991). Cognitive-behavioral therapy for affective disorders in the elderly. In W. Myers (Ed.), *New techniques in the psychotherapy of older clients* (pp. 3–20). Washington, DC: American Psychiatric Press.

Vercruyssen, M. (1997). Movement control and speed of behavior. In A. D. Fist & W. A. Rodgers (Eds.), *Handbook of human factors and the older adult* (pp. 55–86). New York: Academic Press.

Waters, E. B. (1984). Building on what you know: Techniques for individual and group counseling with older people. *Counseling Psychologist, 12,* 81–96.

Waters, E. (1995). Let's not wait until it's broke: Interventions to maintain and enhance mental health in late life. In M. Gatz (Ed.), *Emerging issues in mental health and aging* (pp. 183–209). Washington, DC: American Psychological Association.

Welford, A. T. (1977). Motor performance. In J. E. Birren & K. W. Schaie (Eds.), *Handbook of the psychology of aging* (pp. 450–496). New York: Van Nostrand Reinhold.

Wells, L. E., & Stryker, S. (1988). Stability and change in self over the life course. In P. Baltes & O. Brim (Eds.), *Life-span development and behavior* (Vol. 8, pp. 191–229). Hillsdale, NJ: Erlbaum.

West, R. L. (1989). Planning practical memory training for the aged. In L. W. Poon, D. C. Rubin, & B. A. Wilson (Eds.), *Everyday cognition in adulthood and later life* (pp. 573–597). Cambridge: Cambridge University Press.

Whitbourne, S. K. (1987). Personality development in adulthood and old age: Relationships among identity, health, and well-being. In K. W. Schaie & C. Eisdorfer (Eds.), *Annual Review of Gerontology and Geriatrics* (pp. 189–216). New York: Springer.

Whitbourne, S. K. (1986). *The me I know: A study of adult identity.* New York: Springer-Verlag.

Whitlatch, C. J., & Zarit, S. H. (1989). Sexual dysfunction in aged married couples: A case study of behavioral intervention. *Clinical Gerontologist, 6,* 14–21.

Willis, S. L. (1985). Towards an educational psychology of the older adult learner: Intellectual and cognitive bases. In J. E. Birren & K. W. Schaie (Eds.), *Handbook of the psychology of aging* (2nd ed., pp. 818–847). New York: Van Nostrand Reinhold.

Woodruff, D., & Birren, J. E. (1972). Age changes and cohort differences in personality. *Developmental Psychology, 6,* 252–259.

Wright, R. E. (1981). Aging, divided attention, and processing capacity. *Journal of Gerontology, 36,* 605–614.

Zarit, S. (1996). Interventions with family caregivers. In S. Zarit & B. Knight (Eds.), *A guide to psychotherapy and aging* (pp. 139–162). Washington, DC: American Psychological Association.

Zeiss, A., & Steffen, A. (1996). Behavioral and cognitive-behavioral interventions: An overview of social learning. In S. Zarit & B. Knight (Eds.), *A guide to psychotherapy and aging* (pp. 35–60). Washington, DC: American Psychological Association.

Resources

American Psychological Association: `www.apa.org`

American Journal of Psychotherapy: `www.ajp.org`

American Psychologist: `APEditor@apa.org`

American Psychological Association, Inc.: `www.apa.org/books`

CHAPTER 7

Social Aging

Susan Brown Eve, PhD

Sharon Prentice, RN, MS

Charlie D. Pruitt, Jr., MS

Diana Torrez, PhD

COMPETENCIES

After completing this chapter, the reader should be able to:

- *Describe structural lag theory.*
- *Review data on race and ethnic differences in aging.*
- *Identify the different social roles commonly associated with older adults.*
- *Describe how the role of grandparenthood has evolved into parenthood the second time around.*
- *Discuss how the role of retirement has changed in recent years.*
- *Compare and contrast the differences experienced in widowhood by gender.*
- *Examine special issues of spirituality as it relates to the aging process.*

MAKING THE CONNECTION

Refer to the following chapters to increase your understanding of the social aspects of aging:

Aging and Structural Lag

What is it like to be old? The experience of growing old has varied considerably throughout history and across the different cultures of the world. Even if the discussion is limited to aging at the dawn of the twenty-first century in the United States, there is considerable variation in the experience of aging. Life experiences even within one culture are influenced by one's place in the social structure of a given society.

In the contemporary United States, race, ethnicity, gender, and class as well as age continue to influence how people live their daily lives. This chapter will focus on the influences of these social structural factors on the experience of aging. Discussion will begin with a review of the effects of social structure on **age structure** within society. One of the founders of gerontology, Matilda White Riley, and her colleagues have argued over the course of the transition from the twentieth to the twenty-first centuries. The United States is in the process of moving from a relatively age-segregated society to a more flexible age-integrated society, in which people of all ages are more free than they have ever been to move into and out of jobs, schools, family roles, and community volunteer roles in ways that are best suited to their current needs and abilities rather than rigid age-defined norms. Race and ethnicity specifically affect life changes for older adults. The major **social roles** of the aging process are **grandparenthood, retirement,** and **widowhood.** Spirituality in old age and the ways spirituality can mitigate the problems of aging are important also.

Matilda White Riley, Marilyn Johnson, and Anne Foner are credited with founding the field of sociology of the aging with the publication of the three volume set *Aging and Society* in 1972. Riley pioneered the aging and society approach to the study of aging. The guiding thesis of this approach is that there is a dynamic interplay between people growing older in a society and the social structure of the society (Riley, Johnson, & Foner,

1972). This thesis is illustrated in Figure 7-1, as adapted from Riley & Riley (1994), Foner (1994), and Kahn (1994). The age structure of a society is composed of **age roles, age norms,** and **age values** for age-appropriate behavior within the basic social institutions, including the economy, family, educational system, political system, religion, leisure institutions, and community. The age structure of a society sets the context in which individuals experience aging. Different social roles are open or closed to people of different ages in a given historical period. Norms define appropriate age-related activities for different age groups. Values are statements of what is good and true in a society and underlie the definitions of roles and norms. The Rileys believe that the social structure is changing from an **age-segregated social structure** into a more **age-integrated social structure.** In the age-segregated structure that has characterized U.S. society for most of the latter half of the twentieth century, childhood and youth have been reserved for the pursuit of education, adulthood for work and family responsibilities, and old age for retirement and leisure pursuits. In an age-integrated society, education, work, family, responsibilities, and leisure activities occur *throughout the life course,* with individuals having more flexibility in moving in and out of education, work, family, and leisure roles based on their own needs, desires, and resources at different stages in their lives.

As groups of individuals age within their **birth cohorts** and move through society, they also influence the social structure, causing changes in the roles, norms, and values. Major sociodemographic changes in older cohorts in modern Western societies that are creating pressure on the age structures include increases in life expectancy and improvements in health of older populations (Riley & Riley, 1994). Increases in life expectancy are causing increases in the number and proportions of the old (65 years of age and older) and old-old (85 years of age and older). Kahn (1994) argued that improvements in health status are causing changes in the abilities and capacities of older adults (what they can do) and changes in the needs and goals of the old (what they want to do). For example, as the functioning of the older adult population has improved, older adults are increasingly expressing the desire for more structured activities, including paid part-time employment and unpaid volunteer activities. Riley and Riley (1994) argued that there is currently a mismatch between older adults needs and desires and the social structural opportunities for older adults, a mismatch that they refer to as **structural lag.** Kahn (1994) attributed this lag to a lack of **goodness of fit** between the needs, aspirations, and abilities of individuals and the expectations and opportunities that confront them in the social structure. Although older adults want more opportunities to work part time, for example, there are few structural opportunities for such work available to them.

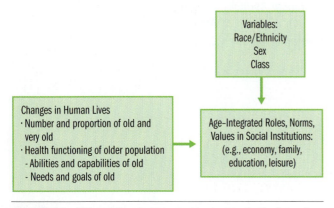

FIGURE 7-1   Effects of sociodemographic changes in the lives of older adults on age-related social structural change

Foner (1994) discussed the three major mechanisms that create change in the social structure. These are **policy changes, cohort norm formation,** and **age conflicts** that result in social movements. Policy change results from deliberate actions of policymakers to create change through the use of the political process. These processes may include enacting specific laws, issuing executive orders, and reallocating societal resources. Cohort norm formation (Riley, 1978; cited in Foner, 1994) occurs when large numbers of individuals reacting independently but in a similar fashion to societal changes produce new patterns of behavior and norms that spread from one cohort to the next. The **baby-boom generation** (e.g., those people born between 1946 and 1964) has created new cohort norms as they have passed through the age structure in society. These new norms range from increases in age at first marriage to longer periods of time reserved for education to increasing periods of full-time employment for women. Age conflicts and social movements have been infrequent in the past and are likely to remain so because of the ties binding the generations together. Some gerontologists have speculated that the issue of *intergenerational equity* over the continued support of Social Security by young people has the potential to create such conflict. Foner (1994) argued that three factors are likely to mitigate against such a conflict developing. First, young people benefit from Social Security incentives that encourage older adults to retire from the labor force and open up jobs for younger people. Second, younger people are spared the responsibility for supporting their older family members as long as the family members are receiving Social Security benefits. Third, by supporting the current generation of Social Security beneficiaries, young people are guaranteeing their own financial security in old age.

Foner also discussed obstacles to change in the social structure. These obstacles include economic conditions, social and economic costs of change, institutional inertia, and basic social values. A current obstacle to increased employment of older adults is the corporate downsizing and exportation of jobs to less costly global wage areas. With fewer jobs for the adult population, society is less likely to encourage increased employment of retirees. Social and economic costs of change may also limit the change society is likely to encourage. Employers, for example, objected to paying employees during family leaves to care for sick family members, and so the family leave legislation in the United States does not require paid leave. Obviously this limits the ability of people with low or moderate income to take advantage of the greater flexibility in allocating their time to family versus work roles that the law allows. Third, there is a built-in institutional resistance to change. Bureaucracies are slow to change, and people with vested interests in the status quo are likely to resist changes that threaten their interests. Robert Kahn (1994) proposed that the U.S. adopt 4-hr work modules as the standard unit of work rather than the 8-hr module to allow workers greater flexibility in allocating their time between education, family, and work. Employers object to the increased costs of fringe benefits for shorter work periods, while others object to the increased hassles involved in scheduling workers using shorter work modules. Finally, deeply held basic values of what is good and true in society may hamper change. The economic system in the United States is based on basic values of economic competition, comparative achievement among individuals, and consumption. Increased flexibility in allocating time to work versus other roles in family, education, or leisure would threaten the primacy of those values.

Cultural, Race, and Ethnic Issues

Riley and Riley (1994) argued that to understand the effects of changing sociodemographic characteristics among the aging population on the age-related social structure in the United States, one must consider the related social structures that are specific to gender, class, and race or ethnicity. They argued that these additional factors affect the age-related social structure, which affects the opportunities available to older adults.

If one is to discuss older Americans in the United States, racial and ethnic diversity within this population must be given serious consideration. Older adults age 65 and older in 1998 accounted for 12.7% of the total population, and minorities comprised 16% of that population (*A Profile,* 1999). Although minorities constitute a small percentage of the older adults today, they are growing at a much faster rate than white older adults. It is projected that by 2030 those age 65 and older will have increased to 20% of the total population. However, the increase among nonwhites will be much greater than among whites during this period. White adults age 65 and older will increase by 79%; while Hispanics will increase by 341%; African Americans 130%; American Indian, Eskimo, and Aleuts 150%; and Asians and Pacific Islanders 323% (*A Profile,* 1999). It is, therefore, essential for gerontologists, policy planners, and the general public to be well informed with respect to minority older adults, including their culture, economic, and social situation. African Americans, Latinos, American Indians, and Asians account for the majority of the minority older adults today and are also the fastest growing groups.

Economic Issues

Because minorities have much higher rates of poverty than their white counterparts, every other aspect of their lives is affected by their economic status. Although in 1992 12.9% of those age 65 and older lived in poverty, 33.8% of African Americans were poor and 11.3% were defined by the U.S. Census as being *near poor,* compared with 6.8% of all races. Hispanics (22%) and Americans Indians (28%) similarly reported higher rates of poverty. Only Asians reported similar levels of poverty (14%) as those of Caucasians (U.S. Bureau of the Census, 1996).

Also, unlike whites, minorities were less likely to receive private pensions. Thirty-one percent of whites as compared with 17% of African Americans and 19% of Hispanics received private pensions. Minorities are more likely to report public assistance as a source of income than whites. Twenty-five percent of African Americans receive public assistance, 22% of Hispanics, and 29% of American Indians (Chen, 1994; John, 1994).

Chen (1994) noted than any discussion of economic security among minorities age 65 and older must include concerns unique to them such as health status, education, and family structure. It is important to note not only how these factors are affected by their economic status but also how their health, education, and family structure affect their economic status.

Education

The income level and poverty status of minorities age 65 and older are in part affected by their educational level. Although the educational attainment of minorities has increased in the past decades, the educational attainment among those age 65 years and older remains low. Sixty-three percent of whites age 65 and older are high school graduates. Only 33.3% of African Americans and 26% of Hispanics age 65 years and older are high school graduates (U.S. Bureau of Census, 1995). As a result of low educational attainment and limited job skills, these older adults were unable to secure well-paying jobs in their adult lives and therefore often are not eligible for retirement benefits. Many of those age 65 and older who live in poverty today have lived in poverty all their lives. Becoming old did not give them economic stability. Although they may be receiving Social Security benefits, their income is often not enough to live on adequately, and therefore, some must also seek public assistance. It is also important to note that research suggests that education extends both total life expectancy and **active life expectancy** (Land et al., 1994). It is also important to realize that because many minority elders have difficulty reading and writing in English and may have only limited proficiency communicating in English, they are often unable to acquire social and health services for which they are eligible.

Health Status

On average, minorities have a shorter life expectancy than their white counterparts. African-Americans have a life expectancy that is 5 years less than that of whites. Asian and Hispanic life expectancies have improved in recent decades and are now approaching that of whites (U.S. Bureau of the Census, 1996). American Indians also report a life expectancy that is 3.3 years less than whites (John, 1994).

The life expectancy differential for African Americans is because of significantly higher **mortality rates** at nearly all ages. African Americans report death rates that are nearly one-and-a-half times greater than that of whites. As noted in Table 7-1, African Americans experience the highest mortality rates. Asian and Pacific Islanders report the lowest rates, even lower than those of whites. Hispanics also report low mortality rates.

American Indians experience slightly higher mortality rates than whites during the ages 55–64. However, after 65 years, they also report lower rates than whites. The lower mortality rates of American Indians age 65 and older are partially attributable to their significantly higher mortality rate at younger ages, particularly between the ages of 5–14 and 24–44. The differences in the mortality rates is reflective of differential life course experience.

Diabetes, although not among the leading causes of death, plays an important role in the lives of African American, Hispanic, and American Indian women. For these women diabetes is the fourth leading cause of death, while for white women it is the seventh leading cause of death, and for white men it is the ninth. Asian women also report diabetes as the sixth leading cause of death. Diabetes is related to obesity, which is disproportionately found among African American, Hispanic, and American Indian women.

Family Structure

There is widespread belief that older minorities are a part of large extended families. These extended kin networks are believed to meet the instrumental and emotional needs of their older members. This was one explanation that was often proposed for the low usage of social services among minority elders. However, recent research suggests that this explanation is somewhat simplistic and that the role of minority elders within the family is much more complex (Chatters & Taylor, 1986; Maldonado, 1989; Torrez, 1998; Williams, 1990).

Studies in the 1970s documented the participation of African-American older adults in informal kinship networks (Aschenbrenner, 1973, 1975; Martin & Martin, 1978; Stack, 1972, 1974). However, more recent research has found that informal support networks among older

TABLE 7-1   Mortality Rates for All Causes, According to Age, Gender, and Race/Ethnicity: 1992 (rate per 100,000)

Population	Age 55–64	Age 65–74	Age 75–84	Age 85+
White				
Female	799.2	1,909.1	4,969.4	14,015.9
Male	1,398.5	3,287.0	7,440.9	17,956.2
Black				
Female	1,405.4	2,796.6	5,483.0	13,264.1
Male	2,493.8	4,746.7	8,744.5	16,717.1
American Indian or Alaskan Native				
Female	912.4	1,743.2	3,307.1	6,878.7
Male	1,384.0	2,604.0	5,239.7	9,381.3
Asian or Pacific Islander				
Female	476.2	1,095.0	2,873.1	9,561.8
Male	766.8	1,962.5	4,919.7	12,628.8
Hispanic				
Female	598.2	1,354.2	3,149.7	8,772.4
Male	1,061.1	2,322.3	4,924.1	10,895.4

Adapted from National Center for Health Statistics. (1995). Health, United States, 1994. Hyattsville, MD: Public Health Service.

African American adults consist of not only family but also friends and church members (Chatters & Taylor, 1986). Family members provide goods and services, financial assistance, and transportation. Friends provide companionship and church members provide spiritual support such as prayers during times of sickness. Research has documented that among African American older adults the preferred source of assistance is children. Shanas (1979) found that whites were more likely to provide assistance to their children and grandchildren, whereas African Americans were more likely to report receiving assistance from their children and grandchildren. Because of the high poverty rates among African American elders, this informal support system is important to their well-being. It is important, however, to note that as a result of the high poverty rate in the general African American population, although children may be the preferred source of assistance, it may not always be possible for children to provide assistance, particularly financial assistance, to their parents. It is for this reason that it is important for African American elders to be aware of and be able to access the formal social service and public assistance programs that are available to them.

Research on Hispanics often has focused on the extended family (Rosenthal, 1986; Starett, Mindel, & Wright, 1983). It was widely believed that the extended family provided assistance with whatever needs the older family members might have (Kaiser, Gibbons, & Camp, 1993). However, research has documented that this support may not be as extensive as previously thought (Dietz, 1995). Torrez (1998) reported that the availability of social and family support networks did not necessarily guarantee adequate support in their daily lives or the assistance they required to apply for social services. It should be noted that although the family continues to be an important component of the Mexican American culture, the extended family support system often associated with Hispanics is no longer the norm (Maldonado, 1989; Williams, 1990).

There also exists the notion that American Indian elders reside in an extended family. It is further suggested that these households continue to function independently and care for their elders. However, recent research suggests that the primary reason for the extended family among American Indians is financial (Manson, 1988). In the context of high unemployment on the reservation, older adults may be the only persons with a stable source of income, modest as their old age pension may be. This may force younger family members to rely on the older person's Social Security and lead to alarming rates of elder abuse (John, 1994).

There is limited research on Asian Americans age 65 and older. There are no national data, and therefore, the majority of what exists is the result of studies on select populations. It is important to note that although the term *Asian Americans* is used, there is extreme diversity among this population, which consists of seven ethnic groups. In addition, there are considerable differences among foreign and native-born Asians. The majority of Asian men age 65 and older are married, while women age 65 and older are widowed. Older Asian men are less likely to live alone (19%) than older white men (30%) (Yee, 1997). However, Lubben and Becerra (1987) found that among Chinese elders the reason they were more likely to live with other family members and receive help from their children is related not only to cultural value but to economic need as well. Although Asian Americans often are referred to as the model minority, referring to their educational and economic success as a group, it is important to be aware that economic bipolarity exists in this population and that 14% of Asians Americans live in poverty.

The previous discussion has highlighted the racial and ethnic diversity that exists among those age 65 and older. It is impossible to refer to the older population in research as though they are a homogenous population. If one is to understand accurately and address the needs of the increasing older population, ethnic diversity in this population must be discussed. Minority older adults have unique problems as a result of their life course experiences that are not found among the white older adult population. Because minority elders are increasing at a much faster rate than white older adults, it does a disservice to refer simply to the elders in research, particularly because this often refers only to white older adults.

Social Roles

Social roles are how individual persons define themselves and their function in society (Atchley, 1997; Moen, 1996). Roles are generally associated with positions, and what is expected of persons depends a great deal on the position occupied (Atchley, 1997). For example, older men commonly held positions as war veterans and primary household breadwinners, while older women

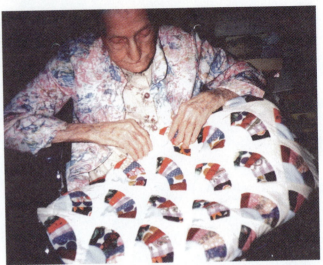

FIGURE 7-2   Older adults may experience new roles as long-term care residents but continue lifelong activities. This woman continues to piece quilts at age 106.

commonly occupied the role of caregiver as housewife and mother (Moen, 1996). The importance of a position is primarily measured by prestige, status, influence, and wealth. In current American society the role of an older adult is often synonymous with low prestige, status, wealth, or influence (Atchley, 1997). The act of aging influences what roles we can act out as well as the way they are acted out (Atchley, 1997; Moen, 1996). Several roles that older adults age 65 and older may experience for the first time include that of older adult, grandparent, retired person, volunteer, caregiver, widowed person, dependent, disabled, patient, and long-term care resident (Figure 7-2). Researchers have added a recent designation for those 85 years old and over, the role of *oldest old* (Johnson & Barer, 1997).

The aging experience itself does not always inflict undesirable roles on older adults, as often roles depend on the social supports one has (Rook, 1997). Research has been devoted to the impact of negative and positive social influences on the well-being of older adults (Ingersoll-Dayton, Morgan, & Antonucci, 1997). Social relationships provide an interlocking network of experiences with resulting positive and negative outcomes (Ingersoll-Dayton et al., 1997; Rook, 1997). What has concerned researchers is that as one ages, the negative social experiences may lead to the disability and illness role (George, 1996). However, it appears that the presence of social and familial support is the deciding factor for whether or not an older adult enters the disability and illness role (Ingersoll-Dayton et al., 1997; Rook, 1997).

Because women live, on average, 7 years longer than men, it is women who are more likely to experience the roles of grandparent, spousal caregiver, widow, and long-term care resident (Moen, 1996). It should be noted that although women live longer than men, they also have higher **morbidity rates** than older men (Allen & Phillips, 1997; Moen, 1996; Pickard, 1995; Taeuber & Allen, 1993). Older women report more physician visits, prescribed medications, and higher rates of chronic illnesses than their male counterparts. When compared to men, women have a disproportionately more variety of chronic illnesses, including, autoimmune disorders, diabetes mellitus, arthritis, digestive disorders, osteoporosis, and chronic obstructive pulmonary disease (Allen & Phillips, 1997). Because of increased longevity, women have a 1-in-2 chance of becoming a long-term care resident (Allen & Phillips, 1997; Moen, 1996; Taeuber & Allen, 1993). Some of the factors that place older women at risk for long-term care placement include widowhood, chronic disability, and survival of sons. Approximately one in four women will outlive her son if the son was born during her early twenties (Arendell & Estes, 1994). Therefore, in addition to women outliving their spouses, they may also outlive their sons, demonstrating the genuine potential for a reduction in available familial support often desired by older adults. Older women constitute almost 80% of the residents in nursing facilities (Allen & Phillips, 1997; Arendell & Estes, 1994; Taeuber & Allen, 1993). See Figure 7-3.

Social roles for older men and women are complex, and while they may occupy the same roles, women and men may experience these roles differently. Older men may experience grandparenthood, but for a shorter duration and most likely with younger grandchildren. Older women are more likely to experience not only grandparenthood but also great-grandparenthood. Older men are more likely to be married and have a wife who can be his caregiver when his health declines. Older women are more likely to be widowed and remain unmarried for the rest of their lives. If older men experience widowhood, they are more likely to remarry. Older men are more likely to have been employed long enough to receive a pension upon retirement. Older women who work often leave the work force several times during their careers to care for children, parents, and spouses and thus have less or no pension and less Social Security benefits.

The perceptions associated with older men's roles and older women's roles also vary greatly. Older men are often viewed as dignified and stoic, while older women are often viewed as meddling, aggressive, shrill, and threatening (Allen & Phillips, 1997; Jacobs, 1993; Pickard, 1995). Many legends and fairy-tales associate older women with witches, hags, crones, and sorceresses (Jacobs, 1993; Pickard, 1995). This Morracan legend is an example of how society can devalue older women, and how older women can feel abandoned.

Think About It

A Morraccan legend states (Gutmann, 1987, p. 174): When a boy is born a hundred evil jinn (devils) are born with him, and when a girl is born there are born with her a hundred angels, but every year a jinn passes from the man to the woman, so that when the man is 100 years old he is surrounded by one hundred angels and when the woman is 100 years old she is surrounded by one hundred devils.

Often the most feared role of aging is that of disability and illness (Allen & Phillips, 1997; Pickard, 1995). Older women fear losing the ability to provide a clean home and providing care for their husbands, while older men fear losing the physical strength needed to be the provider/protector (Pickard, 1995). Both sexes fear loss of autonomy and eventual relocation into a long-term care institution. Placement in a long-term care institution automatically places the older resident at a disadvantage with loss of autonomy (Robbins, 1996).

Grandparenthood

Grandparenthood can be considered a mark of accomplishment, an acknowledgment that one has reached the top of the family tree (Pickard, 1995). The role of grandparent involvement is a relatively recent addition to the American lifestyle and has rapidly become integral to

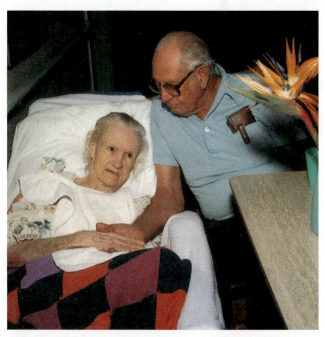

FIGURE 7-3 Eighty percent of nursing facility residents are older women.

the normal aging process (Somary & Stricker, 1998). Although a common assumption has been that the extended family is on the decline, the actual facts are that for the first time in history the vertical extended family exists (Cherlin & Furstenberg, 1997). In historical times,

---

Nursing Tip

It is important for health care providers to remain alert to situations that require ethical decision-making skills (Robbins, 1996). Ethics in health care often involve choosing between two equally good or equally bad alternatives. Health care providers often are faced with dilemmas about deciding to do what is best for someone versus allowing individual autonomy. Health care providers must use their communication skills and listen to individual needs before determining the best course of action.

Research Focus

Citation:
Kelley, S. J., Yorker, B. C., & Whitley, D. (1997). To grandmother's house we go . . . and stay: Children raised in intergenerational families. *Journal of Gerontological Nursing, 23*(9), 13–20.

Purpose:
An estimated 1.1 million children in foster care have been placed with relatives, especially grandparents, where neither biological parent is present in the home. This study focused on the issues older adults' experience when parenting the second time around.

Methods:
Review of U.S. Census Bureau statistics, personal interviews of grandparents with children in prisons, and studies of low-income and minority neighborhoods.

Findings:
There is a severe increase in recent years of grandparents formally and informally becoming the primary caregivers of grandchildren.

Implications:
Health care providers need to be alert to the fact that the most vulnerable grandparents tend to be the ones forced into full-time caregiving. This group needs extensive support with child caregiving responsibilities and monitoring of personal health care.

---

people did not live long enough for grandchildren to know grandparents. The extended families of early America were those of siblings, aunts, and uncles. Grandparenthood is actually a post–World War II event (Cherlin & Furstenberg, 1997). In recent decades life expectancy has increased to the extent that families are typically three generations (80%) and increasingly up to four or five generations (16%) (Szinovacz, 1998).

In earlier times, women were normally at home raising young children, while the oldest child had already married and had a child (Cherlin & Furstenberg, 1997). Grandparents at this stage had very little time to consider themselves grandparents. Declining birth rates and increasing life expectancy have resulted in taking for granted the status of grandparenthood in recent decades (Cherlin & Furstenberg, 1997; Somary & Stricker, 1998). An advantage of increased longevity is that grandparents have extended leisure time through survival into their retirement years (Cherlin & Furstenberg, 1997; Szinovacz, 1998).

Trends in grandparenthood reflect both generational and familial behavior patterns (Szinovacz, 1998). While some families may experience multigenerational benefits, it also needs to be considered that other families are waiting longer to get married and raise children. Therefore, it is still probable that some families will have grandparents around for the first-born grandchildren but not the last born. It has been noted that grandparenthood occurs at younger ages for black and Hispanic women as compared to white women (Somary & Stricker, 1998; Szinovacz, 1998). Over 50% of black women under the age of 55 are grandmothers, compared to 33% of white women in the same age bracket (Szinovacz, 1998).

Another trend to consider with grandparenthood is that grandchildren are more likely to know their grandmothers than their grandfathers. Studies indicate that many adults in their late twenties will have only one surviving grandmother and will frequently have lost their grandfathers prior to reaching age 18 (Szinovacz, 1998). Therefore, grandparent-grandchild interaction is more commonly found with grandmothers (Pearson, Hunter, Cook, Ialongo, & Kellam, 1997). The reasons cited include increased longevity for women; also, women are more likely to assume a caregiving role with their grandchildren (Figure 7-4).

A dramatic phenomenon discovered with the 1990 Census was the finding that **grandparent caregiving** has risen 44% over the previous decades (Fuller-Thomson, Minkler, & Driver, 1997; Jendrek, 1994). Causes cited for this recent phenomenon of grandparent caregiving involve impairment of the biological parents through substance abuse, teen pregnancy, acquired immunodeficiency syndrome (AIDS), incarceration, mental illness, emotional problems, and premature parental death (Burton, 1992;

Dowdell, 1995; Dressel & Barnhill, 1994; Jendrek, 1994; Minkler, Roe, & Price, 1992). The most common reason cited for grandparent caregiving was child maltreatment and neglect, frequently associated with substance abuse by the biological parents (Burton, 1992; Dowdell, 1995; Jendrek, 1994; Minkler et al., 1992). In 1995, a study conducted by Joslin and Brouard among low-income neighborhoods in New York City revealed that 1 out of every 10 children in those neighborhoods was living in foster care, with grandparents being the majority of the foster parents (Kelley, Yorker, & Whitley, 1997).

Approximately one-quarter of black and Hispanic grandmothers live in households with grandchildren compared to less than one-tenth of white grandmothers (Szinovacz, 1998). Again, more than one-quarter of black grandmothers are second-time parents, compared to just over one-tenth of white grandmothers. The group at the highest risk for grandparent caregiving are African American women (Bengston, Rosenthal, & Burton, 1996). This group is most often burdened with caring for teen pregnancy births and grandchildren of substance-abuse parents (Bengston et al., 1996; Minkler et al., 1992). A further burden on grandparent caregivers is that they tend to have significantly more grandchildren living in close proximity that need caregiving than do grandparents who are not thrust in the caregiver role (Fuller-Thomson et al., 1997).

Studies have indicated that grandparent caregivers may be at greater risk for health problems because of their caregiving roles (Burton, 1992; Dowdell, 1995; Jendrek, 1994). Of concern is whether these grandparent caregivers have increased health risks simply because of their caregiving role or because they were already compromised by financial issues (Strawbridge, Wallhagen, Shema, & Kaplan, 1997). Full-time grandparent caregivers are more likely than grandparents who are not caregivers to have financial difficulties, high rates of unemployment, less than a 12th-grade education, one or more chronic illnesses, and to be female, urban dwelling, and African American (Kelley et al., 1997; Pearson et al., 1997; Strawbridge et al., 1997). The highest levels of stress and poor health were associated with those grandparent caregivers that had full custody and child-rearing responsibilities. The other group of grandparent caregivers were assisting part time by watching children in the daytime while parents worked. This second group of grandparent caregivers expressed fewer feelings of stress and better health issues (Strawbridge et al., 1997). Box 7-1 lists a number of resource contacts and support groups for grandparents as caregivers.

With the accepted *normal* lifestyle of grandparenthood, what is the perception of closeness among grandchildren and grandparents? Recent arguments for generational equity may have damaged relationships in that the younger generations feel they are carrying the financial burdens for older generations (Lynott & Roberts, 1997; Moody, 1998). A provocative argument is that American children are now poorer and less healthy than their older American counterparts for whom the age-65-and-older social programs were developed (Atta, 1998; Moody, 1998). Further research indicates that it is not simply a matter of taking from the young to give to the old; however, this perception still exists (Moody, 1998). Even among older adults there is a lack of consensus when all persons age 65 and older are lumped together. Many persons age 65 and older are vitally healthy and active and resent being lumped in with those age 85 and older, whose interests are not the same (Atta, 1998).

In considering the future of the grandparent role, it is important to remember that when baby boomers enter their retirement years many perceptions and ways of organizing will change. The baby boom generation grew up involved with special-interest groups, and there is no reason to expect that will change simply because they are older (Atta, 1998). Society must begin to accept that there are differences among older adults; there are active, healthy younger-old and more ill older-old, with a diverse range between. Another effect on future grandparenthood is that of retirement being pushed back to age 70 or later. With more grandparents remaining in the work force longer (Figure 7-5), it would be prudent to watch that the grandparent-grandchild relationships do not suffer.

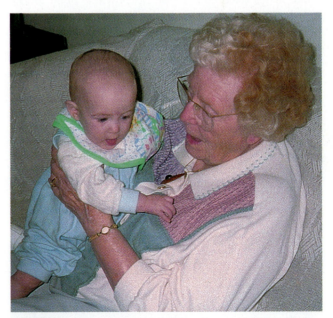

FIGURE 7-4 Older women often assume the caregiver role with their grandchildren.

BOX 7-1   Resources for Grandparents

AARP Grandparent Information Center
Social Outreach and Support
601 E. Street, NW
Washington, DC 20049
202-434-2296, Fax: 202-434-6474

Grandparents as Parents (GAP)
P.O. Box 964
Lakewood, CA 90714
310-924-3996, Fax: 714-828-1375

Grandparents Raising Grandchildren
7301 Miller Road
Rowlett, TX 75088
972-475-3559; Contact: Bob Chandler

Grandparents Who Care
One Rhode Island Street
San Francisco, CA 94103
415-856-3000, Fax: 415-865-3099

National Coalition of Grandparents
137 Larkin Street
Madison, WI 53705
608-238-8751

Pacific Northwest Coalition of Grandparents Raising Grandchildren
Pierce County Health Department
3629 South D Street
Tacoma, WA 98408
206-565-4484, Fax: 206-627-3943

R.O.C.K.I.N.G./Raising Our Children's Kids:
    An International Network of Grandparents, Inc.
P.O. Box 96
Niles, MI 49120
616-683-9038

Second Time Around Parents
Family and Community Service of Delaware County
100 W. Front Street
Media, PA 19065
610-566-7540

Retirement

Retirement from the active work force has become normative for the twentieth century in America (Hayward, Friedman, & Chen, 1998; Moody, 1998), especially for white males (Henretta, 1994). No previous point in history has provided such impetus for withdrawing from full-time work after many decades of service to spend one's days as one chooses. Retirement is taken for granted by current American society and is assumed to be a rite of passage into later life; however, the phenomenon of retirement began fairly recently.

It has only been since the Industrial Revolution that the issue of retirement was introduced (Hayward et al., 1998). It was not until 1935 that the United States developed the **Social Security Act** (Crown, 1998; Moody, 1998). The purpose of the U.S. Social Security Act was actually to create jobs (Crown, 1998). During the height of the Great Depression, the United States chose to move older workers out of the labor force at age 65 to make room for younger workers as one way of creating jobs. This process was accomplished by the Social Security program acting as a retirement income program allowing older adults to receive benefits according to the number of years worked prior to retirement and previous salary or wages, although it should be noted here that the Social Security program was never intended to be the sole income during retirement (Hayward et al., 1998; Moody, 1998).

White male retirees today began their careers following World War II, when the nation was experiencing labor shortages, and consequently, American industries and businesses were under pressure to attract and keep employees by offering increased wages and fringe ben-

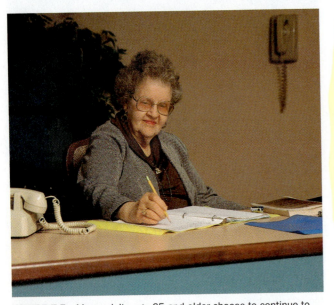

FIGURE 7-5   More adults age 65 and older choose to continue to work.

efit packages. The ideal American work experience involved employment at a young age right after high school or college graduation, advancement up the corporate ladder, and remaining with one company until retirement (Hayward et al., 1998). Employees tended to be life-long employees of one company, often unionized, with regular employment linked to fringe benefits, such as retirement pensions. The development of the Social Security system and retirement pensions led to linking retirement with a specific life stage (Henretta, 1994.)

With economic changes that have included movement to a global, postindustrial economy, American work experiences have come to include many career and occupational changes as a result of company downsizing, obsolescence of job function from technological advancement, and even disability (Couch, 1998). Older workers are not less likely to change jobs than their younger counterparts. Hayward et al. (1998) found that approximately 38% of recent retired workers left a career that was not their job of longest duration. It has been found that both upward and downward mobility seem to be associated with increased retirement rates (Crown, 1998; Hayward et al., 1998). The most frequent career changes were found in blue-collar labor occupations, while the highest rates of occupational retention were found among white-collar professionals. Researchers hypothesized that higher disability rates for blue-collar workers contributed to job mobility (Couch, 1998; Crown, 1998). White-collar professionals retained their career choices because of increased flexibility between upward and downward mobility within their chosen profession. The most distinct factor associated with lower retirement rates is that of the self-employed worker (Couch, 1998).

In contemporary times, policymakers are now trying to encourage older adults to remain in the labor force longer, thereby reducing the length of time retired workers would receive benefits (Crown, 1998; Moody, 1998). This shift in public policy has been caused by the shift in employment away from lifetime employment to contingent employment, including part-time and temporary work. In the contingent labor market, there is not an expectation of a long-term relationship between the employer and employees. Contingent labor jobs do not include fringe benefits such as retirement pensions. This trend may result in increased variability in career patterns and retirement in the future (Henretta, 1994). Henretta suggested that one possible change may be the increased use of *bridge jobs* between the major job during the lifetime and full retirement. These jobs are likely to be in different occupations and industries than the major *career* job and to carry lower wages.

In 1986 the legal practice of mandatory retirement at a specific age was withdrawn; however, there are still a few distinct occupations in private industry allowed to enforce it (Moody, 1998). Withdrawal of the mandatory age retirement does not eliminate informal age discrimination practices. The incidence of **job displacement** among workers aged 55–64 has greatly increased in recent years (Couch, 1998; Gardner, 1995). Other studies have demonstrated that older workers have lower rates of reemployment following job displacement (Crown, 1998; Gardner, 1995). While older workers may have anticipated returning to work in another occupation, employers may not have been willing to hire them (Crown, 1998). An important reason for reviewing job displacement among older workers involves those workers in the 55–60 age category who are not yet age eligible for Social Security retirement benefits, with many more who are not qualified for private pensions (Couch, 1998). Utilizing data from the Displaced Workers' Surveys, job displacement is commonly defined as the loss of a job because of plant closure or layoff in which the worker had been employed for at least 3 years (Couch, 1998). The deleterious effect of job displacement on older workers included loss of earnings, difficulty finding reemployment, and forced early retirement. The effects of job displacement are magnified for minority race and ethnic groups (Couch, 1998; Crown, 1998).

An interesting aspect of retirement involves retirement migration (Carlson, Junk, Fox, Rudzitis, & Cann, 1998). What are the factors that encourage one to move from a specific geographic area once employment ends? Haas and Serow (1993) developed the model of Amenity Retirement Migration Process. This model describes the factors that influence a person's decision to move following retirement. It identified *push* factors that tend to cause one to leave a home, such as the cost of living, population density, crime rates, and location of family members. It also identified *pull* factors, such as lower cost of living, lower population density, and better quality of life. Pull factors tend to cause one to want to move to another location. The sunbelt states, especially Florida, are commonly considered when looking for a high concentration of retired older adults. However, according to research completed by Carlson et al. (1998), Idaho has become a retirement migration center. Using the model of Amenity Retirement Migration Process for understanding this phenomenon, he concluded that the pull factors were strongly related to older retired adults' perceptions about a nonmetropolitan state. Older retired adults appeared drawn to tranquil scenic communities where they could live a short drive outside of an urban center (Carlson et al., 1998).

Recent alterations in the Social Security program were intended to increase the labor reserve of older workers (Honig, 1996). Current trends in retirement reflect the desire of policymakers to increase the average retirement age to 70. Although policymakers may wish to increase the number of working older adults, much depends on two factors. First, whether employers demonstrate a willingness to employ older workers and, second, the opinions of older adults as to whether retirement is more important than working. Future understanding of retirement issues can be enhanced by a comprehension of retirement expectations from a cultural perspective (Honig, 1996). It has been debated that a classification of flexible retirement where workers can gradually reduce their work hours and take longer vacations would provide for work longevity and an adjustment period to retirement (Moody, 1998). If this aspect were added to retirement, employers would have more time to replace departing older workers by allowing new replacements a longer integration time. Retiring employees would benefit from the slower phasing out of their many years of active service in the work force.

Henretta (1994) argued that women and minorities have always been more likely than white males to participate in the contingent labor force. Women's retirement patterns have always been more variable than that of men, and women who are single or divorced are likely to experience greater economic difficulty in retirement than is true of men. African American and Hispanic males have also been more likely to participate in the contingent labor force and have never conformed to the white male patterns of retirement, as a rule. It is difficult to distinguish unemployment from retirement in these minority groups, and William J. Wilson (1987, cited in Henretta, 1994) argued that current economic trends may increase this variability in the future.

Many people look forward to having time for leisure activities, volunteer work, further education, or another career (Moody, 1998) (Figure 7-6). Although retirement can bring relaxing pleasures such as travel and inventive pursuits for some, not all older adults are able to easily adapt to retirement. It has been a common mistaken assumption that retirement brings feelings of rejection, purposelessness, and exclusion. Research has been conducted that largely disproves the assumption of negative consequences of retirement (Moody, 1998). The majority of working Americans appear to look forward to retirement; however, there are a few among those that retire who have not found their comfort zone. Common reasons include loss of work relationships, loss of occupational identity, unanticipated ill health, and loss of structure. For those who remain in good health but feel lost without the structure of work, volunteering has been postulated as a means of overcoming feelings of purposelessness (Caro & Bass, 1997; Johnson & Barer, 1997).

Because the work force was largely dominated by men until recent years, adverse retirement issues have affected men more so than women. Women previously remained at home for significant periods of time and developed networks with family and friends, while the men went to work every day. The man's identity was generally tied up in his occupation, and withdrawal from that occupation resulted in loss of identity and purposelessness. Women, on the other hand, were already familiar with activities such as volunteer work and family interaction that working husbands probably did not do. Now these women had their husbands at home, possibly interfering with the daily activities of shopping, cleaning, family visitation, and charitable routines. With the movement of women into the work force, it will be interesting to observe the changes that will undoubtedly occur with retirement of the baby boomers (Honig, 1996). It is anticipated that women will manage better psychologically because of their continued familial involvement even while working. The downside is that the rate of poverty among older retired women is extremely high if they are divorced, widowed, black, or Hispanic (Honig, 1996).

Widowhood

The experience of aging is very different in American society for men and women (Moody, 1998). Of significance is the fact that while women's average life expectancy is several years greater than men's, many women tend to marry older men. Therefore, it is women who are most likely to be widowed and remain alone in their later years (Moody, 1998; Wortman & Silver, 1990).

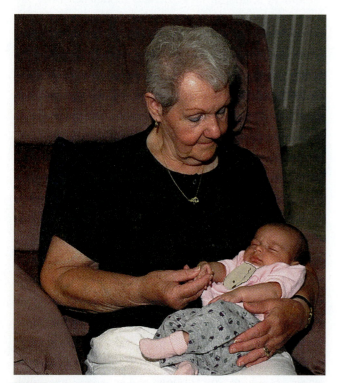

FIGURE 7-6 Volunteering at a child care center provides a sense of purpose for this woman.

Among older Americans under age 75 only half of the women are married and living with a spouse, whereas more than three-fourths of the men are married (Moody, 1998). When comparing the 75 and older age groups, the number of widowed women soar to over four-fifths, and it is women that tend to remain alone the rest of their lives (Atchley, 1997; Moody, 1998; Pickard, 1995; Wortman & Silver, 1990).

Recent literature tends to be insufficient in the area of widowhood (Wells & Kendig, 1997). The recent research that has occurred has been focused on comparing the hardships of widowers and widows, only to discover that both sexes experience difficulties equally in different ways (Johnson & Barer, 1997; Pickard, 1995).

Think About It

Dear Ann Landers:

My husband was diagnosed with Lou Gehrig's disease (amyotrophic lateral sclerosis) at the age of 56. Within 18 months, he was a quadriplegic and on a ventilator. He continued to fight for the best quality of life he could have and managed to live on another 6 years. I cared for him at home.

We never had the chance to enjoy his retirement years. How I would love to have had him follow me around the kitchen, getting in my way, lifting the lids on the pots to see what's for dinner. It would be wonderful if he would rearrange my cupboards and tag along when I go to the supermarket. Women who are lucky enough to still have their husbands should get inventive and find interests and hobbies for the guy. They should also count their blessings and stop complaining. Sign me—Lonely Nights in Washington.

Source: Landers, A. (1998, May 30). Women lucky to have hubby underfoot, widows say. Dallas Morning News, p. C2. Used with permission.

Of special interest is the transition from the spousal caregiver role to that of widowhood. The most stressful life event cited by researchers is that of widowhood (Bradsher, Longino, Jackson, & Zimmerman, 1992; Muller, 1992). However, the aspect of caring for a spouse is also very stressful for different reasons (Wells & Kendig, 1997). Caregiving limits and drains the spouse both physically and mentally to the point that widowhood may actually symbolize freedom from severe constraints (Aldersberg & Thorne, 1990; Johnson & Barer, 1997; Muller, 1992). The majority of previous widowhood research among older adults has centered on women experiencing the death of their husband (Johnson & Barer, 1997). This situation is because of the greater numbers of women in that age group. In terms of bereavement, the significance of the death of a spouse is only rivaled by the death of a mother or a child (Pickard, 1995; Muller, 1992). The most frequent conclusion to spousal caregiving is institutionalization, followed by widowhood (Wells & Kendig, 1997; Johnson & Barer, 1997).

A study of health effects on recently widowed persons resulted in findings that survivors demonstrated poorer appetites, increased smoking, more frequent use of hypnotic drugs, boredom, depression, and loneliness (Wells & Kendig, 1997). These findings were not surprising; however, the researchers were comparing the transition from spousal caregiving to widowhood. It has been a common assumption for many years that widows are susceptible to decreased health status, increased depression, and addictions to both prescribed and easily available habit-forming substances. For some, the combination of major caregiving duties suddenly ending and the loss of the spouse can overwhelm the displaced caregiver (Bradsher et al., 1992). Decreased health compounded by the loss of a spouse can increase an older widow's need to move in with family or into an institution (Bradsher et al., 1992; Johnson & Barer, 1997).

CLINICAL ALERT

Be alert to signs and symptoms of depression and suicidal thoughts in older adults who have been widowed in the previous 1–2 years.

Think About It

Being aware of the severe emotional difficulties of widowhood, what can be done to successfully negotiate through the issues of bereavement in later life?

Many health care professionals regard intense grief as a process that individuals must go through to successfully master bereavement and accept the reality of their loss (Eliopoulos, 1993; Wortman & Silver, 1990). The initial period of loss is the time when the surviving spouse is emotionally weakest and has unreasonably high-cost funeral services (Eliopoulos, 1993). It is actually after the intenseness of the funeral and during the first year after the death of a spouse that health care professionals need to be available to the widowed. This time period is ripe for severe depression and decreased health status (Eliopoulos, 1993; Wells & Kendig, 1997; Wortman & Silver, 1990).

Several means exist to assist widows and widowers through the intense grief period immediately after loss, including familial support, awareness of health care professionals, widowhood support groups, clergy visitation, and social services. If the family had **hospice** services in place prior to the death of the spouse, support services are included for one year after the death has occurred. After the loss of a spouse, it is especially important for health care professionals to monitor the health status of the recently widowed older adult (Figure 7-7). It is during this period of intense grief that the widowed spouse may ignore self-care activities, become malnourished, not take medications appropriately, refuse social interactions, or indulge in substance abuse.

Are there noticeable differences in how older men face widowhood? One large difference is that widowers seldom exist past the age of 75 (Atchley, 1997; Johnson & Barer, 1997; Moody, 1998). The consequence of widowhood on older males has much to do with how the marriage was perceived, the amount of outside activity, and familial and social support (Atchley, 1997). The same factors influence the widowhood role for older females. One very interesting difference in the gender approach to widowhood is that older men are often encouraged to remarry, while many older women are not given the opportunity for remarriage simply because of their increased numbers in the population (Atchley, 1997; Johnson, & Barer, 1997). The loss of intimacy with a partner after many years can impact one's life and health. Being physically and psychologically close to someone is an important part of self-concept and self-esteem, so widowhood after a long marriage can greatly affect one's self-image.

Health has been hypothesized to be linked to social factors such as stress, demographics, social integration, and social support (George, 1996). The loss of a spouse

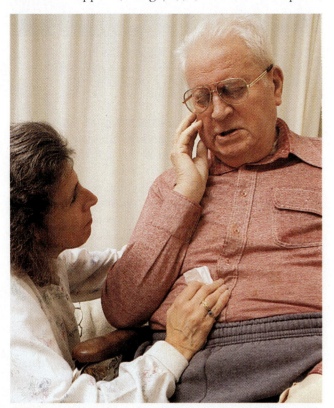

FIGURE 7-7   Recently widowed older adults may need assistance managing their emotions during the acute phases of grief.

and entering into widowhood is generally perceived as a serious life event and classified as severe social stress that affects the health of the widowed individual. It has been reported that older male widowers had more problems with household management after the loss of a wife, while older female widows had increased financial burdens (Atchley, 1997; George, 1996; Moody, 1998). In either case, the health of the widowed spouse potentially decreases, calling for the awareness of health care workers to remain available for health support.

Spirituality

People grow old within a social context. A systems model that is used to develop holistic services in the health care field includes the biological, psychological, and interpersonal. Koenig (1995) suggested adding spirituality to the model to make it a more complete response to health issues of older adults. The biopsychosocial-spiritual model of health states there is a spiritual dimension of the human experience that both interrelates and influences the health of older adults.

Background

The study of spirituality by social gerontologists has a relatively brief history. In a review of past research efforts in spirituality and aging, Barbara Payne (1990, 1995) presented a historical perspective that suggested focus has shifted from religiosity to **spiritual well-being** to spirituality. Spirituality as a concept has a multidisciplinary approach. Interest began to grow in the 1940s along with the awareness of increasing life expectancy. Research interests were focused on the influence of organized religion and the older adult. Researchers generally thought the study of religion in the lives of older adults contributed little to an understanding of the aging process. Little work in spirituality and aging was done prior to the 1970s. That which was done gave more attention to themes of religious activity within organized groups. Interestingly, an effort to avoid the issue of separation of church and state led to the religious section of the 1971 White House Conference on Aging being labeled spiritual well-being. This effort to avoid conflict had an important effect. It brought together those who were interested in the study of religious aspects of spiritual well-being and those who were interested in the study of mental health or psychological well-being.

The background paper that David Moberg (1971) developed for the 1971 White House Conference on Aging created the groundwork for a conceptualization of spirituality. He identified six areas of **spiritual need** as deserving special attention by researchers: (a) sociocultural sources of spiritual need, (b) relief from anxieties and fears, (c) preparation for death, (d) personality integration, (e) personal dignity, and (f) a philosophy of life. While scholars have not reached a consensus regarding spirituality and aging, these six areas of spiritual need have become a focus for research.

Spiritual Well-Being

Another important outcome related to the efforts of 1971 was the institution of the National Interfaith Coalition on Aging (NICA). This ecumenical coalition adapted a definition of spiritual well-being reflecting the views of Roman Catholic, Eastern Orthodox, Jewish, and Protestant religious leaders associated with the NICA. Spiritual well-being is the affirmation of life in a relationship with a God, self, community, and environment that nurtures and celebrates wholeness (National Interfaith, 1975).

Spiritual well-being is a developmental task that must be achieved during the journey of aging. While gerontologists believe spiritual well-being is important, the difficulty in defining conceptual components has produced a lack of literature. Writers on the topic have referenced the work of Dan Blazer (1991) to identify the components that construct spiritual well-being as a developmental concept. He suggested six dimensions of spiritual well-being: (a) self-determined wisdom, by which people know how to influence their environment without upsetting its balance; (b) self-transcendence, by which they cross beyond the boundary of the self being touched by physical and emotional losses; (c) meaning achieved by an understanding of life; (d) accepting the totality of one's life without regret; (e) revival of spirituality through which they become advocates for others; and (f) exit and existence, by which they accept death as a part of human existence.

Similar descriptions for spirituality are included in a review of nursing literature by Martsolf and Mickley (1998). The purpose of their review is to present modern nurse theorists' ideas on spirituality. Five attributes conceptualizing spirituality in nursing theories include (a) meaning derived from purpose in existence; (b) values having to do with truth, beauty, and worth of thought; (c) transcendence through appreciation of dimensions beyond the self; (d) connecting relationships with self, others, God/higher power, and the environment; and (e) becoming through experiencing life and knowing who one is.

Spiritual Activity

What comes clearly into focus from the above-mentioned concepts is that each dimension can be described as an outcome of a working process or mental reflective action on the part of the older adult (Figure 7-8). Each dimension or attribute holds to be an objective reached through

spiritual activity. According to the above conceptualizations, older adults engage in spiritual activities that may not be connected to an organized religious institution or group. Heriot (1992) suggested that spirituality is a broader notion than religion, providing an umbrella concept under which one finds religion and the needs of the human spirit. The dimensions of spirituality are applicable to older adults who are religious, nonreligious, or antireligious (Forbes, 1994). Dyson, Cobb, and Forman (1997) reviewed health-care-related material on the topic of spirituality and nursing. The authors reported an emerging paradigm in the study of spirituality. The new perspective is one that takes a broader view than Judeo-Christian tradition of western society. The literature review indicated an emerging theme in the centrality of the relationship between self, others, and God. The relationship with the self has to do with the strengthening of inner resources. The relationship with others suggests spiritual growth arises in the context of community. Community also involves the importance of giving and receiving love, forgiveness, trust, touch, and commitment within an interdependent relationship. The nature of God is suggested to take many forms according to the individual's highest value in life.

Because the emerging paradigm of spirituality is held as a broader concept providing an umbrella under which religion is found (Heriot, 1992), the assertion is made that religious activity may be a part of one's spirituality and have powerful implications for health (Mickley, Carson, and Soeken, 1995). Religious activity and beliefs are more important to those over the age of 50 (Princeton Religious Research Center, 1993).

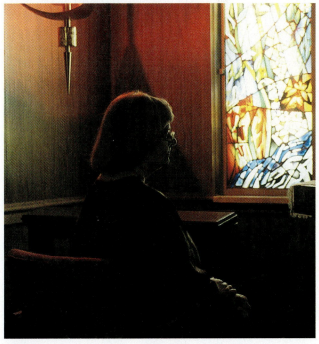

FIGURE 7-8 Spirituality is a working process for the older adult.

Atchley (1995) suggested that people focus religious activity and spirituality differently. Some maintain an inner **continuity focus** on the aspects of spirituality. For these individuals, spirituality is more intellectual. In contrast, others hold an external continuity focus on spirituality. External continuity individuals focus on activities related to geographic location, external aspects of worship, ceremony, music, and religious symbols. One might expect different reactions to late-life losses and challenges depending on the focus. Older people who hold an external continuity may be more troubled when faced with the challenge of not being able to participate with a particular religious congregation.

The spiritual activity of an older individual may involve activity unrelated to organized religious ceremony. Listening to music from the period of life when the older adult fell in love could produce a focus on the client's journey through life with a mate. The mate may have died long before. Story telling may be a form of spiritual life review connecting past events or social roles within the context of the present community members. For Bianchi (1995), the very telling of a story, especially expressing self-vulnerability, represents a spiritual act and a quest for personal meaning. An older resident in a nursing facility who occasionally chooses to sit alone in her room instead of participating in a group activity may be actively reflecting on the meaning of her life. For her, the re-creation of self may be more valuable than the creation of crocheted napkins. Knitting memories together into a beautiful tapestry of life may be a more important activity than weaving potholders. Viewing a rainbow or watching the sunrise maybe a spiritual activity resulting in a deeper relationship with God. Dyson et al. (1997) reviewed literature that indicates happiness, crying, and other expressions of caring within relationships may be spiritual activities expressing connections with oneself, others, and God. Heriot (1992) made a strong point that aging changes are known to affect the body and the mind, but there is no evidence that the spirit succumbs to debilitating physical and mental illness.

Spirituality and Caregiving

How then is the caregiver to respond with help for older adults? Helpful and appropriate response begins with understanding. Aging has long been viewed as a **spiritual journey** on which the sojourner encounters unique spiritual challenges (Bianchi, 1982; Berggren-Thomas & Griggs, 1995). Biological changes, social stereotyping, loss of social bonds, and loss of autonomy are only a few of the obstacles encountered on the journey. Negative stereotypes believed by society, older adults in-

cluded, influence self-concept. Loss of friends and relatives to death produces loss of companionship and introduces an uncertain future. Older survivors may be forced to learn new tasks that were performed previously by a spouse. Reduced income and relocation to different housing arrangements present unique obstacles. Death is one of the greatest spiritual challenges that must be confronted in late life. Impending death may bring other spiritual challenges such as perceived need of forgiveness both for and from others. Death also presses older adults to review their life as it was lived while admitting their journey is about to end (Berggren-Thomas & Griggs, 1995).

Health care professionals may respond to the spiritual needs and concerns of the older adult who is dying. For Missinne (1990), the process of dying is a stage of human development that includes spiritual needs that must receive attention. He gives practical suggestions for providing this attention. It is important to create an atmosphere where people can talk openly about spiritual concerns. The older adult must be able to express beliefs to the caregiver. Because religious ceremony and beliefs do not encompass spirituality, music, poems, art, or flowers may assist the dying in meeting spiritual needs. Older patients may need assistance in making peace with others or even themselves. An unexpected outcome may be a benefit to the caregiver. Health care professionals may experience insight into their own personal spiritual journey as they assist the aging sojourner.

Spiritual Assessment

Health care professionals and researchers who view spiritual well-being as important to the care of older adults have developed assessment instruments to measure components of spirituality. The nursing literature suggests spiritual care is part of the nursing role and that it should be part of nurse education (Ross, 1996). Leetun (1996) suggested a wellness spirituality protocol for assessment and intervention. The protocol includes (a) a clinical presentation of possible responses to illness that challenge the older client; (b) diagnosis and evaluation of the client's spiritual activities; and (c) suggestions for management approaches to support activities that reflect spiritual well-being. Williams (1994) reviewed several epidemiological approaches to measuring religion. He also related the strengths and weaknesses of several instruments used to measure spiritual well-being. Some of the characteristics measured by the scales include relationship with God, relationship with others, purpose in life, direction, satisfaction in life, and perception of being loved by God. A widely used scale is the Spiritual

Well-Being Scale (SWBS; Ellison & Smith, 1991). The SWBS is shown to correlate with a broad range of health status indicators as well as indicators of general well-being, church attendance, and other measures of religious involvement (Ellison & Smith, 1991).

Knowing how central spirituality has been over the life span of a person can give important clues for understanding how specific late-life changes may affect that older adult. To understand how spirituality is integrated into the ideas and behavior of older adults, one must first know how spiritual themes fit for the person in the past. If spiritual identity and religious behavior have been a central theme for the person at a younger age, then one would expect this emphasis to continue (Atchely, 1995).

Caregiving roles require health care individuals to walk alongside older adults as they face unique challenges and crises in their spiritual journey. Insight and perception are required to make connections between the spiritual work in which older adults are engaged and the challenge or obstacle that confronts them.

Summary

Matilda and John Riley have argued that the United States is experiencing a structural lag because of a mismatch between what older adults want to do and are capable of doing and the structural opportunities available to them. This lag is caused by (a) an increase in the life expectancy of older adults that has produced increases in the numbers and proportion of the old and older old in society and (b) an increase in the healthy functioning of older adults. Thus there is pressure for the United States to move from an age-segregated society to a more age-integrated society where people of all ages have greater flexibility to move in and out of social roles in education, work, family, and leisure throughout the life cycle. Foner (1994) discussed the three major mechanisms for creating this change—policy changes, cohort norm formation, and age conflicts among people in different age stages. Foner (1994) also argued that there are powerful barriers to change in the social structure, making sweeping change unlikely. These obstacles include economic conditions, social and economic costs of change, institutional inertia, and threats to basic social values.

Older adults are not a homogeneous group. Life circumstances differ dramatically for groups of older adults, based on their race, ethnicity, social class, and gender. The numbers and proportions of minority elders are increasing at faster rates than those of whites. By the middle of the twenty-first century, one-third of older adults will be members of racial and ethnic minority groups. Older minorities are more likely than older whites to live in poverty or near poverty, less likely to receive private pensions, and more likely to receive benefits from public assistance programs. Older minorities have less education than older whites, which limits income throughout the life cycle, and are more likely to have difficulty reading, writing, and communicating in English. Older African Americans and Native Americans have much poorer health than older whites. It is a common misperception that older minority adults do not use as many social services as older whites because they have extended families that provide for their need. While African American and Hispanic elders do receive support from their families, this support is often not adequate to meet their needs and is by no means the norm, any more than it is for whites. Among Native Americans, living in extended families is most often because of financial necessity, and the older Native American may often be the only family member with a stable source of income because of high rates of unemployment on reservations.

As people age, they are likely to experience a decrease in the prestige, status, influence, and wealth of the roles they occupy. Examples of roles that older adults are likely to experience in old age include grandparent, retiree, volunteer, caregiver, widow(er), disabled person, patient, and long-term care resident. Because women have longer life expectancies than men, and also have higher rates of morbidity, they are more likely to experience these roles and to be in these roles longer.

Grandparenthood is generally seen as a positive role, but the age at which the role occurs and the expectations associated with it vary with race/ethnicity, social class, and gender. Retirement is also a role that many older adults look forward to with anticipation but may find stressful once they have entered the role. Widowhood is a stressful role for both men and women, although women are more likely to be widowed and are less likely to remarry. Older adults who are widowed are at greater risk for depression, suicidal ideation, morbidity, and substance abuse (including alcohol).

Since the 1970s there has been an increased interest in spirituality and aging that brings together those who are interested in the religious aspects of spiritual well-being and those interested in mental health and psychological well-being. Spiritual needs that are receiving research attention are sociocultural sources of spiritual need, relief from anxiety and fear, preparation for death, personality integration, personal dignity, and a philosophy of life.

Review Questions and Activities

1. One participates in many social roles throughout the life span. Historically, older adults have been retirees, housewives, grandparents, widows, and residents of long-term care institutions. What are some role changes you see in the future? With women increasingly involved in the world of work, increases in volunteering and childless couples, increased divorce rates, and increases in longevity, describe social roles you anticipate will exist when you are 80 years old.

2. Grandparenthood is a phenomenon of recent decades. Another recent phenomenon is increased number of grandparents raising grandchildren. Several reasons have caused this occurrence, such as financial instability, substance abuse, and familial instability. Grandparents are feeling pressed to continue working to support and raise their grandchildren at a time in their lives when they were anticipating retirement, relaxation, and family visitation. What are some alternatives to grandparents raising families all over again? Or, is this an acceptable arrangement because they obviously did not raise their own child right, so now they are obligated to raise the grandchildren? What are some solutions to lighten the load of caregiving for grandparents?

3. Since the introduction of the Social Security Act in 1935, Americans have come to believe in paid retirement as a right. Write a brief letter to your congressperson presenting your ideas and suggestions for solving the retirement dilemma, considering both the pros and cons of keeping older adults in the work force longer. Be very scholarly in your approach and consider carefully how future legislation will affect you when you consider retirement.

4. In the section on widowhood, the subject of suicide was briefly mentioned. Think about an older couple age 80. The wife has a terminal illness and wishes to commit suicide "when the time is right." Without coercion, the husband wishes to commit suicide along with his wife, stating "we've been together all our lives, we will not be separated now." Both appear to be healthy at the moment and mentally alert. You are an only child of this couple and cannot believe they are considering such an act. Going against their wishes, you contact a psychiatrist and an attorney, who determine the couple to be in rational control of the situation. In the meantime, the city has been contacted about the poor state of the house and yard. Regardless of the psychiatrist and attorney, the city public health officials begin to intervene. You determine, after all, that it is your parents' right to live eccentrically, but the issue has been taken out of your hands now by the city public health officials. What would you do? If the couple are not permitted to end their lives at a time of their choosing, their house will be taken, finances seized, and in all likelihood they will be placed in a long-term care institution "for their own good." This is exactly what they were trying to avoid. What insights or suggestions do you have?

5. What are five dimensions of spiritual well-being?

6. How can wanting to be alone be explained as a health spiritual activity?

7. What is meant by aging as a spiritual journey?

8. What are the spiritual needs of older adults?

9. Apply the concept of spiritual focus to an older adult who is unable to leave home and attend public religious activities.

References

Aldersberg, M., & Thorne, S. (1990). Emerging from the chrysalis: Older widows in transition. *Journal of Gerontological Nursing, 16*(1), 4–8.

Allen, K. M., & Phillips, J. M. (1997). *Women's health across the lifespan: A comprehensive perspective.* Philadelphia: Lippincott.

A profile of older Americans: 1999. (1999). Washington, DC: American Association of Retired Persons and Administration on Aging, the Department of Health and Human Services.

Arendell, T., & Estes, C. L. (1994). Older women in the post-Reagan era. In E. Fee & N. Krieger (Eds.), *Women's health, politics, and power: Essays on sex/gender, medicine, and public health* (pp. 333–349). Amityville, NY: Baywood.

Aschenbrenner J. (1973). Extended black families in America. *Journal of Comparative Family Studies, 4,* 250–268.

Aschenbrenner, J. (1975). *Lifelines: Black families in Chicago.* New York: Holt, Reinhart, and Winston.

Atchley, R. C. (1995). The continuity of the spiritual self. In M. A. Kimble, S. H. McFadden, J. W. Ellor, & J. J. Seeber (Eds.), *Aging, spirituality, and religion* (pp. 68–73). Minneapolis: Fortress Press.

Atchley, R. C. (1997). *Social forces and aging* (8th ed.). Belmont, CA: Wadsworth.

Atta, D. V. (1998). *Trust betrayed: Inside the AARP.* Washington, DC: Regenery.

Bengston, V., Rosenthal, C., & Burton, L. (1996). Paradoxes of families and aging. In R. H. Binstock & L. K. George (Eds.), *Handbook of aging and the social sciences* (4th ed., pp. 253–282). San Diego, CA: Academic Press.

Berggren-Thomas, P., & Griggs, M. J. (1995). Spirituality in aging: Spiritual need or spiritual journey. *Journal of Gerontological Nursing, 21*(3), 5–9.

Bianchi, E. (1982). *Aging as a spiritual journey.* New York: Crossroad.

Bianchi, E. (1995). A catalyst for crafting elderhood. *Aging and Spirituality, 7*(2), 1–3.

Blazer, D. G. (1991). Spirituality and aging well. *Generations, 15*(1), 61–65.

Bradsher, J. E., Longino, C. F., Jackson, D. L., & Zimmerman, R. S. (1992). Health and geographic mobility among the recently widowed. *Journal of Gerontology: Social Sciences, 47*(5), S261–S268.

Burton, L. M. (1992). Black grandparents rearing children of drug-addicted parents: Stressors, outcomes, and social service needs. *Gerontologist, 32*(6), 744–751.

Carlson, J. E., Junk, V. W., Fox, L. K., Rudzitis, G., & Cann, S. E. (1998). Factors affecting retirement migration to Idaho: An adaptation of the Amenity Retirement Migration Model. *Gerontologist, 38*(1), 18–24.

Caro, F. G., & Bass, S. A. (1997). Receptivity to volunteering in the immediate postretirement period. *Journal of Applied Gerontology, 16*(4), 427–444.

Chatters, L., & Taylor, R. J. (1986). Intergenerational support: The provision of assistance to parents by adult children. In J. S. Jackson, L. M. Chatters, & R. J. Taylor (Eds.), *Aging in Black America.* Newbury Park: Sage.

Chen, Y-P. (1994). Improving the economic security of minority persons as they enter old age. In *Minority elders: Five goals toward building a public policy base* (2nd ed.). Washington, DC: Gerontological Society of America.

Cherlin, A. J., & Furstenberg, F. F. (1997). The modernization of grandparenthood. In A. S. Skolnick & J. H. Skolnick (Eds.), *Family in transition* (9th ed., pp. 419–425). New York: Longman.

Couch, K. A. (1998). Late life job displacement. *Gerontologist, 38*(1), 7–17.

Crown, W. H. (1998). Social Security and employment policy: Retirement incentives and disincentives [Review of the book *Social Security in the 21st century*]. *Gerontologist, 38*(1), 132–135.

Dietz, T. (1995). Patterns of intergenerational assistance within the Mexican American family: Is the family taking care of the older generations' needs? *Journal of Family Issues, 16*(3), 344–356.

Dowdell, E. B. (1995). Caregiver burden: Grandparents raising their high-risk children. *Journal of Psychosocial Nursing, 33*(3), 27–30.

Dressel, P. L., & Barnhill, S. K. (1994). Reframing gerontological thought and practice: The case of grandmothers with daughters in prison. *Gerontologist, 34*(5), 685–690.

Dyson, C., Cobb, M., & Forman, D. (1997). The meaning of spirituality: A literature review. *Journal of Advanced Nursing, 26*(6), 1183–1188.

Eliopoulos, C. (1993). *Gerontological nursing* (3rd ed.). Philadelphia: Lippincott.

Ellison, C. W., & Smith, J. (1991). Toward an integrative measure of health and well-being. *Journal of Psychology and Theology, 19*(1), 35–48.

Foner, A. (1994). Endnote: The reach of an idea. In M.W. Riley, R.L. Kahn, & A. Foner (Eds.), *Age and structural lag: Society's failure to provide meaningful opportunities in work, family and leisure.* New York: Wiley.

Forbes, E. J. (1994). Spirituality, aging, and the community-dwelling caregiver and care recipient. *Geriatric Nursing, 5*(6), 297–302.

Fuller-Thomson, E., Minkler, M., & Driver, D. (1997). A profile of grandparents raising grandchildren in the United States. *Gerontologist, 37*(3), 406–411.

Gardner, J. M. (1995). Worker displacement: A decade of change. *Monthly Labor Review, 118*(4), 45–57.

George, L. K. (1996). Social factors and illness. In R. H. Binstock & L. K. George (Eds.), *Handbook of aging and the social sciences* (4th ed., pp. 229–252). San Diego, CA: Academic Press.

Gutmann, D. (1987). *Reclaimed powers.* New York: Basic Books.

Haas, W. H., & Serow, W. J. (1993). Amenity retirement migration process: A model and preliminary evidence. *Gerontologist, 33*(2), 212–220.

Hayward, M. D., Frieman, S., & Chen, H. (1998). Career trajectories and older men's retirement. *Journal of Gerontology: Social Sciences, 53B*(2), S91–S103.

Henretta, J. C. (1994). Social structure and age-based careers. In M.W. Riley, R.L. Kahn, & A. Foner (Eds.), *Age and structural lag: Society's failure to provide meaningful opportunities in work, family and leisure.* New York: Wiley.

Heriot, C. S. (1992). Spirituality and aging. *Holistic Nursing Practice, 7*(1), 22–31.

Honig, M. (1996). Retirement expectations: Differences by race, ethnicity and gender. *Gerontologist, 36*(3), 373–382.

Ingersoll-Dayton, B., Morgan, D., & Antonucci, T. (1997). The effects of positive and negative social exchanges on aging adults. *Journal of Gerontology: Social Sciences, 52B*(4), S190–S199.

Jacobs, R. H. (1993). Expanding social roles for older women. In J. Allen & A. Pifer (Eds.), *Women on the front lines: Meeting the challenge of an aging America* (pp. 191–219). Washington, DC: The Urban Institute.

Jendrek, M. P. (1994). Grandparents who parent their grandchildren: Circumstances and decisions. *Gerontologist, 34*(2), 206–216.

John, R. (1994). The state of research on American elders' health, income security, and social support networks. In *Minority elders: Five goals toward building a public policy base* (2nd ed.). Washington, DC: The Gerontological Society of America.

Johnson, C. L., & Barer, B. M. (1997). *Life beyond 85 years: The aura of survivorship.* New York: Springer.

Kahn, R. L. (1994). Opportunities, aspirations and goodness of fit. In M.W. Riley, R.L. Kahn, & A. Foner (Eds.), *Age and structural lag: Society's failure to provide meaningful opportunities in work, family and leisure.* New York: Wiley.

Kaiser, M. A., Gibbons, J.E., & Camp, J. J. (1993). Long-term care: Development of services for Latino elderly. In M. Sotomayor & A. Garcia (Eds.), *Elderly Latinos: Issues and solutions for the 21st century.* Washington, DC: National Hispanic Council on Aging.

Kelley, S. J., Yorker, B. C., & Whitley, D. (1997). To grandmother's house we go . . . and stay: Children raised in intergenerational families. *Journal of Gerontological Nursing, 23*(9), 13–20.

Koenig, H. G. (1995). Religion and health in later life. In M. A. Kimble, S. H. McFadden, J.W. Ellor, & J. J. Seeber (Eds.), *Aging, spirituality, and religion* (pp. 8–29). Minneapolis: Fortress Press.

Land, K., Guralnik, C., & Blazer D.G. (1994). Estimating increment-decrement life tables with multiple covariates from panel data: The case of active life expectancy. *Demography, 31*(2), 297–319.

Landers, A. (1998, May 30). Women lucky to have hubbies underfoot, widows say. *Dallas Morning News,* p. C2.

Leetun, M. C. (1996). Wellness spirituality in the older adult: Assessment and intervention protocol. *Nurse Practitioner, 21*(8), 60–70.

Lubben, J. E., & Becerra, R. M. (1987). Social support among Black, Mexican and Chinese elderly. In D. E. Gelfand & C. M. Barresi (Eds.), *Ethnic dimensions of aging.* New York: Springer.

Lynott, P. P., & Roberts, R. E. L. (1997). The developmental stake hypothesis and changing perceptions of intergenerational relations, 1971–1985. *Gerontologist, 37*(3), 394–405.

Maldonado, D. (1989). The Latino elderly living alone: The invisible poor. *California Sociology, 2*(1), 8–21.

Manson, S. M. (1988). Provider assumptions about long-term care in American Indian communities. *Gerontologist, 29,* 355–358.

Martin, E. M., & Martin, J. M. (1978). *The Black extended family.* Chicago: University of Chicago.

Martsolf, D. S., & Mickley, J. R. (1998). The concept of spirituality in nursing theories: Differing world-views and extent of focus. *Journal of Advanced Nursing, 27*(2), 294–303.

Mickley, J. R., Carson, V., & Soeken, K. L. (1995). Religion and adult mental health: State of the science in nursing. *Issues in Mental Health Nursing, 6*(4), 345–360.

Minkler, M., Roe, K. M. & Price, M. (1992). The physical and emotional health of grandmothers raising grandchildren in the crack cocaine epidemic. *Gerontologist, 32*(6), 752–761.

Missinne, L. E. (1990). Death and spiritual concerns of older adults. *Generations, 14*(4), 45–47.

Moberg, D. O. (1971). *Spiritual well-being.* Washington, DC: White House Conference on Aging.

Moen, P. (1996). Gender, age, and the life course. In R. H. Binstock & L. K. George (Eds.), *Handbook of aging and the social sciences* (4th ed., pp. 171–187). San Diego, CA: Academic Press.

Moody, H. R. (1998). *Aging: Concepts and controversies* (2nd ed.). Thousand Oaks, CA: Pine Forge Press.

Muller, J. T. (1992). The bereaved caregiver: A prospective study of changes in well-being. *Gerontologist, 32*(5), 673–683.

National Center for Health Statistics. (1995). *Health United States, 1994.* Hyattsville, MD: Public Health Service.

National Interfaith Coalition on Aging. (1975). Spiritual well-being definition: A model of ecumenical work product. NICA Inform 1 (August 25), 4.

Payne, B. P. (1990). Research and theoretical approaches to spirituality and aging. *Generation, 14* (4), 11–14.

Payne, B. P. (1995). The interdisciplinary study of gerontology. In M. A. Kimble, S. H. McFadden, J. W. Ellor, & J. J. Seeber (Eds.), *Aging, spirituality, and religion* (pp. 558–567). Minneapolis: Fortress Press.

Pearson, J. L., Hunter, A. G., Cook, J. M., Ialongo, N. S., & Kellam, S. G. (1997). Grandmother involvement in child caregiving in an urban community. *Gerontologist, 37*(5), 650–657.

Pickard, S. (1995). *Living on the front line; a social anthropological study of old age and aging.* Aldershot, England: Avebury.

Princeton Religious Research Center. (1993). *Religion in America,* Princeton, NJ: Gallup Poll.

Riley, M. W. (1978). Aging, social change and the power of ideas. *Daedalus, 107,* 39–52.

Riley, M. W., & Riley, J. W., Jr. (1994). Structural lag: Past and future. In M. W. Riley, R. L. Kahn, & A. Foner (Eds.), *Age and structural lag: Society's failure to provide meaningful opportunities in work, family and leisure.* New York: Wiley.

Riley, M. W., Johnson, M., & Foner, A. (1972). *Aging and society: Vol. III. A sociology of age stratification.* New York: Russell Sage.

Robbins, D. A. (1996). *Ethical and legal issues in home health and long-term care: Challenges and solutions.* Gaithersburg, MD: Aspen.

Rook, K. S. (1997). Positive and negative social exchanges: Weighing their effects in later life. *Journal of Gerontology: Social Sciences, 52B*(4), S167–S169.

Rosenthal, C. (1986). Family supports in later life. Does ethnicity make a difference? *Gerontologist, 26,* 19–24.

Ross, L. A. (1996). Teaching spiritual care to nurses. *Nurse Education Today, 16*(1), 38–43.

Shanas, E. (1979). *National survey of the elderly.* Washington, DC: Department of Health and Human Services. Administration on Aging.

Stack, C. B. (1972). Black kindreds: Parenthood and personal kindreds among urban Blacks. *Journal of Comparative Family Studies, 3,* 194–206.

Stack, C. B. (1974). *All our kin.* New York: Harper & Row.

Starett, R. A., Mindel, C. H., & Wright, R. (1983). Influence of support systems on the use of social services by the Hispanic elderly. *Social Work Research and Abstracts, 19*(4), 34–30.

Strawbridge, W. J., Wallhagen, M. I., Shema, S. J., & Kaplan, G. A. (1997). New burdens or more of the same? Comparing grandparent, spouse, and adult-child caregivers. *Gerontologist, 37*(4), 505–510.

Szinovacz, M. E. (1998). Grandparents today: A demographic profile. *Gerontologist, 38*(1), 37–52.

Taeuber, C. M., & Allen, J. (1993). Women in our aging society: The demographic outlook. In J. Allen & A. Pifer (Eds.), *Women on the front lines: Meeting the challenge of an aging America* (pp. 11–45). Washington, DC: The Urban Institute.

Torrez, D. J. (1998). Health and social service utilization patterns of Mexican American older adults. *Journal of Aging Studies, 12*(1), 83–99.

U.S. Bureau of the Census. (1995, May). *Sixty-five plus in the United States. Statistical brief.* U.S. Department of Commerce.

U.S. Bureau of the Census. (1996). *Current Population Reports, Special Studies, 65+ in the United States* (pp. 23–190). Washington, DC: U.S. Government Printing Office.

Wells, Y. D., & Kendig, H. L. (1997). Health and well-being of spouse caregivers and the widowed. *Gerontologist, 37*(5), 666–674.

Williams D. R. (1994). The measurement of religion in epidemiologic studies: Problems and prospects. In J. S. Levin (Ed.), *Religion in aging and health* (pp. 125–148). Thousand Oaks: Sage.

Williams, N. (1990). *The Mexican American family: Tradition and change.* Dix Hills, NY: General Hall.

Wilson, W. J. (1987). *The truly disadvantaged.* Chicago, IL: University of Chicago Press. Cited in Henretta, J. C. Social structure and age-based careers. In M.W. Riley,

R.L. Kahn, & A. Foner (Eds.), *Age and structural lag: Society's failure to provide meaningful opportunities in work, family and leisure*. New York: Wiley.

Wortman, C. B., & Silver, R. C. (1990). Successful mastery of bereavement and widowhood: A life-course perspective. In P. B. Baltes & M. M. Baltes (Eds.), *Successful aging: Perspectives from the* *behavioral sciences* (pp. 225–264). New York: Cambridge University Press.

Yee, D. (1997). Issues and trends affecting Asian Americans, women and aging. In J. M. Coyle (Ed.), *Hand book on women and aging*. Westport, CT: Greenwood Press.

Resources

Institute on Aging (University of Pennsylvania): **www.upenn.edu/aging**

White River Area Agency on Aging (Aging Related Issues & Links): **www.wraaa.com**

CHAPTER 8

Successful Aging

Janis M. Fleming, PhD, RN

COMPETENCIES

After completing this chapter, the reader should be able to:

- *Discuss the essential components of successful aging.*
- *Distinguish between the characteristics of successful and unsuccessful aging.*
- *Discuss the importance of a nutritious diet for older adults.*
- *Describe a diet that promotes successful aging.*
- *Discuss the importance of support systems for older adults.*
- *Identify the ways older adults can engage in specific activities that promote healthy lifestyles.*
- *Evaluate the advantages and precautions of a regular exercise program for older adults.*

MAKING THE CONNECTION

Refer to the following chapters to increase your understanding of the successful aspects of aging:

- **Chapter 6** *Psychological Aspects of Aging*
- **Chapter 9** *Geriatric Nutrition*
- **Chapter 10** *Informal Support Systems*
- **Chapter 24** *Community Organizations and Services*

Essential Components of Successful Aging

In 1997, individuals reaching age 65 had an average life expectancy of an additional 17.6 years (*A Profile*, 1999). However, living longer does not necessarily mean **successful aging.** The far-reaching effects of good health practices and health care teaching are important for successful aging. To age successfully, healthy living and daily lifestyle activities need to be integrated to maintain optimal health. A number of authors have found that **nutrition, exercise,** and a **support system** are the most important factors for successful aging (Bender & Bender, 1997; Chandler & Halley, 1996).

Although aging occurs through a long, gentle process, the inevitable and irreversible passage of time can have certain effects on organ functions. Such changes vary with individuals, and decisions made throughout life affect how successful aging is experienced (Sugar & Marinelli, 1997). Everyone experiences the gradual physiological, psychological, and social process of aging that is universal and unidirectional from conception to death. But, successful aging requires active pursuit, effort, and continual involvement.

In a study that examined **self-help** and **help-seeking behaviors** related to depressive cognition, adaptive functioning, and life satisfactions (Zauszniewski, 1995), the author concluded that there was an association between the two strategies. Resourceful older adults maintain independence despite normal changes and losses associated with aging. Medical science has been successful in increasing the older adult's life span and is addressing ways to increase quality of life. There are gaps in the knowledge of aging, such as the physiological mechanism that promotes a continuous ongoing aging process. Successful aging is multidimensional and depends on many factors that should be considered early in life. This chapter will discuss ways to utilize the advantages of aging and minimize its drawbacks for a satisfying, enjoyable life growing old.

Most people do not consider the effects of aging until well into middle age, when physiological changes begin to become apparent. But, the best time to prepare and take action toward successful aging is during childhood, when healthy habits are formed, reinforced, and encouraged. In youth, most individuals give little thought to the process of aging or consider it so far in the future that it is something that always happens to someone else. Younger individuals find it difficult to view aging objectively and without pessimism. But, growing old can be an enriching experience. Successful aging requires an adjustment, positive attitude, planning, and work. To grow old successfully, individuals must be committed to work at the process. A design for successful aging aims toward a satisfying and productive longer life.

Older adults are the largest consumers of health care and have more interactions with **health care providers** than any other age group. Any change in their health status could affect their lifestyle, living arrangements, or ability to carry out **physical activities of daily living (PADL).** Even with preparation for advancing chronological years, there will be some physical, psychological, and social decline. A major consideration of older adults is the maintenance of independence through good health and by reducing health problems related to physical and cognitive decline that result in dramatic changes in their life. Successful aging transcends race, class, and ethnic issues and instead places the responsibility on each individual.

Studies have shown that older adults generally consider themselves to be well as long as they can carry out activities of daily living even when they have multiple **chronic health problems** (Allison & Keller, 1997). As a collective group, older adults usually do not dwell on their health as long as they are mobile. Restricted mobility affects all aspects of a client's life and leads to rapid deterioration of health status.

Aging occurs within a biological context and is affected by individual environmental and social circumstances. Identifying a single factor or factors that relate to successful aging is difficult. Genetic background plays an important part in the make-up of individuals and longevity. However, three things that are within the control of older adults that impact significantly on successful aging are nutrition, exercise, and a support system (significant others).

Biological and psychological changes do occur as an individual ages. However, extensive deterioration of cognitive functioning does not normally occur as an individual ages. Physiological and sociological changes may mediate the changes experienced by older adults and affect the changes observed. Such factors as nutrition, health, emotions, environment, educational level, and culture play a role in cognitive functioning.

Think About It

How can health care providers best promote the three successful components of aging?

Nutrition

Practicing good health habits is one of the best approaches to successful aging. Good nutritional habits are prerequisite for maintaining and promoting optimal health. Although changing a diet to be more nutritious may not alter the aging process, it can help older adults stay healthy longer. As with any age, nutrition is fundamental to healthy and successful aging for older adults. The essential nutritional requirements for older adults are the same as any age group except that the calorie intake diminishes because of a decrease in lean body mass as aging occurs (Phillips, Cassmeyer, Sands, & Lehman, 1995). Older adults are subject to the possibility of developing malnutrition or vitamin deficiency because of normal age-related changes such as gastrointestinal changes; reduction in taste, vision, smell, dentition, and financial resources; and the psychological impact of loneliness on eating. Eating with others can improve appetite (Figure 8-1).

Aging and stress impact on the biochemical defenses that cause vitamins and metabolites to be lost from the body (Bender & Bender, 1997). By maintaining good nutritional habits and reducing stressors, the body has better protection from infections and organ function depletion. Some authorities consider aging to be a stressor that can be controlled through health habits such as exercise and proper diet (Bender & Bender, 1997). Recent research suggests that certain substances work to protect the body from stressors and include such elements as vitamin E and beta-carotene, omega-3 fatty acids, and minerals like magnesium, zinc, boron, and molybdenum. Antioxidant defenses need the intake of antioxidants in the diet that include certain B vitamins, ascorbate (vitamin C), tocopherol (vitamin E), beta-carotene, cysteine, taurine, and coenzyme Q10 (Bender & Bender, 1997). Health care providers should encourage older adults to read labels of containers for contents that contain important ingredients for health. Foods high in antioxidants are carrots, spinach, and other greens.

Eating a balanced, moderate, nutritious diet helps prevent the onset of diseases and disabilities and increases feelings of well-being. Physiological and psychosocial aspects of aging affect nutrition in a variety of ways. Older adults also may have poor lifelong nutritional intake habits, misunderstand the importance of certain foods in their diet, lack access to nutritious foods, and lack the knowledge or ability to prepare nutritional meals. Many of these issues can be easily addressed through educational programs and experimentation with different substances. A thorough assessment of nutritional status is essential with proper referral to health care providers when needed. By the time an individual reaches older age, habits and routines have been established for a long period of time. Therefore, teaching programs need to be aimed toward meeting the nutritional needs of older adults, including the preparation, shopping, storage, and purchasing of foods. Health care providers can make arrangements for dental visits or encourage good oral hygiene in addition to regular dental care. Numerous organizations such as churches offer hot meals for older adults that are nutritious and offer companionship during mealtime.

Income could be a major obstacle in selecting, purchasing, and preparing nutritious meals. The median income of people age 65 and older in 1998 was $18,166 for males and $10,054 for females, and 36% reported incomes less than $10,000 (*A Profile*, 1999). Health care providers have to know foods that are inexpensive but nutritious and that can be purchased on a low income.

Older adults can experience a deficiency in water intake because they usually have a reduced thirst sensation mechanism. Water is necessary for body function and temperature regulation. With a reduction in caloric intake, the amount of fluid ingested with food is reduced. Along with reduced levels of physical exercise, older adults can experience bowel elimination problems when water and fiber intake are decreased. Fiber is an important constituent in an older adult's diet for a number of reasons. It adds bulk to the diet and may play a role in reducing the chances of developing serious conditions in the gastrointestinal tract.

Some older adults are thinner than they were when they were younger because of calorie decreases or medication reactions. Obesity may be a problem accompanied by additional problems of malnutrition, immobility, diabetes, heart problems, and respiratory problems. The National Institutes for Health divided obesity into three levels based on the **body mass index (BMI).** This index is determined by dividing measured body weight in kilograms by the height in meters squared (Phillips et al., 1995). Normal BMI is 20–25 kg/m². They further divide obesity into mild BMI, 27.5–30 kg/m²; moderate BMI, 30–40 kg/m²; and morbid obesity BMI, >40 kg/m².

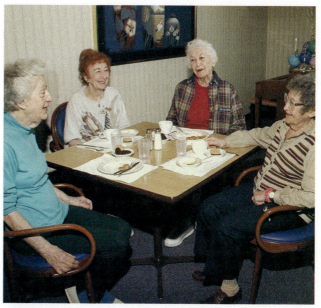

FIGURE 8-1 Many older adults enjoy dining out or sharing a meal at their local senior center.

An obesity state affects self-image and self-concept in an individual whose appearance has changed with aging. Added to the normal occurrence of aging on the external physiological changes, obesity has a detrimental effect on the psychological feelings of overweight individuals.

A gradual weight reduction program coordinated by health care providers can lead to positive effects. Not only will the individual feel better psychologically but there will be less burden on the musculoskeletal system, cardiovascular system, kidneys, and liver. Loss of weight with a planned exercise program can reduce blood pressure and improve mobility. Health care providers can offer planned weight reduction programs that include a daily food diary, weekly weights, and evaluation of nutritional intake. Weight reduction provides a visual means to promote positive reinforcement to continue with a planned program. Generally, a change in the type of foods ingested will lead to a decrease in weight rather than a reduction in the amount of intake. It is important to teach about reading food labels, making the right choices in foods, selecting nutritious foods when dining out, and knowing what foods are nutritious. When collecting data about nutrition, the health care provider should phrase questions so that the person describes a typical eating pattern or 24-hour recall diet rather than saying what they think they should eat. Also, a description of the amount of food and number of meals and snacks ingested is helpful in determining the total picture.

As aging occurs, changes in the gastrointestinal tract can lead to indigestion and an inability to tolerate spicy foods, and interactions with medications may limit the type of foods ingested. Dietary requirements may call for a change in the way foods are cooked. Older adults can learn to cook using different substances such as herbs that can add flavor but do not cause gastrointestinal problems or problems related to interactions with medications. Taste does not have to be sacrificed by cooking differently. Box 8-1 summarizes some basic nutritional guidelines for older adults.

Nutritional Needs of Older Adults

Physiological changes in aging include sensory, gastrointestinal, and metabolic. Health problems and medications alter nutritional needs and requirements. Many of the medications taken for chronic diseases cause an increase or decrease in appetite, anorexia, or a decrease in absorption of important nutrients.

The Food Guide Pyramid (U.S. Department of Agriculture, 1992, revised 1996) and the more recent food exchange list commonly used to control diabetes mellitus are easy guides to follow. Table 8-1 outlines exchange lists for meal planning. Both are practical approaches to organizing food intake and meeting a balanced diet. Established dietary requirements and individual needs

are more important to follow than trying fad diets. Health care providers can give the guidance that prevents using potentially harmful fad diets or self-determined diets. Diet also may be affected by factors unrelated to physiological changes. Psychosocial changes often cause inadequate or poor dietary habits. Diet intake could be affected by income, loss of functional activities, transportation problems, immobility, eating alone, and cooking and storage facilities.

Exercise

Physical activities are important to the physiological and psychological welfare of each person. Exercise can produce a variety of beneficial physiological changes and slow the progressive decline in functions that inevitably occurs with inactivity and aging. Older adults may have to face physical limitations, but adapting to changes can lead to successful aging. It is well documented and evident that physical exercise is beneficial, but only 30% of older adults report exercising regularly (Allison & Keller,

---

BOX 8-1 Nutritional Guidelines for Older Adults

- Reduce calories 5% per decade for individuals 51 years of age or older (Harris, 2000).

- Increase complex carbohydrates from fruits, vegetables, cereals, and whole wheat breads.

- Reduce protein intake from beef and substitute fish, poultry, and plant foods.

- Limit fats to 30% of daily calories.

- Obtain vitamins and minerals primarily from food intake, but nutritional vitamin and mineral supplements usually are also needed.

- Include adequate fluids in the diet, especially water (eight 8-ounce glasses daily).

- Eat four to five small meals a day rather than three large ones.

- Eat a variety of foods.

- Maintain ideal body weight for age and height.

- Avoid saturated fat and cholesterol.

- Eat foods with adequate starch and fiber.

- Avoid excess sugar (desserts and candy).

- Reduce salt intake (do not add salt at the table).

- Drink alcohol in moderation, if at all.

TABLE 8-1	Exchange Lists for Meal Planning

Starch Exchange List

One starch exchange equals 15 g carbohydrate, 3 g protein, 0–1 g fat, and 80 kcal.

Bread/Starches

Bagel	½ (1 oz)
Bread, reduced-calorie	2 slices (1½ oz)
Bread, white, whole-wheat, pumpernickel, rye	1 slice (1 oz)
Bread sticks, crisp, 4 in. long × ½ in.	2 (⅔ oz)
English muffin	½
Hot dog or hamburger bun	½ (1 oz)
Pita, 6 in. across	½
Raisin bread, unfrosted	1 slice (1 oz)
Roll, plain, small	1 (1 oz)
Tortilla, corn, 6 in. across	1
Tortilla, flour, 7–8 in. across	1
Waffle, 4½ in. square, reduced-fat	1

Beans, Peas, and Lentils

(Count as 1 starch exchange, plus 1 very lean meat exchange.)

Beans and peas (garbanzo, pinto, kidney, white, split, black-eyed)	½ cup
Lima beans	⅔ cup
Lentils	½ cup
Miso*	3 tbsp

= 400 mg or more sodium per exchange.

Cereals and Grains

Bran cereals	½ cup
Bulgur	½ cup
Cereals	½ cup
Cereals, unsweetened, ready-to-eat	¾ cup
Cornmeal (dry)	3 tbsp
Couscous	⅓ cup
Flour (dry)	3 tbsp
Granola, low-fat	¼ cup
Grape-Nuts®	¼ cup
Grits	½ cup
Kasha	½ cup
Millet	¼ cup
Muesli	¼ cup
Oats	½ cup
Pasta	½ cup
Puffed cereal	1½ cups

(continues)

TABLE 8-1   Exchange Lists for Meal Planning   *continued*

Cereals and Grains   *continued*

Rice milk	½ cup
Rice, white or brown	⅓ cup
Shredded Wheat®	½ cup
Sugar-frosted cereal	½ cup
Wheat germ	3 tbsp

Crackers and Snacks

Animal crackers	8
Graham crackers, 2½ in. square	3
Matzoh	¾ oz
Melba toast	4 slices
Oyster crackers	24
Popcorn (popped, no fat added or low-fat microwave)	3 cups
Pretzels	¾ oz
Rice cakes, 4 in. across	2
Saltine-type crackers	6
Snack chips, fat-free (tortilla, potato)	15–20 (¾ oz)
Whole-wheat crackers, no fat added	2–5 (¾ oz)

Starchy Vegetables

Baked beans	⅓ cup
Corn	½ cup
Corn on cob, medium	1 (5 oz)
Mixed vegetables with corn, peas, or pasta	1 cup
Peas, green	½ cup
Plantain	½ cup
Potato, baked or boiled	1 small (3 oz)
Potato, mashed	½ cup
Squash, winter (acorn, butternut)	1 cup
Yam, sweet potato, plain	½ cup

Starchy Foods Prepared with Fat

(Count as 1 starch exchange, plus 1 fat exchange.)

Biscuit, 2½ in. across	1
Chow mein noodles	½ cup
Corn bread, 2 in. cube	1 (2 oz)
Crackers, round butter type	6
Croutons	1 cup
French-fried potatoes	16–25 (3 oz)
Granola	¼ cup
Muffin, small	1 (1½ oz)

(continues)

TABLE 8-1 Exchange Lists for Meal Planning *continued*

Starchy Foods Prepared with Fat *continued*

Pancake, 4 in. across	2
Popcorn, microwave	3 cups
Sandwich crackers, cheese or peanut butter filling	3
Stuffing, bread (prepared)	⅓ cup
Taco shell, 6 in. across	2
Waffle, 4½ in. square	1
Whole-wheat crackers, fat added	4–6 (1 oz)

Meat and Substitutes List

Very Lean Meat and Substitutes List

One exchange equals 0 g carbohydrate, 7 g protein, 0–1 g fat, and 35 kcal

- One very lean meat exchange is equal to any one of the following items.

Poultry: Chicken or turkey (white meat, no skin), Cornish hen (no skin)	1 oz
Fish: Fresh or frozen cod, flounder, haddock, halibut, trout; tuna fresh or canned in water	1 oz
Shellfish: Clams, crab, lobster, scallops, shrimp, imitation shellfish	1 oz
Game: Duck or pheasant (no skin), venison, buffalo, ostrich	1 oz
Cheese with 1 g or less fat per ounce:	
Nonfat or low-fat cottage cheese	¼ cup
Fat-free cheese	1 oz
Other: Processed sandwich meat with 1 g or less fat per ounce, such as deli thin, shaved meats, chipped beef*, turkey ham	1 oz
Egg whites	2
Egg substitutes, plain	¼ cup
Hot dogs with 1 g or less fat per ounce*	1 oz
Kidney (high in cholesterol)	1 oz
Sausage with 1 g or less fat per ounce	1 oz

- Count as one very lean meat and one starch exchange.

Beans, peas, lentils (cooked)	½ cup

*= 400 mg or more sodium per exchange.

Lean Meat and Substitutes List

One exchange equals 0 g carbohydrate, 7 g protein, 3 g fat, and 55 kcal

- One lean meat exchange is equal to any one of the following items.

Beef: USDA Select or Choice grades of lean beef trimmed of fat, such as round, sirloin, and flank steak; tenderloin; roast (rib, chuck, rump); steak (T-bone, porterhouse, cubed), ground round	1 oz
Pork: Lean pork, such as fresh ham; canned, cured, or boiled ham; Canadian bacon*; tenderloin, center loin chop	1 oz
Lamb: Roast, chop, leg	1 oz
Veal: Lean chop, roast	1 oz

(continues)

TABLE 8-1   Exchange Lists for Meal Planning *continued*

Lean Meat and Substitutes List   *continued*

Poultry: Chicken, turkey (dark meat, no skin), chicken (white meat, with skin), domestic duck or goose (well-drained of fat, no skin)	1 oz
Fish:	
Herring (uncreamed or smoked)	1 oz
Oysters	6 medium
Salmon (fresh or canned), catfish	1 oz
Sardines (canned)	2 medium
Tuna (canned in oil, drained)	1 oz
Game: Goose (no skin), rabbit	1 oz
Cheese:	
4.5%-fat cottage cheese	¼ cup
Grated Parmesan	2 tbsp
Cheeses with 3 g or less fat per ounce	1 oz
Other:	
Hot dogs with 3 g or less fat per ounce*	1½ oz
Processed sandwich meat with 3 g or less fat per ounce, such as turkey pastrami or kielbasa	1 oz
Liver, heart (high in cholesterol)	1 oz

Medium-Fat Meat and Substitutes List

One exchange equals 0 g carbohydrate, 7 g protein, 5 g fat, and 75 kcal

• One medium-fat meat exchange is equal to any one of the following items.

Beef: Most beef products fall into this category (ground beef, meatloaf, corned beef, short ribs, Prime grades of meat trimmed of fat, such as prime rib)	1 oz
Pork: Top loin, chop, Boston butt, cutlet	1 oz
Lamb: Rib roast, ground	1 oz
Veal: Cutlet (ground or cubed, unbreaded)	1 oz
Poultry: Chicken (dark meat, with skin), ground turkey or ground chicken, fried chicken (with skin)	1 oz
Fish: Any fried fish product	1 oz
Cheese: With 5 g or less fat per ounce	
Feta	1 oz
Mozzarella	1 oz
Ricotta	¼ cup (2 oz)
Other:	
Eggs (high in cholesterol, limit to 3 per week)	1
Sausage with 5 g or less fat per ounce	1 oz
Soy milk	1 cup
Tempeh	¼ cup
Tofu	4 oz or ½ cup

(continues)

TABLE 8-1 Exchange Lists for Meal Planning *continued*

High-Fat Meat and Substitutes List

One exchange equals 0 g carbohydrate, 7 g protein, 8 g fat, and 100 kcal

Remember these items are high in saturated fat, cholesterol, and calories and may raise blood cholesterol levels if eaten on a regular basis.

- One high-fat meat exchange is equal to any one of the following items.

Pork: Spareribs, ground pork, pork sausage	1 oz
Cheese: All regular cheeses, such as American*, cheddar, Monterey Jack, Swiss	1 oz
Other: Processed sandwich meats with 8 g or less fat per ounce, such as bologna, pimento loaf, salmai	1 oz
Sausage, such as bratwurst, Italian, knockwurst, Polish, smoked	1 oz
Hot dog (turkey or chicken)*	1 (10/lb)
Bacon	3 slices (20 slices/lb)

- Count as one high-fat meat plus one fat exchange.

Hot dog (beef, pork, or combination)*	1 (10/lb)
Peanut butter (contains unsaturated fat)	2 tbsp.

= 400 mg or more sodium per exchange.

Fruit Exchange List

Fruit

One Fruit exchange equals 15 g carbohydrate and 60 kcal

The weight includes skin, core, seeds, and rind.

Apple, unpeeled, small	1 (4 oz)
Applesauce, unsweetened	½ cup
Apples, dried	4 rings
Apricots, fresh	4 whole (5½ oz)
Apricots, dried	8 halves
Apricots, canned	½ cup
Banana, small	1 (4 oz)
Blackberries	¾ cup
Blueberries	¾ cup
Cantaloupe, small	⅓ melon (11 oz) or 1 cup cubes
Cherries, sweet, fresh	12 (3 oz)
Cherries, sweet, canned	½ cup
Dates	3
Fruit cocktail	½ cup
Grapefruit, large	½ (11 oz)
Grapefruit sections, canned	¾ cup
Grapes, small	17 (3 oz)
Honeydew melon	1 slice (10 oz) or 1 cup cubes

(continues)

TABLE 8-1   Exchange Lists for Meal Planning   *continued*

Fruit   *continued*

Kiwi	1 (3½ oz)
Mandarin oranges, canned	¾ cup
Mango, small	½ cup
Nectarine, small	1 (5 oz)
Orange, small	1 (6½ oz)
Papaya	½ fruit (8 oz) or 1 cup cubes
Peach, medium, fresh	1 (6 oz)
Peaches, canned	½ cup
Pear, large, fresh	½ (4 oz)
Pears, canned	½ cup
Pineapple, fresh	¾ cup
Pineapple, canned	½ cup
Plums, small	2 (5 oz)
Prunes, dried	3
Raisins	2 tbsp
Raspberries	1 cup
Strawberries	1¼ cup whole berries
Tangerines, small	2 (8 oz)
Watermelon	1¼ cup cubes

Fruit Juice

Apple juice/cider	½ cup
Cranberry juice cocktail	⅓ cup
Cranberry juice cocktail, reduced-calorie	1 cup
Fruit juice blends, 100% juice	⅓ cup
Grape juice	⅓ cup
Grapefruit juice	½ cup
Orange juice	½ cup
Pineapple juice	½ cup
Prune juice	⅓ cup

Milk Exchange List

Fat-Free and Very Low Fat Milk

Each item on this list contains 12 g of carbohydrate, 8 g of protein, a trace of fat, and 90 kcal. One exchange is equal to any one of the following items:

Fat-free	1 cup
½% milk	1 cup
Low-fat milk (1%)	1 cup
Low-fat buttermilk	1 cup

(continues)

TABLE 8-1 Exchange Lists for Meal Planning *continued*

Fat-Free and Very Low Fat Milk *continued*

Evaporated fat-free milk	½ cup
Dry nonfat milk	⅓ cup
Plain nonfat yogurt	¾ cup
Nonfat or low-fat fruit-flavored yogurt sweetened with aspartame	1 cup

Low-Fat Milk

Each item on this list contains 12 g of carbohydrate, 8 g of protein, 5 g of fat, and 120 kcal. One exchange is equal to any one of the following items:

Reduced-fat milk (2%)	1 cup
Plain low-fat yogurt (with added nonfat milk solids)	¾ cup

Whole Milk

Each item on this list contains 12 g of carbohydrate, 8 g of protein, 8 g of fat, and 150 kcal. One exchange is equal to any one of the following items:

Whole milk	1 cup
Evaporated whole milk	½ cup
Whole plain yogurt	8 oz

Fat Exchange List

Each item on this list contains 5 g of fat and 45 kcal.

One exchange is equal to any one of the following items:

Unsaturated

Avocado	⅛ medium or 1 oz
Margarine	1 tsp
Margarine, diet	1 tbsp
Mayonnaise	1 tsp
Mayonnaise, reduced-calorie	1 tbsp
Nuts and seeds:	
Almonds, dry roasted	6 whole
Cashews, dry roasted	6 whole
Pecans	2 whole
Peanuts	10 nuts
Peanut butter	2 tsp
Seeds, pine nuts, sunflower	1 tbsp
Oil (canola, corn, cottonseed, safflower, soybean, sunflower, olive, peanut)	1 tsp
Olives, ripe; black	8 large
Olives, green, stuffed	10 large
Salad dressing, mayonnaise type	2 tsp
Salad dressing, mayonnaise type, reduced-calorie	1 tbsp
Salad dressing (all varieties)	1 tbsp
Salad dressing, reduced-calorie	2 tbsp

(continues)

TABLE 8-1   Exchange Lists for Meal Planning   *continued*

Saturated

Butter	1 tsp
Bacon	1 slice
Chitterlings, boiled	$\frac{1}{2}$ oz
Coconut, shredded	2 tbsp
Cream (light, coffee, table)	2 tbsp
Cream, sour	2 tbsp
Cream (half and half)	2 tbsp
Cream cheese	1 tbsp
Salt pork	$1'' \times 1'' \times \frac{1}{4}''$ if eaten

Other Carbohydrates Exchange List

One exchange equals 15 g carbohydrate, or 1 starch, or 1 fruit, or 1 milk.

Food	Serving Size	Exchanges Per Serving
Angel food cake, unfrosted	$\frac{1}{12}$ cake	2 carbohydrates
Brownie, small, unfrosted	2 in. square	1 carbohydrate, 1 fat
Cake, unfrosted	2 in. square	1 carbohydrate, 1 fat
Cake, frosted	2 in. square	2 carbohydrates, 1 fat
Cookie, fat-free	2 small	1 carbohydrate
Cookie or sandwich cookie with creme filling	2 small	1 carbohydrate, 1 fat
Cranberry sauce, jellied	$\frac{1}{4}$ cup	$1\frac{1}{2}$ carbohydrates
Cupcake, frosted	1 small	2 carbohydrates, 1 fat
Doughnut, plain cake	1 medium ($1\frac{1}{2}$ oz)	$1\frac{1}{2}$ carbohydrates, 2 fats
Doughnut, glazed	$3\frac{3}{4}$ in. across (2 oz)	2 carbohydrates, 2 fats
Fruit juice bars, frozen, 100% juice	1 bar (3 oz)	1 carbohydrate
Fruit snacks, chewy (pureed fruit concentrate)	1 roll ($\frac{3}{4}$ oz)	1 carbohydrate
Fruit spreads, 100% fruit	1 tbsp	1 carbohydrate
Gelatin, regular	$\frac{1}{2}$ cup	1 carbohydrate
Gingersnaps	3	1 carbohydrate
Granola bar	1 bar	1 carbohydrate, 1 fat
Granola bar, fat-free	1 bar	2 carbohydrates
Honey	1 tbsp	1 carbohydrate
Hummus	$\frac{1}{3}$ cup	1 carbohydrate, 1 fat
Ice cream	$\frac{1}{2}$ cup	1 carbohydrate, 2 fats
Ice cream, light	$\frac{1}{2}$ cup	1 carbohydrate, 1 fat
Ice cream, fat-free, no sugar added	$\frac{1}{2}$ cup	1 carbohydrate
Jam or jelly, regular	1 tbsp	1 carbohydrate
Milk, chocolate, whole	1 cup	2 carbohydrates, 1 fat
Pie, fruit, 2 crusts	$\frac{1}{6}$ pie	3 carbohydrates, 2 fats
Pie, pumpkin or custard	$\frac{1}{8}$ pie	1 carbohydrate, 2 fats

(continues)

TABLE 8-1 Exchange Lists for Meal Planning *continued*

Food	Serving Size	Exchanges Per Serving
Potato Chips	12–18 (1 oz)	1 carbohydrate, 2 fats
Pudding, regular (made with low-fat milk)	½ cup	2 carbohydrates
Pudding, sugar-free (made with low-fat milk)	½ cup	1 carbohydrate
Salad dressing, fat-free*	¼ cup	1 carbohydrate
Sherbet, sorbet	½ cup	2 carbohydrates
Spaghetti or pasta sauce, canned*	½ cup	1 carbohydrate, 1 fat
Sugar	1 tbsp	½ carbohydrate
Sweet roll or Danish	1 (2½ oz)	2½ carbohydrates, 2 fat
Syrup, light	2 tbsp	1 carbohydrate
Syrup, regular	1 tbsp	1 carbohydrate
Syrup, regular	¼ cup	4 carbohydrates
Tortilla chips	6–12 (1 oz)	1 carbohydrate, 2 fats
Vanilla wafers	5	1 carbohydrate, 1 fat
Yogurt, frozen, low-fat, fat-free	⅓ cup	1 carbohydrate, 0–1 fat
Yogurt, frozen, fat-free, no sugar added	½ cup	1 carbohydrate
Yogurt, low-fat with fruit	1 cup	3 carbohydrates, 0–1 fat

*= 400 mg or more sodium per exchange.

Source: The American Diabetes Association and the American Diabetic Association.

1997). Regular physical exercise minimizes and prevents chronic problems and increases muscle strength, flexibility, range of motion, balance, endurance, and functional ability, and causes relaxation and improves sleep. Exercise is essential to good health and to a sense of well-being. Each program should be tailored to the individual's physical makeup so the program does not negatively affect acute or chronic illnesses.

Biological changes are unavoidable, and some are related to hereditary, lifestyle, or individual differences. The biological decline that occurs has little impact on mental capability to problem solve. Exercise serves many functions for older adults. Aging of body systems occurs at different rates with measurable decline in oxygen uptake in the lungs, maximum strength of muscle contraction, and decline in the autonomic nervous system. Individuals' rates of aging are variable and related to a number of factors. Health care providers should teach ways to preserve muscle strength to help the older adult maintain self-care activities to prevent loss of muscle strength (Blaylock, 1991).

Regular exercise is part of an older adult's involvement in a continuing interrelated series of health-promoting behaviors. Physical exercise should be a planned activity, and older adults should talk to their physicians, nurses, social workers, physical therapists, and other health care professionals about the benefits

of planned programs and what is best for their individual needs. Exercise programs need to be geared to a form that is beneficial, safe, and consistent with an individual's lifestyle. Physical exercise programs are geared to reducing activity intolerance using aerobic training. Individuals should be carefully tested and exercises prescribed that are tailored to each person's physiological response to activity.

Physical inactivity has been linked with managing age-related chronic conditions, such as hypertension, heart disease, diabetes, obesity, and osteoporosis. Lack of exercise increases the risk of developing these conditions. Only 8% of all adults in the United States currently exercise at a recommended level. According to the **Centers for Disease Control and Prevention** (1997), an estimated 92% of American retirees do not participate in meaningful exercise and half of all retirees are completely sedentary. Part of the problem is the myths surrounding aging and physical activity, physical attractiveness, vitality, and health (see Box 8-2). Negative images hamper the development of exercise programs when in fact most older adults stay active, vital, contributing members of society.

When health care providers assume the myths are true, it can be a costly mistake both in economic and human aspects. Programs that encourage and help older adults to exercise and be physically active are necessary. However, an evaluation of current physical status is

Research Focus

Citation:

Connelly, D. M., & Vandervoort, A. A. (1995). Improvement in knee extensor strength of institutionalized elderly women after exercise with ankle weights. *Physiotherapy Canada, 47,* 15–23.

Purpose:

To determine if simple resisted exercise at moderate intensity improved the quadriceps muscle strength of frail, older women.

Methods:

Ten female nursing home residents with a mean age of 81.6 years completed an 8-week strengthening program consisting of three sets of 10 repetitions per leg at three group sessions per week. The exercises were held at a constant intensity between 30% and 50% of their one-repetition maximum.

Findings:

Significant improvement was seen in strength and self-paced walking speed. The researchers recommended further investigation into the clinical implication of this type of exercise for both functional rehabilitation and fall prevention.

Implications:

The results of this preliminary study indicate that frail, older women may derive significant benefits from exercise. These benefits include improved strength and mobility.

BOX 8-2   Myths About Aging and Exercise

- Older adults do not have the energy or strength to exercise.

- Exercise cannot help after age 65 or 70.

- Exercise is dangerous for older adults.

- Older adults do not like to exercise.

exercise and other natural chemicals help control pain by functioning as natural tranquilizers and antidepressants.

Many of the age-related losses are caused by the lack of the use of different physiological systems. This is particularly pertinent to muscle function related to lack of exercise. Exercise is beneficial for many purposes, but especially for the musculoskeletal and cardiovascular systems. Exercise programs may play a role in reducing loneliness and depression at the same time it reduces the chances of heart disease, obesity, and other health problems. It reduces sleep disturbances and reduces the effects of stress. A regular exercise program helps improve appearance and enhances self-image and self-concept.

Exercise, when combined with periods of rest, aids all body functions and almost all organ systems. Adequate rest is needed for the body, mind, and spirit to function properly. When individuals sleep, the body releases melatonin, which has its highest peak around midnight and causes a deeper, more restful sleep. During deep sleep the body's healing and immune-building processes regenerate cells and cellular functions. By promoting the functioning of the immune system and decreasing stress, an individual improves the chances of slowing down the aging process. Chronic illness in older adults may not be preventable in some cases, but many such conditions can be reduced or minimized through diet and exercise.

Exercise programs should start slowly and increase according to individual tolerance levels. Most programs begin with 5 minutes of exercise or until the individual reaches a tolerance level. Rest periods and exercise periods can be alternated until 20–30 minutes of sustained activity can be generated.

Because mobility has a profound effect on an individual's perception of well-being, a careful initial assessment of PADL must be made. Clients often consider themselves well as long as they do not require personal care. Evaluating PADL is an important component of the nursing assessment. Assessment tools such as the Katz Index of Independence in Activities of Daily Living (Katz et al., 1970) and the Instrumental Activities of Daily Living (IADL) Scale (Lawton & Brody, 1969) are valuable, regardless of the setting, in determining the extent of an older adult's mobility. Some tools measure PADL in-

essential before an exercise program begins. Physical examination begins with an assessment of general appearance, behavior, motor activity, and body language. The client's appearance gives clues to adaptation and coping with possible physical problems. Physical aspects of activities of daily living can be evaluated easily and include respiratory functioning, circulation, nutrition, elimination, mobility, and sleep patterns. Older adults may have problems finding exercise programs that are geared to functional limitations related to aging, available transportation, individual attitudes, reasonable cost, and accessibility of programs.

Loss of muscle strength is especially problematic for older adults who experience illness, but it is important for all older adults to keep active and prevent immobility with all the accompanying problems (Figure 8-2). Immobility leads to age-related decline in force-generating capacity in muscle fibers, while exercise and resistance training on the neuromuscular system increases older adult's functional capacity (Hopp, 1993). Endorphins released during

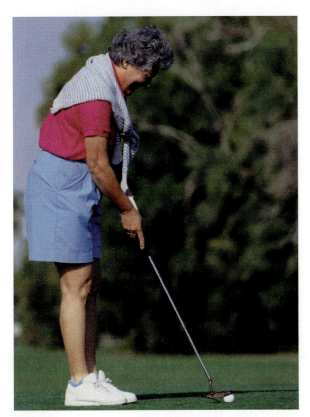

FIGURE 8-2 A regular exercise program helps promote successful aging.

directly and do not include observed behavior but instead include the client's perceptions of capabilities. In 1994–1995, over 4.4 million older people needed assistance with PADL, and 52.5% of the older population reported having at least one disability that limited carrying out PADL (*A Profile,* 1999). Often, clients will answer positively about their PADL for fear of being placed in a nursing home when they may not be functioning as well as stated (Allison & Keller, 1997). Asking them to perform simple tasks will assist in evaluating their ability to perform PADL tasks. Verbal or written reports require validation. Some older people are frightened of making mistakes and will try to please the interviewer and respond in a way perceived as positive. Alleviation of anxiety will help them to relax. This may be accomplished with a short conversation to relax them.

Instrumental activities of daily living (IADL) assess task performance at a higher level. These tasks are more complex than PADL and focus on clients' ability to interact with their environment. The tasks include shopping, cooking, housekeeping, laundry, use of transportation, managing money, managing medications, use of telephone, reading ability, home maintenance, forms of communication, and use of time (Lawton & Brody, 1969).

Fitness Centers

Fitness centers offer an opportunity to engage in a planned exercise program within a controlled environment. In addition, the chance to socialize with other older adults and people of all ages is enhanced in a fitness center. A fitness center may be located in a variety of places that could be accessible to older adults: hospital, retirement center, assisted-living facility, church, commercial fitness center, or YMCA/YWCA. The companionship during an exercise program can serve as a psychological stimulant that provides the incentive to continue with a program.

Aging eventually does cause some change in physiological system functioning. This change may be a result of aging or physical deconditioning. The degree to which decreases occur with aging can be impacted by physical activity. The best types and examples of physical exercise can have a profound effect on older adults' physical fitness. The best exercises are those that strengthen large muscles and include aerobic activities. Simple walking is probably the best and safest exercise for older adults. Walking around the house, around the yard, or at the mall are all helpful. Weight-training exercises such as lifting 5-pound weights are also recommended to maintain upper arm strength. There is mounting evidence that aerobic exercise serves as a preventive measure in the same ways that it affects younger people. Experts have found that exercise can prevent or reverse up to half the physical decline problems associated with aging. Lack of muscle use leads to atrophy and exercise can be beneficial for physiological changes and slow the progressive decline in function. The major benefits of exercise are shown in Table 8-2. Suggested exercises for older adults are listed in Box 8-3.

TABLE 8-2 Benefits of Exercise

• Normalize glucose tolerance	• Decrease the effects of arthritis
• Improve gait and balance	• Promote weight loss
• Improve cardiovascular function	• Reduce blood pressure
• Increase energy	• Lower cholesterol
• Promote bone mineral density	• Promote rest and relaxation
• Improve mobility	• Improve sleep

BOX 8-3   Suggested Exercises for Older Adults

- Walking
- Dancing
- Gardening and yard work
- Swimming
- Weight lifting

Low-intensity activities for at least 20 minutes three or more times a week are needed to produce health benefits. In addition to walking, dancing and swimming are good exercises for older adults that help prevent osteoporosis and may relieve the discomforts of osteoarthritis. Other exercises that can be beneficial are gardening, golfing, cycling, and aerobic dancing (Figure 8-3). Many chronic diseases develop insidiously and can be prevented with early planned programs of exercise.

Exercise has a profound impact on the cardiovascular system. Studies have demonstrated that cardiac rehabilitation plays a role in minimizing disability associated with myocardial infarction and coronary artery bypass surgery (Hellman & Williams, 1994). Exercise improves functional capacity and reduces myocardial workload.

CLINICAL ALERT

Absolute contraindications for physical activity include such conditions as severe coronary heart disease, decompensated congestive heart failure, uncontrolled arrhythmia, valvular disease, uncontrolled hypertension, acute myocarditis or infectious illness, recent pulmonary embolism, and deep vein thrombosis.

Nursing Tip

Assess for the following before recommending a specific exercise program:
- Heart disease or heart attack
- Pains or pressure in left or midchest area, left neck, shoulder, or arm
- Faintness, dizziness, or extreme breathlessness with mild physical exercise
- High blood pressure
- Musculoskeletal problems such as osteoarthritis
- All prescription and over-the-counter medications

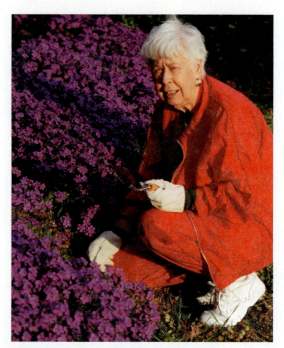

FIGURE 8-3   Gardening is a beneficial form of exercise.

Precautions

An exercise program should not be started without careful assessment by a health care provider and identification of possible contraindications. The risk of injury from moderate exercise is insignificant. Older adults need careful assessment before beginning any planned exercise program, especially individuals who have not been physically active. This assessment includes functional ability, exercise tolerance, physical limitations, and psychological and social support. Exercise should be prescribed for intensity, frequency, and duration.

Support Systems

Aging is a unidirectional process in that an individual can never grow younger. However, there are many older adults who have not or do not want to be identified with a chronological age. These individuals have friends at all ages but also tend to identify with others who are going through the same sequence of roles. An older adult's social relationships, the amount and quality of contacts with support persons, the number of social roles compared with previous social roles at a younger age, economic resources to meet changing needs, and capability to perform activities of daily living are all important considerations in the overall assessment of current and potential future functioning. Regardless of the age of an individual, older adults need human interaction to feel needed, appreciated, and useful.

Socialization with others assists in maintaining cognitive status and preventing boredom and depression. Research has demonstrated that women have more friends than men and seem to fare better as widows than men do as widowers. Women have a special relationship with other women. It is not uncommon to see older women showing affection, spending time with each other, or providing emotional support. Women have traditionally been the caregivers, widows, or single members of society. Men may have one or two friends and most consider their spouse as their best friend. Also, older adults seem to get the same satisfaction from friends as they do from family members' interactions.

Studies have demonstrated that individuals with more social support involvement have high morale and better life satisfaction, personal adjustment, and mental health than those with less involvement. Support systems are influential in helping older adults view life more calmly and relax and focus their minds on important matters.

Families provide older adults with physical and emotional support that comes in many forms. The family is the greatest source for affection and emotional support (Figure 8-4). Family members are the primary source of caregiving for disabled or dependent older adults.

A social support system provides an older adult with attachments that help cope with life changes, stresses, and promotion of a feeling of well-being. Support systems provide a source of identity, material and emotional assistance, and communication with the outside world. Support systems may be family, friends, neighbors, religious organizations, pets, health care agency personnel, and voluntary organizations. These support systems become increasingly more important as individuals become more physically dependent on assistance. There are times when caregiving services are needed from the community for older adults who are unable to be cared for by family members.

Support systems within the same age group are highly regarded as current life tasks are shared. Because older adults have had some similar experiences, they often have common interests. The ease of communication within age groups facilitates mutual support systems. As within other age groups, most older adults feel comfortable with others who have the same values,

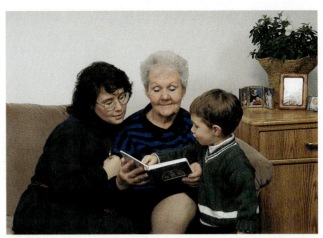

FIGURE 8-4 Spending time with family members promotes a sense of well-being and provides emotional support.

experiences, and interests. However, this does not preclude the interest in associating with other age groups and family members who are often separated by social and/or physical distance.

Sibling relationships are important to older adults even when there is only psychological closeness. Sibling relationships stretch over a lifetime of special and shared experiences with common perceptions of such events as school, religion, parents, home, and growing up. Although family members, especially grandchildren, are loved and cherished, most sibling relationships are enduring.

Community Service Agencies

There are many community organizations that health care providers can use to help families arrange for services for older adults. Some of the agencies are low cost, no cost, or covered by Medicare or Medicaid. Table 8-3 identifies a number of resources available to the older adult through community service agencies.

Older adults need social interaction for their well-being. Emotional care of family and friends helps an older adult maintain and adjust to physiological changes related to aging. Social support is needed on a daily basis, but it is especially important during a crisis. During

---

TABLE 8-3 Community Resources

• Mobility-impaired transportation services	• Home-delivered meals
• Support groups	• Hospice care
• Adult day services	• Companion services
• Home health care	• Respite care
• Churches/synagogues	• Benefits counseling (financial guidance)
	• Errand and assurance programs

crisis periods, a single confidante may be enough to maintain an older adult's morale, while the lack of an intimate friend may lead to progressive social withdrawal.

Activities Important to Successful Aging

There are many individual and group activities for older adults that provide exercise, enjoyment, and socialization with others. Exercise programs are especially successful when older adults are able to participate in group activities. A number of problems can be addressed in group exercise programs, such as socialization, friendship, shared programs, and motivation to continue with a planned program. When exercise positively affects appearance, self-concept improves. Group contact promotes social activities that enhance human responses of belonging, communication, and encouragement.

Individual and Group Activities

Many older adults enjoy reminiscing, and this gives health care providers an opportunity to gain insight into lifestyles and health histories. A **life review** is a conscious, systematic evaluation of life events, including successes and failures, with the guidance and support of a professional health care provider. The objective of the task is to gain a sense of integrity in reviewing one's life as a whole and to prepare for death. Encouraging reminiscence demonstrates interest in the person and is a valuable source of information. A life review gives data regarding the present health issues as background for the development of the many health concerns. As a person discusses life review and reminiscences about the past, the interviewer gathers data about memory, decision making, preferences, patterns of living, reactions of life's situations, and developmental stage accommodation. Efforts have to be made to balance an older adult's need to engage in life review and reminiscence and the need to collect data.

Focusing the conversation on the task at hand will keep the person on the topic. The vast experience of older adults may lead to long explanations of the events leading to a situation. The very nature of the chronicity of health conditions requires a long time to explain the development of the condition, course of the problems, and the treatment regimen.

Age influences social life, which filters individual experience, group life, and societal institutions. Older adults uniquely experience life changes, individual behavior, power and status relations, and social supports. Social aging is not unidirectional, and there are no increments to social reward. There may be a reduction

or loss of some rewards that can lead to despair until an individual assumes an active role in pursuing new avenues for expression and personal rewards.

Intimacy

Social support systems are important to older adults for emotional security, help, communication, sexual intimacy, and loyalty. Satisfying social relationships and intimacy are essential to adaptation and successful aging (Figure 8-5). Gratifying reciprocal relationships provide social and psychological support needed to continue feelings of affinity. Sexual activities continue into the later years if health is good and there is an acceptable partner.

Type of intimacy may change for older adults. They value emotional security and companionship and place less emphasis on physical appeal, status, and standard of living. As adults move to older ages, there may be a shift in friendships and self-identity. The most important people in an older adult's life in descending order are their spouse, children, siblings, other kin, friends, neighbors, and community workers. Social relationships continue even though retirement may sever ties with work associates and declining health may reduce or end community activities.

Think About It

How would you begin to assess how satisfied an older adult is with his or her intimate relationships?

Education

The educational level of older adults is increasing with each cohort group. As the educational level increases, more older adults will want access to continuing education in either a formal or an informal format. The better use of leisure time for older adults may come in the form of (a) opportunities to complete a college education, (b) programs geared to increased adaptability to a rapidly changing economy, and (c) increased choices of educational options. A system of lifelong education has been part of the present older adults' environment and attitude since their middle years. Older adults' continued education and learning are ways to assume meaningful roles at a time when they would otherwise face a loss of role with few if any alternatives to take their place.

According to U.S. government statistics, the percentage of older adults who completed high school rose from 28% in 1970 to 67% in 1998. Completion of high school among older adults varies by race and ethnic group, as demonstrated by 1998 statistics: 69% whites, 43% African Americans, and 30% Hispanics. In 1998, 15% of all older adults had a bachelor's degree or higher

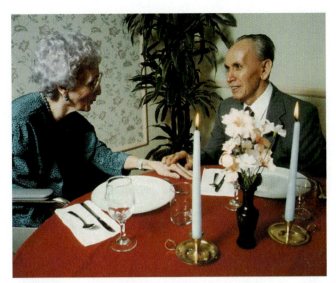

FIGURE 8-5 Older adults still experience the need for companionship and intimacy.

(*A Profile,* 1999). Educational levels and health status are major intervening factors in failing memory, declining language skills, and other cognitive problems often thought to be an inevitable consequence of aging (Morley, Flood, Perry, & Kumar, 1997).

A system of lifelong learning provides older adults with a means to education as a continuous process to be experienced at all stages of the life cycle and integrated into their lives. Many states have made provisions for older adults to attend educational institutions at a reduced rate or no fee. Older individuals can move freely in and out of educational settings, with some finishing degrees in their eighties and nineties. International **Elderhostel** programs provide informal to formal educational opportunities and a chance to travel. The barriers to educational institutions have been eliminated or reduced for older adults to take advantage of continuing education. Accommodations should be made for older adults when attending any educational program, including teaching methods and environmental factors. Printed material should be large enough to be seen easily.

Responses to verbal requests may take time for an individual to process because a normal aging symptom is the slowing of the response time. This slowing is related to the impulses being sent to the brain and the transmission of response. Older adults process information based on life experiences, sensoriperceptual capabilities, and modification of instructional material to meet the needs for pacing instructions (Norton, 1998). The setting where learning is supposed to take place has a major impact on an individual's ability to process information. However, allowing sufficient time for response will result in the needed information. Coupled with physical impairments, chronic illnesses, and medications, many older adults experience fatigue that further impacts their ability to process information in a timely manner.

Not allowing time for this normal process to occur conveys to the older adult the lack of understanding of aging. Slowed responses may also be related to language, terms, or words used that may be confusing or not clear to the client. Health care programs should be tailored to older adult needs and use of different techniques to present materials. Proper instruction may lead to clear improvements in memory processing and problem solving.

Employment

Successful aging means making plans that include continued employment, semiretirement, or retirement. Planning and setting priorities reduces stress. Retirement can be a time of enjoyment when activities are planned that balance solitary and group work. Adapting to physiological, social, and emotional changes can be accomplished through planning.

Employment has a different meaning for different individuals, but work usually has a special focal point for meeting many of life's needs. Older adults need support in their decisions to retire completely from the work environment or seek employment. The outcome depends on each person's view of retirement (Pritchard, 1996). Individuals who worked as unskilled workers often viewed their job as primarily a means of income and friendships, while professionals and skilled workers often valued their jobs as a chance for personal rewards, enhanced self-concept, and self-expression. Work fulfills the need for income but also for social relationships and a sense of identity and personal worth. The type of job an individual had often affects that person's desire to seek employment opportunities after retirement. It may also affect the way retirement is perceived: as a crisis or a welcome relief from work. Because work affords material, psychological, and social satisfaction, retirement can make individuals feel lonely and depressed.

According to U.S. government statistics, about 3.7 million older Americans (12%) were in the labor force in 1998, including 2.2 million men and 1.6 million women. More older adults are in some employment, but many prefer part-time employment after retirement. In 1998, approximately 54% of workers over age 65 were employed part time: 48% of the men and 62% of the women (*A Profile,* 1999). Although the policy for retirement has changed and raised the age from 65 to 67 by the year 2022 for full Social Security benefits, many older adults are retiring early with pension plans that encourage early retirement. The potential for remaining in the work force longer is possible because of the low unemployment rates in 2000.

Many older adults are willing and able to participate in volunteer work as a means to provide a community service and to fulfill unmet self-esteem needs not found in retirement. Because work may have played a pivotal role in an older adult's life, retirement may adversely affect feelings of well-being. Volunteering services offer many opportunities to provide skills without the continuous commitment of employment and meet the developmental level of generativity. Many communities have a federal initiative called a **Retired Senior Volunteer Program (RSVP)** in which older adults can select and be trained for specific volunteer activities.

Social and Political Activities

Older adults can find social involvement and social support from a variety of groups in various locations. Participation in such groups offers both physiological and psychological benefits. Many communities or agencies provide transportation to senior centers or for other events that are government supported, free, or a low fee. Older adults can be involved in as many activities as they choose. Many health-promoting community events are planned for the older adults and encourage their participation. Older adults adapt best when they exercise personal selection and control over the events they attend.

Older adults can be a powerful political force. People age 65 and older vote more than any other age group (Senior Watch, ND). Older adults have varied political interests, and as the educational level of older adult cohorts increases, so will their involvement in social and political issues. The AARP is very active, at both the state and federal levels, in influencing legislation that will affect older people.

Think About It

Why are many older people active and influential in social political issues?

Summary

Successful aging is a part of a planned health program. Essential components of successful aging are nutrition, exercise, support systems, and various types of activities. The nature of aging is multidimensional and can be utilized by health care providers as a means to promote a healthy lifestyle.

As the fastest growing segment of the American population, successful aging of people age 65 and older challenges health care providers to promote living a quality life. Older adults are the most diverse group of individuals in our society; yet, some of their health needs are universal. The biological, social, and physical environment and sensory functioning are issues that can be approached by healthy interventions.

Review Questions and Activities

1. What are the major components of successful aging?

2. Discuss ways to promote successful aging in an older adult population.

3. How are nutritional needs different for older adults?

4. What are the effects of a regular exercise program?

5. What effect does a support system or significant other have on successful aging?

6. What are two major factors that determine whether an older adult will want to be employed?

7. What role does formal and informal education have in the life of an older adult?

8. What kinds of group activities are helpful to older adults?

9. Describe the roles health care providers can assume in relation to nutrition, social support systems, activities, and exercise.

10. Develop an exercise program for an older adult using the principles of adult learning and taking into consideration their unique physiological changes.

References

Allison, M., & Keller, C. (1997). Physical activity in the elderly: Benefits and intervention strategies. *Nurse Practitioner: American Journal of Primary Health Care, 22*(8), 53–54, 56, 58.

A profile of older Americans: 1999. (1999). Washington, DC: American Association of Retired Persons and the Administration on Aging, U.S. Department of Health and Human Services.

Bender, D. A., & Bender A. E. (1997). *Nutrition: A reference handbook.* New York: Oxford University Press.

Blaylock, B. (1991). Mobility and ambulation: Not easy tasks for all older adults. *Advancing Clinical Care, 6*(6), 20–21.

Centers for Disease Control. (1997). Years of potential life lost before age 65. United States 1990 and 1991, *Morbidity and Mortality Weekly Report 42*(13), 252–253.

Chandler, J. M., & Hadley, E. C. (1996). Exercise to improve physiologic and functional performance in old age. *Clinics in Geriatric Medicine, 12*(4), 761–784.

Harris, N. G. (2000). Nutrition in aging. In L. K. Mahan & S. Escott-Stump (Eds.), *Food, nutrition & diet therapy* (pp. 287–305). Philadelphia: Saunders.

Hellman, E. A., & Williams, M. A. (1994). Outpatient cardiac rehabilitation in elderly patients. *Heart and Lung: Journal of Critical Care, 23*(6), 506–514.

Hopp, J. F. (1993). Effects of age and resistance training on skeletal muscle: A review. *Physical Therapy, 73*(6), 361–373.

Katz, S., Down, T. D., Cash, H. R., et al. (1970). *The Gerontologist, 10,* 20–30.

Lawton, M. P., & Brody, E. M. (1969). Assessment of older people self-maintaining and instrumental activities of daily living. *The Gerontologist, 9,* 179–185.

Morley, J. E., Flood, J. F., Perry, H. M., & Kumar, V. B. (1997). Peptides, memory, food intake and aging. *Aging, 9*(4), 17–18.

Norton, B. (1998). From teaching to learning. Theoretical foundations. In D. M. Billings & J. A. Halstead (Eds.), *Teaching in nursing: A guide for faculty* (pp. 211–245). Philadelphia: Saunders.

Phillips, W. J., Cassmeyer, V. L., Sands, J. K., & Lehman, M. K. (1995). *Medical-surgical nursing: Concepts and clinical practice* (pp. 73–74). St. Louis: Mosby.

Pritchard, P. (1996). There is life after work. *Practice Nurse, 11*(6), 373–375.

Sugar, J., & Marinelli, R. D. (1997). Healthful aging: A social perspective. *Activities, Adaptation and Aging 21*(4), 1–11.

U.S. Department of Agriculture. (1992, revised 1996). *Food guide pyramid: A guide to daily food choices.* Washington, DC: USDA/HNIS.

Who votes? Older Americans! (N.D.) *Senior Watch.* Families USA Foundation.

Zauszniewski, J. A. (1995). Self-help and help-seeking behavior patterns in healthy elders. *Journal of Holistic Nursing, 14*(3), 223–236.

Resources

American Dietetic Association: **www.eatright.org**

Extended Care: **www.elderconnect.com**

UNIT 3

Holistic Health Care

PERSPECTIVE...

Mrs. J. is a 50-year old mother of seven children. Four of her children are married and have children of their own. Three of them are teenagers living at home. Both Mrs. J. and her husband are employed full time. Mrs. J.'s mother, who is 70, had been healthy until recently, when she had a mild heart attack, and is recovering in the home of her daughter and husband. Mrs. J.'s mother had been under stress for several years because she had been caring for her mother, who is 92, in her own home. All of these circumstances demonstrate the increasing prevalence of five-generation families living in one home. Mrs. J. will need to care for her grandmother and mother as well as provide the needs and supervision of her three teenagers at home and a grandchild who recently had an accident requiring surgery. Reflect on the needs of this family, especially Mrs. J. This is a typical example of some of the problems and concerns of the sandwich generation syndrome and informal caregiving, which are discussed in this unit.

CHAPTER 9

Geriatric Nutrition

Dianne M. Chiu, RD, LD

COMPETENCIES

After completing this chapter, the reader should be able to:

- *Discuss the role of nutrition in maintaining a healthy body.*
- *Evaluate the energy requirements, realizing that kilocalorie needs may decrease with inactivity and increasing age.*
- *Evaluate the importance of meeting the nutrient requirements for the older adult.*
- *Identify standards and food guides available for promotion of healthy eating.*
- *Explore the impact of socioeconomic, psychological, cultural, religious, and physiological factors on food intake.*
- *Identify chronic diseases that may occur as a result of inadequate nutrition in older adults.*
- *Provide suggestions for feeding patients who cannot feed themselves.*
- *Identify resources available that can assist in supplying food and other help to those who need assistance.*
- *Provide guidelines for planning healthy meals.*
- *Identify ideas for making the food dollar go further while not reducing calories.*

MAKING THE CONNECTION

Refer to the following chapters to increase your understanding of geriatric nutrition:

- **Chapter 11** *Wellness and Health Promotion*
- **Chapter 12** *Health Education*
- **Chapter 13** *Assessment, Diagnosis, and Planning*
- **Chapter 14** *Major Diseases of Older Adults*
- **Chapter 15** *Acute-Care Issues*
- **Chapter 16** *Chronic Illness*
- **Chapter 17** *Management of Medications*
- **Chapter 18** *Mental Health Issues*
- **Chapter 24** *Community Organizations and Services*

Nutritional Considerations

The nutrition and health status of the older population has become a great concern of health care professionals. The focus on nutrition for this population has become significant because of the predicted increase in the number and proportion of the older population and the increase in life expectancy. Concern about malnutrition in older adults is growing as health care providers and researchers realize how poorly many older Americans eat. It has been estimated that one-third to one-half of the health problems experienced by older individuals are directly or indirectly related to nutritional problems (Food and Nutrition for Life, 1994). Adequate nutritional care for the older adult deserves considerable emphasis, because the well-nourished older adult will not only be more comfortable and energetic but will also be better able to tolerate medical and surgical treatment when it is necessary.

Nutrition is important in the aging process. It is not enough merely to survive into the years from 60 to 100; they should be years of health, enjoyment, and mental vigor. The intake of food is one of the greatest variables in life. People have an instinctive appetite for the pleasure of eating, but the desire for food does not necessarily ensure availability, adequate intake, or nutritional balance. The food eaten must furnish the building materials from which muscles, organs, teeth, blood, and all other body components are made and repaired. Regardless of a person's age, it is necessary for nutrients to be converted into energy, supply substrates for enzymes and hormones, and regulate and control body functions. Because people do not age physically at the same rate as chronologically, the older population cannot be classified as a homogeneous group. Each older adult is an individual, and the health professional must be very careful to avoid stereotyping older adults (see Figure 9-1).

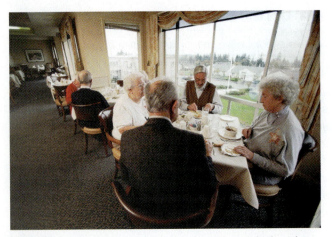

FIGURE 9-1 Nutritional considerations are important in the aging process.

Energy

Although nutritional requirements remain similar no matter what one's age, the kilocaloric requirements decrease with age. However, disease and ill health in many older adults may actually increase their need for some nutrients while reducing the efficiency of their nutrient digestion, absorption, and metabolism. The unit for measuring energy is the **kilocalorie** (commonly referred to as the **calorie**), the amount of heat or energy required to raise the temperature of one kilogram of water one degree Celsius. The number of calories needed is determined by (a) the number of calories necessary for basal metabolism, (b) the number of calories needed for muscular activity, and (c) the number of calories required for the digestion and absorption of food.

The calorie requirements decrease with age because of a reduction in the number of metabolically active cells. This is because of an increase in the proportion of body weight that is adipose tissue, along with the reduction in **lean body mass,** such as muscle tissue and bone. The calorie requirements are usually diminished by 10% in people aged 51–75 and 20%–25% in those older than 75 (Roe, 1991a). However, there are large variations in the need for calories according to age, size, occupation, environment, physical activity habits, and the presence or absence of chronic illness. The Harris Benedict Equation—**basal energy expenditure (BEE)**—is sometimes used to estimate basal calories needed for older individuals (Box 9-1). This equation has factors for both age and gender and is therefore a more accurate method for calculating needed calories (Taaffe, Thompson, & Butterfield, 1995). The basal calorie result is multiplied by a factor, depending on the individual's physical status and activity level to obtain recommended energy intake (calories):

BOX 9-1   Harris-Benedict Equation

Female: $BEE = 65.1 + (9.6 \times \text{weight in kg}) + (1.8 \times \text{height in cm}) - (4.7 \times \text{age})$

Male: $BEE = 66.5 + (13.8 \times \text{weight in kg}) + (5 \times \text{height in cm}) - (6.8 \times \text{age})$

W = weight in kilograms (kg)
  (weight in pounds ÷ 2.2 = kg)
H = height in centimeters (cm)
  (height in inches × 2.54 = cm)
A = age in years

If averages are used, the **recommended dietary allowance (RDA)** for calories beyond age 60 for men of reference size (77 kg) is 2,300 calories per day; for women of reference size (65 kg) it is 1,900 calories per day. The normal variation plus or minus 20% is accepted (*Recommended dietary allowances,* 1989).

There is obviously a need for further reduction in the calorie intake of an immobilized older adult in bed. The lower intake of calories poses the problem of obtaining sufficient nutrients (protein, carbohydrate, fat). The diet of the geriatric client has much less room for so-called **empty calories** received from high-calorie, low-nutrient dense foods. These foods may be inexpensive, easy to eat, and well liked, but foods containing large amounts of sweets, fats, and alcohol are examples of empty-calorie foods that should be consumed in limited quantities. It has been determined that for each 3,500 calories eaten and not burned, a person gains 1 pound of body weight. There must be a constant awareness of slight increases in weight, because it is much easier to maintain normal weight than to decrease it after the gain occurs. Obesity, characteristic of adult populations, persists into old age. After the age of 60, approximately 40% of all women and 30% of all men are overweight (Andres, 1990).

Increased physical activity is important for any person interested in maintaining good health. Not only does exercise help control weight, it also increases blood flow to all body organs, helping to keep them healthy; it helps maintain good muscle mass and slows atrophy associated with chronic disease; it helps avoid constipation problems; it allows for the consumption of more food that will provide more nutrients; it lowers blood sugar levels, often improving glucose tolerance; it is stimulating; and it may serve to lift an individual's spirits (Barry & Eathorne, 1994).

Proteins

Protein requirements must be met to maintain healthy tissue. Twelve to 14% of the calories in the average daily diet should be derived from protein. Foods such as meat, fish, eggs, poultry, milk, and cheese provide high-quality protein. Together with other protein foods (vegetables and grains) in the diet, this high-quality protein should meet the requirements of all older adults. If vegetable and grain proteins are served exclusively, it is necessary to check the amino acid composition of the foods. Good examples of complementary proteins are cornbread served with pinto beans, cereal with milk, bread with peanut butter, macaroni with cheese, and spaghetti with meat sauce. The daily RDA for protein of 0.8 g/kg body weight is accepted to be the same for the older adult as for young adults. Because of the difference in body composition, this allowance is higher per unit of lean body mass in an older adult and should allow for some decrease in utilization efficiency (*Recommended dietary allowances,* 1989). Clinical conditions

such as severe infections, fever, surgery, or skin breakdown (pressure ulcers) lead to increased protein requirements (Campbell, Crim, Dallal, Young, & Evans, 1994). The five important syndromes that result in part from protein deficiency in older adults are hunger, edema, nutritional liver disease, pellagra, and nutritional macrocytic anemia.

Fats

The Food and Nutrition Board of the National Research Council has been reluctant to make a dietary recommendation for fat. However, some fat must be included in the diet to (a) ensure the presence of essential fatty acids; (b) allow an adequate intake and utilization of the fat-soluble vitamins A, D, E, and K; and (c) serve as a lubricating agent (Food and Agriculture Organization, 1994). Fats are the most efficient (concentrated) form of energy with twice the energy content per gram as carbohydrates and proteins. Dietary fat is primarily responsible for the feeling of being satiated by food. It also

Research Focus

Citation:
Diehr, P., Bild, D. E., Harris, T. B., Duxbury, A., Siscovick, D., & Ross, M. (1998). Body mass index and mortality in non smoking older adults: The Cardiovascular Health Study. *American Journal of Public Health, 88*(4), 623–629.

Purpose:
To study the relationship between body-mass index (BMI) and 5-year mortality.

Methods:
Body-mass index and 5-year death rate for 2,410 women and 1,907 men age 65–100 (mean age 73) were analyzed using logistic regression analysis.

Findings:
Women with the lowest BMI at the beginning of the study (≤20) had the highest 5-year mortality rate (17%) and those with a BMI between 30 and 32 had a 6.9% mortality rate. Substantial and unintended weight loss after age 50 could indicate poor prognosis. There was no significant association for men.

Implications:
Obesity may provide some protection for women in old age because of the nutritional reserve it provides when stress occurs and protection from acute injury and trauma.

improves the flavor of many foods, making them more appetizing and appealing, which can be important for those who have a decreased appetite.

The desirable fat intake for older adults does not differ from that of younger adults. To retard atherogenesis, the American Heart Association (1994) recommends that the total fat intake be limited to 30% or less of the total energy intake, the saturated fat intake be limited to 10%–15% of the total energy intake, and cholesterol intake be limited to 300 mg/day or less.

Carbohydrates

There must be an adequate intake of carbohydrates (a) to prevent the breakdown of tissue protein, (b) to maintain normal levels of blood glucose for the central nervous system, and (c) to make up calorie deficits. Dietary guidelines published for the public by various agencies recommend that carbohydrates contribute 50%–58% of the total energy intake. Concentrated (simple) sweets should account for no more than 10% of the total calories. Food intake studies have demonstrated that most older adults do not choose to eat fresh fruits and vegetables. It is not known whether this is related to early dietary habits, expense, or difficulty in storage and preparation. It is important that the diet of the older individual include more complex carbohydrates such as fruits, vegetables, cereals, and breads and fewer simple sugars such as candy, sugar, jams, jellies, preserves, and syrups.

Older adults are susceptible to the development of diabetes, pancreatic malfunction, decreased cellular sensitivity to insulin, and glucose intolerance. Lactose in milk products poses a difficult problem; intolerance to this disaccharide is being recognized more frequently in older adults, although the reason is unknown. One should always ascertain if an older adult can drink milk and eat dairy products without intestinal discomfort (Lee & Krasinski, 1998).

Fiber

Fiber can play a crucial role in bowel maintenance in the older adult. Decrease in gastrointestinal (GI) motility is a common physical change during the aging process. This decrease can contribute to gastrointestinal distress and constipation. Coupled with a diet low in fiber, decreased GI motility can lead to GI problems such as constipation and **diverticulosis.** The recommended daily intake of fiber is 25–35 g. The average American consumes only about 11 g of fiber daily. Many older individuals can increase the fiber in their diets by following the simple guidelines shown in Box 9-2. The older adult should make any of these changes slowly. Adding too much fiber or not drinking enough fluid can cause bloating, gas, and other uncomfortable symptoms.

Vitamins

Vitamins are unrelated compounds needed in minute amounts in the diet. They are essential for specific metabolic reactions in the cells and for normal growth and maintenance of health. Vitamins regulate metabolism, help convert fat and carbohydrate into energy, and assist in forming bones and tissues. Vitamin deficiencies can be one of the most frequent and serious nutritional problems affecting older adults. Adequate intake of vitamins is essential at all age levels for optimal mental, emotional, and physical health. Older adults with a food energy intake of less that 1,500 calories should probably take a vitamin-mineral supplement (Whitney, Hamilton, & Rolfes, 1990). Taking supplements in quantities that exceed the recommended amount of each vitamin is of no value, and excessive dosages may actually be harmful.

Many older adults use vitamin and mineral supplements. Studies on vitamin supplementation in this population revealed that the supplements taken were not always the nutrients that were most likely to be deficient in the diet. The most often supplemented vitamins and minerals are vitamin C, magnesium, vitamin E, and calcium (Schellhorn, Doring, & Stieber, 1998). Patients should be warned against self-medication with high-potency vitamin preparations. Long-term megadosing with vitamins A and D can result in toxicity and should be discouraged.

Attention should be directed to the amount of money being spent on vitamin supplements, because older adults who have limited incomes may be spending money that would be better spent on nutritious food. They need to keep in mind that food is the best source of nutrients for everyone and that supplements should be used only as supplements to food, not substitution for it. Administration of specific vitamins should be based on need, defined by clinical and biochemical assessment of nutritional status. Older adults should then be given specific instructions about taking vitamin supplements and not just told to take a multivitamin pill.

Fat-Soluble Vitamins

Vitamins A, D, E, and K are **fat-soluble vitamins.** These vitamins are soluble in lipids and insoluble in water. They are absorbed along with dietary fats. Conditions interfering with fat absorption will also interfere with absorption of the fat-soluble vitamins. They can be stored in the body and are not normally excreted in the urine; therefore, excessive supplementation can lead to toxicity.

Vitamin A (retinol)

It is not surprising that dietary surveys and biochemical investigations of older clients have indicated inadequate intakes of vitamin A. Vitamin A, one of the fat-soluble vitamins, is derived either from preformed vitamin A

(retinol) or from provitamin A **(carotenoids).** Vitamin A performs important functions in the body, such as maintaining the skin and mucous membrane (lining of the nose and mouth) and protecting against night blindness. The overt manifestations of vitamin A deficiency occur only after the disease is moderately well advanced. The main external target sites are the eyes and the skin. Loss of visual acuity in dim light (night blindness) and drying of the surface of the conjunctiva **(xerophthalmia)** usually are the only eye changes associated with vitamin A deficiency in older adults. The dermatologic changes resulting from vitamin A deficiency create a dry, rough skin.

Until recently the activity of vitamin A was expressed in **international units (IU),** but this value has been changed to **retinol equivalents (RE).** This unit of measure allows for the variable absorption and conversion of the carotenoids, which were not considered in the previous method. During a period of transition, both IU an RE will be used. The daily RDA for vitamin A is 1,000 RE (5,000 IU) for men and 800 RE (4,000 IU) for women (*Recommended dietary allowances,* 1989). The best food sources of vitamin A are liver, fortified margarine, eggs, butter, and whole milk. Dark green and yellow vegetables, such as broccoli, chard, collard greens, spinach, turnip greens, carrots, pumpkin, sweet potatoes, winter squash, apricots, and cantaloupe are the best sources of carotene, which the body converts into vitamin A. There is no danger of a toxic level of vitamin A from food sources.

The habitual use of mineral oil as a laxative has been known to decrease the absorption of fat-soluble vitamins and results in a vitamin A deficiency. However, excessive vitamin A can also be dangerous. Since such excesses are not excreted by the body and are degraded slowly, they are stored and can have a serious toxic effect. Symptoms of hypervitaminosis A are headache, nausea, and irritability. Other symptoms include enlargement of the liver and spleen, hair loss, and rheumatic pain. Large doses of vitamin A can lead to the development of intracranial pressure that mimics a brain tumor. Toxic levels are reached not by the intake of food but from excessive supplementation.

Vitamin D

Vitamin D is known to aid in the absorption of calcium and phosphorus in bone formation, which is an important aspect of bone integrity for older adults. The deficiency disease is **osteomalacia** (adult rickets), which results in softening of bones causing weakness and fractures. People exposed to sunlight need no other source of vitamin D because it can be formed in the skin by ultraviolet rays. Foods fortified with vitamin D are intended mainly for infants and for older adults who cannot be exposed to sunlight. Vitamin D also aids in

the absorption of calcium. Too much vitamin D causes nausea, weight loss, excessive urination and calcification of soft tissue. Good sources are milk and sunlight and the RDA is 400 IU daily.

Vitamin E (tocopherol)

Vitamin E belongs to a group of compounds called **tocopherols,** which are naturally occurring alcohols that have antioxidant and specific biologic properties. Recent research on vitamin E suggests that there may be a relationship between vitamin E supplementation and reduced colon cancer risk (White, Shannon, & Patterson, 1997); that vitamin E may have a role in the maintenance of the immune system (Beharak, Redican, Leka, & Meydani, 1997); and that the aging, physically active person may benefit from vitamin E supplementation (Meydani et al., 1998). Additionally, new research also suggests a strong link between vitamin E supplementation and prevention of atherosclerosis by retardation of low-density lipoprotein (LDL) oxidation, inhibition of platelet adhesion, and aggregation and attenuation of synthesis of leukotrienes (Chan, 1998). One study suggested that coronary artery

---

BOX 9-2 Suggestions for Increasing Fiber in the Diet

- Eat fresh fruits and vegetables. If the older adult has difficulty chewing raw fruits and vegetables, gently steamed vegetables and soft fruits are appropriate.

- Eat some of the skins of potatoes, apples, pears, and other fruits or vegetables. The outer portion of these foods contains fiber and valuable nutrients.

- Use whole-grain breads and cereals instead of refined white bread and sugary cereals. Instead of meat, add beans (navy, lima, kidney, pinto), all of which are high in fiber and can also be a less expensive source of protein. Beans can also be used in casseroles, soups, stews, and other dishes.

- Try unbuttered air-popped popcorn or the reduced/low-fat versions of microwave popcorn for a snack.

- Remember how important it is to increase the water in the diet when the fiber content is increased. At least eight cups of liquid are needed each day.

- Keep moving; being active helps bowel regularity.

disease clients have existing suboptimal tocopherol levels compared to normal controls, which may be an important risk factor for atherogenesis and coronary artery disease (Dube, Khalsa, Gupta, Singh, & Sharma, 1998). All researchers recommend additional study as to the mechanism and dosage of vitamin E that may be effective. The daily RDA of vitamin E is 8 mg of α-tocopherol equivalent (TE) for women and 10 mg of TE for men (*Recommended dietary allowances,* 1989). Because vitamin E is a fat-soluble vitamin, it can be stored in the liver; however, the commonly recommended 800–1,000 IU daily is generally considered safe. The long-term effect of this dose is currently under investigation. Vitamin E is present in vegetable oils, whole grains, dark, leafy vegetables, nuts, and legumes.

Vitamin K

Vitamin K is essential for the formation of prothrombin and is necessary for proper clotting of blood. There are several forms of vitamin K. Vitamin K_1 is found in foods of animal and vegetable origin. Foods rich in vitamin K_1 include liver and green leafy vegetables, such as spinach, broccoli, and brussels sprouts. Vitamin K_2 is synthesized by the intestinal bacteria. Antibiotics interfere with the synthesis of vitamin K_2. Prolonged use of mineral oil interferes with the absorption of vitamins K_1 and K_2. The human requirement for vitamin K is 1 g/kg body weight/day (*Recommended dietary allowances,* 1989). If older adults eat a variety of foods, including green vegetables, and are not on prolonged use of antibiotics or mineral oil, there is no evidence to indicate a need for vitamin K supplementation (Roe, 1987).

Water-Soluble Vitamins

Water-soluble vitamins are not normally stored in the body in significant amounts; a daily supply is desired to avoid depletion and interruption of physiologic functions. Water-soluble vitamins include the B vitamins and vitamin C. Most water-soluble vitamins are components of essential enzyme systems and are normally excreted in small quantities in the urine. Toxicity is generally not a problem with water-soluble vitamins because they are not stored in appreciable quantity in the body.

Thiamin

Thiamin has an important role in the process that changes glucose to energy. It functions as a part of a **coenzyme** that is necessary for the action of enzymes and is indispensable in carbohydrate metabolism, providing a supply of energy to the nerves and brain. Thiamin also appears to be essential for fat and protein metabolism. The most common signs of thiamin deficiency are mental confusion, peripheral paralysis, loss of ankle and knee-jerk reflexes, weakness, painful calf

muscles, edema, and enlarged heart. Poorly balanced or highly refined diets, stress, alcoholism, and impaired intestinal absorption are most often the precipitating factors in thiamin deficiency. Based on dietary recall studies, thiamin intakes of most healthy independent older adults in the United States have been judged adequate. The daily RDA is 0.5 mg of thiamin per 1,000 calories (*Recommended dietary allowances,* 1989). Important food sources of thiamin are whole-grain products, enriched flour, organ meats, pork, and legumes.

Riboflavin

Riboflavin is an essential component of enzymes important in energy metabolism. A deficiency of riboflavin results in dermatitis, lesions around the mouth and nose, hypersensitivity to light, and reddening of the cornea. The best food sources of riboflavin are liver, milk, leafy vegetables, whole grains, and enriched breads. The daily RDA is 0.6 mg of riboflavin per 1,000 calories (*Recommended dietary allowances,* 1989). Deficiency of riboflavin is often associated with high-carbohydrate diets lacking in animal protein milk and vegetables.

Niacin

Niacin is a functional component of coenzymes that is essential for the release of energy from carbohydrates, fats, and proteins. It also plays a significant role in the synthesis of fats and proteins. Niacin is best known for its prevention of pellagra. Pellagra affects the gastrointestinal tract, the skin, and the nervous system. The symptoms of deficiency include fatigue, listlessness, headache, loss of weight, loss of appetite, diarrhea, dermatitis, and mental confusion.

Vitamin B_6 (pyridoxine)

Vitamin B_6 is actually three closely related chemical compounds—pyridoxine, pyridoxal, and pyridosamine—that serve as coenzymes for biological functions involving amino acid metabolism and protein synthesis. It is poorly absorbed by persons with liver disease and is commonly deficient in people with uremia and gastrointestinal disease. Because these conditions are often present in older adults, these relationships should be monitored.

The drug dihydroxyphenylalanine (L-dopa), a neurotransmitter, is used in the treatment of Parkinson's disease. Pyridoxine enhances the conversion of L-dopa to dopamine. Because dopamine cannot cross the blood-brain barrier, such conversion may result in nullification of the therapeutic effects of the drug. Therefore persons on L-dopa drug therapy should avoid taking vitamin supplements containing vitamin B_6. The daily RDAs are 1.6 mg for women and 2.0 mg for men (*Recommended dietary allowances,* 1989). Sources of vitamin B_6 are rice, bran, beans, potatoes, and bananas.

Vitamin B₁₂ (Cyanocobalamin)

The most severe form of vitamin B₁₂ deficiency is pernicious anemia. An absence of the intrinsic factor and free hydrochloric acid in gastric juice in some older clients prevents the intestinal absorption of vitamin B₁₂. The deficiency state is characterized by weakness, glossitis, numbness and tingling of the extremities, and macrocytic anemia. If a vitamin B₁₂ deficiency becomes evident because of changes in gastric acidity, a malabsorption syndrome with partial or total removal of the stomach or ileum, or taking drugs that interfere with the uptake of vitamin B₁₂, the vitamin should be administered by injection (intramuscularly).

The daily RDA is 2 μg (*Recommended dietary allowances,* 1989). The best food sources of the vitamin are beef, liver, kidney, whole milk, eggs, oysters, fresh shrimp, pork, and chicken. Because plants are unable to synthesize vitamin B₁₂, it can be found only in food of animal origin.

Folacin (Folic Acid)

Folic acid (or folacin) is important in the metabolism of a number of amino and nucleic acids and especially in hemoglobin synthesis. This vitamin's activities are interrelated with those of vitamin B₁₂. The most notable effect of folic acid deficiency is macrocytic anemia stemming from changes in the bone marrow megaloblasts. A low serum folic acid level is associated with mental disorders. Folic acid intake is frequently reported as low among older adults.

Anticonvulsant drugs frequently used by older adults are antagonistic to folic acid. Research indicates that approximately 80% of all alcoholics are deficient in folic acid (Shils, Olson, Shike, & Ross, 1999). There is no good evidence that alcohol has a direct effect on folic acid metabolic pathways. Evidence does show that alcohol produces transitory malabsorption of folate (Shils et al., 1999).

The daily RDA for folic acid is 200 μg for men and 180 μg for women (*Recommended dietary allowances,* 1989). Folic acid is available in liver, kidney, yeast, and deep green, leafy vegetables.

Vitamin C (Ascorbic Acid)

The requirement for vitamin C for the geriatric client is still being researched. Because the body cannot synthesize vitamin C, the deficiency state in the older population could be critical. Some people develop an aversion to *acid foods* that brings on heartburn and thus restricts their intakes of vitamin C (Hamilton, Whitney, & Sizer, 1991). There are some reports of low vitamin C intake among older adults (Food and Nutrition for Life, 1994).

The primary function of vitamin C is to promote growth and repair of tissues, including the healing of

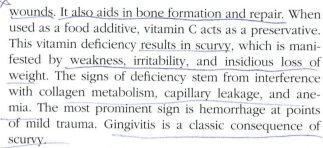

wounds. It also aids in bone formation and repair. When used as a food additive, vitamin C acts as a preservative. This vitamin deficiency results in scurvy, which is manifested by weakness, irritability, and insidious loss of weight. The signs of deficiency stem from interference with collagen metabolism, capillary leakage, and anemia. The most prominent sign is hemorrhage at points of mild trauma. Gingivitis is a classic consequence of scurvy.

The RDA is 60 mg for men and women (*Recommended dietary allowances,* 1989). Food sources rich in vitamin C are citrus fruits, tomatoes, strawberries, and green vegetables such as cabbage, broccoli, collards, mustard greens, and turnip greens. This vitamin has received much publicity. Research studies that large amounts of vitamin C can cure or prevent the common cold have not been validated.

Minerals

Minerals are elements in simple inorganic form found in the body. They include calcium, phosphorus, magnesium, sodium, potassium, iodine, iron, and zinc. Minerals compose approximately 4 to 5 percent of body weight. There are 22 mineral elements known to be essential in human nutrition. Minerals have many essential roles in the body, including regulation of metabolism via enzymes, maintenance of acid-base balance and osmotic pressure, facilitation of membrane transfer of essential compounds, and maintenance of nerve and muscular irritability. Some mineral elements are building components of body tissues and are indirectly involved in the growth process.

Calcium

Calcium is the most abundant mineral in the human body. Ninety-nine percent of the body's calcium is found in bones and teeth as calcium salts (hydroxyapatite). The remaining 1% exists in the blood, other body fluids, and various soft tissues. Calcium is necessary for the proper mineralization of bone. It is important in the growth and maintenance of the skeleton and also plays an important role in blood clotting, cell wall permeability, muscle contractility, micromuscular transmission, and cardiac function. The function of calcium is closely related to that of phosphorus and vitamin D. The ratio of calcium to phosphorus in the diet should be 1:1 and certainly no greater than 1:2. If phosphorous levels are too high, the calcium is withdrawn from the bone to restore equilibrium. Vitamin D must be present for calcium to be absorbed. The daily RDA of calcium for people 60 years of age and above is 1,200 mg (Food and Nutrition Board, 1997); see Table 9-1 for current recommendations for calcium intake. A number of age-related physiological and lifestyle

TABLE 9-1   Recommended Calcium Intake (mg/day)

National Academy of Sciences (1997)		National Institutes of Health (1994)	
Age	**Recommended Calcium Intake**	**Age**	**Recommended Calcium Intake**
Birth–6 months	210	Birth–6 months	400
6 months–1 year	270	6 months–1 year	600
1–3 years	500	1–10	800–1,200
4–8 years	800	11–24	1,200–1,500
9–13 years	1,300	25–50 (women and men)	1,000
14–18 years	1,300	51–64 (women on hormone therapy and men)	1,500
19–30 years	1,000	51+ (women not on hormone therapy)	1,500
31–50 years	1,000	65 or older	1,500
51–70 years	1,200		

From Dietary Reference Intakes for Calcium, Phosphorus, Magnesium, Vitamin D, and Fluoride *(pp. 71–144)*, by the Food and Nutrition Board, Institute of Medicine, 1997, Washington, DC: Author; Optimal Calcium Intake, *by the National Institutes of Health, 1994, Washington, DC: Author.*

changes can increase the need for calcium. Menopause, illness, drug-nutrient interactions, low exposure to sunlight, lactose deficiency, and a decrease in physical activity either directly or indirectly decrease the intestinal absorption of calcium and effectively increase the requirements for this mineral.

Osteoporosis (loss of bone mass), osteomalacia (demineralization of bone, known as adult rickets), and hypertension may all be related in part to calcium deficiencies. Although the cause of osteoporosis is not understood completely, there is substantial evidence that the disease involves marked changes in calcium and vitamin D metabolism. For example, postmenopausal women do not absorb dietary calcium as efficiently as do younger women. There is also a drop in calcium absorption in men, but this is less significant and occurs at a later age.

One of the best ways to prevent or treat diseases related to calcium deficiency is to increase the consumption of calcium-rich foods. Milk and other dairy products are the major dietary sources of calcium. For individuals who cannot consume milk and other dairy products, calcium supplementation may be recommended.

Phosphorus

The daily RDA for phosphorus is 800 mg for men and women (*Recommended dietary allowances,* 1989). The 1:1 ratio of calcium to phosphorus with the updated recommendations for calcium daily would increase this amount. Phosphorus is available from a variety of foods; deficient intakes are unlikely. Older adults taking large amounts of antacids may have increased excretion of phosphorus, which could result in deficiency.

Magnesium

The daily RDA for magnesium is 350 mg for men and women (*Recommended dietary allowances,* 1989). No evidence exists for an increased need with aging. Severe loss of body fluid, malabsorption, and liver disease are the conditions that may lead to a deficiency. Dehydration is the most likely factor in older adults. Magnesium is widely available from the food supply, so a deficiency is unlikely to occur.

Sodium

Sodium is the principal electrolyte in extracellular fluid for the maintenance of normal osmotic pressure and water balance. Sodium intake requires particular attention because many older adults have hypertension and are taking antihypertensive medications. Such persons are usually cautioned to reduce their intake of sodium. An adequate intake of sodium is 1,100–3,300 mg daily, about half the amount that most adults generally ingest. Recent research suggests that sodium restriction may only be necessary for those individuals considered "sodium sensitive" or approximately 10%–30% of hypertensive individuals (Elliott et al., 1996).

Potassium

Potassium is required for enzymatic reactions within the cell. Potassium deficiencies are not primarily dietary in origin. They may occur in malnutrition, chronic alcoholism, or any illness that seriously interferes with appetite. Any condition that reduces the availability of nutrients for absorption, such as prolonged vomiting, gastric drainage, or diarrhea, may lead to a potassium deficiency.

Diuretic drugs sometimes release the sodium in the extracellular fluid, in turn depleting the potassium within the cell. On the other hand, rapid infusions of glucose and insulin used in treating diabetic acidosis bring about such rapid shifts of potassium into the cell that the plasma potassium content may be reduced to levels that could bring about cardiac failure. Meat, poultry, fish, oranges, bananas, and celery are rich sources of potassium.

Iodine

Iodine is an essential nutrient that must be available for the synthesis of the thyroid hormones (thyroxine and triiodothyronine). The public health measure of adding iodine to table salt has helped protect people from developing endemic goiter. The daily RDA for iodine in both men and women is set at 150 μg (*Recommended dietary allowances,* 1989).

Iron

Iron deficiency is relatively common in older adults because of decreased intake or absorption or both (Shils et al., 1999). The most common symptom of iron deficiency in older adults is nutritional anemia, which is characterized by fatigue, weakness, irritability, dizziness, pale skin color, and sore mouth and tongue. The daily RDA for iron is 10 mg for men and women age 60 and older (*Recommended dietary allowances,* 1989).

There appear to be considerable differences in the absorption of iron from different foods. Iron is more efficiently absorbed from muscle and hemoglobin (e.g., red meats and organ meats) than from vegetables and eggs. Iron in whole wheat is better absorbed than iron from enriched bread in spite of the phytate content. Conversely, iron in eggs is poorly absorbed, but its absorption can be enhanced by the addition of orange juice. A superimposed iron deficiency anemia can be a serious handicap in an older adult with an already impaired, atherosclerotic circulation. The need for iron may be increased in the older adult because of mild bleeding from hemorrhoids or other gastrointestinal lesions. Sufficient iron-containing foods such as green leafy vegetables, meat, and egg yolk should be incorporated into the daily diet.

Zinc

Zinc is a component of more than 80 metalloenzymes and proteins that may have catalytic or structural functions. It is an important factor in the synthesis of deoxyribonucleic acid, ribonucleic acid, and protein. It is thought to stabilize cell membranes. It is essential for growth and cell division, reproduction, taste acuity, wound healing, and normal immune function.

The daily RDA for adult men is 15 mg. The allowance for adult women, because of their lower body weight, is set at 12 mg (*Recommended dietary allowances,* 1989).

Although zinc is available from many foods, decreased absorption occurs with aging. Stresses, such as physical trauma, wounds (including surgery), burns, and muscle-wasting disease, all result in dramatic increases in urinary zinc losses. Many medications (both those sold over the counter and by prescription) used by older adults can affect zinc status. Diuretics, chelating agents, antacids, laxatives, and iron supplements may decrease absorption or increase excretion of zinc from the body (Chernoff, 1991).

Counseling of older adults should emphasize a varied diet of high nutrient density. Consumption of red meats, poultry, and fish will help ensure adequate zinc intake, because bioavailability of this nutrient is greater from animal foods than from those of plant origin. Among plant foods, legumes and grains are the most significant sources of zinc. For those on a vegetarian diet, consumption of these should be emphasized; vegetables and fruits have significantly lower levels of zinc.

Water

Although water is not often thought of as a food, it has been described as the indispensable nutrient. Without water, survival of a human being is considered limited to 4 days (Bidlack, 1996). Insufficient consumption of fluids, for whatever reason, may precipitate disaster in the organism more quickly than the lack of any other component. Maintenance of fluid balance is essential for the distribution of nutrients to the cellular units, the elimination of water, and the multiple physiochemical processes of life. Total body water decreases with age. In young males, 60% of total body weight is water, compared to 52% in the older male. In younger females 52% of total body weight is water, compared to 45% in older females. The normal adult gains and loses approximately 2,400 ml of fluids each day (Jaffe, 1991).

Six to eight 8-oz glasses of fluid per day will generally satisfy the water requirement. Older adults often find liquids more acceptable in soups, fruit juices, milk products, soft drinks, tea, and coffee. If the client has difficulty swallowing thin liquids, especially water, foods with the consistency of gelatin, fruit ices, yogurt, custards, or puddings may be more desirable. Also, a powdered substance may be obtained to thicken thin liquids so that they can be more easily swallowed. Water is still the best choice if it can be swallowed easily without choking.

Nutrient Standards and Food Guides for Health Promotion

Several standards are used to determine the amounts of nutrients, vitamins, minerals, and fluids individuals should consume to maintain health. These standards include the Recommended Dietary Allowances (RDA), the United States Recommended Daily Allowances (USRDA), the Food Guide Pyramid, and the Dietary Guidelines for Americans.

Recommended Dietary Allowances

The Food and Nutrition Board was organized in 1940 as a division of the National Academy of Sciences National Research Council. One of the projects of this group has been to establish a set of figures for human needs in terms of specific nutrients. *Recommended dietary allowances,* which has been referred to throughout the chapter, was first published in 1943. The most recent edition was published in 1989. *Recommended dietary allowances* lists the levels of intake of essential nutrients that, on the basis of scientific knowledge, are judged by the Food and Nutrition Board to be adequate to meet the known nutrient needs of practically all healthy persons.

Adults are divided into two age categories: 25–50 years and 51 years upward. The researchers agree that the older age groups need to be addressed separately. However, the committee concluded that data are insufficient at this time to establish separate RDAs for people 70 years of age and older.

This does not mean not that the RDAs should be rejected in terms of planning diets for older adults but that their limitations should be recognized and that the older adult's specific health status and problems should be considered. The RDAs are expressed in nutrients rather than in specific foods because these recommendations can be fulfilled by a variety of different food patterns.

United States Recommended Dietary Allowances

Recommended dietary allowances should not be confused with the U.S. recommended dietary allowances (USRDA). The USRDA standards were established by the Food and Drug Administration for the purpose of regulating nutrition labeling (Figure 9-2). Although the USRDA standards are derived from the National Research Council's dietary allowance, they encompass just a few broad categories. The guidelines for nutrition labeling are currently being revised, and there are strong indications that the guidelines will not be called the USRDA, to avoid the confusion between RDAs and USRDAs.

The Food Guide Pyramid

Because most people are not going to take the time to calculate their nutrient intake in terms of calories, proteins, fats, carbohydrates, minerals, and vitamins, *the food guide pyramid* (see Figure 9-3) has been prepared as a guide.

Each food group provides some but not all of the nutrients one needs. Foods in one group cannot replace

those in another. No one food group is more important than another—for good health one needs them all. It is a convenient plan designed to help a person plan an adequate diet. The food guide pyramid allows the menu planner to evaluate the daily intake of milk and milk products, meat, fruits, vegetables, and bread, grains, and cereals. Most older adults can name the food groups but are unable to give quantities of food that should be consumed within each group (see Table 9-2).

Dietary Guidelines for Americans

There has been increasing concern that overnutrition may be contributing to the illnesses many people have

Nutrition Facts
Serving Size 1/2 cup (114g)
Servings Per Container 4

Amount Per Serving

Calories 90	Calories from Fat 30

	% Daily Value
Total Fat 3g	**5%**
Saturated Fat 0g	**0%**
Cholesterol 0mg	**0%**
Sodium 300mg	**13%**
Total Carbohydrate 13g	**4%**
Dietary Fiber 3g	**12%**
Sugars 3g	
Protein 3g	

Vitamin A	80%	¥	Vitamin C	60%
Calcium	4%	¥	Iron	4%

¥ Percent Daily Values are based on a 2,000 calorie diet. Your daily values may be higher or lower depending on your calorie needs:

		Calories	2,000	2,500
Total Fat	Less than		65g	80g
Sat Fat	Less than		20g	25g
Cholesterol	Less than		300mg	300mg
Sodium	Less than		2,400mg	2,400mg
Total Carbohydrate			300g	375g
Fiber			25g	30g

Calories per gram:
Fat 9   ¥   Carbohydrate 4   ¥   Protein 4

FIGURE 9-2 Food labels, like this one, are the result of USRDA standards. *(Courtesy of the Food and Drug Administration)*

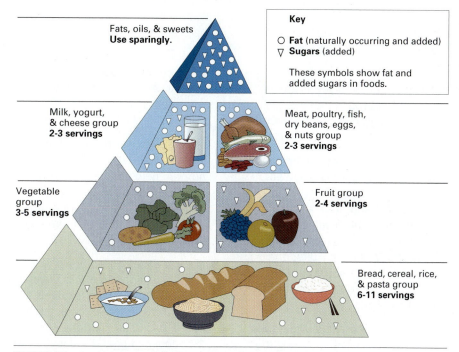

FIGURE 9-3 Food guide pyramid. *(Courtesy of the U.S. Department of Agriculture and the Department of Health and Human Services, 1992, revised 1996)*

TABLE 9-2 How Many Servings Do You Need Each Day?

Calorie Level*	Women and Some Older Adults: About 1,600	Children, Teen Girls, Active Women, and Most Men: About 2,200	Teen Boys and Active Men: About 2,800
Bread group	6	9	11
Vegetable group	3	4	5
Fruit group	2	3	4
Milk group	2–3†	2–3†	2–3†
Meat group	2	2	2
	for a total of 5 oz	for a total of 6 oz	for a total of 7 oz

*These are the calorie levels if you choose low-fat, lean foods from the five major food groups and use foods from the fats and sweets group sparingly.
†Women who are pregnant or breastfeeding, teenagers, and young adults to age 24 need three servings.
From Dietary Guidelines for Americans 2000 (5th ed.), Home and Garden Bulletin 232, by the U.S. Department of Agriculture and U.S. Department of Health and Human Services, 1999, Washington, DC: Author. Adapted from The Food Guide Pyramid, Home and Garden Bulletin 252, by the U.S. Department of Agriculture, Center for Nutrition Policy and Promotion, 1996, Washington, DC: Author.

BOX 9-3 Dietary Guidelines for Americans

- *Eat a variety of foods daily.* Get the many nutrients your body needs by choosing different foods you enjoy eating from these five groups daily: vegetables, fruits, grain products, milk and milk products, and meats and meat alternatives.

- *Maintain a healthy weight.* Check to see if you are at a healthy weight. If not, set reasonable weight loss goals and try for long-term success through better habits of eating and exercise.

- *Choose a diet low in fat, saturated fat, and cholesterol.* Have your blood cholesterol level checked, preferably by a physician. If it is high, follow the physician's advice about diet and, if necessary, medication. If it is at the desirable level, help keep it that way with a diet low in fat, saturated fat, and cholesterol. Eat plenty of vegetables, fruits, and grain products. Choose lean meats, fish, poultry without skin, and low-fat dairy products most of the time. Use fats and oils sparingly.

- *Choose a diet with plenty of vegetables, fruits, and grain products.* Eat more vegetables, including dry beans and peas, fruits, and breads, cereals,

pasta, and rice. Increase your fiber intake by eating more of a variety of foods that contain fiber naturally.

- *Use sugars only in moderation.* Use sugars in moderate amount, sparingly if your kilocalorie needs are low. Avoid excessive snacking. Brush and floss your teeth regularly.

- *Use salt and sodium only in moderation.* Have your blood pressure checked. If it is high, consult a physician about diet and medication. If it is normal, help keep it that way; maintain a healthy weight, exercise regularly, and try to use less salt and sodium. (Normal blood pressure for adults: systolic—less that 140 mm Hg; diastolic—less than 85 mm Hg.)

- *If you drink alcoholic beverages, do so in moderation.* If you drink alcoholic beverages, do not drive. For individuals who drink, limit all alcoholic beverages (including wine, beer, liquors, and so on) to one or two drinks per day. "One drink" means 12 ounces of beer, 5 ounces of wine, or 1½ ounces of distilled spirits (80 proof).

Source: Nutrition and your health: Dietary guidelines for Americans (3rd ed.). (1990). Washington, DC: U.S. Department of Agriculture and Department of Health and Human Services.

today: heart disease, cancer, diabetes, liver disease, and others. Therefore the Dietary Guidelines for Americans (U.S. Dietary Guideline Committee, 1995), as shown in Box 9-3, places emphasis on prevention of overnutrition and disease.

Factors Influencing Nutritional Status of Older Adults

Because the health status of a person is influenced by a variety of socioeconomic, psychological, cultural, religious, and physiological factors, the nurse should understand these factors and their influence on nutritional needs before adequate health care can be provided.

Socioeconomic Factors

Limited income is a major problem among older adults. There is a relationship between income and poor nutritional status in the population now institutionalized (Chernoff, 1991). Income usually decreases sharply with

age. The income of persons 55–64 years old is about twice that of the corresponding 65-and-over age group. Not only do many older adults have a decrease in income, they must also cope with inflation. As income decreases, people buy less meat and more high-carbohydrate foods, resulting in insufficient nutrients to maintain normal weight (Food and Nutrition for Life, 1994).

Many older adults live in substandard housing without adequate food preparation and storage facilities, refrigeration space, and other essentials. The nurse will find that a visit to the home may be more useful than an inquiry into diet in evaluating a patient's ability to purchase a balanced diet. Some older adults are too proud to admit they are destitute and would rather starve than ask for help. A discussion of food costs, food preparation, use of leftovers and information on meals provided by agencies to the home may be helpful in improving the patient's nutrition.

Dependence on others for transportation is another problem older adults face. The lack of transportation may force the older adult to shop at a neighborhood grocery store where prices are higher and there is limited selection of foods. It is difficult for a person who is taken from familiar surroundings to live with other family members, or for one who lives in a retirement home or nursing home to make adjustments in eating patterns. When an older adult is separated from family, friends, or community, such changes often lead to apathy, depression, and loss of appetite (Morley & Solomen, 1994). Therefore, malnutrition can be a major problem in nursing facilities because of the many changes in environment and types of food available. Routine assessment and recording of amounts eaten daily and weight gain or loss at least monthly are essential to detect early nutritional problems that could affect overall health status.

In seeking relief from chronic aches, an older adult is particularly susceptible to the food faddists who claim to have a "miracle cure" that is likely very expensive. Older adults often lack nutrition information because they may have received little or no formal nutrition education. In their youth, nutrition was just beginning to emerge as a science.

Think About It

A resident in a nursing facility gradually decreases the percentage of food eaten from 90% to 25%, although there seems to be no physical cause for it. What are some of the reasons for this change in appetite? What can the nurse do about it?

Psychological Factors

Authorities believe that malnutrition among older adults is associated with loneliness (Food and Nutrition for Life, 1994). The older client can experience loneliness, boredom, anxiety, fear, bereavement, or general unhappiness, which leads to isolation and depression. The client may react to loneliness and depression either by refusing to eat, which leads to malnutrition, or by overeating, which results in obesity, another form of malnutrition. It is important for such older adults to avoid isolation. Eating should not become a chore or a dietary experiment. It should remain a genuine pleasure at any age. Mealtime should be one of the highlights of each day.

Socially, food and eating serve as a mode of communication and socialization. Food eaten in solitude lacks these aspects. Socially isolated persons have decreased incentive to prepare and eat food. There is a strong link between isolation and nutrition (isolation can lead to malnutrition). The lonely person who eats little food becomes increasingly apathetic and listless, failing to reach out for social contact (Food and Nutrition for Life, 1994).

Failure to Thrive

When a medically diagnosed cause for malnutrition cannot be found, other causes psychosocial in nature are sought. Malnutrition in the absence of a tangible, physio-

logical reason signals a closer analysis of other factors. The concept called **failure to thrive (FTT)** was recognized in the late 1980s as a syndrome depicting the presence of malnutrition in combination with a diminished will to live in older adults (Braun, Wycle, (Cowling, 1988). The concept was derived from the work of Spitz in the 1940s and Bowlby in the 1950s in research on FTT in infants (Bowlby, 1958; Spitz, 1945). In infants FTT was related to lack of maternal attachment. Whether mothers held, touched, talked to, and made eye contact with their babies made a difference in the infants' weight gain, growth, and development. Mothers who failed to bond with their babies deprived them of the necessary contact needed for the baby to thrive. Similarly, older adults who are not touched, loved, and nurtured manifest progressive weight loss and psychological distress. The self and the social dimension of the older adult's life become fragmented. Weight loss and depression become symptoms of the disintegration of self. An overall giving up pervades FTT (Zembrzuski, 1999).

Depression and dehydration are discussed in the literature as often accompanying FTT (Egbert, 1996; Grossberg & Nakra, 1986; Sarkisian & Lachs, 1996; Zembrzuski, 1999). Upon admission to the hospital with a diagnosis of FTT, it has been found that older adults have other diagnoses: dehydration, impaired cognition, dementia, impaired ambulation, and difficulty with at least two activities of daily living. Neglect, behavioral problems, family stress, and substance abuse comprise nearly 8% of diagnoses of older adults admitted for FTT (Egbert, 1996).

Health care providers must analyze FTT in older adults not only from a physiological perspective but also from a psychosocial and especially a spiritual perspective (Newbern & Krowchuk, 1994; Groom, 1993; Zembrzuski, 1999). The approach to what initially appears to be a physiological disorder with unknown medical cause is a complex syndrome requiring the intervention of the interdisciplinary team, including nutritionist, nurse, physician, social worker, psychologist, and clergy. Research on this syndrome is greatly needed.

Cultural-Religious Factors

By middle age, eating patterns have become relatively fixed and change may be difficult. Familiar food patterns serve as a security blanket. Distinctive ethnic, racial, and regional characteristics are still prevalent among older adults. Ethnic or racial identity can be reaffirmed by suggesting the use of traditional foods.

To determine the cultural-religious influence on the client's diet, the caregiver should start with an in-depth history of the client's dietary habits. The client should be questioned closely on food likes and dislikes, ethnic preferences, and general nutritional knowledge. The client may eat too much of one type of food and neglect other essential foodstuffs. It is best to encourage the good food habits of the client's particular cultural group and to make improvements gradually rather than impose too many changes at once. A knowledge of the food customs plays an important part in establishing good relationships with a client (see Tables 9-3 and 9-4).

When working with cultural and religious food patterns—whether they be Chinese, Japanese, Mexican-American, Italian, Indian, Jewish, or any other—the health care professional must have a thorough understanding of the client's cultural and religious preferences. These could significantly impact their food intake and nutritional status.

Physiological Factors

Body composition changes with age. In later years there is a cell loss as well as reduced cell metabolism. For example, the cell mass may decrease form 47% of the total body mass at age 25 to 36% at age 70. The physiological changes that occur may vary considerably from one person to another, and the aging process may even vary within the same individual. For example, a 70-year-old man may have the cardiac output typical of a 60-year-old and the renal function of an 80-year-old. It is important to realize that when acute illness occurs, the older adult, because of less lean body mass, will have deple-

tion of muscle protein to a proportionally greater degree than someone with normal lean body mass. Consequently, when a person becomes ill, the nutritional status must be assessed. Because of the decrease in basal metabolic rate, there is a need to decrease the number of kilocalories to avoid weight gain; at the same time, care must be taken to include the necessary nutrients.

Perceptual ability changes with age. Of particular importance to patterns of nutrient intake are changes in hearing, vision, taste, and smell. Loss of hearing may translate into an aversion to talking to grocery clerks, pharmacists, waiters, social workers, or anyone else who might otherwise provide guidance, direction, or helpful information (Roe, 1991b).

The visual change that accompanies aging is familiar, as most people require eyeglasses for reading and close work after 40 years of age. Because of visual changes, some older adults may restrict social activities because they cannot or do not want to drive. Reduced peripheral vision may restrict driving ability; make it difficult to read labels, prices, recipes, and directions; and make it difficult to operate appliances to cook food.

Nutrition and age are two major factors that affect the number of taste cells and the ability to taste and smell is altered with age (Bartoshuk & Duffy, 1995). Taste and smell are closely related. In lieu of taste, the smell of food is a key factor in acceptability. Although most gerontologists agree that a decline in taste bud

TABLE 9-3 Ethnic Dietary Preferences

The Netherlands	Germany	Italy
Smoked fish	Smoked meat	Pasta
Rich pastry	Fruit	Olives (oil)
Cheese	Beans	Tomatoes
Lamb	Pickled vegetables	Meat, poultry
Shellfish		Parmesan cheese
Dairy products		Anise, tarragon, oregano, bay leaves, basil, spices

Near East	South Africa	Southeast Asia
Lamb	Bredie (stew of meat/fish and vegetables/chilies)	Rice
Rice		Hot, dry curries
Poultry	Pickled/curried fish	Chili
Cracked wheat foods	Corn as porridge	Shell fish
Fish	Corn on cob	Soy sauce
Lemon juice, garlic	Cloves, garlic, cinnamon	Garlic, citronella
Spices	Spices	Spices
Perfumed sweets		

TABLE 9-4 Religious Dietary Practices

Restricted Food	Christian Science	Roman Catholic	Latter Day Saints (Mormons)	Seventh Day Adventist	Some Baptist	Greek Orthodox (on Fast Days)	Jewish Orthodox	Moslem Islam	Hinduism	Buddhism
						Faith				
Coffee	•		•	•	•					
Tea	•		•	•	•					
Alcohol	•		•	•	•					
Pork/pork products				•			• Also shellfish	•		
Caffeine-containing foods			•	•						
Dairy products						•	Certain holy days			
All meats		1 hour before communion, Ash Wednesday, Good Friday				Fasting from meat and dairy products on Wednesday/Friday during Lent and other holy days	Forbids the serving of milk and milk products with meat. Regulates food preparation. Forbids cooking on the Sabbath.	Fasting during Ramadan during day, feasting at night	Some are vegetarians.	Meat must be blessed and killed in special ways. Some sects are vegetarians.

sensitivity is part of the aging process, some believe that it is caused by other factors such as smoking and disease. The diminishing senses of taste and smell result in less desire to eat and may lead to malnutrition. Diminishing taste is also accompanied by a decline in salivary flow that accompanies aging. The taste buds are sensitive to sweet, sour, salt, and bitter. Although some taste sensations probably decline with age, the sensitivity to sweet is apparently higher, which may account for the older adult's preference for sweet-tasting foods. Some loss of sour and bitter taste sensation occurs with new dentures because the palate is covered. However, perception often improves as the client becomes adjusted to wearing dentures. The client accepts food better if it is well seasoned. Herbs and spices can be used to season the food, but overuse of table salt should be avoided because of its sodium content. Because flavor perception decreases at very hot or cold temperatures, food served at body temperature (about 95°F) is more acceptable.

Abnormalities that increase or decrease sensitivity to one or more of the four basic tastes include nutritional deficiencies such as those of niacin, vitamin A, and trace metals (zinc, copper, and nickel); various disease states such as cancer, renal failure, and diabetes; radiotherapy to the head or neck for cancer; and drug therapy such as tranquilizers, some anesthetic agents, and some amphetamines. Some cancer patients who are undergoing radiotherapy or chemotherapy require as much as five times the usual amounts of sugar for cereal to taste sweet. Cheese and eggs are often more acceptable as a protein source for such clients because meat tastes bitter to them.

Another obvious change in older adults is the loss of teeth **(edentulous).** The failure to replace lost teeth with dentures or the use of ill-fitting dentures makes it difficult to bite or chew food. The loss of natural teeth and poorly fitting dentures cause many older adults to resort to soft, high-caloric foods such as breads and pastries that lack protein, vitamins, minerals, and fiber. When the loss of teeth and poorly fitting dentures cause older adults to avoid important foodstuffs, it is best to encourage them to return to the dentist for a proper fit. If this suggestion is not successful, they should receive a list of nutritious soft foods. Cheese, sauces, eggs, beans, yogurt, and ground meat are good sources of protein. Whole-grain cereals, either the cooked or cold varieties softened with milk, provide excellent nourishment, as do cooked vegetables. Some vegetables, such as tomatoes and avocados, are soft enough to be eaten raw. Raw bananas and berries as well as cooked fruit make excellent soft desserts. Aging causes a decrease in the secretion of hydrochloric acid as well as of the digestive enzymes of the stomach, intestine, liver, and pancreas, so that the absorption of many nutrients is diminished, con-

tributing to borderline malnutrition in some older clients.

The majority of older adults have one or more chronic diseases. Among the chronic diseases most frequently observed in the older population that are related to nutrition are obesity, cardiovascular diseases, diabetes mellitus, osteoporosis, hypertension, hiatal hernia, constipation, and dysphagia.

Chronic diseases may alter food intake in different ways. If a modified diet has been prescribed, the nurse should check with the client to determine if he or she understands and accepts the diet. If the client does not understand the importance of the diet or refuses to eat the prescribed foods, in a short time the client will return to former eating habits. It is important to determine if the prescribed diet includes the required nutrients. If it does not, a dietary supplement should be recommended. It is best to meet dietary needs by serving a variety of foods. But if variety is not possible, supplementary feedings must be considered.

> ### *Nursing Tip*
>
> An adequate amount of nutritious food is essential for life. Although this statement seems so obvious, it is especially important in the oldest-old, who may have a sudden acute illness in addition to multiple coexisting chronic conditions. For example, when an older adult has a stroke or a fractured hip, that person may not be able to eat and/or have a decreased appetite, thus delaying recovery because of the lack of fluids, vitamins, and minerals essential to the healing process. In the later stages of Alzheimer's disease, the person either does not want to eat and/or forgets how to eat or swallow. People with Alzheimer's disease do not die of the disease but of the consequences of the disease, such as malnutrition and immobility, which lead to other complications such as pneumonia and heart failure.

Obesity

Obesity is the most common nutritional problems of public health in the United States. Older adults should be encouraged to maintain a normal weight by eating a well-balanced diet with caloric restrictions and by engaging in a planned activity, with walking being the most highly recommended exercise.

Recent research (Diehr et al., 1998) has suggested that obesity may provide some protection for women in old age. The additional weight provides a nutritional reserve when stress and acute illness occur. For example, a 90-year-old woman weighing 140 pounds who fractures a hip may do better than a 90-year-old woman weighing only 90 pounds. The added tissue also provides some protection from acute trauma and injury.

Cardiovascular Diseases

Cardiovascular diseases, including heart attack and stroke, are major causes of death. Factors that have been researched and associated with cardiovascular disease include (a) personal factors (heredity, sex, and age), (b) lifestyle factors (obesity, smoking, stress, and diet), (c) pathological factors (other diseases), and (d) environmental factors (air and water pollutants). Recent research has increased the number of dietary links to cardiovascular diseases, especially lipid metabolism, trace-element imbalances, excess sugar and refined carbohydrates, and dietary fiber. Refer to the section on vitamin E for a discussion of this vitamin and prevention of heart disease. The American Heart Association has published easy-to-follow dietary guidelines for the prevention and treatment of cardiovascular disease.

Diabetes Mellitus

Diabetes mellitus is a chronic metabolic disease characterized by a deficiency in the production and utilization of the pancreatic hormone insulin. The most important aspect of dietary treatment of maturity-onset diabetes is reduction of weight. The American Diabetes Association (1994) and the American Dietetic Association (1998) revised the Diabetic Exchange List in 1994, so anyone giving diet instructions for the diabetic should be familiar with the revised Exchange List for Meal Planning and carbohydrate counting. Often weight reduction is necessary to promote successful treatment of primary conditions such as diabetes or arthritis (Stunkard, 1996).

Osteoporosis

Osteoporosis, which means porous bones, is a disease caused by loss of bone mass. Osteoporosis is a major public health threat for 28 million Americans (10 million have osteoporosis, 18 million have low bone mass), 80% of whom are women. Peak bone mass is achieved at age 30–35 years and declines thereafter. This gradual decrease in bone mass is particularly accelerated in women after menopause (Galsworthy & Wilson, 1996). Osteoporosis can involve most of the bones of the skeleton, but most disability and pain are because of vertebral osteoporosis. Certain risk factors are linked to the development of osteoporosis (Osteoporosis and Related Bone Diseases, 1997) and are listed in Box 9-4.

Treatments for osteoporosis focus on slowing or stopping the demineralization of the bone, preventing bone fractures, and controlling pain associated with the disease. **Hormone replacement therapy (HRT)** such as estrogen and progestin beginning at menopause can slow or stop bone loss and reduce the rate of hip fracture up to 50%. However, there are side effects and precautions with their use. **Calcitonin** is a medical treatment approved by the Food and Drug Administration (FDA) for reducing bone loss and for pain relief. It is a peptide hormone that increases deposition of calcium and phosphate in bone. As a medication, however, there are side effects such as nausea and appetite loss. **Alendronate** (Fosamax) is a drug classified as a biophosphonate, which has been approved for both the prevention and treatment of osteoporosis. It increases bone density in both spine and hip, reduces bone loss, and also reduces the risk of both spine and hip fractures. Side effects from alendronate can include abdominal pain, heartburn, nausea, or irritation of the esophagus. **Raloxifene** (Evista) is a drug that was recently approved for prevention of osteoporosis. It comes from a new class of drugs called selective estrogen receptor modulators (SERMs), which appear to prevent bone loss at the spine, hip, and total body. However, this effect on the spine does not appear to be as powerful as either HRT or alendronate, but its effect on the hip and total

BOX 9-4   Risk Factors for Osteoporosis

- Gender: Females are at higher risk for osteoporosis than males.

- Age: The older the person is, the greater the risk for development of osteoporosis.

- Body size: Small, thin-boned women are at highest risk.

- Ethnicity: Caucasian and Asian women are at highest risk. African-American women have a lower, but still significant risk.

- Family history: The susceptibility to fracture may be, in part, hereditary.

- Sex hormones: Abnormal absence of menstrual periods (amenorrhea), low estrogen level (menopause), and low testosterone level in men.

- Anorexia.

- A lifetime diet low in calcium and vitamin D.

- Use of certain medications, such as thyroid, corticosteroids, or some anticonvulsants.

- An inactive lifestyle or extended bed rest.

- Cigarette smoking.

- Excessive use of alcohol.

body are comparable. Eating a diet high in calcium and vitamin D can also slow or stop excessive bone loss. The aging body is less efficient at absorbing calcium and other nutrients; therefore postmenopausal women and older men need to consume more calcium. While some older individuals may resist calcium-rich dairy foods because of lactose intolerance, there are other sources of calcium such as dark green, leafy vegetables (broccoli, collard greens, bok choy, spinach), sardines and salmon with bones, tofu, almonds, and foods fortified with calcium such as orange juice, cereals, and breads. If an older individual does not get enough calcium in food daily, a calcium supplement may be needed. Studies have also shown that vitamin D production decreases in older adults (Francis, 1997); therefore, an older individual may also need a vitamin D supplement of between 400 and 800 IU daily. Massive doses of vitamin D are not recommended because of possible toxicity.

Hypertension

Hypertension is identified as high blood pressure. Clinical evidence now indicates that mild sodium restriction can lower blood pressure. A no-added-salt (4-g-sodium) diet with use of a diuretic is the approach used by many current practitioners. The no-added-salt diet provides a wide variety of foods, limiting foods naturally high in salt such as bacon, lunchmeat, dill pickles, chips, or foods with visible salt such as pretzels. The 4-g-sodium diet also limits the use of salt at the table (removal of the salt shaker) but does allow for some salt in cooking. This diet is more appetizing and better tolerated by the older individual who may have many other restrictions or whose taste acuity is diminished.

Constipation

Constipation may be caused by lack of exercise, psychological stress, or a diet low in fiber. After the possi-

CLINICAL ALERT

Choking on food can and does cause death in people who have difficulty swallowing. Essential nursing interventions are:

- *Assess for ability to swallow before eating.*
- *Check to verify the type of diet ordered and served.*
- *Assist in feeding the client, if needed.*
- *If the client has any difficulty swallowing, do not leave alone during meals.*
- *Be sure the client is sitting upright and remains upright for 1–2 hr after eating.*
- *Suggest an evaluation by a speech pathologist if possible.*

bility of disease is ruled out, a modified diet should be planned. Increasing dietary fiber, fluid intake, and physical exercise can prevent constipation. Diets generous in fiber produce larger, softer stools and more frequent bowel movements. High-fiber diets are also used in the treatment of hemorrhoids, diverticulosis, and other colon-related diseases.

Dysphagia

Dysphagia is associated with problems in swallowing. This is a result of changes in esophageal motility and decreased secretion of saliva or may happen as the result of a stroke. If the problem is severe, food may be rejected as swallowing becomes difficult. Aspiration into the lungs may occur if the swallowing problem is caused by a stroke and leads to pneumonia. Heartburn from backflow of stomach acid into the esophagus is frequent when the esophageal sphincter has lost control because of disease or medication side effects. Dry mouth resulting from reduced secretion of saliva or general dehydration adds to the difficulty in swallowing. Certain drugs such as antidepressants, anticonvulsants, and amphetamines can cause dry mouth, as can dentures, anxiety, or breathing through the mouth.

Feeding Issues

The older adult may have several physiological problems and, as a result, several dietary restrictions when under the care of a physician. A person with diabetes may, for instance, also be sodium restricted, texture modified, and fat restricted. These limited foods can lead to lower intake and undernutrition. For that reason, it is now recommended that some liberalization of diet be allowed to encourage adequate intake of a variety of foods. If the older individual has a need for controlled carbohydrate intake (diabetes) and sodium and also has difficulty chewing and swallowing, the least restricted diet possible, such as consistent carbohydrate with texture modification, may be the best alternative. Choosing the most physiologically important food limitation instead of using double or triple restrictions can be less confusing for the client while allowing for better compliance and intake, with avoidance of undernutrition (American Dietetic Association, 1998).

Suggestions for Feeding Clients

Older adults who are dependent, seriously ill, or recovering from illness sometimes are unable to feed themselves. Some suggestions for feeding clients who cannot help themselves are given in Box 9-5.

BOX 9-5   Suggestions for Feeding Clients

- Provide an environment free of odors, clean, and orderly, with appropriate temperature and ventilation.

- Have the client in a comfortable, upright position. Reclining interferes with chewing and swallowing.

- Before feeding, assess the client's ability to swallow. Never attempt to feed a client who cannot swallow.

- Sit across from the client. Have the client look straight ahead and introduce the food straight into the mouth. It is difficult for a person to swallow with head turned at a 45-degree angle.

- Test the temperature of the food by placing a drop on the back of the wrist. Soups, coffee, and other hot items should not be allowed to burn the person's mouth.

- Start by offering liquids or thin soups served in a container with a covered lid.

- Identify each food as it is given.

- Ask the client to smell the food to encourage chewing and salivating reflexes.

- Do not mix foods together.

- Allow time for eating at a slow pace, giving the client sufficient time to chew and swallow between bites.

- Blot the mouth. Do not wipe. Wiping stimulates the rooting reflex which opens the mouth, making swallowing more difficult.

- Have the person use the upper lip (not upper teeth) to scrape food from utensil. Scraping with the teeth stimulates the bite reflex, which interferes with chewing.

- Place food well into the person's mouth to avoid tongue thrust, which pushes food out of the mouth.

- Keep food moist. Salivation in older adults is frequently reduced. Lack of fluid makes chewing and swallowing more difficult. Give sips of fluid frequently during the meal.

- If the person is paralyzed on one side of the body, place food in the side of the mouth that is not paralyzed.

- Observe which textures are easiest to chew and swallow.

- Encourage the person to think swallow, if swallowing is difficult, by repeating the word swallow.

- Allow for and accept the person's feelings of frustration, anger, and embarrassment.

Nursing Tip

If an older adult eats in bed, keep the head of the bed up for at least 1 hr after the meal to prevent possible regurgitation of food from the stomach up into the esophagus.

It is not pleasant for an adult to be fed. The attitude of the person feeding the older adult often sets the mood and is the single most important factor in the amount of food consumed by the older adult who requires feeding. Feed slowly. Be positive and show enthusiasm and encouragement at mealtime. An individual's attitude toward both food and mealtime is likely to be more positive if self-feeding is possible. Achieving this level of independence supports both physical and mental well-being. Problems in self-feeding may be caused by weakness in the hand or arm, making it difficult to lift a cup or spoon. Partial paralysis and effects of Parkinson's disease can limit range of motion or make it difficult to flex the fingers and hand to grasp a cup or fork.

Various devices have been developed to help disabled individuals feed themselves. In many cases, only a slight modification of existing utensils facilitates food handling. A cup with a partial lid or small opening (plastic travel cup) or a straw helps prevent spills. Lightweight plastic cups are easier to handle when filled with liquid than are glass or china cups. Covering a standard utensil (fork or spoon) with foam rubber increases the friction and aids in holding. A suction device on the bottom of the dish or a plate with a broad edge helps those with limited motor skills. Special aids are often available from local hospital supply companies or can be ordered by mail.

Careful selection of food served and a positive approach facilitate progress and encourage effort. A soft diet rather than pureed foods not only is more palatable but also requires less skill in eating (Figure 9-4). Finger foods require less effort and energy for eating. Ideas for making difficult items into finger foods include putting

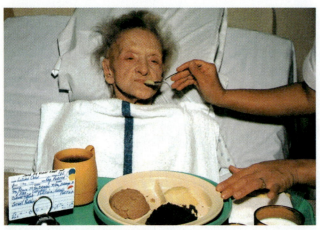

FIGURE 9-4   Ensuring client safety and comfort when assisting with a meal.

ground meat in a roll, folding a pancake in half so it can be picked up, or serving hard-cooked eggs or small fruit slices.

Nutrition Programs for Older Adults

There has been an increased social concern for the concerns of older Americans. In 1965 Congress passed the Older Americans Act, which provides for various programs designed to improve the quality of life for older adults. One of the programs provided under this legislation is the Nutrition Program for the Elderly. This pro-

gram has been referred to in the past as the Title VII Meal Program because it came under Title VII of the Older Americans Act. As a result of amendments to the act in 1978 the program is now referred to as the Title III Meal Program. The congregate meal program is designed to provide inexpensive, nutritionally balanced meals for older adults. Low-cost meals are served in group settings to people who are 60 years or older and to their spouses. Meals are designed to provide at least one-third of the RDAs. Older adults are not required to pay, but they may contribute voluntarily toward the meals. In addition to food, various supportive services are also provided as part of the program. Transportation to and from the meal, information and help for other services, health counseling, nutrition education, and recreation activities are some of the other services. Information about the program and how to participate in it are also provided to eligible older adults.

The Title III Meal Program helps meet the nutritional needs of many older adults through the **Meals-on-Wheels** program. This program provides hot meals that are delivered to older adults unable to leave home. This service is provided at the community level. The extent of the services varies from one to three meals daily (one hot and one or two cold) for a varying number of days per week (three to seven). Cost is based on the ability to pay.

Many older people qualify for the **Food Stamp Program.** This program allows the person on a very limited budget to purchase more food.

Program aides, who are trained through the Expanded Food and Nutrition Program of the U.S. Depart-

---

BOX 9-6   Recommended Guide for Menu Planning

- Serve meals on a regular schedule.

- Include a variety of foods.

- Serve smaller amounts of food more frequently.

- Be aware of new trends in nutrition education.

- Make older adults aware that money spent on nutritional food is money well spent.

- Recognize food and drug interactions.

- Prepare and serve food attractively.

- Increase fluid intake.

- Include fibrous foods for proper elimination.

- Recognize social, economic, cultural, and religious factors.

- Season foods to stimulate taste buds.

- Use polyunsaturated oils and margarine.

- Select complex carbohydrates.

- Learn to identify intolerances.

- Use meat substitutes such as cheese, dried beans, and peanut butter.

- Use various forms of milk—skim milk, nonfat dry milk, or buttermilk.

- Serve fresh fruits and vegetables.

- Serve whole-grain or enriched breads and cereals.

- Follow instructions for therapeutic diets.

- Check the menu against a daily food guide, suggested serving guide, or the food guide pyramid (refer to Figure 9-1).

BOX 9-7 Money-Stretching Ideas to Make the Food Dollar Go Further

- Plan menus and shop from a prepared list. Be careful to avoid foods containing large amounts of fat and sugar.

- Avoid costly, instant, or convenience items. They are generally higher in sodium and sugar.

- Take advantage of vegetables and fruit in three forms: fresh, canned, and frozen. Select fruits and vegetables that are in season and locally grown.

- Select juices for vitamin C content. Rule out fruit-flavored choices supplying only sugar.

- Meat generally requires the larger part of the food dollar. Lower cost cuts can be as nutritious but must be cooked and stored properly to prevent shrinkage. Serve more fish and chicken. Avoid frying.

- Avoid prepackaged, sliced, or processed meats. They are usually more expensive and higher in sodium than bulk meats.

- Check the price of canned meats such as tuna, chicken, and fish, noting that the boneless meat could be the most economical. Avoid canned meats packed in oil.

- Buy cereals that require cooking rather than ready-to-serve cereals. Avoid presweetened cereals.

- Use nonfat dry milk solids in cooking. These may be used dry in recipes for bread and cake but should be in liquid form for recipes such as gravies, sauces, and puddings. Use larger amounts of nonfat dry milk than recommended on the package to increase nutrient density.

---

ment of Agriculture, are providing basic nutrition to low-income families. While the program aides' focus is families with young children, they also work with other families as their priorities permit. Aides provide information on wise shopping, basic food needs, and food preparation techniques. Teaching is done on a one-to-one basis, with the aide going to the home. Box 9-6 provides a recommended guide for menu planning for older adults and Box 9-7 presents some ideas about how to stretch the food dollar.

CARE PLAN

Case Study

Dom Delgado has been living at home alone for the past 10 years. He is an 83-year-old man who has no living or available family. He is the oldest of six children and a World War II veteran. Two of his brothers died in World War II. Two sisters died of diabetes. One sister resides in a nursing facility in Florida. Mr. Delgado has a nephew who lives 50 miles away and visits three times yearly.

The case manager at the state Agency on Aging follows Mr. Delgado's overall status under Protective Services, acknowledging his potential for decline and self-neglect. Mr. Delgado receives federal and state aid. He has home-delivered meals provided by community services. His medications for diabetes and hypertension are partially covered by a state and federally administered program for older adults. The home care nurse visits weekly, reinforcing all aspects of diabetic management, including foot care, medication side effects, diet, and blood glucose monitoring. A home health aide visits three times weekly to assist him with personal care.

Lately, the case manager noted significant changes in Mr. Delgado's attitude. He expressed feelings of loneliness and despair. Upon the home care nurse's assessment, findings showed a 25-pound weight loss over the past 6 months. The home health aide noticed progressive decline in strength and motivation. Statements like "I wish I could go to sleep and not wake up" and "Why should I get dressed everyday? For what!" were frequent. The home health aide also noticed that the home-delivered meals were being thrown in the garbage. Was Mr. Delgado's will to live diminishing?

Assessment

Physical decline may accompany psychological and spiritual distress in older adults who no longer have a purpose to live. When meaningful social contact in the form of family and friends is lacking over long periods of time, an individual gives up on life. This syndrome has been labeled failure to thrive (FTT). This

(continues)

CARE PLAN *continued*

syndrome was noted in the 1960s in infants who lacked human contact. In older adults, the syndrome was recognized in the late 1980s. Weight loss, loneliness, hopelessness, and isolation are classic symptoms. Advocating and correcting a situation like Mr. Delgado's are not simple matters and require coordinated efforts of the interdisciplinary team, including nurse, dietitian, social worker, mental health specialists, and physician. Even with a team effort, Mr. Delgado's will to live is a determining factor in the outcome. An aggressive care plan is necessary to influence his health—and life.

NURSING DIAGNOSIS

Failure to thrive related to ability to live and cope with everyday activities, as evidenced by rejecting daily meals, weight loss, and physical and psychosocial decline

Outcomes:

Mr. Delgado will:
- *Express feelings about his circumstances.*
- *Gain 2 pounds per month.*
- *Make one or two positive comments about life and living on a weekly basis.*
- *Identify one positive aspect of his life.*
- *Attend adult day programs at the Veterans Affairs (VA) center at least once weekly.*
- *Motivate himself to conduct his (nighttime) care.*

Planning/Interventions:

The nurse will:
- *Prompt Mr. Delgado to express his feelings about his situation.*
- *Listen attentively and sincerely to Mr. Delgado's concerns.*
- *Assess Mr. Delgado's mental and nutritional status, especially weights at least weekly.*
- *Explain the day program to Mr. Delgado and coordinate the services at the Veterans Affairs Hospital three times weekly.*
- *Demonstrate to Mr. Delgado how to perform nighttime care for himself, with returned demonstration.*
- *Contact Mr. Delagado's nephew to explore whether he is able to visit more than three times yearly.*
- *Collaborate with the case manager at the State Agency on Aging to ensure maximum benefits for Mr. Delgado.*

Evaluation:

Mr. Delgado will verbalize his feelings about his situation. He will express his perception of life. The nurse will listen nonjudgmentally and respond supportively. Mental status will return to baseline. Mr. Delgado will agree to try the adult day program two times each week at the VA center. He will also perform nighttime care adequately. As the nurse advocates for Mr. Delgado, she or he will facilitate the nephew's visit to five times annually. Because of Mr. Delgado's critical situation, he will receive a home health aide four times per week.

NURSING DIAGNOSIS

Risk for fluid volume deficit related to vascular dehydration, as evidenced by fluid intake less than 1,500 cc, change in mental status, change in weights, or signs and symptoms of dehydration

Outcomes:

Mr. Delgado will:
- *Describe the amounts of fluid which he needs to ingest.*
- *Ingest at least 1,500 mL of fluid, preferably water.*

(continues)

CARE PLAN *continued*

- *Manifest no symptoms of dehydration.*
- *Manifest no changes in mental status.*
- *Manifest no weight loss.*

Planning/Interventions:

The nurse will:

- *Assess Mr. Delgado's hydration status.*
- *Obtain baseline electrolytes, serum osmolality, and vital signs.*
- *Explain the importance and amounts of fluids needed.*
- *Teach Mr. Delgado how to monitor his own intake and output.*
- *Observe for signs and symptoms of dehydration.*
- *Assess for mental status changes.*
- *Monitor for weight loss.*
- *Collaborate with physician/advanced practitioner.*

Evaluation:

Mr. Delgado will ingest at least 1,500 mL daily. This is necessary to prevent acidosis and late stages of dehydration. Baseline laboratory values (electrolytes) and vital signs will be obtained and will remain within normal limits, although some older adults maintain high normal limits for electrolytes. He will monitor his own I&O and identify fluids he enjoys. No-sugar Popsicle's, no-sugar lemonade, and no-sugar Jell-O in a variety of flavors will be prepared with the help of the home health aide.

NURSING DIAGNOSIS

Hopelessness related to decreased appetite, weight loss, lack of motivation, and sense of abandonment

Outcomes:

Mr. Delgado will:

- *Express a desire to live; express anger as opposed to depressive, passive comments.*
- *Diminish verbalization of comments on wanting to die.*
- *Become involved in an adult day program.*
- *Look forward to his nephew's visit or one other event.*
- *Eat two of three home-delivered meals.*

Planning/Interventions:

The nurse will:

- *Encourage Mr. Delgado to express his feelings.*
- *Explore further Mr. Delgado's desire not to live.*
- *Encourage a trial attendance at the adult day program.*
- *Facilitate Mr. Delgado's nephew's additional visits; examine other events that Mr. Delgado could attend and view as important, such Memorial Day or Labor Day veterans' events.*
- *Explain the value of nutritional meals and allow Mr. Delgado to describe how he perceives home-delivered meals.*
- *Pursue Mr. Delgado's likes and dislikes of foods.*
- *Determine fluid I&O.*
- *Assess and monitor weight, hygiene, foot care, blood sugars, and hypertension.*
- *Collaborate with physician/advanced practitioner, social worker, and case manager.*

Evaluation:

Mr. Delgado's "failure to thrive" emanates from psychosocial and physiological circumstances, grounded in chronic illness, lack of social support, and social isolation. Case management from multiple disciplines is

(continues)

CARE PLAN *continued*

necessary and could prevent nursing facility admission. With aggressive intervention, Mr. Delgado will remain at home. He will gain at least 2 pounds/month. He will have fluids readily available, which he enjoys. He will express a desire to live, with special attention on his nephew's visits and veterans' contact, adult day program, and companion visits. With psychiatric nursing, social work, and perhaps clergy involvement, Mr. Delgado will seek solace and peace as opposed to despair and hopelessness as he reflects on his life.

NURSING DIAGNOSIS

Social isolation relate to aloneness, absence of significant others, and sad, dull affect

Outcomes:
Mr. Delgado will:
- *Attend an adult day program at least once weekly.*
- *Visit with nephew more frequently.*
- *Agree to addition of a home companion through the VA.*
- *Verbalize positively about his new social situation.*
- *Agree to try a mild antidepressant.*

Planning/Interventions:
The nurse will:
- *Arrange for an adult day program and a VA companion one to two times weekly.*
- *Contact nephew to support increased visits as critical to Mr. Delgado's welfare.*
- *Encourage expression of feelings about this new social situation.*
- *Assess for depression (Beck Depression Scale or other instrument).*
- *Discuss use of a mild antidepressant with physician/advanced practitioner.*

Evaluation:
Mr. Delgado will agree to a mild antidepressant. He will attend an adult day program and agree to a companion. His nephew will increase contacts and visit more frequently. These are steep goals for Mr. Delgado, and his situation is not as easily solvable as this care plan might indicate. It is important that the nurse strives to be an advocate for Mr. Delgado—aggressively pursuing his nephew to spend more time with him, the VA for services, and the case manager to maintain his health and well-being.

Summary

The increasing number of older Americans presents health care professionals with a unique challenge. Adequate nutritional care for the older adult deserves considerable emphasis because the well-nourished older adult not only is more comfortable and energetic but also is better able to tolerate medical and surgical treatment.

The daily RDAs, the food guide pyramid, and the dietary guidelines for Americans are designed to be beneficial in planning a diet that will furnish the needed nutrients. Factors contributing to nutritional deficiencies in older adults include poor food habits, reduced income, racial and cultural patterns, poor dental health, and chronic diseases.

Nutrition education during the entire lifespan as well as during later life is needed. People who have accurate knowledge of nutrition and are motivated to use it can best achieve good food habits.

The nurse must emphasize to the older adult the importance of good nutrition. Although the nurse cannot reverse the effect of poor nutritional habits developed early in life, nutrition education can positively influence the quality of life for the older adult.

Review Questions and Activities

1. In what ways does physical activity contribute to nutritional balance in older adults?

2. What are the major problems associated with carbohydrates, fats, and protein among older adults?

3. Discuss the pros and cons of vitamin supplements for older adults.

4. Identify the role and some of the major problems among older adults with regard to fat-soluble vitamins, B complex vitamins, and vitamin C.

5. Why is the absorption of minerals inefficient?

6. Identify the role and some of the major problems among older adults with regard to calcium, phosphorus, magnesium, sodium, potassium, iodine, iron, and zinc. Include an in-depth discussion of current views regarding osteoporosis.

7. Discuss the role of water and major problems associated with water imbalance among older adults.

8. Explain the purpose of having RDAs, USRDAs, the food guide pyramid, and dietary guidelines for Americans.

9. Visit a congregate meal site. Evaluate the menu and observe the activities of the participants.

10. Volunteer to the local Meals-on-Wheels program to deliver meals to older adults in their homes.

References

American Diabetes Association. (1994). Nutrition recommendations and principles for people with diabetes mellitus. *Journal of the American Dietetic Association, 94,* 504–506.

American Dietetic Association. (1998). Position of the American Dietetic Association: Liberalized diets for older adults in long-term care. *Journal of the American Dietetic Association, 98,* 201.

American Heart Association. (1994). *Dietary guidelines for healthy American adults: A statement for physicians and health professionals by the nutrition committee.* Dallas, TX: American Heart Association.

Andres, R. (1990). Mortality and obesity: The rationale for age-specific height-weight tables. In W. Hazzard, R. Andres, E. Rierman, & J. Blass (Eds.), *Principles of geriatric medicine and gerontology* (pp. 759–765). New York: McGraw-Hill.

Barry, H. C., & Eathorne, S. W. (1994). Exercise and aging. Issues for the practitioner. *Medical Clinics of North America, 78,* 357–376.

Bartoshuk, L. M., & Duffy, V. B. (1995). Taste and smell in aging. In E. F. Masoro (Ed.), *Handbook of physiology* (pp. 363–375). New York: Oxford University Press.

Beharak, A., Redican, S., Leka, L., & Meydani, S. N. (1997). Vitamin E status and immune function. *Methods of Enzymology, 282,* 247–263.

Bidlack, W. R. (1996). Interrelationships of food, nutrition, diet and health: The National Association of State Universities and Land Grant Colleges White Paper. *Journal of the American College of Nutrition, 15*(5), 422–433.

Bowlby, J. (1958). The nature of the child's tie to his mother. *International Journal of Psychoanalysis, 39,* 350–373.

Braun, J. V., Wycle, M. N., & Cowling, W. R. (1988). Failure to thrive in older persons: A concept derived. *Gerontologist, 28,* 809–812.

Campbell, W. W., Crim, M. C., Dallal, G. E., Young, V. R., & Evans, W. J. (1994). Increased protein requirement in elderly people; New data and retrospective reassessments. *American Journal of Clinical Nutrition, 60*(4), 501–509.

Chan, A. C. (1998). Vitamin E and atherosclerosis. *Journal of Nutrition, 128*(10), 1593–1596.

Chernoff, R. (1991). *Geriatric nutrition.* Gaithersburg, MD: Aspen.

Diehr, P., Bild, D. E., Harris, T. B., Duxbury, A., Siscovick, D., & Rossi, M. (1998). Body mass index and mortality in nonsmoking older adults: The cardiovascular health study. *American Journal of Public Health, 88*(4), 623–629.

Dube, A., Khalsa, A., Gupta, S. K., Singh, U., & Sharma, P. (1998). Serum tocopherols and lipids in patients with coronary artery disease. *Indian Heart Journal, 50*(3), 292–294.

Egbert, A. M. (1996). The dwindles: Failure to thrive in older patients. *Nutrition Reviews, 54*(1), S25–S30.

Elliott, P., Stamler, J., Nichols, R., Dyer, A. R., Stamler, R., Kesteloot, H., & Marmot, M. (1996). Intersalt revisited: Further analyses of 24-hour sodium excretion and blood pressure within and across populations. *British Medical Journal, 312,* 1249–1253.

Food and Agriculture Organization.(1994). *Fats and oils in human nutrition: Report of a joint expert consultation* (WHO.FAO Paper No. 57). Rome: Food and Agriculture Organization.

Food and Nutrition Board. (1997). *Dietary reference intakes for calcium, phosphorus, magnesium, vitamin D, and fluoride.* Press release, August 13, 1997.

Food and Nutrition for Life. (1994). *Malnutrition and older Americans.* Report by the Assistant Secretary for Aging, Administration on Aging, DHHS. Available: <http://www.fiu.edu/~nutreldr/malisspa.htm>.

Francis, R. M. (1997). Is there a differential response to alafacalcidol and vitamin D in the treatment of osteoporosis? *Calcified Tissue International, 60* (1), 111–114.

Galsworthy, T. D., & Wilson, P. L. (1996). It steals more than bone. *American Journal of Nursing, 96*(6), 27–34.

Groom, D. D. (1993). A diagnostic model for failure to thrive. *Journal of Gerontological Nursing, 19*(6), 12–16.

Grossberg, G. T., & Nakra, B. R. (1986). Treatment of depression in the elderly. *Neuropsychiatry, 12*(10), 16–22.

Hamilton, E., Whitney, E., & Sizer, F. (1991). *Nutrition concepts and controversies* (5th ed.). St. Paul, MN: West Publishing.

Jaffe, M. (1991). *Geriatric nutrition and diet therapy.* El Paso, TX: Skidmore-Roth Publishing.

Lee, M. R., & Krasinski, S. D. (1998). Human adult-onset lactase decline: An update. *Nutrition Reviews, 56*(1, pt 1), 1–8.

Meydani, M., Lipman, R. D., Han, S. N., Wu, D., Beharka, A., Martin, K. R., Bronson, R., Cao, G., Smith, D., & Meydani, S. N. (1998). The effect of long-term dietary supplementation with antioxidants. *Annals of the New York Academy Sciences, 854,* 352–360.

Morley, J. E., & Solomon, D. H. (1994). Major issues in geriatrics over the last five years. *Journal of the American Geriatrics Society, 42,* 218–225.

Newbern, V. B., & Krowchuk, H. V. (1994). Failure to thrive in elderly people: A concept analysis. *Journal of Advanced Nursing, 19,* 840–849.

Nutrition and your health: Dietary guidelines for Americans (3rd ed.). (1990). Washington, DC: U.S. Department of Agriculture, Department of Health and Human Services.

Osteoporosis and Related Bone Diseases, National Resource Center. (1997). *Osteoporosis and co-morbid conditions* (Vol. III, No. 6). Available: <http://www.osteo.org/comorbid.htm>.

Recommended dietary allowances (10th ed.). (1989). Washington, DC: National Academy Press.

Roe, D. A. (1987). *Geriatric nutrition* (2nd ed). Englewood Cliffs, NJ: Prentice-Hall.

Roe, S. N. (Ed.). (1991a). *Geriatric patient education resource manual* (Vol. 1). Gaithersburg, MD: Aspen.

Roe, S. N. (Ed.). (1991b). *Dietician's patient education manual* (Vol. 1). Gaithersburg, MD: Aspen.

Sarkisian, C. A., & Lachs, M. S. (1996). "Failure to Thrive" in older adults. *Annals of Internal Medicine, 124,* 1072–1078.

Schellhorn, B., Doring, A., & Stieber, J. (1998). Use of vitamins and minerals all food supplements from the MONICA cross-sectional study of 1994/95 from the Augsburg study region. *Zeitschrift fur Ernahrungswissenschaft, 37*(2), 198–206.

Shils, M., Olson, J., Shike, M., & Ross, A. C. (1999). *Modern nutrition in health and disease* (9th ed.). Baltimore, MD: Williams & Wilkins.

Spitz, R. (1945). Hospitalization: An inquiry into the genesis of psychiatric conditions in early childhood. *Psychoanalytic Study of Childhood, 1*(1), 53–74.

Stunkard, A. J. (1996). Current views on obesity. *American Journal of Medicine, 100,* 230–236.

Taaffe, D. R., Thompson, J., Butterfield, G., & Marcus, R. (1995). Accuracy of equations to predict basal metabolic rate in older women. *Journal of the American Dietetic Association, 95*(12), 1387–1392.

U.S. Department of Agriculture and Department of Health and Human Services. (1992). *The food guide pyramid.* Home and Garden Bulletin Number 252.

U.S. Dietary Guideline Committee, Department of Agriculture, and Department of Health and Human Services. (1995). *Nutrition and your health: Dietary guidelines for Americans* (4th ed). Home & Garden Bulletin Number 232.

White, E., Shannon, J. S., & Patterson, R. E. (1997). Relationship between vitamin and calcium supplement use and colon cancer. *Cancer Epidemiology Biomarker Preview, 6*(10), 769–774.

Whitney, E. N., Hamilton, E. M. N., & Rolfes, S. R. (1990). *Understanding nutrition* (5th ed.). St. Paul, MN: West Publishing.

Zembrzuski, C. D. (1999). *Malnutrition, depression and dehydration in older people*. Unpublished paper, New York University at New York City.

Resources

www.webring.org

American Dietetic Association: **www.eatright.org**

Novartis Foundation for Gerontology: **www.healthandage.com**

CHAPTER 10

Informal Support Systems

Mildred O. Hogstel, PhD, RN, C

*A special acknowledgement to JoAnn Wedig, MA, RN
for her contribution on Parish Nursing.*

COMPETENCIES

After completing this chapter, the reader should be able to:

- *Identify sources of social support for older adults living in the community.*
- *Describe the process of family caregiving.*
- *List the benefits and burdens of family caregiving.*
- *Identify the major problems of family caregivers.*
- *Explain the reasons for family caregiver problems.*
- *Discuss the definition, purpose, and process of respite care for family caregivers.*
- *Explore the role of the church and synagogue in meeting the needs of older adults in the community.*
- *Relate the role and functions of the parish nurse to eldercare issues.*
- *Evaluate availability of social support groups for older adults in the community.*
- *Discuss the nursing role in identifying and using community social support services in the community.*

MAKING THE CONNECTION

Refer to the following chapters to increase your understanding of informal support systems:

- **Chapter 1**   *Aging Yesterday, Today, and Tomorrow*
- **Chapter 3**   *Changes in the Health Care Delivery System Affecting Older Adults*
- **Chapter 8**   *Successful Aging*
- **Chapter 20** *Home Health Care*
- **Chapter 24** *Community Organizations and Services*
- **Chapter 26** *End-of-Life Decisions and Choices*

Informal Caregiving

As the aging population increases in numbers and longevity in the twenty-first century, the need for health care services and social support assistance also will increase. There is increasing national concern about how these numbers will affect governmental programs such as Medicare, Medicaid, Social Security, and other types of similar supportive services for older adults. Some national leaders and others have stated that the needs of chronically ill and dependent older adults will have to be met by family, church, and other types of support in the local community. In recent years, older adults and their family members have depended more on governmental resources for care rather than family and local community support like many years ago. However, the family is still the *major* source of support for older adults with needs (Hey, 1997). It is important to note that the structure and lifestyles of family members also have changed since the early to mid-part of the twentieth century, so having family caregivers available in the home is a problem.

Women have been the traditional family caregivers in the past, perhaps because of their historical nurturing nature, their role as homemaker, and/or their personal and emotional feelings of commitment to older family members. With the large majority of working-age women away from the home during the day and with younger family members in school or at work, there are fewer family members in the home to provide essential supervision and care to older family members. It is not likely that this trend for women will change because of the financial need to work and the personal satisfaction of an active rewarding career. It is yet to be seen if churches, synagogues, and other community groups and agencies will be able to provide the types of programs and services needed by an increasing aging population in the future.

When multiple health problems and long-term care needs begin to occur, especially for those people in their late 80s, 90s, and 100s, independent living and functioning may not be possible for physical, safety, psychological, and/or financial reasons. Family members often need to take on more and more caregiving responsibilities such as shopping, housekeeping, help in paying bills, transporting for medical appointments, and important socialization. With progress of the disease or disability, more direct care may be needed, such as assisting with bathing, dressing, feeding, taking medications, and toileting. Help with these tasks requires a competent willing caregiver, either an employee (reliable 24-hour help is difficult to find and expensive) or a family member or friend.

Informal caregivers may be family members, neighbors, or close friends. The most typical family caregivers are spouse, daughter, sister, daughter-in-law, grandchild, son, or brother. According to Stoller (1992), a spouse is the most likely to willingly accept the caregiver role and to be the only care provider. Occasionally a close friend or a long-term neighbor may become the primary caregiver, especially if there is no surviving relative. The latter situation is especially true for people who live to be 95 or 100 because they have often outlived not only their spouse but also their siblings and children as well.

The Caregiver Role

Informal caregiving is a broad term that implies providing a variety of services and assistance to a family member or close friend, generally without payment. When the **care recipient** becomes immobile, incontinent, and confused or disoriented, the person often is unable to leave home except for essential trips for medical care. When this situation occurs, the caregiver usually cannot leave the home either because it is not safe to leave the care recipient alone. Sometimes there are adequate financial resources for paid assistance or other family members are available and willing to be part-time caregivers (sometimes causing family conflicts in deciding a shared responsibility plan).

Caregiving ranges from occasional social visits to full-time 24-hour care for a dependent ill older adult in the home with many needs. See Table 10-1 for a description of the caregiver role as it changes over time and as the status of the care recipient changes. Therefore, caregiving may occur in any setting from the older adult's own private home or apartment to a retirement center to an assisted-living facility to a nursing facility. For example, the *social* and *assistive* roles of the caregiver may occur while the older family member is still living in his or her private home or retirement center. The *transitional* role will predominate when the older family member is living in an assisted-living facility or nursing facility. Variations of the *care role* will be needed when the older family member is living in the caregiver's home or in a nursing facility.

Ask Yourself

Who will care for your parents, grandparents, or great-grandparents if and when they are unable to care for themselves?

Benefits and Burdens

The informal caregiving role has several **benefits** but also **burdens** that accompany the changing caregiver roles, as noted in Table 10-2. There are benefits of developing a new kind of relationship with an older family member. This relationship is termed **filial maturity,**

TABLE 10-1 Family/Informal Continuum of Caregiver Roles

Social Role →	Assistance Role →	Transitional Role →	Care Role
Makes personal visits	Takes to bank or grocery store	Assists with IADL	Assists with PADL
Involves in preferred social activities	Assists with or arranges for house cleaning	Provides or arranges housing	Manages all financial resources and uses personal resources when needed
Takes out for a meal	Accompanies to physician's office	Does all shopping as needed, including medications	Cannot leave care recipient alone at home
Goes on trips together	Reminds care recipient when and how to take medications	Writes checks to pay bills and balances checkbook	Provides physical and emotional support and care
Makes telephone calls to care recipient	Runs errands	Arranges for health care and/or companion services	
	Receives frequent care recipient telephone calls		

Abbreviations: IADL, instrumental activities of daily living such as shopping, cooking, and cleaning; PADL, physical activities of daily living such as bathing, dressing, grooming, and eating.

which implies a mature person-to-person relationship rather than, for example, a parent-child relationship. An excellent example of this concept has been expressed in a *Time* article by a caregiver daughter. Booth (1999) described her relationship with her 83-year-old father after her mother died. She stated that she and her father ate out three times a week and "we clink our glasses and connect—more than we ever connected before . . . we hug and kiss—things we never did when I was growing up" (p. 48). See Figure 10-1.

It is essential that the adult family caregiver, who may range in age from 30 to 70 years or more, does not talk to or treat the older adult like a child. Disrespectful and demeaning terms such as *childish* and *childlike* should never be used to refer to a person who is becoming more dependent because of a medical condition such as a stroke or dementia. An adult child never becomes a parent to a parent and a daughter never

TABLE 10-2 Benefits and Burdens of Caregiving

Benefits	Burdens
Being near the older adult, perhaps not since a long time ago	Lack of time
Getting to know the older adult better as an individual human being	Anxiety
	Fear
	Worry
Knowing that the person is safe, comfortable, and well cared for	Fatigue
	Guilt
Learning about aging and the normal aging process	Depression
	Increased expenses
Receiving appreciation and thanks from other family members and friends for what you do	Family conflicts
	Decreased social contacts
Feeling a personal satisfaction, now and in the future, for a job well done	Loss of other relationships

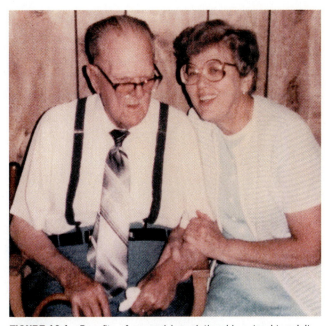

FIGURE 10-1 Benefits of a caregiving relationship extend to adult children as well as to older adults.

becomes a mother to her mother. There are other benefits of caregiving such as a personal feeling of satisfaction or reward that an older family member who is loved is being cared for very well in a safe and secure environment.

Some of the burdens of caregiving can be stressful and dangerous to the caregiver's physical and emotional health status (Pearlin, Mullan, Semple, & Skaff, 1990). Feelings of stress can cause an increase in blood pressure and a decreased functioning immune system, thus making the caregiver more prone to common infectious diseases. Lack of time to do everything that needs to be done for the older family member and the caregiver's family can be very stressful and cause fatigue and depression. Caregiving also differs among various countries, cultures, and ethnic groups. For example, in a study by Fredman, Daly, and Lazur (1995), African American caregivers had taken on more caregiving responsibilities but said that they felt less burden. The cycle of caregiver feelings is shown in Figure 10-2.

Problems and Needs

When one member of the family experiences an illness or other problem, it has an effect on all of the other members of the family. Family members of older adults, therefore, also experience loss, grief, and especially guilt that often lasts for years. Nurses should be aware of these family concerns and needs, include the family in the plan of care, and be caring and supportive as much as possible. Support and assistance for these family members will ultimately mean their continued support and caring for the older adult.

> ### Nursing Tip
>
> Be aware of the needs of family members of your older clients and include them in your plan of care.

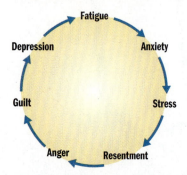

FIGURE 10-2   Cycle of informal caregiver's feelings. *[From Community Resources for Older Adults: A Guide for Case Managers (p. 254), by M. O. Hogstel (Ed.), 1998, St. Louis: Mosby. Reprinted with permission.]*

Figure 10-3 lists the most common intergenerational family problems and conflicts related to family caregiving as well as how the feelings of both the caregiver and the care recipient are affected by the most common problems that occur. Often called the **sandwich generation syndrome,** family caregivers find that use of time is probably one of the most difficult, especially if 24-hour care is needed and/or if there are other family responsibilities (Silverman, Brache, & Zielinski, 1981; Hansen, 1991). Mace and Rabins (1999) have perceptively titled their book on family caregiving for persons with dementia as *The 36-Hour Day.*

Think About It

What do you think are the pressures on a middle-aged adult-child employed full time who is the primary and only family caregiver for a dependent older parent?

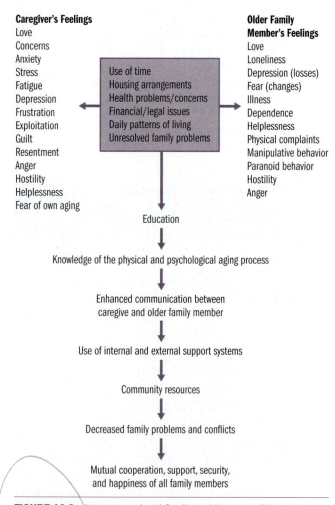

FIGURE 10-3   Intergenerational family problems, conflicts, and interventions. *[Adapted from Geropsychiatric Nursing (2nd ed., p. 326), by M.O. Hogstel, 1995, St. Louis: Mosby. Adapted with permission.]*

Where the care recipient will live is also a difficult decision. Most older adults prefer to live in their own home or apartment as long as possible, but sometimes that becomes unsafe if not impossible. The caregiver may decide to live in the older adult's home, but that may not be possible if the caregiver's other family members are involved. More often the older adult will move into the home of a family member, perhaps a daughter, son, sister, or brother. It is best if the older adult has individual private space where he or she can use some favorite furniture and other furnishings from a previous home (Figure 10-4). Older adults should make or participate in the decision about where to live before a move has to be made if at all possible because of later changing physical conditions or mental status. There are many alternative types of facilities today, however, so the older adult should make the decision if at all possible.

Health problems and changes in condition are usually the reasons for a change in living arrangements. These issues may cause fear, anxiety, fatigue, and depression for the caregiver. If the care recipient does not have adequate financial resources to pay for needed housing and care, the caregiver must plan for how the needs are to be met. If there is a critical and/or dementing illness, the caregiver will probably need legal assistance regarding financial and health care decisions such as preparing a will, Medical Power of Attorney, and/or Directive to Physician.

If there are several generations living in the home where the older adult is being cared for, many differences of opinions and conflicts can occur about simple daily activities such as type of food, television viewing, temperature of the environment, and hours of sleep and activity.

Perhaps the most difficult problem is the issue of unresolved family problems. For example, there may have been major conflicts between the mother and the adult child caregiver when the caregiver was young. The adult child may have been abused or neglected when young and now has the responsibility to care for the person who was the abuser. All families have some conflicts at times, but conflicts and bad feelings among family members that were never resolved in the past will affect relationships between the older adult and adult child when the child is the caregiver of the parent. Sometimes this situation can lead to **neglect** or **physical abuse** and/or **psychological abuse.** Nurses in home health care need to especially look for signs or symptoms of possible abuse when they are doing assessments and/or providing care in the home. New or healing bruises, especially around the face or eyes, burns, loss of weight, and a client who does not want to talk could be signs of possible abuse and/or neglect (Hogstel & Curry, 1999).

Ask Yourself

What would you do as a nurse if you witnessed or discovered a caregiver daughter yelling at her ill mother or a son hitting his father?

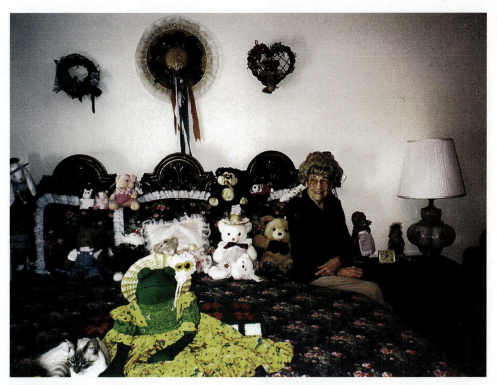

FIGURE 10-4 Feeling at home in her room with personal belongings.

The nurse, therefore, needs to be aware of these caregiver conflicts and attempt to intervene and assist families in obtaining essential facts and information so that the entire family can make wise choices. Figure 10-3 also includes some possible resolutions to assist caregivers, such as increased knowledge about the normal aging process and sources for personal and family assistance in the community. Young and middle-aged adult caregivers often do not understand what normal aging is

and believe, as part of society does, that aging is a disease. Therefore, family caregivers need to learn what is normal and what is not normal aging and where and how to seek health care and supportive services when the need arises. In addition to seeking help for the care recipient, the caregiver also has unique needs. Some of these needs are **respite care** and education and support for the caregiver.

Research Focus

Citation:
Campbell, D. D., & Travis, S. S. (1999). Spousal caregiving. *Journal of Psychosocial Nursing, 37*(8), 20–25.

Purpose:
To determine what informal support systems are used by spousal caregivers on the weekends when formal day services are not available, how much caregivers miss the formal services, and how likely they would use such weekend services if available.

Methods:
Twenty-seven spousal caregivers using adult day services completed and returned study questionnaires for an 82% response rate. The questionnaire included questions about amount and type of respite time needed as well as how they used the time, would they miss it if not available, and if they would use it if available.

Findings:
Age of respondents ranged from 55 to 83 and were primarily well-educated white females who were unemployed or retired and provided 100% of the care to their spouses. The majority (60%) had no respite time available on the weekend. Only 37% of the caregivers said that they would not miss weekend respite care if not available. About 33% were not likely to use weekend day services if available.

Implications:
These results were surprising, but other factors were not considered, such as additional costs for weekend services, transportation issues, and other working family members who could help on the weekend. For example, spousal caregivers, especially men, were receiving weekend respite time from other sources than formal adult day services, such as adult children or grandchildren and home health care assistants for an average of 3 hours a week.

Respite Care

It is obvious from Table 10-2 and Figures 10-2 and 10-3 that the informal/family caregiver experiences many potential problems and stresses, especially if caregiving continues for months and years. One of the most helpful types of assistance, therefore, is respite or relief from those caregiving responsibilities periodically.

Respite care involves programs and services that provide rest and relief for family members who are caring for a loved one in the home. Respite care is "a convenient, socially sanctioned break from the round-the-clock care of a dependent family member" (Campbell & Travis, 1999, p. 21). Types of services include:

- Arrangements to have the older family member stay in a hospital (for example, hospice patient) or a nursing facility for a weekend or week while the family caregiver(s) are out of town, ill, or need rest.

- Working family members can take the older adult to a local **adult day services** agency for needed care and supervision while the family members work or rest. This type of respite is especially important for caregivers whose older family member has some type of dementia. The person may be able to eat, drink, dress, and care for self, but it may be unsafe to leave the person alone at home during the day for fear of wandering away from the home and being injured. The person with dementia could receive essential care and supervision in an adult day services agency.

- **Home health aides** or **personal care attendants** may provide respite care for an hour or so in the home while providing direct care to the older adult. The time may be short, but the caregiver can at least take a walk and get out of the house.

However, even when one or all of these respite care services are available, the care recipient still may need care 24 hours a day, 7 days a week, often for years. Therefore, short-time respite care on a regular basis can be very helpful so that the caregiver can get out of the house at least 1–3 hours once or twice a week. This type of respite care will help the care recipient, possibly preventing institutionalization, by helping the caregiver. With the prospect of decreasing federal funds, especially for home health care agencies and nursing facilities, the family and community will have a much greater responsibility in meeting the needs of disabled older adults.

Volunteers such as friends, neighbors, and church members can provide short-term respite care in the home. In one community, a church organization has developed a training program and provided 4–6 hours of training on respite care for volunteers in churches. A few hours of respite care a week can decrease a family caregiver's burden to some extent and also provide the care recipient with some friendly outside assistance and stimulation. Volunteer respite care services are greatly needed in many communities. A structured program consisting of specific guidelines and training will help volunteers to feel more secure in providing this type of service safely (*Respite care,* 1997).

Education and Support

Almost everyone will be a caregiver to some degree for an older adult at some time. The care recipient may be a spouse, parent, parent-in-law, grandparent, sibling, or friend. In recent years there has been increased emphasis on the caregiver role and support for informal caregivers. Specific programs have evolved to help meet this need.

As People Grow Older

One of the first specific programs, developed in the early 1980s at the University of Michigan, was a program called As Parents Grow Older (Sliverman et al., 1981). More recently some groups have revised the title to be **As People Grow Older (APGO),** because the care recipient may be someone other than a parent. This program involves education about a variety of topics helpful to family caregivers as well as serves as a support group where caregivers can openly share their thoughts, concerns, and problems about their caregiver role (see the example in Box 10-1). After the 6-week 12-hour course, participants may decide to continue attending a monthly caregiver support group. Ideal membership for such groups should be limited to about 8–10 people. Some of these support groups have been called **Children of Aging Parents (CAPs).** Nurses or social workers with special education and interest in the field of aging are ideal group facilitators, although others can be taught to lead the APGO classes and support groups.

Box 10-2 lists some very practical and helpful suggestions for informal caregivers. These are some of the suggestions discussed in caregiver support groups, although topics can be anything the members need to

discuss. One primary purpose of any kind of support group is to help members realize that they are not the only people with similar feelings, needs, and concerns. Local chapters of the Alzheimer's Association also offer various types of support groups for family caregivers, with special focus on learning and sharing more knowledge about Alzheimer's disease and related caregiving issues. Booth (1999), a caregiver herself, has provided "some tips for navigating this difficult rite of passage: don't wait . . . seek support . . . shop around . . . take care of yourself" (p. 51).

A Caregiver Coalition

One local community has developed a caregiver coalition. The mission statement and specific goals of the coalition are listed in Box 10-3.

BOX 10-1 A Series of Programs for Adults with Aging Family Members

If you have concerns about:

- Living arrangements for your aging family members
- Psychological and emotional aspects of aging
- Chronic illnesses of older adults and how to manage them
- Community services for older adults
- Your ability to manage stressful time with your aging family member

Then As People Grow Older will benefit you!

As People Grow Older is a series of six sessions designed to give information and support to adults caring for an aging family member. The sessions enable family caregivers to better understand the physical and psychological aspects of aging, identify their family needs, locate helpful community resources, and share feelings and coping strategies. The following topics are discussed:

Week 1 Understanding the psychological aspects of aging
Week 2 Chronic illness and behavioral changes with age
Week 3 Sensory loss and improving communication
Week 4 Living arrangements and shared decision making
Week 5 Availability and use of community resources
Week 6 Understanding our feelings

BOX 10-2   Ten Tips for Caregivers

- Accept the fact that feelings experienced are normal or at least common.

- Learn as much factual information as you can about the condition(s) of the older family member needing care.

- Ask physicians and other health care providers specific questions until you get clear satisfactory answers.

- Learn about the best treatment and care needed.

- Seek assistance from sources of support such as family members, friends, religious leaders, support groups, and professionals.

- Accept assistance from others. You probably have or will return the favor someday. Being too independent is not necessarily a virtue if it harms yourself and/or others.

- Take time for personal essential health practices and adapt them based on your schedule (for example, nutritious food, adequate exercise, enough rest and relaxation, and regular physical examinations).

- Recognize that you are doing a good job, or at least the best you can and perhaps better than most, in a difficult situation.

- Reward yourself occasionally by buying something you really do not need or by doing something different and interesting.

- Do not attempt to give total care 24 hours a day alone. The intensity of problems will increase for both the caregiver and the family member needing care.

This coalition was organized by individual representatives from nine different community groups who meet regularly. The agencies represented are:

- County home care association

- Local Alzheimer's association

- Local area agency on aging

- Alzheimer's association research and special care facility

- County senior citizens services

- Local community of churches

- County gerontological society

BOX 10-3   Mission Statement and Goals of a Caregiver Coalition

Mission
The caregiver coalition will serve as a centralized clearinghouse for caregiving information, referral, and advocacy.

Goals
- Encourage a greater community dialogue about family caregiving.

- Enhance advocacy and accessibility of services for caregivers.

- Promote the development and dissemination of appropriate caregiving educational materials within the community.

- Stimulate the development of countywide caregiver support groups.

- Serve as a clearinghouse for caregiving information.

- Identify the need for eldercare support and education in the workplace.

- Assist in the development of a countywide caregiver center.

- School of Nursing in a local university

- Home-delivered meals agency

The first activities of the coalition were to survey the needs of informal caregivers in the area and to prepare a resource list of community programs specifically for caregivers. A telephone number is available 24 hours a day for caregivers to call about their questions and concerns. Volunteers, several of whom are nurses, social workers, or case managers, return the calls as soon as they can. A long-term goal was to fund, open, and staff a caregiver center where information about community resources, education, and support would be available to caregivers throughout the local area 24 hours a day. These types of centers are located in universities in some areas of the country. This concept is ideal because not only are information, education, and services available to informal caregivers, but the setting is also an ideal place for faculty research on caregiving issues and student experience and learning (refer to Box 10-4). Because gerontology and caregiving are interdisciplinary in focus, faculty and students in nursing, nutrition, sociology and social work, religion and ethics, business and economics, and education can be directly involved in the center activities.

BOX 10-4 Suggested Topics for Caregiving Research

- Reliability of community support services

- Instruments to measure caregiver burden

- Differences in family caregiving in diverse populations, including age, gender, and ethnicity

- Costs of family caregiving

- Physical and emotional effects of caregiving

- Stress factor on one-person family caregiving and several people responsible for caregiving

- Caregiving for single disabled people as they age

Adapted from "Literature of Some Review of Social Support and Suggestions: Caregiver Burden, 1980–1995," by N. J. Vrabec, 1997, Image: Journal of Nursing Scholarship, 29(4), p. 383.

Other Voluntary Community Resources

As previously mentioned, there are expectations that care for dependent older adults in need should be met by the community. This section describes some of those community resources that provide care primarily on a volunteer basis.

Churches and Synagogues

Churches and synagogues have traditionally been concerned about the spiritual and perhaps personal needs of their members. These services have usually been somewhat general, although effective, and performed by church staff and/or church volunteers. However, recently more specific programs and services have been developed that go beyond the spiritual and personal needs to include psychosocial, emotional, financial, and physical needs based on the belief that spirituality involves the whole person. Three programs with a more specific and holistic approach to members are:

- **Eldercare programs**

- **Parish nursing**

- **Stephen ministry**

Eldercare Programs

Eldercare, which could have other names or titles, is a program based on the nursing model in that a designated staff member, lay leader, and/or specific organized group identify those older members in the church who have special

BOX 10-5 Characteristics of a Successful Program

- The program is intentional, planned, and somewhat formal.

- It is part of a specific organization or structure in the church.

- Needs of older members are assessed.

- Records are kept.

- Leadership is available.

- Training is provided for volunteers.

- Volunteers are supported.

- The program has a budget.

- Community resources are known and used.

- The program connects to the neighborhood.

- It involves interfaith cooperation.

- It has support from the parent religious body.

- Community agencies are supportive.

Adapted from "Principles of Integrating Spiritual Concerns into Programs for the Aging," by C. J. Fahey and M. A. Lewis, 1990, Generations, 14(4), pp. 59–62.

"Given the current and future health needs of aging Americans, and the limited governmental resources being made available, there is great opportunity (and responsibility) for the religious community to demonstrate their own faith and trust by supporting and ministering to the emotional, spiritual, and sometimes physical needs of this population."

Source: Aging and God (p. 508), by H. G. Koenig, 1994, New York: Haworth Pastoral Press.

needs. This list may include those 60, 70, or 80 years of age and older; those in nursing facilities; those who have no close family members or friends; and those who have acute and/or chronic illnesses. Lay church members are recruited and trained as volunteers to visit and/or telephone an assigned older adult in need once a month or more. Individual needs of older members are identified and met as far as possible, either by members of the church or by community agencies that the staff and special volunteers learn about through training (Hogstel, 1998; Hogstel, Smith, & Reckling, 2000). These types of programs can be very helpful in providing support and assistance to older church members who have special need, possibly preventing premature institutionalization. Characteristics of a successful program are described in Box 10-5.

Some of the specific activities of an organized eldercare program in churches other than routine visiting, flowers, and food are listed in Box 10-6.

Eldercare church volunteers also can be very important in providing respite care to caregivers who are church members, friends, or neighbors. The eldercare program coordinator and/or parish nurse can provide training for volunteers for this type of service. See Box 10-7 for guidelines for respite care by volunteers and Box 10-8 for determining eligibility of respite care by a volunteer.

Parish Nursing

Holistic health care is often described as promoting the health of spirit, mind, and body. Parish nursing is a sig-

nificant practice model providing nurses the opportunity to practice within a holistic framework. The concept of parish nursing is an outgrowth of the work of Granger Westberg, a clergyman with many years of experience working in hospitals and universities. Throughout his career, he promoted the concept of holistic health and wellness in body, mind, and spirit. Nurses play a critical role in holistic health care because they are knowledgeable in both the sciences and the humanities (Westberg, 1990). All priority areas of *Healthy People 2000* are important for parish nurses, who should be aware of the priority objectives for all age groups.

Parish nursing is community-based nursing practice positioned in communities of faith. Faith communities refer to intentional communities where members of a congregation live and worship (Brown, Congdon, & Magilvy, 1996). The biblical mandate to heal the sick gave priority to sanitation and disease prevention in the Old Testament,

---

BOX 10-6   Activities of a Church Eldercare Program

- Provide large-print reading materials such as church bulletins and devotional booklets to those confined to their home.

- Provide individual hearing devices that can be worn during church services.

- Arrange for an emergency response system (ERS) for an older adult with some mobility or other physical problems who is living alone in the community.

- Provide transportation to church activities, especially at night.

- Deliver audiotapes of complete church services each week. Music as well as the sermon should be included.

- Provide handyman services in the home (for example, changing light bulbs).

- Provide educational sessions for older members and/or family caregivers on topics related to health care or similar matters (for example, normal aging, geriatric pharmacology, Alzheimer's disease).

- Arrange for special church services, lunch following the service, and corsages or boutonnieres for all members age 80 and older once a year.

- Arrange for special parking places close to the church entrance.

- Install grab bars by the toilets

- Paint the edges of outside steps yellow to prevent falling.

BOX 10-7   Guidelines for Volunteer Respite Care Training

- Respite care can be provided from 30 minutes to 3 hours once or twice a week (the volunteer cannot provide extensive periods of time).

- Volunteers cannot provide any kind of personal or nursing care such as transferring a person from bed to wheelchair or taking the person to the bathroom.

- Volunteers can provide food and fluids by mouth if the care recipient can eat and drink safely and if the caregiver has left clear instructions in writing.

- Volunteers should not be asked to go into homes that are not safe (for example, smoking or high-crime area).

- The older adult should not be receiving continuous intravenous fluids or medications at the time of the respite care, be dependent on a ventilator for breathing, have a tracheostomy, have a permanently placed tube for feeding by electric pump, be critically ill or near death, or have an infectious or contagious disease.

- The name and phone number of the primary caregiver and one other contact person will be readily available at all times in case of an emergency.

- Volunteers should attend initial and ongoing training sessions by the eldercare coordinator, parish nurse, and/or guest speakers on topics related to respite care.

and numerous stories of physical, emotional, and spiritual healing are found in the New Testament. "The potential contribution that churches and other religious organizations can make to health promotion and disease prevention efforts is largely untapped," according to *Healthy People 2000* (U.S. Department, 1991, p. 261). The concept of parish nursing supports the philosophy of *Healthy People 2000* (U.S. Department, 1991). Parish nursing facilitates public and private partnerships.

> ### Nursing Tip
>
> With recent attention on spiritual health, it is important that nurses assess and link clients to internal and external spiritual resources.

Different models of parish nursing exist. The two most common models are the institution-based model and the congregation-based model. The institution-based model is characterized by a faith-based health care system employing the nurse and providing administrative, educational, supervision, and support for the parish nurse. The congregation-based model is characterized by the infrastructure of support, supervision, education, and salary coming from the congregation. Variations of these two basic models exist and volunteer and/or paid nurses work in both models. There are congregations where all services are provided by volunteers, depending on their resources (Henderson & Holstrom, 1995; Lloyd & Solari-Twadell, 1994; Solari-Twadell & Westberg, 1991).

The concept of parish nursing draws on the role that the church has historically held in health care. The goal of the program is to provide support, promote wellness, and

---

BOX 10-8 Initial Assessment of Care Recipient Needs and Environment to Determine if a Volunteer Can Provide Respite Care

During the first visit by a prospective respite care volunteer to an older care recipient, the following information will be obtained to determine (1) if the person meets the eligibility requirements and (2) what kind of volunteer assistance will be needed.

	Yes	No
1. Is the person age 60 or older?	____	____
2. Does the person smoke?	____	____
3. Can the person walk without assistance?	____	____
4. Does the person use a wheelchair?	____	____
a. Occasionally?	____	____
b. All of the time?	____	____
5. Can the person speak well enough to be heard and understood?	____	____
6. Can the person see to read?	____	____
7. Can the person hear a normal tone of voice?	____	____
8. Can the person feed himself/herself?	____	____
a. Food?	____	____
b. Fluids?	____	____
c. Special diet?	____	____
9. Does the person have any difficulty swallowing?	____	____
10. Does the person take any medications?	____	____
a. Will any medications be needed during the time of the respite care?	____	____
b. Can he/she take his/her own medications without any assistance?	____	____
11. Does the person have any unusual behavior (for example, tries to leave the house, is aggressive or combative)?	____	____
12. Can the person go to the toilet alone?	____	____
13. Does the person have any of the following:		
a. Tracheostomy?	____	____
b. Feeding tube?	____	____
c. Artificial ventilation?	____	____
d. Intravenous fluids or medications?	____	____
e. Infectious or contagious disease?	____	____
14. Is the person critically ill or near death?	____	____
15. Is there a telephone in the home?	____	____

enhance the feeling of caring among the members of the congregation. Faith communities are excellent settings to learn about health promotion, discuss health care concerns, and develop an understanding of the emotional and spiritual aspects involved in healing. Parish nursing offers nurses a great opportunity to promote healthier communities (Solari-Twadell, Djupe, & DeDermott, 1990).

The role of the parish nurse is complex, incorporating both health promotion and health care management activities. Parish nurses work with individuals, families, and the congregation, often extending services to the larger community through educational offerings and health fairs.

The goals of a parish nurse program are to:

- Assess and identify congregational health needs and plan appropriate programs.

- Promote health and well-being.

- Encourage lifestyle changes.

- Improve access and utilization of needed health services.

- Enhance quality of life for members of the congregation.

- Increase client satisfaction with health care (McDermott & Burke, 1993; Westberg, 1990).

Parish nursing addresses the health care needs of people in communities of faith where people live and worship together. Parish nursing offers nurses the opportunity to contribute to healthier communities. The roles of the parish nurse include educator, counselor, referral agent, and advocate/facilitator (Schank, Weis, & Matheus, 1996). Examples of some selected activities performed by the parish nurse can be found in Table 10-3.

Stephen Ministry

The Stephen ministry involves church member volunteers who have had special training in working with others who are in or have been in an acute crisis such as depression (Stephen Series Training Manual, 1991). The eldercare program coordinator can refer to the Stephen ministry for assistance that is needed beyond the scope of the eldercare training and the Stephen ministry can refer an older adult who is more apt to have a long-term chronic problem to the eldercare program. Both of them can refer people in need to the parish nurse. Each program serves a different goal.

Another similar church program is Christ Care, which involves small groups studying the Bible and applying the beliefs and practices in society today. This program focuses on small-group interaction, assistance, and prayers for those in need (Basic Training Manual, 1994).

All of these programs are nondenominational and can be found in a variety of congregations.

Telephone Reassurance

Older adults who live alone sometimes become lonely or depressed and/or have accidents such as falls that result in a fracture. Therefore, some contact with another person, even if by telephone on a periodic basis, can be very reassuring to the older adult and the older adult's family members if they live out of the area. Group members are assigned to call one or more vulnerable older adults at a specific time every day. If there is no response, they call a close neighbor or friend to check on the person. If they have no success, they go to the person's house. Telephone reassurance is an ideal activity for church groups who may already have a prayer chain for telephoning members to pray for those having surgery or who have developed other acute illnesses. Other groups such as women's social groups or American Association of Retired Persons chapters also do telephone reassurance. All of these are volunteer groups, but some agencies or individuals provide this telephone service for a fee. Some computer programs can be set up to automatically call a person at a specific time every day.

Errand and Assurance Programs

A similar program provides personal assistance with errands and assurance. One of the priority problems of older adults in the community is transportation because some people cannot purchase, maintain, and/or drive a car. Therefore, a church, social group, and/or individual can offer to run errands to purchase groceries and medicines or do other essential shopping. This type of assistance and support also provides reassurance for the person. Other types of assistance that can be very helpful to a vulnerable older adult living in the home alone are home maintenance tasks such as:

- Mowing the yard, clearing snow

- Changing light bulbs in ceiling lights

- Changing furnace and air conditioner filters

- Doing light housekeeping

- Making minor house repairs

- Installing grab bars in the bathroom

- Making and installing a wheelchair ramp

There are volunteer organizations in some communities that receive financial support from churches, businesses, and foundations to pay for essential costs, although most of the work is performed by volunteers.

TABLE 10-3	Activities Performed by the Parish Nurse

Nursing Role	Activity
Education	Health promotion • Blood pressure checks • Articles for a bulletin and newsletter • Screening for diabetes, cancer, strokes • Growth and development screenings • Other community agencies that serve as site for flu shots or immunization clinics • Group education for various health issues
Counselor	• Conduct private consultations regarding health issues • Support groups: grief, cancer, weight loss • Guide persons to use existing community resources • Act as spokesperson when an individual cannot act on own behalf • Assist families in time of crisis • Incorporate spiritual values into health education • Meet with families to plan care of individuals or to counsel members • Communicate with clergy, church staff, church council, wellness committee, and volunteers
Referral agent	• Coordinate plan of care following discharge from hospital/nursing facility • Contact physician's office for individuals who need assistance
Advocate facilitator	• Coordinate volunteers to assist with various programs and needs of individuals • Provide transportation • Pick up prescription medications • Prepare meals • Provide respite care for family caregivers • Work with the wellness committee to meet the needs of the congregation • Record statistical information • Document health information on the client's record

Nursing Roles and Responsibilities

Nurses need to become aware of changes in the health care delivery system that clearly indicate that they need to perform major roles in the community, either as their primary employment or as a volunteer in one of the organizations described in this chapter. Nurses are ideal to become eldercare coordinators, parish nurses, and Stephen ministers as well as to participate in volunteer activities in other organizations. Nursing schools are increasingly requiring a specific amount of volunteer work in the community as a part of a specific course. These activities increase students' knowledge about community resources for older adults as well as stimu-

late ideas about possible future roles of nurses as entrepreneurs. Nurses in the future must look beyond medical diagnoses, physical needs and care, and technology to become more aware of the home and community where patients and clients live, including *all* of the present and future resources that are available to assist families and their older members. As noted in other chapters in this book, more and more health care and long-term care will be provided in the community as opposed to acute-care hospital settings. Therefore, nurses need to be aware of those community resources so that they can help clients and their family members find the resources that they need. Nurses must be strong **advocates** for their older clients, friends, and family members.

Summary

With the increasing number of older adults in the twenty-first century and a decreased amount of money for health care and social service programs for older adults, it has been suggested that the family and community need to meet more of those needs. The family has not been replaced as the primary source of assistance and support for older adults, but it has become more difficult to provide care, especially over a period of many years, for young and middle-aged adult children who also have other family, work, and community responsibilities.

Even though there are benefits of caregiving, the role of informal/family caregivers can become very difficult at times. There are an increasing number of community programs that provide information, education, and support to caregivers of older adults. Some of these are a national program called As People Grow Older, eldercare in the church and synagogue programs, parish nursing, the Stephen ministry, telephone reassurance, and errand and assurance programs.

Nurses need to assess and assist informal/family caregivers who are caring for older adults by referring them to appropriate community services and by being a strong advocate for them in the health care delivery system.

Review Questions and Activities

1. What are four major caregiver roles?

2. Who are the most common informal family caregivers?

3. What are the benefits and burdens of family caregiving?

4. What are the major problems of family caregiving?

5. Why is respite care for family caregivers needed?

6. What are some dangers of volunteers providing respite care in the home?

7. What are the differences in church eldercare programs, parish nursing, and the Stephen ministry?

8. Visit a church that has one or more of the programs listed in question 7. Suggest an eldercare program or parish nurse for your church.

9. Why is errand and telephone reassurance a need for older adults who live alone in their home?

10. How can the content presented in this chapter be used by a nurse employed in a hospital?

References

Basic Training Manual (1994). Division of Education and Ministry, National Council of Churches of Christ in the USA.

Booth, C. (1999, August 30). Taking care of our aging parents. *Time,* pp. 48–50.

Brown, N. J., Congdon, J. G., & Magilvy, J. K. (1996). An approach to care management for rural older adults. *Parish Nursing, New Horisons, 5*(27), 7.

Campbell, D. D., & Travis, S. S. (1999). Spousal caregiving when the adult day services center is closed. *Journal of Psychosocial Nursing, 37*(8), 20–25.

Fredman, L., Daly, M. P., & Lazur, A. M. (1995). Burden among white and black caregivers to elderly adults. *Journal of Gerontology: Social Sciences, 50B,* S110–S118.

Hansen, S. (1991). "Sandwich generation" faces triple-decker squeeze. *Lutheran Brotherhood Bond, 67*(5), 4–5.

Henderson, G., & Holstrom, S. (1995). Parish nurse collaboration: Two churches, two models. In *Proceedings of the ninth annual Westberg parish nurse symposium, parish nursing: Ministering through the arts* (pp. 217–218). Northbrook, IL: National Parish Nurse Resource Center.

Hey, R. P. (1997). Families are taking care of each other. *AARP Bulletin, 38*(5), 4.

Hogstel, M. O. (Ed.). (1998). *Community resources for older adults. A guide for case managers.* St. Louis: Mosby.

Hogstel, M. O., & Curry, L. C. (1999). Elder abuse revisited. *Journal of Gerontological Nursing, 25*(7), 10–18.

Hogstel, M. O., Smith, H. N., & Reckling, D. M. (2000). *Eldercare/faith in action program training manual for church volunteers* (5th ed.). Fort Worth, TX: Tarrant Area Community of Churches.

Koenig, H. G. (1994). *Aging and God.* New York: Haworth Pastoral Press.

Lloyd, R. C., & Solari-Twadell, P. (1994). Organizational framework, functions and educational preparation of parish nurses: A comparison of national survey results. In *Proceedings of the Eighth Annual Westberg Symposium on Ethics and Values: A framework for parish nursing practice* (pp. 105–115). Northbrook, IL: National Parish Nurse Resource Center.

Mace, N. L., & Rabins, P. V. (1999). *The 36-hour day* (rev. ed.). Baltimore: Johns Hopkins University Press.

McDermott, M., & Burke, J. (1993). When the population is a congregation: The emerging role of the parish nurse. *Journal of Community Health Nursing, 10*(3), 179–190.

Pearlin, L. L., Mullan, J. T., Semple, S. J., & Skaff, M. M. (1990). Caregiving on the stress process: An overview of concepts and their measures. *Gerontologist, 30,* 583–594.

Respite care training manual. (1997). Fort Worth: Tarrant Area Community of Churches.

Schank, M. J., Weis, D., & Matheus, P. (1996). Parish nursing: Ministry of healing. *Geriatric Nursing, 17*(1), 11–13.

Silverman, A. G., Brahce, C. I., & Zielinski, C. (1981). *As parents grow older.* Ann Arbor, MI: University of Michigan.

Solari-Twadell, P. A., Djupe, A. M., & DeDermott, M. A. (Eds.). (1990). *Parish nursing: The developing practice.* Park Ridge, IL: National Parish Nurse Resource Center.

Solari-Twadell, P., & Westberg, G. (1991). Body, mind and soul. *Health Progress,* pp. 24–28.

Stephen Series Training Manual (1991). St. Louis, MO: Stephen Ministries.

Stoller, E. P. (1992). Gender differences in the experiences of caregiving spouses. In J. W. Dwyer & R. T. Coward (Eds.), *Gender, families, and elder care* (pp. 49–64). Newbury Park, CA: Sage.

U.S. Department of Health and Human Services. (1991). *Healthy people 2000: National health promotion and disease prevention objectives* (DHHS Publication No. PHS 91-50213). Washington, DC: Government Printing Office.

Vrabec, N. J. (1997). Literature review of social support and caregiver burden, 1980 to 1995. *Image: Journal of Nursing Scholarship, 29*(4), 383–388.

Westberg, G. (1990a). A historical perspective: Wholistic health and the parish nurse. In P. A. Solari-Twadell, A. M. Djupe, & M. A. McDermott (Eds.), *Parish nursing: The developing practice* (pp. 27–39). Park Ridge, IL: National Parish Nurse Resource Center.

Westberg, G. E. (1990b). *The parish nurse.* Minneapolis, MN: Augsburg Fortress Press.

Resources

www.nursefriendly.com

www.nurseweek.com

Advocate Health Care: www.advocatehealth.com

CHAPTER 11

Wellness and Health Promotion

Margaret C. Basiliadis, DO
Mildred O. Hogstel, PhD, RN, C

COMPETENCIES

After completing this chapter, the reader should be able to:

- State the reason for the increasing emphasis on wellness and health promotion for older adults.
- Differentiate primary, secondary, and tertiary prevention.
- List the major types of health screenings recommended for people age 65 and older.
- Identify sites where older adults can obtain free or inexpensive health screening tests.
- Differentiate screening tests from diagnostic tests.
- Discuss simple screening tests that can be performed in the home setting.
- Identify the types of immunizations recommended for older adults.
- Identify barriers to wellness and health promotion in older adults.
- Explore the importance of individual responsibility and assertiveness in obtaining and maintaining health and wellness.
- Discuss how to assist older clients select health care providers.
- Discuss the role of the nurse in assisting older adults to maintain wellness.
- Give realistic examples of the advocacy role of the nurse.

MAKING THE CONNECTION

Refer to the following chapters to increase your understanding of wellness and health promotion:

Overview

Older adults are not only living longer but are also healthier. Some of the reasons for this rather recent phenomenon are:

- Medical technology (for example, surgery innovations and new pharmaceuticals)

- Better nutrition and more exercise

- More focus on geriatric medicine (for example, **geriatricians**)

- More specialists in gerontology (for example, gerontological nurses)

- Increasing **assertiveness** of older adults concerning health care issues

A goal for the future is **compressed morbidity,** which means that people ultimately should be able to live independent healthy lives until about the age of 110 or 120 and, because life is eventually mortal, die after being ill for a few days. Because of the prevalence of multiple chronic illnesses in the later years, many older adults now live for 5 or 10 years or more with the problems that accompany their illnesses, such as chronic pain, decreased mobility, dependency, and social isolation. These problems often require medical care, supervision, and assistance that is often expensive as well as depressing because they last so long and reduce the quality of life. With improved medical technology, greater individual responsibility, and improved knowledge gained through education, older adults can stay healthier longer (see Figure 11-1).

Focus of Health Care Changing

Not only may earlier diagnosis prevent death, but also early treatment of diseases may prevent the long-term complications of specific diseases (for example, hypertension, glaucoma, and diabetes). Much of the health care in the United States in the past has been primarily centered on treatment of diseases, except possibly for prenatal care, infant immunizations, and dental care. However, the focus of health care is slowly changing to more emphasis on preventing disease and promoting health. According to Waltzer (1998), "the best preventive care consists of a combination of office-based services, patient education, lifestyle counseling, clinical vigilance through routine checkups, and the administration of timely screening" (p. 65).

While a broad-based focus on preventive health care will cost more initially because of the cost of screening and **diagnostic tests,** money will be saved eventually when there are fewer complications and less need for acute and long-term care, both of which are extremely expensive. The focus of this chapter, therefore, is to present specific recommendations for action that will help older adults to live longer and healthier lives. Nurses should actively teach their older clients in all settings about these recommendations. Refer to Box 11-1 for recommendations from the National Institute on Aging (NIA).

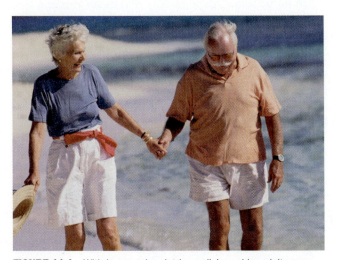

FIGURE 11-1   With improved geriatric medicine, older adults can look forward to longer, healthier lives.

BOX 11-1   Ten Tips for Healthy Aging

1. Eat a balanced diet.

2. Exercise regularly.

3. Get regular check-ups.

4. Don't smoke. It's never too late to quit.

5. Practice safety habits at home to prevent falls and fractures. Always wear your seatbelt when traveling by car.

6. Maintain contacts with family and friends, and stay active through work, recreation, and community.

7. Avoid overexposure to the sun and the cold.

8. If you drink, moderation is the key. When you drink, let someone else drive.

9. Keep personal and financial records in order to simplify budgeting and investing. Plan long-term housing and financial needs.

10. Keep a positive attitude toward life. Do things that make you happy.

Source: *National Institute on Aging. (N.D.). Rockville, MD: National Institutes of Health.*

Primary, Secondary, and Tertiary Prevention

Public health officials have long emphasized the importance of preventing diseases by means of **primary prevention,** which involves measures to prevent an illness or disease from occurring. Immunizations, proper nutrition, and regular fluoride dental treatments are simple examples of primary prevention. **Secondary prevention** refers to methods and procedures to diagnose the presence of disease in the early stages so that effective treatment and cure are more likely. Routine **mammograms,** hypertension screening, and **prostate specific antigen (PSA)** blood tests are a few examples. **Tertiary prevention** is needed after the disease or condition has been diagnosed and treated in an attempt to return the client to an optimum level of health and wellness despite the disease or condition. Physical, occupational, and speech pathology services following a cerebrovascular accident (CVA) are typical examples that attempt to return the client to as near the prestroke status as possible (Shi & Singh, 1998).

Primary Prevention

Primary prevention is synonymous with health promotion, that is, the encouragement of healthy habits and lifestyles known to maximize one's quality of health. Public health efforts have been made to educate the community on the benefits of practices such as eating a low-fat diet, regular exercise, and accident prevention. There is increasing evidence in the medical literature of the impact of health behaviors on morbidity and mortality at all ages. Smoking is the most preventable cause of death in the United States, including cancer, coronary artery disease, cerebrovascular disease, and pulmonary disease. Physical inactivity and dietary factors have been linked to coronary atherosclerosis, cancer, diabetes, and **osteoporosis.** Failing to use safety belts and driving intoxicated are major contributors to motor vehicle injuries and deaths.

It is time to shift focus from decreasing mortality to one of compressing morbidity. Human lifespan can be prolonged, but at what cost to the health of caregivers and the health care system? Primary prevention provides an opportunity to decrease risky behaviors to avoid unnecessary disability and promote independence. This should be the major function of a health care system facing an aging population. Most older adults do not want to live as long as possible in a debilitated state. Invariably, elders say if they cannot do for themselves, they do not want to burden their family. In a recent telephone survey of more than 2,000 people age 18 and older, 63% said that they did not want to live to be 100. Those with more education hoped to live longer (92%) than those with less formal education (89%), and those who are actively trying to stay healthy (for example, exercising) expected to live to 81 and the others to 76 (Crowley, 1999). However, health care providers still have difficulty letting go and not equating death with their own failure. Maximizing one's quality of life by compressing the time spent in an impaired state is an important goal.

Another important area in health promotion that is often forgotten or neglected by health practitioners is that of emotional and spiritual health. There are many anecdotal examples of the power of the mind and positive thinking on the healing process. The effect of prayer on health has been accepted by people from the beginning of time, when the *doctors* of the tribe were also the spiritual leaders of the tribe. The sense of wellness that comes from having a positive outlook on life and an inner source of spiritual energy is a tremendous force in health promotion. Yet in the Western practice of medicine, these two powerful sources of energy and the benefits they can have are often overlooked. Because this type of energy is not readily measurable, it is neglected in studies of health promotion. Perhaps future qualitative research can better define the benefits of emotional and spiritual health forces on physical health status.

The concept of health promotion cannot be fully considered without a discussion of holistic health and the movement toward alternative practice. Holistic health is defined as the view of a person as a biopsychosocial and spiritual being (Cohen, 1998). In an effort to incorporate the multiple human dimensions, a movement toward alternative therapy has evolved. It is important to note that in a *New England Journal of Medicine* report, 34% of adults surveyed had visited at least one holistic practitioner in the past year (Eisenberg et al., 1993).

One of the greatest advances in primary prevention and public health has been the use of immunizations to prevent disease. People age 65 and older and persons of all ages with chronic diseases are at increased risk for complications from influenza infections. During epidemic outbreaks, more than 90% of deaths attributed to pneumonia and influenza occurred among persons aged 65 and older. The few controlled studies of efficacy in persons age 65 and older suggest that when there was a good antigenic match between vaccine and virus, influenza vaccination prevented about 40% of hospitalizations and deaths caused by respiratory illness. The effectiveness of pneumococcal vaccine in the general U.S. population has not been determined with certainty. However, there is some evidence—and the U.S. Preventive Task Force has recommended—that the pneumococcal vaccine be used in immunocompetent individuals age 65 and older or at otherwise high risk for pneumococcal disease. In contrast, the effectiveness of tetanus and diphtheria toxoids is established on the basis of clinical studies and decades of experience. Currently, adults ages 50 and older account for the majority of cases of tetanus, with persons age 70 and older having a 26% case-fatality rate. The Td vaccine series should be completed for all clients who have not received the primary series, and all adults should receive periodic Td boosters. The optimal interval for booster doses is not established, but the standard regimen suggests a booster about every 10 years (*Guide to clinical,* 1996).

Secondary Prevention

Secondary prevention, or the early detection and treatment of disease, is the next level of preventive medicine. Health screening is one weapon in the battle for the practice of preventive medicine. It is most effective when coupled with counseling interventions, immuniza-

tion programs, and chemoprophylactic regimens. Preventive services for the early detection of disease have been associated with substantial reductions in morbidity and mortality. Age-adjusted mortality from stroke has decreased, a trend attributed in part to earlier detection and treatment of hypertension. Dramatic reductions in cervical cancer mortality have occurred since the use of **Papanicolaou testing** to detect cervical dysplasia.

Health Screening

The primary purpose of health screening is to detect diseases early when they are more treatable and possibly curable. A **screening test** is usually relatively simple, noninvasive, and economical. These tests can be performed by the **health care provider** using equipment and supplies designed for that specific test (Figure 11-2). Frequency depends upon the client's family history and high-risk status and discussion between the physician and the patient. Screening tests do not provide a specific diagnosis but instead indicate that further testing is needed to determine a definite diagnosis. One elevated blood pressure reading, for example, does not diagnose hypertension. A series of at least three elevated readings (as determined by the health care provider) will lead to a specific diagnosis. A high PSA laboratory test score may not indicate cancer of the prostate (it could mean some other prostate condition such as benign prostatic hyperplasia), so other tests such as a rectal exam and a

Research Focus

Citation:

Goldberg, T., & Chavin, S. (1997). Preventive medicine and screening in older adults. *Journal of the American Geriatrics Society, 45,*(3) 344–354.

Purpose:

To review important current issues, studies, recommendations, and controversies relating to preventive medicine and screening in older adults.

Methods:

MEDLINE searches for literature on prevention and screening with regard to older adults as well as each individual condition were reviewed: bibliographical reviews of textbooks, journal articles, government and advocacy organization task force reports, and recommendations. Important information was synthesized and discussed qualitatively.

Findings:

Attempts to prevent diseases of old age should start in youth; the older the client, the less likely the possibility or value of primary and secondary prevention, and the greater the stress must be on tertiary prevention.

Implications:

Age 85 is proposed as a general cutoff range beyond which conventional screening tests are unlikely to be of continued benefit; however, care must always be individualized. Emphasis should be on offering the best proven and most effective interventions to the individuals at highest risk for conditions such as cardiovascular diseases, malignancies, infections and endocrine diseases, and other important threats to function in older adults.

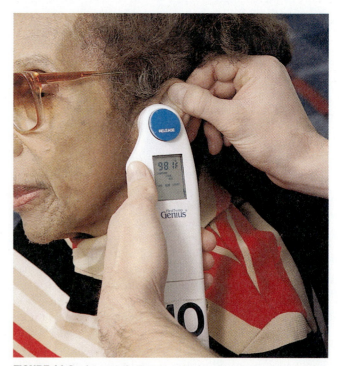

FIGURE 11-2   A tympanic thermometer is an example of an easy-to-use, noninvasive screening tool.

biopsy of the prostate gland may be necessary for a specific diagnosis. A diagnostic test, therefore, will be more extensive, involve more skill, be performed by a health care provider, and be more expensive.

Types of Screening

The various types of health screening tests most important for adults age 65 and older, considering the major causes of death in people age 65 and older (heart disease, cancer, and stroke) (see Box 11-2) and morbidity (diabetes, cataracts, and fractures), are listed in Table 11-1. It is important that older adults keep a personal written record of the dates and results of all screening and diagnostic tests. This information may be needed when traveling, when seeing a specialist, or when the primary health care provider retires or leaves the person's health insurance plan and a new provider is selected. Several of the assessment tools used in various health screening exams are shown in Figure 11-3.

Strategies for screening for medical conditions need to be appropriate for the specific population, in this case the older adult. Considerations of functional status and quality of life become increasingly important and may outweigh the importance of prolonging life at any cost. For example, it would not be reasonable to screen an 85-year-old man with severe heart failure for prostate cancer, which has a long preclinical stage. The impact of his cardiac condition on morbidity and mortality will far outweigh that of prostate cancer. Second, consideration of what the clinical course of action would be if disease is discovered should be made prior to screening. Not everyone desires to have aggressive chemotherapy or surgery, but the client should be clearly informed of his or her choices. Sometimes treatment decisions can be made without the client enduring the time and cost of another test.

If reasonable treatment does exist, the disease must have an asymptomatic period during which detection

and treatment significantly reduce morbidity and/or mortality. It is from this perspective that screening for hypertension, cancers, mental health disorders, and osteoporosis is discussed. Blood pressure screening with a sphygmomanometer remains the most appropriate screening test for hypertension in the asymptomatic population. Although the test is highly accurate when performed correctly, errors may result from instrument, observer, environment, or client factors.

Breast cancer is the most common diagnosed cancer in women. Routine screening for breast cancer every year with mammography is recommended for women

TABLE 11-1 Recommended Screening Tests for the General Population of People Age 65 and Older

Test	Frequency*
Blood pressure	Every visit or at least yearly
Pulse	Every visit or at least yearly
Electrocardiogram	Clinician's judgment
Cholesterol	Yearly if high risk
Blood sugar	Clinician's judgment
Urinalysis	Yearly as appropriate
Clinical breast exam	Every year after age 40
Mammogram	Every year after age 50
Papanicolaou test	Every 1–3 years based on risk
Pelvic exam	Every year
Fecal occult blood test	Every year after age 50
Digital rectal exam	Every year after age 40
Sigmoidoscopy	Every 3–5 years after age 50
Vision exams	Every year after age 65
Hearing	Periodic after age 65
Bone mineral density (BMD)	At least once after menopause (men if high risk)
Prostate specific antigen (men)	Every year after age 50

*Different organizations have different recommendations. These frequencies are sample recommendations. Frequency will depend upon the clinician's judgment and risk factors of the client.
Adapted from Guide to Clinical Preventive Services, Report of the U.S. Preventive Task Force, 1996, The Clinician's Handbook of Preventive Services, 1994, Alexandria, VA: International Medical Publishing; Practical Guide to Health Assessment Through the Lifespan, by M. O. Hogstel & L. C. Curry, 2001, Philadelphia: F. A. Davis.

BOX 11-2 Leading Causes of Death in Persons Age 65 and Older

- Heart disease
- Malignant neoplasm
- Cerebrovascular disease
- Chronic obstructive pulmonary disease (COPD)
- Pneumonia and influenza

Source: *National Center for Health Statistics, U.S. Department of Health and Human Services, 1994.*

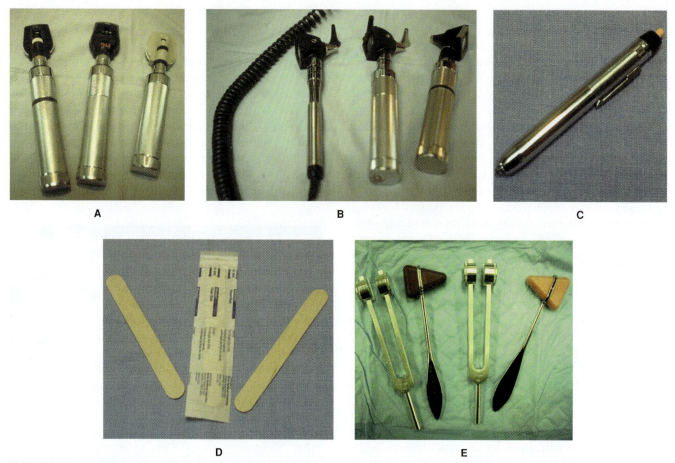

FIGURE 11-3 (a) Opthalmoscope, (b) otoscope, (c) penlight, (d) tongue depressors, and (e) tuning forks and reflex hammers.

aged 50–69 years of age. Currently there is insufficient research to recommend for or against routine mammography in healthy women ages 70 and older, although it seems reasonable to continue for women who have a moderate life expectancy.

Colorectal cancer is the second most common form of cancer in the United States and has the second highest mortality rate. Screening for colorectal cancer is recommended for all persons aged 50 and older with annual fecal occult blood testing. **Sigmoidoscopy,** barium enema, and/or colonoscopy should also be considered based on the patient's risk factors. There is insufficient evidence to determine which of these screening methods is preferable or whether the combination of procedures produces greater benefit than either test alone.

Routine screening for lung cancer with chest x-ray or sputum cytology in asymptomatic persons is not recommended primarily because of unnecessary radiation exposure. All clients should be counseled against tobacco use. Routine screening for prostate cancer with digital rectal examinations, serum tumor markers (for example, PSA), or transrectal ultrasound is controversial, not because they are ineffective, but because there is

some question of their cost effectiveness in our expensive current health care delivery system. Screening to detect problem drinking is recommended for all adult clients. Screening should involve a careful history of alcohol use and/or the use of standardized screening questionnaires.

Routine screening for cervical cancer with Papanicolaou testing is recommended for all women who are or have been sexually active and who have a cervix. Pap smears should be repeated every 1–3 years. There is insufficient evidence to recommend for or against an upper age limit, but this probably could be discontinued in women after age 65 if they have had regular screenings that have been consistently negative and do not have other risk factors (*Guide to clinical,* 1996).

The **bone mineral density (BMD)** and the PSA tests are relatively new. The National Osteoporosis Foundation advises "all women over age 65 to have a bone density test" (Who needs, 1998, p. 5). This test is now "widely available and is covered by Medicare for women at risk" (Who needs, 1998, p. 5). Men are at less risk for osteoporosis than women because they generally have larger bones with more bone mass. However, if they have risk factors such as small stature, are Caucasian, smoke, and use excessive alcohol, sodium, and/ or caffeine, they also need to be screened for osteoporosis (Siddiqui, Shetty, & Duthie, 1999).

The PSA test may indicate conditions other than cancer. For example, levels above 10 ng/ml usually mean cancer, but a finding of 4 and 10 ng/ml is called a "diagnostic gray zone" that may or may not indicate cancer (Prostate cancer, 1998, p. 5). Newer versions of the test are becoming more accurate.

Sites

Most of the screening tests can be performed in any setting where the essential personnel and equipment are available. Examples are:

- Physicians' offices
- Hospitals
- Assisted-living facilities
- Nursing facilities (homes)
- Community clinics
- Mobile screening units
- Health fairs at malls or other businesses such as pharmacies or grocery stores
- Churches

> **Nursing Tip**
>
> Plan and coordinate a blood pressure, glaucoma, and/or bone mineral density measurement screening for the older members of your community or church.

The sponsoring organization and/or institution has the legal responsibility for ensuring that correct procedures are followed, personnel are trained, the equipment is safe, and follow-up reporting is accurate. For example, the American Red Cross sponsors community hypertension screening clinics using criteria and guidelines developed by a medical staff member or consultant. The American Council of the Blind, through local agencies, may conduct glaucoma screening clinics in senior citizen centers. The American Cancer Society may provide a mobile van for mammogram screening at churches arranged by a parish nurse.

Think About It

Do you see more older adults or younger people smoking? At whom is the advertising for cigarettes aimed?

Providers

Health care providers are beginning to place more emphasis on wellness by discussing nutrition, exercise, and the dangers of smoking with their clients. However, their time is limited, and often they cannot spend as much time on health education as is needed, especially in a busy medical office or in an acute-care setting. Gerontological nurse practitioners, who may be in independent practice or work with a physician group, focus on health education and promoting health as well as assessing and treating certain health problems. They are the ideal health care provider to implement more health promotion activities in retirement centers, assisted-living facilities, and nursing facilities. Unfortunately, there are not enough of these types of providers in many areas of the country.

Costs

Another important factor to consider is the cost of screening. Is it possible or even essential that all citizens have all the recommended screening tests done at the intervals recommended? Are the recommendations by various national organizations (for example, the American Cancer Society or the National Osteoporosis Foundation) based on thorough research? Recommendations on who should have screening how often vary, so it is sometimes difficult to determine what is best. One criterion to consider is the cost benefit of a particular screening test. For example, is the cost of the screening worth the benefit? See Boxes 11-3 and 11-4 for the principal

> **BOX 11-3** **Principal Findings of the U.S. Preventive Task Force**
>
> - Interventions that address clients' personal health practices are vitally important.
> - The clinician and client should share decision making.
> - Clinicians should be selective in ordering tests and providing preventive services.
> - Clinicians should take every opportunity to deliver preventive services, especially to persons with limited access to care.
> - For some problems, community-level interventions may be more effective than clinical preventive services.
>
> *Adapted from* Guide to Clinical Preventive Services, Report of the U.S. Preventive Task Force, *1996, Alexandria, VA: International Medical Publishing.*

BOX 11-4   Criteria to Justify Screening for a Disease

- The disease must have a significant effect on quality or quantity of life.

- Acceptable methods of treatment must be available.

- The disease must have an asymptomatic period during which detection and treatment significantly reduce morbidity and/or mortality.

- Treatment in the asymptomatic phase must yield a therapeutic result superior to that obtained by delaying treatment until symptoms appear.

- The incidence of the condition must be sufficient to justify the cost of screening.

Adapted from Guide to Clinical Preventive Services, Report of the U.S. Preventive Task Force, *1996, Alexandria, VA: International Medical Publishing.*

findings of the U.S. Preventive Task Force and for a list of criteria to justify screening for a disease.

Self-monitoring Tests

Height and Weight

Older adults should be encouraged to take and record their weight monthly as an indicator of possible malnutrition and/or fluid retention. Height should be measured and recorded about every 6 months because decreased height is an early indication of osteoporosis and/or compression fractures of the spinal vertebrae.

Blood Pressure and Pulse

Considering that heart disease and cerebrovascular disease are two of the three major causes of death in people age 65 and older, frequent monitoring of the blood pressure and pulse is essential. Blood pressure equipment that is easy to use can be purchased in most community pharmacies. If desired, the person can purchase an aneroid sphygmomanometer and stethoscope in a local medical supply store. Nurses in physicians' offices, hospitals, or clinics should teach their clients how to take their own blood pressure. The procedure is not that difficult, and most can manipulate the equipment when taught by a willing person. The client can practice several times with the nurse observing and then the nurse can check the blood pressure after each reading for evaluation, recognizing that there will always be minor fluctuations. There may be some difficulties if the client has a major hearing deficit or arthritic fingers.

Clients who are diagnosed as hypertensive should take their blood pressure daily to help monitor the effectiveness and perhaps dosage of their regular hypertensive medication.

The procedure for taking the pulse should be much easier. After discussing the essential sites and degree of pressure on the artery, the nurse can take the pulse at one site at the same time as the client takes the pulse at a separate site for evaluation purposes. Clients should be told to record daily blood pressure and pulse readings and take the written record with them each time they visit their primary care provider (PCP). Initial blood pressure and pulse findings in the physician's office or hospital are sometimes abnormally high (for example, **white coat hypertension**) because of anxiety or stress. Therefore, it is very helpful to the physician to see readings taken under normal circumstances.

Guaiac Stool Test

Cancer of the colon increases with increasing age in both men and women. Therefore, one of the easiest and least expensive screening tests is to check for undetected blood in the feces. The physician, clinic, or other health care provider may send the testing slides home with the client to collect small samples of feces each day for 3 days. These slides are then returned to the physician or clinic by mail for testing. Instructions are clearly provided with the testing materials. Some older adults may have blood in the feces but not be able to see it because of poor eye sight or lack of knowledge about what to look for. Although blood in the feces could be caused by other factors (for example, hemorrhoids, especially if the person has problems with constipation), a series of 3 days testing is a good screening test for possible cancer.

Blood Glucose Monitoring

There are many kinds of equipment that can be purchased in medical supply stores and/or pharmacies for monitoring the blood glucose level in clients who have diabetes. The glucose monitors, test strips, and lancets for finger stick are covered by Medicare for non-insulin-dependent diabetics. Learning these skills is somewhat more difficult and requires a patient nurse who can teach the client and family how to perform the finger stick, how to test the blood on the monitor, what the results mean, and what action to take based on the results and the physician's orders.

Barriers to Health Promotion

Although most physicians intuitively understand/believe the benefits of preventive medicine, studies have shown that physicians often fail to provide recommended clinical preventive services. This problem may be related to a variety of factors, including inadequate reimbursement for preventive services, fragmentation of health care delivery, and insufficient time allowed with clients to deliver the range of suggested services. Also, the traditional medical model taught in medical schools in the past has primarily focused on illness and disease rather than primary prevention. But even when these barriers are accounted for, clinicians' performance of preventive measures is woefully shy from ideal practice (see Box 11-5).

Other barriers are potential factors that relate to adherence to health promotion activities of the older adult. See Box 11-6.

Ageism

Another barrier to health promotion is **ageism,** which is discussed in several other chapters. Some health care providers, family members of older adults, and older adults themselves may think that it is not necessary to have screening tests or medical treatment because they think their physical and/or mental problems are part of the normal aging process. Physicians may not be as likely to suggest certain screening and/or diagnostic tests for older adults (for example, mammograms, bone mineral density measurements, or PSA blood tests), believing that health status will not change and that they are not necessary or helpful. Some older adults may not be aware of newer tests (such as the PSA) and not request it (see section on attitudes and assertiveness).

Think About It

Why are many older adults reluctant to ask their physicians specific questions about prevention measures such as new screening methods they have read about in the media?

Cultural

Because of traditional family and/or personal practices, some older adults may believe that one seeks care from a health care provider only when ill and do not think that health promotion is important. They follow practices of past and current family members from a time when routine annual health examinations were not practiced. Some religious beliefs may even prevent the full use of the health care delivery system for prevention of disease and promotion of health (for example, the Christian Science Church, which believes in prayer and other spiritual methods alone for well-being). Also, some people do not think it is necessary to see a health care provider when they feel well and have no specific symptoms. Others believe that if the person thinks about some problem, it will happen, so screening is avoided.

Ask Yourself

What is your responsibility as a nurse when a client refuses a specific treatment based on spiritual or cultural belief systems?

Financial

One of the most prevalent barriers to health promotion is probably financial. Health care, even preventive care, can be very expensive. Medicare, the primary source of health care coverage for people age 65 and older,

BOX 11-5 Barriers to the Practice of Health Promotion/Disease Prevention

- Inadequate reimbursement for preventive medicine practices
- Fragmentation of health care delivery system
- Insufficient time spent with clients
- Confusion resulting from conflicting recommendations by the various health experts/panels
- Health providers' concerns over risk versus benefit of screening procedures
- Health providers' concern about the cost-effectiveness of preventive efforts
- Prejudices toward client populations
- Medical school focus on illness and disease

BOX 11-6 Potential Factors Affecting Patient Adherence

- Health-seeking behavior
- Belief in the efficacy of screening
- Cost of screening program (and subsequent testing)
- Anticipated feelings of anger, fear, and shame
- Availability of transportation
- Availability of a companion
- Lack of a regular physician

does not cover an annual examination for health promotion. There has to be a specific diagnosis for the physician to do an annual assessment under Medicare benefits (Self, 1998). However, Medicare benefits have gradually changed, and although the fee for the health care provider's office visit may not be covered, additional preventive benefits were added in the Federal Balanced Budget Act (BBA) of 1997. See Table 11-2 for a description of Medicare preventive services covered by Medicare.

As noted elsewhere in this chapter, some of these preventive tests can be performed by the individual or a family member in the home (for example, blood pressure and fecal occult blood tests) and at health fairs in malls or other sites where older adults participate in activities such as churches (for example, blood glucose monitoring and vision screening).

Gender

There is a common perception that women visit their health care provider more frequently than men. Perhaps that begins because women make regular visits to their obstetrician when pregnant during their earlier years. Although there certainly are individual differences, older men may feel reluctant to make an appointment with a health care provider for a routine examination when they have no specific symptoms. In one survey (Erwin, 1998), it was found that about 10% of men had not had a routine health examination for more than 10 years. About 15 million men have not had a checkup in more than 5 years. Perhaps men just do not want to admit they have a need, believe they are strong and indestructible, or do not want to spend money on something they do not think is important. However, women generally live 7 or so years longer than men (*A profile,* 1999) probably for a variety of reasons, so men need to be encouraged to have routine physical examinations and diagnostic tests to detect diseases in earlier treatable stages.

Think About It

Why do you think men are less likely to routinely have annual physical examinations? How can they be encouraged to do so?

Lack of Information

The mass media, newspapers, television, radio, magazines, and the Internet are increasingly including more articles and information on wellness and health promotion. Many people also receive multiple advertisements in the mail or by fax for health newsletters and magazines offering alternative therapies such as herbs or vitamins. However, sometimes people need help in evaluating what part of that information is realistic, appropriate, and safe for them.

Nurses, therefore, are in an ideal situation to help older adults separate fact from marketing for useless or even dangerous products. Telemarketing fraud of older adults about health care products is a major threat to physical health and financial resources. See the role of the nurse in health education later in this chapter.

Attitudes and Assertiveness

Older adults, like all other age groups, have different attitudes about health care. Many are very independent, despite multiple obstacles such as poverty, personal losses, and presence of acute or chronic illnesses. Some would rather live and die in an old home needing repair in a neighborhood with increasing criminal activity than ask for or accept help. These people may not have access to primary prevention or, because of a lack of formal education and finances, not be aware of what prevention strategies are available. That is why inexpensive screening examinations in community settings such as churches and malls are so important.

Others may not have received recent information about newer screening examinations such as a PSA or a bone mineral density measurement. For these reasons, education by the nurse regarding primary prevention is so important in every setting where older adults receive care and support.

Assertiveness in seeking quality health care is another issue. Although some older adults are very assertive in some areas of their lives, others are less likely to be assertive, especially in relation to health care. People in the past trusted their family physician, whom they knew well because of a long-term relationship, perhaps from childhood through the child-bearing years and into middle age. But, as their family physician retired and they selected a new physician as a Medicare client or were assigned a primary care physician (PCP), perhaps in a health maintenance organization (HMO), they continued to trust the physician but the same relationship might not exist because of the changing health care environment.

In the new environment of **Independent Practice Associations (IPAs),** multiple-physician groups, hospital mergers, and managed care insurance plans, older clients need to be more assertive to be sure that they and their family members receive the quality care that they need and deserve. See Box 11-7 for a list of suggestions on how nurses can teach older adults how to be more assertive when seeking and receiving health care.

TABLE 11-2 Medicare Part B Covered Preventive Services

Medicare Part B Covered Preventive Services	Who is Covered	Client Payments
Bone mass measurements: Varies with health status.	Certain people with Medicare who are at risk for losing bone mass.	Twenty percent of the Medicare-approved amount after the yearly Part B deductible.
Colorectal cancer screening: • Fecal occult blood test—once every 12 months. • Flexible sigmoidoscopy—once every 4 years. • Colonoscopy—once every 2 years if at high risk for cancer of the colon. • Barium enema—doctor can substitute for sigmoidoscopy or colonoscopy.	All people with Medicare age 50 and older. However, there is no age limit for having a colonoscopy.	Nothing for the fecal occult blood test. For all other tests, 20% of the Medicare-approved amount after the yearly Part B deductible. Costs may be different when services are received in a hospital.
Diabetes monitoring: Includes coverage for glucose monitors, test strips, and lancets. Diabetes self-management training.	All people with Medicare who have diabetes (insulin users and nonusers). If requested by the physician or other provider.	Twenty percent of the Medicare-approved amount after the yearly Part B deductible.
Mammogram screening: Once every 12 months. One baseline mammogram between ages 35 and 39.	All women with Medicare age 40 and older.	Twenty percent of the Medicare-approved amount with no Part B deductible.
Pap smear and Pelvic examination (includes a clinical breast exam): Once every 36 months. Once every 12 months if at high risk for cervical or vaginal cancer or of childbearing age and have had an abnormal Pap smear in the preceding 36 months.	All women with Medicare.	Nothing for the Pap smear lab test. For Pap smear collection, pelvic, and breast exams, 20% of the Medicare-approved amount (or a set coinsurance amount) with no Part B deductible.
Prostate cancer screening: • Digital rectal examination—once every 12 months. • Prostate specific antigen (PSA) test—once every 12 months.	All men with Medicare age 50 and older.	Generally, 20% of the Medicare-approved amount after the yearly Part B deductible. No coinsurance and no Part B deductible for the PSA test.
Vaccinations: • Flu shot—typically given once a year in the fall or winter. • Pneumonia shot—one may be all one will ever need; physician should be consulted. • Hepatitis B shot—if at medium to high risk for hepatitis.	All people with Medicare.	Nothing for the flu and pneumonia shots if the doctor accepts assignment. For hepatitis B shots, 20% of the Medicare-approved amount (or a set coinsurance amount) after the yearly Part B deductible.

Adapted from Medicare and you: Your Medicare Benefits *(p. 7), 2000, Baltimore, MD: U.S. Department of Health and Human Services, Health Care Financing Administration.*

BOX 11-7   Suggestions for Teaching Older Adults About Individual Responsibility and Assertiveness for Maintaining Wellness

- Learn to do some of the simple health checks yourself (for example, pulse, blood pressure, breast exam). Ask your physician or nurse to teach you how.

- Stop smoking.

- Keep active, both mentally and physically. Reduce stress.

- Take as few medicines as possible, but do not stop taking any without discussing it with your physician. Discuss the possible need for vitamin, mineral, and calcium supplements with your physician.

- Ask your physician about the benefits and risks of specific medicines, treatments, and surgeries. Ask for clear information in writing.

- Prepare for all physicians' office visits by writing down all of your questions and concerns a few days before the visit and do not leave until you get answers to your questions from the physician and/or nurse. Ask at least one question of your physician even if you think you know the answer.

- Keep your own written record of the dates of physician visits, immunizations, and blood pressure readings.

- Select physicians and hospitals that have the special services, staff, and equipment to give quality care to older adults. A quality to look for in a physician and nurse is the ability to listen well.

- When in a hospital, clinic, or physician's office, ask if the nurse caring for you is a registered nurse. A registered nurse must wear a name tag with the label RN (state laws differ).

- Do not let anyone tell you that symptoms or problems are due to age. Aging is not a disease. It is normal to be physically and mentally healthy into the 100s. Problems should be diagnosed and treated.

- Be assertive in seeking quality health care for yourself and your family.

- If you believe that your care has not been good, report it to the appropriate person or agency.

- Take responsibility for your own health and that of your family and insist on quality care.

- Do not change your health insurance unless you can obtain better benefits at the same or lowest cost. Be sure you understand exactly what the benefits are. Ask questions.

- Do not sign anything that you do not completely understand.

Individual Responsibility

Older adults also have an individual responsibility to take action for maintaining their own health. Some of these activities are simple, but still difficult to follow at times. Essential components of wellness are good nutrition, essential safe physical exercise and mental activity, and maintaining a strong social support system such as family members. See Figure 11-4. Most older adults are probably vaguely aware of these components of wellness but will probably need help with details related to diet adaptation, types of safe, appropriate exercises, and referrals or assistance when needed.

Selection of Health Care Providers

Although physicians who specialize in the medical care of older adults (geriatricians) are not available in many areas, that should be one of the characteristics to consider when choosing a primary care physician. Nurses can provide older clients, family, and friends the names of such physicians and/or private practice gerontological nurse

practitioners in the area. If not available, the nurse can recommend several physicians or nurse practitioners who have the specialized knowledge, experience, and communication skills to provide quality medical care to older adults. See Box 11-8 for suggestions for the older adult to use in communicating with the primary care provider.

Physical Resources

Hospitals, clinics, home health agencies, and nursing facilities that have special services and programs for older adults should also be recommended if needed. A hospital or other facility that has a certified gerontological clinical nurse specialist and/or gerontological nurse practitioner should be high on the list of suggestions. The largest hospital with the most extensive marketing and advertising program is not always the best one.

Appeals and Complaint Process

One of the characteristics of assertiveness in health care is the importance of the **appeals process.** If older adults

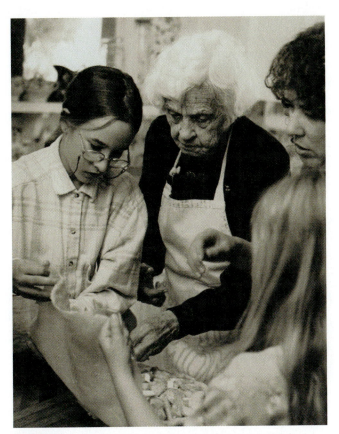

FIGURE 11-4 Contact with family members helps to maintain wellness.

BOX 11-8 Suggestions for the Older Adult to Use When Communicating with the Primary Care Provider

- Bring all medications with you for the PCP to review. Make an effort to know all of your medications' names and dosages and why they were prescribed. Include any vitamin or mineral supplements and any herbs or other similar substances you are taking.

- Make notes of any symptoms or concerns you have had since your last visit. Try to be as specific as possible with details of timing, associations with food or medication, attempts to alleviate the problem, and severity or impact on your lifestyle.

- Be conscientious of scheduled time. If there are multiple problems or new problems to discuss, notify the office ahead of time so that the allotted physician time is sufficient to address your needs.

- Do not be afraid to ask questions. If you do not understand, it is all right to say so. Ask if there is any educational material that you could review and discuss later.

- It is okay to say "no." Just because a PCP suggests a test or treatment, you have a right to consider the risks and benefits for yourself and decide what is right for you. You are not obligated to agree with everything and should feel comfortable to ask for time or further information.

- Ask for final instructions to be written for you. It is not reasonable to expect someone to remember everything discussed months later. (Even the PCP has his or her notes to refer to at the next visit.)

do not believe that they have received essential quality preventive health care, whether from a physician, nurse, or other health care provider, they should be encouraged to be more assertive to seek what they need and/or be informed and assisted with the appeals process.

Role of the Nurse

The role of the nurse has always been holistic to meet or facilitate meeting the overall needs of clients. Disease prevention and health promotion are included in that holistic perspective. However, except for some community settings where health promotion and disease prevention are the primary goals, nurses in other settings such as acute care, physicians' offices, and long-term care have not always had the time or information to implement specific health promotion interventions. Three major roles of the nurse in any setting should be health education, client advocacy, and referral to the appropriate place at the right time for further care if needed.

Health Education

Nurses are in a position to determine needs for health education because of their focus on assessing total needs and their close proximity to clients. The topics for health education are endless. For example, the nurse can teach about good nutrition, breast self-examination, the need for influenza and pneumonia vaccinations, and pertinent screening tests appropriate for specific clients. The nurse will need to determine the best time and content depending on the site and the condition of the client.

Nurses can also volunteer to assist with screening tests and present health education programs in community sites such as churches and other meetings of groups

BOX 11-9　Topics for Health Education Programs for Older Adults

- Arthritis
- Alternative therapies (herbs, acupuncture, music)
- Cancer (breast, prostate, lung, colon)
- Dementia (including Alzheimer's disease)
- Health maintenance organizations
- Heart disease
- Hypertension
- Immunizations
- Incontinence
- Medicare and Medicare Supplement Insurance (Medigap)
- Medications
- Mental health (especially depression)
- Normal aging (ageism and myths)
- Nutrition
- Osteoporosis and fractures
- Sexuality
- Skin problems
- Vision problems (cataracts, glaucoma, and macular degeneration)

of older adults such as the American Association of Retired Persons (AARP). See Box 11-9 for a list of health education topics helpful to older adults.

Advocacy

Another important role of the nurse is advocacy. When clients tell the nurse about problems receiving adequate

CLINICAL ALERT

Postmenopausal women are at highest risk for osteoporosis. The other risk factors include family history of the disease, early menopause, Caucasian or Asian ethnicity, thin or small bone structure, and lifestyle factors such as smoking, excessive alcohol use, and inactivity.

health care such as essential screenings, the nurse should intervene and make suggestions about actions including other resources. The nurse should offer alternative choices and solutions so that the client can make informed choices.

Referral Process

The nurse needs to be familiar not only with the wellness and health promotion needs of older adults but also with the community resources where these needs can be met (Hogstel, 1998). If the individual's regular health care provider has not met the older adult's need for information about maintaining wellness, such as discussion on nutrition and exercise, or if essential screenings have not been recommended, the nurse could suggest alternatives.

Summary

Older adults need to focus on wellness and health promotion as much as any other age group. Although some chronic illnesses do increase with increasing age, early diagnosis and treatment can prevent many of the disabling effects of chronic disease. Primary prevention (good nutrition and exercise), secondary prevention (screening for various types of cancer), and tertiary prevention (rehabilitation following a stroke or fracture) are essential to prevent the development and/or long-term effects of injury and illness.

Screening tests can be performed easily in a variety of settings in the community to detect the possibility of a health problem so that further diagnostic tests can be done to determine a specific diagnosis and treatment. Mammograms, colon tests, vision tests, and prostate specific antigen (PSA) blood tests are especially important for older adults. Medicare now covers many more preventive benefits such as influenza and pneumonia immunizations as well as screening tests, especially for those who are high risk for specific diseases.

Some of the barriers to health promotion activities in older adults are ageism, cultural beliefs, cost of care, male reluctance, and lack of information. Older adults need to be better informed, especially about recent research on health promotion, including new screening tests, and take more responsibility in being assertive to obtain what they need. The nurse has a responsibility to teach health-promoting behaviors to all older clients in all settings and be an advocate for them if needed to receive the best and latest information and techniques available.

CARE PLAN

Case Study

Mr. and Mrs. O'Connor are in their early seventies. They met at law school in their college years and have had long, successful careers as lawyers. Although over the years they admit to "making some bad financial decisions," they are thankful for their good health. They live modestly in a condominium in the northeast.

Both have remained very active over the years. Mrs. O. loves the water. She swims at the pool on a daily basis in good weather. In the winter, she goes to the town's indoor pool. In addition, as a child she enjoyed horseback riding, something she misses. Mr. O. enjoyed a very active childhood full of competitive sports. His favorite sports were basketball and wrestling, both of which he learned to appreciate from his mother. Over the past 20 years, he has played golf and even won a few trophies.

Mr. and Mrs. O'Connor do not have children because of Mrs. O.'s history of endometriosis and subsequent infertility. They have coped with the void through community involvement and volunteer work at a summer camp specifically aimed at children with cancer. Annual donations over the years have supported muscular dystrophy, juvenile diabetes, and bone marrow transplant. Mrs. O. sits on the board of a nearby children's hospital.

Mr. O. has a family history of prostate cancer and MI (myocardial infarction). His only brother died of a heart attack at the age of 62. His father had "hardening of the arteries" and died at 73. Mrs. O. has a history of cystic breasts and severe endometriosis. Her 90-year-old mother (still alive) was hospitalized for PID (pelvic inflammatory disease). All deliveries of the four children were "agonizing and long," according to Mrs. O.'s mother. One of Mrs. O.'s sisters died of uterine cancer, the other two are alive and living on the West Coast. Mrs. O. misses them.

As part of their overall philosophy of health and wellness, the O'Connors embrace traditional medicine supplemented by alternative medicine. Both are informed on some of the conflicting issues with alternative medicine. They are aware that the use of herbal therapies can enhance or detract from medication effectiveness, even causing life-threatening interactions. Mrs. O. takes ginkgo biloba for memory stimulation, plus a vitamin prescribed by her physician-nutritionist. Mr. O. takes Kavatrol (kava kava) for relaxation, along with specifically prescribed vitamins from the same physician-nutritionist.

Mr. and Mrs. O'Connor want to improve upon their good health and have sought your expertise.

Assessment

These are two healthy older adults who enjoy a fulfilling life. They are active and well informed. They take their health seriously—as a lifetime job—and cope with shortcomings in a productive manner. Reflect on how their health history affects their health outcome. What other steps could they take to stay at optimal health? Each has a family history of concern to the clinician. The following care plan reflects some preventive measures aimed at health screening and disease prevention.

NURSING DIAGNOSIS

Health-seeking behaviors related to desire for enhanced health, movement toward a higher level of health, and disease prevention.

Outcomes:

Mr. O. will:
- *Control and screen for risk factors of cardiac and prostate disease.*
- *Learn anxiety-reducing exercises and possibly using biofeedback.*

Mrs. O. will:
- *Control and screen for uterine, breast, and other reproductive-related disorders.*
- *Enhance social well-being by visiting her sister.*

(continues)

CARE PLAN *continued*

Planning/Interventions:

The nurse will:

- *Explain facts as we know them on cardiac disease and prostate, uterine, and breast cancer.*
- *Provide associated recommended reading list on men's and women's health.*
- *Discuss screening procedures and recommended frequencies of associated diagnostic tests. Explain related laboratory/screening tests and frequency (most are annually): lipid profile, HDL/LDL ratio, triglycerides, PSA, rectal examination, testicular self-examination, Pap test, breast self-examination procedure, and mammography screening.*
- *Offer dietary and vitamin information related to cardiac, prostate, uterine, and breast health; follow up with discussion on actual research findings.*
- *Explain the relationship between social interaction and well-being and physical health.*

Evaluation:

Mr. and Mrs. O. will arrange for appropriate disease prevention diagnostic screening and laboratory tests, most of which are due annually. They will remain physically active. Mrs. O. will plan to visit with her sister on the West Coast. Mr. O. will try nonpharmacological strategies to reduce his anxiety. Both will increase their knowledge of current findings on diseases for which they are at risk.

NURSING DIAGNOSIS

Knowledge deficit related to diagnostic screening tests for high-risk diseases and information on those diseases.

Outcomes:

Mr. and Mrs. O. will:

- *Describe relevant screening and laboratory tests specific to their risk profile.*
- *Discuss associated readings on high-risk diseases and prevention.*
- *Explain dietary and vitamin information relative to their lifestyle.*

Planning/Interventions:

The nurse will:

- *Present information on screening and laboratory testing.*
- *Provide information on high-risk diseases.*
- *Give information on dietary and vitamin therapy.*
- *Consult with dietitian, American Cancer Society, and American Heart Association resources.*

Evaluation:

Mr. and Mrs. O. will increase their knowledge about health screening, laboratory tests, and high-risk diseases pertinent to their health. They will demonstrate accurate and adequate knowledge about diet and vitamin therapies and will build upon their readings associated with disease prevention and aging.

Review Questions and Activities

1. What is meant by compressed morbidity?

2. Define and give examples of primary, secondary, and tertiary prevention.

3. What are the essential immunizations that older adults should have?

4. What is the difference between a screening test and a diagnostic test?

5. What is the purpose of a bone mineral density test?

6. Which screening tests are covered by Medicare?

7. How does ageism relate to health promotion?

8. Are most older adults assertive in seeking quality health promotion care? Why or why not?

9. What is the role of the nurse in health promotion and education?

References

A profile of older Americans 1999. (1999). Washington, DC: Association of Retired Persons and Administration on Aging (AA), U.S. Department of Health and Human Services.

Cohen, J. (1998). Holistic health strategies. In C. Edelman & C. L. Mandle (Eds.), *Health promotion throughout the lifespan.* St. Louis: Mosby.

Crowley, S. L. (1999). Live to 100? No thanks. *AARP Bulletin, 40*(7), 6–7.

Eisenberg, D. M., Kessler, R. C., Foster, C., Norlock, F. E., Calkins, D. R., & Delbanco, T. L. (1993). Unconventional medicine in the United States: Prevalence, costs and patterns of use. *New England Journal of Medicine, 328*(4), 246–252.

Erwin, J. (1998). Macho men: Helping men take control of their health. Dallas, TX: *Dallas/Fort Worth Health Week.*

Guide to clinical preventive services, Report of the U.S. Preventive Task Force (2nd ed.). (1996). Alexandria, VA: International Medical Publishing.

Hogstel, M. O. (1998). *Community resources for older adults: A guide for case managers.* St. Louis: Mosby.

Hogstel, M. O., & Curry, L. C. (2001). *Practical guide to health assessment through the life span.* Philadelphia: F. A. Davis.

Medicare and you: Your Medicare benefits. (2000). Medicare preventive services (Publication No. HCFA-10116). Baltimore, MD: U.S. Department of Health and Human Services.

Prostate cancer test becomes more accurate. (1998). *Health News, 4*(8), 5.

Self, D. (1998). Medicare + choice = health care gamble? *Geriatrics, 53*(11), 71.

Shi, L., & Singh, D. A. (1998). *Delivery health care in America.* Gaithersburg, MD: Aspen.

Siddqui, N. A., Shetty, K. R., & Duthie, E. H. (1999). Osteoporosis in older men: Discovering when and how to treat it. *Geriatrics, 54*(9), 20–32.

Waltzer, K. B. (1998). Simple, sensible preventive measures for managed care settings. *Geriatrics, 53*(10), 65–68, 75–77, 81–82.

Who needs bone screening? (1998). *Health News, 4*(5), 5.

Resources

Health Care Financing Administration: `http://www.hcfa.gov`

Administration on Aging: `http://www.aoa.dhhs.gov`

National Institutes of Health: `http://www.nih.gov`

`http://www.elderconnect.com`

CHAPTER 12

Health Education

Jan W. Weaver PhD, RN

COMPETENCIES

After completing this chapter, the reader should be able to:

- *Describe how the future shift in demographics will affect the health care delivery system.*
- *Explain the relationship of health education and healthy aging.*
- *Compare health care of older adults in the United States to that of other developed countries.*
- *Describe the purposes of health education for older adults.*
- *Explore the role of the nurse in health education in various settings where older adults receive health care.*
- *Identify two major learning theories.*
- *Differentiate geragogy from pedagogy.*
- *Discuss learning principles important in teaching older adults.*
- *Discuss barriers to learning in older adults.*
- *Identify factors that facilitate learning in older adults.*

MAKING THE CONNECTION

Refer to the following chapters to increase your understanding of health education:

Shifts in the U.S. Population

Americans are more concerned than ever about the nation's health care system because of the shift in the age and health characteristics of the U.S. population. Since the beginning of the century, the older population has become a larger and more influential segment of American society. As a result of this shift, the current system is under strain and Americans are questioning the availability and quality of future health care and social services.

The political climate of the United States is deeply influenced by the economic status of older adults. In the past two decades, health, pension coverage, and home equity values have improved significantly for older Americans. At the same time, there are dramatic differences in health and social well-being among subgroups and a significant number of older adults are living in or near poverty (Moody, 1998). The diversity of the older population, combined with personal lifestyle choices and political/economical factors, produces challenges for policy planners in the twenty-first century. Although there "certainly is not cause to be gloomy about the coming of an aging society" (Moody, 1998, p. 63), health and social needs mandate effectiveness and efficiency in aging services and programs.

Research in the past decade has confirmed the value of education for older adults. Evidence indicates that individuals, as well as society, benefit from formal and informal learning opportunities. Education has proven to be an integral component of healthy aging and "as critical to the quality of life as income assistance or affordable housing" (Cusack, 1998, p. 1). The new century offers the potential of significant reductions in preventable death and disability as well as improved health status for Americans of all ages.

Think About It

Do you think older adults are more concerned about their health than younger adults? Do they smoke and drink less and eat better and exercise more?

Demographic Characteristics

The United States contains the second largest population of people age 65 and older in the world, numbering 31.6 million individuals. China has the world's largest population of persons 65 and older, numbering 63.4 million (U.S. Bureau of the Census, 1987). Since 1900, a shift in the proportion of older and younger individuals has occurred in the U.S. population. At the beginning of the twentieth century, 4.1% of Americans were 65 and older while 40% of the population was comprised of people under age 18. Between 1990 and 2030, the 65 and older

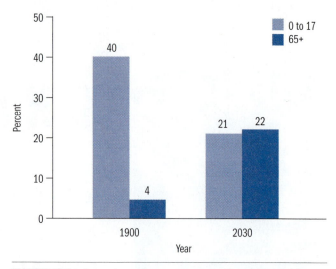

FIGURE 12-1   Percentage of persons younger than 18 and older than 65 in the population: 1900 and 2030. *[From* Aging America: Trends and Projections, *DHHS Publication No. (FcoA) 91-28001, 1991, Washington, DC: U.S. Department of Health and Human Services.]*

population will double and the 85 and older population, as the fastest growing age group, will triple in size. Because of the aging of the baby boomers and people living longer, there will be proportionately more elders than young people by the year 2030 (see Figure 12-1).

During the years between 1946 and 1964, the United States experienced the highest birth rates in its history. The large number of individuals born during these years will become 65 years old between the years of 2011 and 2029. The population will not only contain a greater proportion of older adults, but will also be comprised of more people living longer. However, not all of the years a person lives will be active and independent ones.

Although the diversity of the population has come to be recognized as a national strength, health care programs in the United States are characterized by unacceptable disparities linked to racial and ethnic groups (U.S. Department, 1990). These disparities are summarized in the 1985 *Report of the Secretary's Task Force on Black and Minority Health* (U.S. Department, 1985). See Figure 12-2.

One compelling disparity in health care for older adults relates to socioeconomic status. In 1989, 11.4% of people age 65 and older were below the poverty level. The poverty rate of the oldest-old (people who are 85 years and older) was 18.4% in 1989—more than twice the 8.8% rate of the young-old (ages 65–74) (U.S. Bureau of the Census, 1990). Women were substantially more likely to be poor than men: only 7.8% of men age 65 and older were below the poverty level, compared with 14% of the women. Poverty rates also were higher for people not living in families. Change in marital status, particularly because of the death of a spouse, was an important reason contributing to differences in income among older

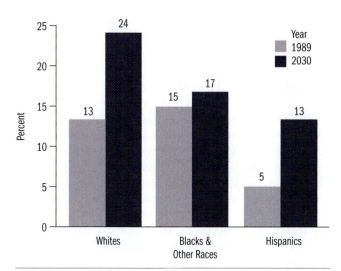

FIGURE 12-2 Percentage of persons 65 and over by race and Hispanic origin. *[From* Aging America: Trends and Projections, *DHHS Publication No. (FcoA) 91-28001, 1991, Washington, DC: U.S. Department of Health and Human Services.]*

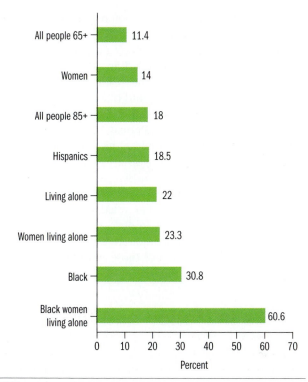

FIGURE 12-3 Percentage of older adults below the poverty level by select characteristic (unless otherwise noted data are for age 65+). *(From* Current Population Reports, *Series P-60, No. 168, 1990, Washington, DC: U.S. Bureau of the Census.)*

adults. More than half of the population age 65–74 was married, while nearly three-quarters of people 85 and older were widowed (U.S. Bureau of the Census, 1990). The greater the accumulation of these factors (age, gender, race/ethnicity, and living arrangements), the greater the risk of poverty. As shown in Figure 12-3, poverty rates were much higher among minority elders than among white older adults, and higher among people who were not living in families. The highest poverty rates were among older black women living alone: three of every five had incomes below the poverty level.

Health Status

In addition to the change in the age of the U.S. population from young to old, the morbidity pattern shifted during the twentieth century. Although acute conditions were prevalent at the beginning of the century, chronic conditions were the predominant health problem for older individuals in the late part of the century. Scientific advances and public health efforts have largely conquered the high rate of acute conditions (for example, life-threatening communicable diseases and injuries caused by accidents) that were prevalent among older adults a century ago. The leading chronic conditions for older adults in 1989 were arthritis, hypertension, hearing impairments, and heart disease (U.S. Department, 1991). Because chronic conditions lead to disabilities and functional impairment, a sharp rise is expected in the number of older adults in need of institutional and community-based care in conjunction with the changes in the size and characteristics of the older population.

Disability associated with chronic conditions is measured by determining limitations in major activities such as physical activities of daily living (PADL—for example, bathing, dressing, using the toilet, eating, and transferring) and instrumental activities of daily living (IADL—for example, shopping, using the telephone, and preparing meals). The role of perceived health is also an important factor because knowledge of underlying disease, recognition of physical disabilities, and awareness of functional limitation all negatively affect individuals' perceptions of their health status (Johnson & Wolinsky, 1994). Because some individuals adapt better than others to chronic health problems and associated limitations, the relationship between disability and functional limitation is variable.

Older adults are diverse in health and chronic conditions. The majority of older adults living in the community (71%) view their health as excellent or good (National Center for Health Statistics, 1990). People age 65 and older tend to take better care of their health than the young. Although they exercise less, elders are not as likely as the younger people to smoke, be overweight, drink, or report that stress has adversely affected their health (U.S. Department, 1991).

The growth in the number of older adults with functional difficulties will have a dramatic impact on health care and social services in coming years. In 1988, 22.6% of people age 65 and older had a limitation in major activity. The 1987 National Medical Expenditure Survey

(NMES) identified 19.5% of the noninstitutionalized population age 65 and older as having either PADL or IADL limitations. The likelihood of having a chronic condition increases rapidly with advanced age. While 5.9% of all persons aged 65–69 experience difficulty with at least one ADL, 34.5% of those 85 and older have ADL limitations (Leon & Lair, 1990). Gender differences are significant for all areas of functional status and increase with advancing age. Consistently higher proportions of women have ADL limitations in all age groups (Leon & Lair, 1990). Older adults who live with a spouse have less PADL/IADL limitations when compared to those who live alone or with other relatives. Almost 8% of older adults living with a spouse experience one or more PADL limitations, compared with 13.3% of those who live alone and 15.6% of those who live with other relatives (Leon & Lair, 1990).

Shifts in Policy and Practice

Care for older adults in the United States took a slow start in comparison to other countries with comparable levels of socioeconomic development. Social Security was not established until 1935 and Medicare, Medicaid, and the Older Americans Act did not appear until 1965. In comparison to the limited social support, income, and services provided for older adults in the United States, countries such as Sweden, Denmark, and Holland have a long history of providing high levels of income support, health care, sheltered housing in a variety of forms, and social services designed to prevent social isolation for their older citizens (Gill & Ingman, 1994).

Health promotion practices in the United States range from self-directed alterations in eating or exercise habits to extensive public policy initiatives such as federally endorsed fitness programs. Initiatives such as *Healthy People 2000* recognize that a better quality of life for older citizens can be achieved through modification of certain harmful practices and behaviors. *Healthy People 2000* (U.S. Department, 1990) has evolved from a health strategy initiated in 1979 with the publication of *Healthy People: The Surgeon General's Report on Health Promotion and Disease Prevention* (U.S. Public Health Service) and expanded in 1980 with the publication of *Promoting Health/Preventing Disease: Objectives for the Nation* (U.S. Public Health Service). Thus, a major objective of *Healthy People 2000* is to "increase to at least 90% the proportion of people aged 65 and older who had the opportunity to participate during the preceding year in at least one organized health promotion program through a senior center, life care facility, or other community-based setting that serves older adults" (U.S. Department, 1990, p. 259). Attaining this objective depends on the involvement of professionals, private organizations, public agencies, and individuals in these and other strategies.

Health Education

Health education, by health professionals for their clients, involves both formal and informal methods. Nurses and other health providers have always recognized the importance and value of client education and have included client teaching as an intervention. As previously mentioned, health education is a major objective of the *Healthy People 2000* initiative. The **Joint Commission on the Accreditation of Healthcare Organizations (JCAHO)** and the **Health Care Financing Administration (HCFA)** mandate client education for hospitals and long-term care facilities that are accredited or participating in Medicare/Medicaid programs. Nurses employed in these facilities must provide education to their clients and document instructions in clients' records. However, nurses need to remember that learning new content during an acute illness and hospitalization may not be retained because of the presence of anxiety and effects of anesthesia and/or medications. Therefore, providing clear readable instructions to both the client and family to take home is extremely important. Teaching is one of the major responsibilities of all nurses, whether they specialize in clinical, community, or administrative practice. They must be skilled in providing learning opportunities that will facilitate their clients' and employees' acquisition of knowledge, attitudes, skills, and new behaviors.

Education as a health promotion intervention is utilized with people of all ages and typically involves teaching about health care information or procedures. More than any other age group, older adults are actively seeking health information and are willing to make changes to maintain their health and independence (U.S. Department, 1990). Health education for older adults is commonly viewed as a means of improving quality of life. However, it serves many additional purposes. It can be a vehicle for self-fulfillment, retraining older employees to technological changes, or personal and group empowerment (Glendenning, 1992). The educational process can help older adults explore their social and political rights and raise their consciousness about their role in society (Glendenning, 1992). Learning promotes health, maintains or enhances mental vigor, and serves as an important life extender (Fischer, Blazey, & Lipman, 1992). Health promotion and mental vigor are strongly correlated with the capacity to survive. Education can foster older adults' self-reliance and independence, thereby reducing the demand for public and private resources. It also strengthens the older adult's actual or potential contribution to society.

A popular ageist myth claims that older adults are a social problem and a disadvantaged group with special needs. Society often marginalizes elders and assumes them to be dependent on others for care (Glendenning, 1992). Within this context, society should examine the treatment of older adults and view them as a heterogeneous group. Social class, gender, and experiential or ethnic differences are not erased by age or by participation in educational programs (Glendenning, 1992). Older learners bring special strengths of age and experience to the learning encounter.

> ### Nursing Tip
>
> Topics to focus on when preparing clients for discharge home are:
> - Medication regimen
>   - What
>   - Purpose
>   - Amount
>   - When
>   - How
>   - Side and adverse effects
>   - Effect on quality of life
> - Dietary adaptations based on condition
> - Mobility and safety factors
>   - Use of assistive devices such as wheelchairs and walkers
>   - Timing and type of exercise
> - Treatments and care required/needed based on the client's current and ongoing medical diagnoses
> - All PADL, such as bathing and toileting

Nurses educate their clients about standard health practices and about treatment regimens necessitated by medical problems. Client education involves the dissemination of knowledge intended to develop and maintain positive health attitudes and habits that contribute to personal well-being and productivity. Effective teaching requires an understanding of the complex internal and external forces that shape people's lives and create barriers to successful change. The goal of client teaching is for the client to adopt desirable health practices that will improve or maintain health and reduce disease prevalence. The nurse is responsible for ensuring that clients have access to the tools and resources they need to participate in decision making regarding their care (see Figure 12-4). Thus, client education is central to professional standards of nursing care that promote the individual's empowerment.

Changes in the health care environment have increased demands on nurses and challenged them to provide the most effective client education possible. Chronic diseases, such as diabetes, arthritis, and hypertension, require client education to achieve adequate

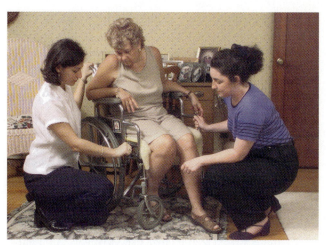

FIGURE 12-4 These community health nurses are instructing a client on the safe use of a wheelchair in the home.

control and prevent adverse health outcomes (Williams, Baker, Parker, & Nurss, 1998). The increase in the older population places additional demands on nurses to provide public education to promote health. It is imperative, therefore, that nurses identify the most efficient methods for enhancing learning and health promotion among their clients and the general public.

Educational Settings

Older adults utilize a number of traditional and technologically advanced educational methods in a variety of individual or group settings. A study of formal and informal learning practices in individuals past retirement age (Lamdin & Fugate, 1997) revealed that older adults seek numerous resources and programs for their educational needs. More than half of the survey's 860 respondents preferred a style of learning that incorporated reading, classes, workshops, seminars, travel, group meetings, and discussion sessions (Lamdin & Fugate, 1997). Respondents who pursued information independently utilized resources at home (76.2%) such as the Internet, through travel (55%), and in libraries (47.2%); those who preferred group settings used community-based resources such as libraries, churches, social clubs, hospitals, health centers, and senior centers (Lamdin & Fugate, 1997). The Internet is an increasing source of information for older adults who have the equipment and interest in learning and using something new in a comfortable home environment.

The choices of older adults in this study reflect the wide array of educational alternatives available to them. These options have come about because of a demographic revolution that has manifested marked improvements in the health and vitality of the older population and the awareness that lifelong learning, work, and social involvement have replaced **disengagement** as the norm for postretirement. The typology presented in Figure 12-5 helps to define the various learning options for older adults.

The programs listed in Figure 12-5 represent educational alternatives commonly used by older adults, including for-credit and noncredit options and programs that are **teacher directed** vs. **learner directed.** The term teacher directed refers to traditional offerings planned by expert educators for groups of learners. Learner directed refers to more individualized, self-paced learning sessions designed or implemented by the learners themselves (Eisen, 1998, p. 44).

The settings for educational programs for older adults are as varied as the curricula. Hospitals and health facilities have expanded their services in recent years to include health promotion and prevention programs. Many health centers now offer diet and exercise programs, nutrition counseling, cardiac rehabilitation programs, and various classes including disease prevention, relaxation techniques, and stress reduction. Such programs are typically available for group and/or individual instruction and utilize trainers, counselors, or video programs that provide information on a broad spectrum of diseases and injuries (Lamdin & Fugate, 1997). Many physicians refer their clients to health facilities or wellness centers for education or training about various

health or disease topics to ensure that the information is delivered completely and accurately.

Community-based educational alternatives are provided in senior centers, adult day centers, support groups, community centers, volunteer programs [such as a **Retired Senior Volunteer Program (RSVP)**], service organizations, clubs, and churches. The programs offered in these sites are usually teacher-directed group sessions that provide socialization as well as information. Social interaction, combined with intellectual stimulation, was reported as a strong preference in the Elderlearning Survey (Lamdin & Fugate, 1997). Group learning gives the older adult the opportunity for social exchange with peers as well as the mental exercise of testing their **cognitive** powers in peer group discussion (Lamdin & Fugate, 1997).

Institutions of higher education provide an additional location for older adult education. Colleges and universities are becoming increasingly popular among older learners for both noncredit and for-credit programs. Aging baby boomers, particularly, are having a growing presence on U.S. campuses, not only because of their desire for intellectual stimulation and participation in lifelong learning activities, but also because of social and economic factors associated with the demographic shift. By the year 2010, the United States will boast the largest and best-educated proportion of the

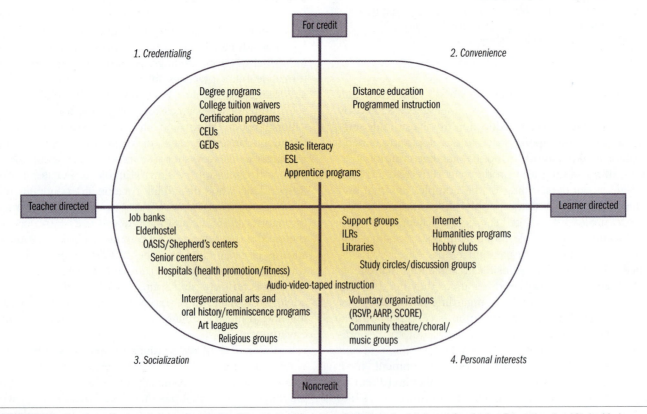

FIGURE 12-5 Typology of educational programs for older adults. [*From* New Directions for Adult and Continuing Education *(p. 43), by M. J. Eisen, 1998, San Francisco: Jossey-Bass Inc. Publishers. Reprinted with permission.*]

population reaching retirement age in history. The increase in retirement-age persons will exacerbate dramatic shortages of workers in the American labor pool. Industrial and labor-intensive fields, such as education, health, and retailing, will need to seek ways to attract and train older adults for a host of entry-level positions. In addition, the declining stability of the traditional family unit and a rise in the number of two-profession families will shape attitudes and options toward the role of retirement and older adults. All of these changes increase pressures on higher education to develop new models for serving older learners.

A few universities across the country offer such programs as **Elderhostel, Institutes for Learning in Retirement (ILR),** and **University of the Third Age (U3A)** or tuition waivers for older adults. Elderhostel was founded in 1970 and the University of the Third Age (U3A) began in France in 1973. Great Britain modified the U3A concept by allowing the members to determine curricula and administer the program. New instructional and nontraditional education systems evolved from U3A as member-driven Institute for Learning in Retirement. The ILR model empowers its members to determine their curricula, administer and market the program, and engage in self-governance under the auspices of a local university. More than 200 ILRs are known to exist across the country, representing the newest and fastest growing educational mode serving older adults.

Trends indicate that older adult education will increase substantially in the future. In 1984, 2.7 million people age 55 and older had taken adult education courses and that number continues to rise. The greatest predictor of participation in lifelong learning activities is prior education. Between 1970 and 1994, the proportion of persons 65 and older who had completed high school rose from 28% to 62% (Moody, 1998). After the year 2000, older Americans will have close to the same number of years of schooling as the general adult population (Moody, 1998).

Age-Integrated Versus Age-Segregated Educational Programs

Health education in group settings is often attended by people of all ages. Community centers, health facilities, and colleges and universities, for example, provide educational programs for anyone interested in attending, regardless of age. In addition to the educational objectives achieved in such settings, studies have shown that **age-integrated** services and programs help to reduce ageism and intergenerational conflict (Moody, 1998). Some researchers suggest that programs designed exclu-

sively for older adults promote social integration, self-expression, a sense of security, and a peer network that helps them cope with the problems of aging (Moody, 1998).

When health education involves people of all ages, one of the objectives of the session should be to promote **generational equity.** To ensure that an age-integrated program supports intergenerational contact and unity, administrative policies, curricula, and class activities should not promote **age segregation** or stigmatize students as a result of age. In addition, the facilitator should involve members of all age groups in policy-making and program design activities. A successful age-integrated program can be accomplished only by eliminating the barriers (that is, attitudes, traditions, policies, regulations, and environmental features) that foster ageist views. Education can help facilitate this goal by ensuring that curricula portray all age groups appropriately and realistically. In addition, education must be accessible to all age groups and provide opportunities where students of all ages are brought together in an organized manner for intergenerational interaction. Learning experiences should assist students in becoming better prepared to deal with their own aging and aging issues in their family experiences.

Educational Theories and Methods

Education assists people in coping with their problems as they adapt to circumstances. It involves both teaching and learning. The term *teaching* suggests the educator's assessment of the need for knowledge and the utilization of techniques for transferring knowledge to the individual (Holli & Calabrese, 1991). *Learning,* on the other hand, refers to the process stemming from an educational experience through which individuals change their behavior as a result of the knowledge and skills acquired (Holli & Calabrese, 1991). Theories about learning are described primarily in the field of psychology where two major schools (**behaviorist** and **cognitive**) have developed. Behaviorist psychologists concentrate on methods of strengthening or weakening new habits through the presence or absence of stimuli intended to produce a response. Satisfying the consequences resulting from the response to the stimulus increases the likelihood of a behavior recurring while annoying or aversive consequences reduce the frequency of the behavior. Thus, positive reinforcement can be used to condition responses, while punishment results in a lack of response or undesirable behavior (Holli & Calabrese, 1991). The behaviorist school offers the learning principles shown in Box 12-1.

Unlike behaviorist approaches, cognitive theories recognize that **human insight** is often a factor in

BOX 12-1 Behaviorist Learning Principles

- Ensure learning success by using positive responses to reinforce the activity to be learned. Negative responses will cause the person to avoid the learning activity.

- Follow every correct response with a reward or satisfier.

- Ignore incorrect responses. Always wait for the person to demonstrate the desired behavior or knowledge and then reward it.

- Make sure that rewards immediately follow the positive response. Do not delay.

- In the early stages of learning, reinforce every desired response. Later, use an intermittent schedule of rewards. When reward is overused, it loses its effect, so that after a learner has had some rewarded successes, rewards should be given less frequently.

- For learning sequential activities, determine the need for practice at each step. Schedule the practice, including reinforcement at each step.

- Strengthen the retention of the learned activity through repetition.

- Practice the activity in a variety of contexts to ensure generalization of learning to similar situations.

- Keep learners informed of their progress. Knowledge of results is an important secondary reinforcer.

- Do not reinforce undesirable behaviors or responses. Ignore them.

- Do not use any form of punishment to foster learning. It causes the learner to avoid the situation.

- Ensure that positive conditions exist and that the individual is not tired, irritable, preoccupied, or disinterested in the learning situation.

- Recognize and resolve any barriers to learning such as conflicts or frustrations.

- Avoid the use of *trick* questions in testing the learner unless he or she has been taught the tricks.

- Try role playing or modeling to enhance learning of certain activities to see if they are acceptable and of interest.

learning: "The learner perceives a relationship, which leads to the solution of problems. Learning is discontinuous and sudden, with behavior changing when insight occurs" (Holli & Calabrese, 1991, p. 176). Cognitive learning principles are presented in Box 12-2.

Cognitive theories view learning as an active, goal-directed process rather than as a passive response to a stimulus. Although positive reinforcement is a very important skill, teachers should allow their students to reflect and participate in decision making and information processing.

Constructivist approaches to teaching and learning have derived from a blend of cognitive and behaviorist theories. Constructivism is an educational approach based on the premise that cognition results when students apply new information to what they already know. Thus, learning is influenced by beliefs, attitudes, and the context in which an idea is taught. Constructivism principles are shown in Box 12-3.

The teaching environment for students of all ages should therefore employ realistic, experiential approaches to solving real-world problems. To ensure the effectiveness of educational delivery, instructors should not only understand the principles of constructivist learning models but also develop learning objectives pertaining to instructional materials. Traditionally, these criteria have been developed by teachers for determining performances they wish their students to exhibit to be considered competent (Allen & Belzer, 1997). Teachers often

BOX 12-2 Cognitive Learning Principles

- Ensure an active, rather than passive, learning environment in which the learner actively participates as a listener, viewer, or responder.

- Assist the learner in setting goals as an important motivation for learning.

- Carefully analyze the tasks that confront learners. Display the problem in a way that is clear to the learner.

- Plan in advance the way knowledge is organized.

- Ensure that learners understand what they are learning. Rote learning is not as permanent and transferable as learning that has meaning.

- Always ensure that the learner is left with the correct answer by providing cognitive responses to confirm knowledge or correct faulty learning.

- Help the learner maintain a high level of motivation and drive to ensure purposive behavior.

follow techniques developed by Mager (1984) in writing educational objectives. Mager's guidelines include (a) determining the learner's performance, (b) identifying the conditions imposed on the learner, and (c) determining criteria for success. The instructor should discuss these objectives with adult learners and obtain their active participation in setting and evaluating criteria.

There are three learning domains in which educational objectives can be developed. Bloom (1956) described a taxonomy that includes the cognitive, **affective,** and **psychomotor** domains. Cognitive learning involves knowledge recall and intellectual skills (for example, comprehension, organization of ideas, analysis and synthesis of data, problem solving, application of knowledge, and evaluation of ideas). Affective learning relates to emotions, attitudes, and personal values. It

occurs when the learner exhibits awareness, interest, attention, concern, responsibility, interaction, or acceptance of the subject matter. Psychomotor learning is concerned with fine or gross motor skills and is demonstrated by physical skills, coordination, dexterity, strength, or speed.

> ### Nursing Tip
>
> Remember that psychomotor learning (skills such as taking a blood pressure or blood glucose testing) may be more difficult for older adults who have severe arthritis in their hands.

Bloom's taxonomy, which utilizes a hierarchy of knowledge attainment and utilization, provides a useful structure for categorizing a variety of learning styles and evaluating competency (see Table 12-1). The skills specified for each level can be used for identifying an individual's preferred style of learning and developing learning objectives. People perceive and process information in different ways.

Differences in ways people learn have been a popular topic of educational research in recent decades. One of the most notable projects, **multiple intelligence theory,** was first described in 1983 by Harvard psychologist Howard Gardner. The theory is based on cognitive research that documented the extent to which students learn, remember, perform, and understand in different ways. According to the theory (Gardner, 1983, p. 83):

> We are all able to know the world through language, logical-mathematical analysis, spatial representation, musical thinking, the use of the body to solve problems or make things, an understanding of other individuals, and an understanding of ourselves. Where individuals differ is in the strength of these intelligences—the so-called profile of intelligences—and in the ways in which such intelligences are invoked and combined to carry out different tasks, solve diverse problems, and progress in various domains.

These differences, according to Gardner, "challenge an educational system that assumes that everyone can learn the same materials in the same way and that a uniform, universal measure suffices to test student learning" (1983, p. 83). He also pointed out that traditional educational systems are biased toward linguistic and logical-quantitative modes of instruction and assessment.

Since Gardner's research, a number of other theories have developed on learning styles. Newer theories tend to be summarized in broader categories (for example, visual, auditory, and kinesthetic learning). A number of assessment tools and inventories have been developed. A teacher or facilitator can determine an individual's

---

BOX 12-3   Constructivist Learning Principles

- The brain simultaneously processes many different types of information, including thoughts, emotions, and cultural knowledge.

- Learning involves all body functions, not just the intellect.

- The search for meaning is innate; students comprehend subject matter based on their unique experiences.

- Learning is influenced by emotions, feelings, and attitudes.

- Learning is influenced by the environment, culture, and climate.

- Humans possess at least two types of memory: spatial and rote. Excluding teaching that does not promote spatial (experiential) learning can inhibit comprehension.

- Learning is enhanced when facts and skills are embedded in natural, spatial memory. Experiential learning is more effective than rote memorization.

- Learning involves both conscious and unconscious processes. Students need time to process what they have learned.

- Learning is enhanced by challenge and inhibited by threat.

- Each brain is unique. Thus, teaching must be multifaceted to promote learning for all students.

TABLE 12-1 Levels of Abstraction in Bloom's Taxonomy

Competence	Skills Demonstrated	Evaluation Cues	
Knowledge	• Observe and recall information. • Know dates, events, places, and major ideas. • Master subject matter.	List Define Tell Describe Identify Show	Label Collect Examine Tabulate Quote Name
Comprehension	• Understand information. • Grasp meaning. • Translate knowledge into new context. • Interpret facts. • Compare, contrast. • Order, group. • Infer causes. • Predict consequences.	Summarize Describe Interpret Contrast Associate Distinguish	Differentiate Discuss Extend Predict Estimate
Application	• Use information. • Use methods, concepts, theories in new situations. • Solve problems using required skills or knowledge.	Apply Demonstrate Calculate Complete Illustrate Show Experiment	Solve Examine Modify Relate Change Classify Discover
Analysis	• Recognize patterns. • Organize parts. • Decipher hidden meanings. • Identify components.	Analyze Separate Order Explain Connect Classify	Arrange Divide Compare Select Infer
Synthesis	• Use old ideas to create new ones. • Generalize from given facts. • Relate knowledge from several areas. • Make predictions. • Draw conclusions.	Combine Integrate Modify Rearrange Substitute Plan Create	Invent Compose Formulate Prepare Generalize Rewrite Design
Evaluation	• Compare and discriminate between ideas. • Assess value of theories and presentations. • Make choices based on reasoned argument. • Verify value of evidence. • Recognize subjectivity.	Assess Decide Rank Grade Test Measure Recommend Convince	Select Judge Explain Discriminate Support Conclude Compare Summarize

Adapted from Taxonomy of Educational Objectives: Cognitive Domain, *by B. Bloom, 1956, New York: McKay.*

preferred learning style by administering a learning style inventory, observing how the person learns, or asking questions about preferences, such as, "Do you prefer to listen, read, view, or experience the topic?" (Holli & Calabrese, 1991, p. 202).

From Pedagogy to Geragogy

Nurses encounter a variety of clients in their professional roles, including children; adolescents; young, middle-aged, and older adults; and people with terminal illnesses or cognitive impairment. Different approaches often are necessary for teaching and learning within these groups, and special strategies are helpful when designing educational interventions (Nemshick, 1997). **Pedagogy,** defined as the art and science of teaching children, is the traditional approach in formal education. It emphasizes teaching functions and is teacher centered, with the student being passive and in a dependent relationship to the teacher. The instructor determines the nature and extent of the subject matter to be delivered and evaluates the students' comprehension of the content. The student maintains a competitive relationship with his or her peers. **Andragogy,** the art and science of teaching adults, places the student at the center of the learning environment and emphasizes learning, rather than teaching, functions. Andragogy produces collaborative relationships among students and between the student and the instructor.

Knowles (1970) was one of the first researchers to describe the theory of andragogy. He based his research on observations that adults are goal oriented and prefer to learn through problem-solving activities. Knowles noted that adults have internal incentives and specific purposes for learning. He also observed that adults are willing to assume responsibility for acquiring information on their own. The primary responsibility of the instructor, therefore, is to facilitate the learning process by selecting appropriate activities and encouraging application of the content. Knowles based his theory on the assumptions that as individuals mature:

- Their self-concept evolves from a state of dependency to one of being a self-directed human being.

- They accumulate a growing reservoir of experiences that serves as a resource for learning.

- There is a strong correlation between their readiness to learn and the developmental tasks associated with their social roles.

- Their time perspective changes from one of postponed application to one of immediate application of what they have learned.

Educational programs for adults, therefore, should be designed in accordance with these basic assumptions. Knowles (1970) recommended that adult education programs:

- Maintain a climate of respect.

- Involve collaboration among students, teachers, and other resources.

- Help learners achieve empowerment and self-direction.

- Capitalize on learners' experiences.

- Foster participation.

- Foster critical and reflective thinking.

- Involve learning for action.

- Pose problem-solving opportunities.

By the 1960s, scholars recognized the need to further develop an andragogy for older learners. Driven by the new phenomenon of increased longevity, the emphasis on education for older adults related primarily to health, social, and recreational needs. The term **geragogy** was used for the first time in 1956 by West German gerontologist Hans Mieskes. Mieskes recommended geragogy (or geragogics as he called it) in both gerontological and educational arenas (Zych, 1992, p. 33):

> The pedagogy of aging and old people includes geragogics on the one hand in gerontological sciences (along with geriatrics and its branches, gerontopsychology and sociology of aging) and on the other in the theory of education . . . which also includes pedagogy of children and youth, and andragogy, which is concerned with pedomorphosis, i.e., changes in human nature throughout all phases of life until old age.

The blend of human development studies and educating older adults has important implications. As Battersby (1990) explained, positive outcomes could result because "learning and teaching in later life can do more for older people than simply provide a form of mental stimulation or exercise for the intelligence. . . . it may prompt people to realize their full developmental potential" (p. 437).

Think About It

- Do you think older adults learn better in groups or in a one-to-one learning situation?
- Do older adults seem to be interested in learning about maintaining wellness?

Adults of all ages will have a more successful learning experience if they are involved in planning about teaching methods and content for the session. They should be allowed the opportunity to assign and achieve their educational goals (Nemshick, 1997, p. 331). Geragogy, distinct from andragogy and pedagogy, is a process of education that is liberating for the older learner. It utilizes a humanist, developmental approach and refers to issues and practices that are relevant to aging, such as retirement planning, nutrition, exercise, memory, cognitive development, coping with transitions in later life, and teaching/learning theories (Glendenning, 1992).

The distinctions between geragogy and andragogy are delineated by theorists who view later life as a unique developmental stage, rather than as an extension of middle age. As Moody (1990) pointed out, a lifetime of experience makes older learners capable of understanding philosophical and spiritual matters that younger learners cannot grasp. Learning in later years is influenced by learning across the lifespan. It includes all formal and informal learning and life events that have occurred throughout one's lifetime. Thus, a principal strategy in geragogy involves eliciting dialog about life's experiences from course participants.

Barriers to Learning for Older Adults

Perhaps the greatest barrier to educational opportunities for older adults is the pervasive myth that people past retirement age are too old to learn. Contrary to this belief, research shows that learning in later years can and does occur and that people of all ages are quite capable of broadening their minds. Although the conditions for successful learning differ between older and younger people, fears of age-related loss in mental function are often exaggerated. Current estimates, for example, suggest that no more than 10% of persons age 65 and older have Alzheimer's disease (Rowe & Kahn, 1998). Studies indicate that "three key factors predict strong mental function in old age: (1) regular physical activity; (2) a strong social support system; and (3) belief in one's ability to handle what life has to offer" (Rowe & Kahn, 1998, pp. 19–20).

Another factor that prohibits older adults' participation in education relates to their personal attitudes about life-long learning. Unfortunately, people are not conditioned during childhood to pursue learning throughout their lifespan. Some older adults avoid educational programs because of embarrassment, fear of failure, or apprehension about modern technological tools. Others accept the stereotype that they are too old to learn. Studies have demonstrated, however, that older adults easily learn computer systems and programs and come to value computer use as a means of social interaction

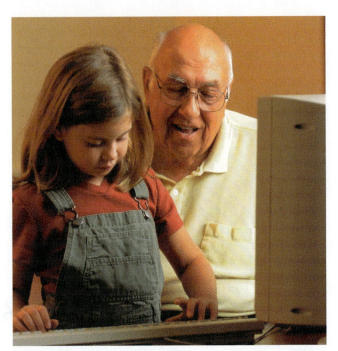

FIGURE 12-6 This man enjoys learning about the Internet with his granddaughter.

(refer to Figure 12-6) (Czaja, Guerrier, Nair, & Landauer, 1993; Cole, 1996; Furlong & Lipson, 1996; Moody, 1998).

Physiological changes that occur with aging, particularly vision and hearing changes, can adversely impact learning. Instructors should be aware of these barriers and take appropriate steps to minimize them. Bright, indirect lighting should be available in the classroom area and glare should be eliminated. Reading materials should be made available in large print with appropriate spacing and font selection (see Box 12-4 for guidelines on the readability of printed materials).

Hearing loss occurs in 25% of people between the ages of 65 and 74 and 50% of people age 75 and older. Many hearing deficits are aggravated by background noise and higher pitches (Allen & Belzer, 1997). The classroom environment should include noise absorbancy materials and sound equipment to help older learners understand the information being discussed. The facilitator should arrange the seating to maximize the number of seats available in the first two rows for hearing-impaired learners to sit closer to the speaker. In addition, the facilitator should speak slowly, face the audience, and repeat information as needed.

Low self-esteem, depression, chronic illness, and altered mental state can also negatively affect an older adult's involvement in educational activities. Such problems often impede the person's motivation to learn and reduce willingness to accept recommendations offered during the learning activity. Facilitators should be aware of signs and symptoms of depression and recommend clinical assessment and intervention as appropriate. Only 31% of people who have a major depressive dis-

---

BOX 12-4 Guidelines on the Readability of Teaching Tools

Printed materials:
- Fifth- to eighth-grade reading level
- Twelve- to 16-point type
- Serif font
- High contrast (black on white)
- Use boldface, italics, and large font size to emphasize main ideas
- Age-appropriate illustrations
- Avoid violet, blue, and green colors

Display boards, charts, bulletin boards:
- Eighteen- to 24-point type (easily viewed from a distance of 4 feet)
- High contrast
- Use bullets or arrows
- Limit to one or two concepts

Audiovisual displays (slides, overhead transparencies):
- Large, black font on white or pastel background
- Age-appropriate illustrations and graphics
- Limit to one concept or idea per slide
- Decrease or omit background music

Adapted from "Implications of Issues in Typographical Design for Readability and Reading Satisfaction in an Aging Population," by J. M. Adams and L. Hoffman, 1994, Experimental Aging Research, 20, pp. 61–69, and "Education in the Elderly: Adapting and Evaluating Teaching Tools," by S. P. Weinrich and M. Boyd, 1992, Journal of Gerontological Nursing, 18, 1, pp. 15–20.

BOX 12-5 Guidelines for Developing Educational Programs for Adults

- Safe, accessible, and comfortable environment
- Adequate and accessible parking
- Good lighting in the parking area
- Compliance with guidelines specified in the Americans with Disabilities Act
- Adequate, indirect lighting, without glare, in the classroom area
- Not-crowded, large-print posters; overhead transparencies; slides; and handouts
- Environmental features that help reduce background noise
- Sound equipment that allows all classroom participants to be heard
- Comfortable room temperature

---

order in any 6-month period receive treatment of any kind. This is primarily because of the failure to recognize that a problem exists. Yet, appropriate treatments have been found to be effective in 8 out of 10 cases (U.S. Department of Health and Human Services, 1990).

Educational Strategies

One of the most important considerations in planning and developing educational programs for older adults is the format. The lecture approach should be abandoned and replaced with a more informal, learner-centered format. As previously discussed, older adults should be allowed the opportunity to participate in educational programs and teachers should incorporate activities that appeal to various learning styles. For one-to-one instruction, the teacher should determine the individual's preferred style and utilize strategies that encompass that style. For group instruction, facilitators should offer a variety of experiences that allow group members to listen, share ideas, reflect, solve problems, experiment, and participate in hands-on activities (Holli & Calabrese, 1991).

Strategies that provide guidelines for planning and developing educational programs for older adults are listed in Box 12-5.

In addition to ensuring appropriate physical conditions, the teacher should utilize a seminar, rather than a lecture, format and incorporate the teaching skills shown in Box 12-6.

Perhaps the most important consideration in educational program planning and design is that older adults are as diverse, if not more diverse, than any age group in the population. Levels of education, socioeconomic status, ethnicity, health status, learning styles, and other characteristics vary extensively from person to person. Thus, in a group setting, the teaching environment, methods, and tools should incorporate a number of strategies to accommodate the needs of the group's participants. Box 12-7 provides a sample lesson plan for an educational program on Alzheimer's disease for a group of community-based older learners.

BOX 12-6   Skills Helpful When Teaching Older Adults

- Offer positive reinforcement for every attempt by the older learner to participate (see Figure 12-7).

- Use silence as a reflective tool to allow older learners additional time to process information.

- Encourage contemplation and reflection, particularly when sensitive issues are being discussed.

- Stimulate both visual and auditory senses in the presentation of material to increase the probability that content matter will be retained.

- Use a variety of teaching methods, such as role playing, games, examples, open discussion, charts, and reading material.

- Use true/false, multiple choice, or open-ended questions to evaluate progress.

- Ask specific questions designed to illicit a response from participants. Avoid general inquiries such as, "Do you have any questions?"

- Utilize the older learner's experience and expertise.

BOX 12-7   Sample Lesson Plan: Alzheimer's Disease

Introduction

Contrary to popular belief, memory loss is not a normal part of the aging process. Most older people *do not* have serious memory loss unless they suffer from a disease or injury. During this session, participants will discuss reasons for memory decline other than clinical dementia and consider diagnostic and treatment protocols when dementia has been diagnosed.

Key Terms: Alzheimer's disease; dementia; cognitive impairment

Objectives

Following this session, participants will:

- Identify at least three causes of reversible memory loss.

- Describe the differences between dementia and changes that could occur in normal aging.

- Discuss ways for ensuring proper diagnosis and treatment in persons with memory loss.

- Describe, in lay terms, the changes that occur in the brain of a person with Alzheimer's disease.

- Describe how Alzheimer's disease progresses.

- Discuss current treatment modalities for a patient with dementia.

Materials

- Transparency: *Beetle Bailey* cartoon

- Handout: "Confusion and Memory Loss in Old Age: It's Not What You Think"

- Transparency: brain map

- Video: *Alzheimer's: A Personal Story* (Terra Nova Films, 1990)

Procedures

- 5 minutes: *Beetle Bailey* cartoon; review objectives.

- 10 minutes: Short-term memory exercise (telephone numbers).

- 10 minutes: Discuss various causes of reversible/irreversible dementia.

- 15 minutes: Read and discuss handout.

- 10 minutes: Overview of Alzheimer's pathology and progression of disease.

- 30 minutes: Video.

- 10 minutes: Questions/answers; discussion.

Technology in Older Adult Education

The increase in computer use among older adults is not an American phenomenon. A recent European study confirmed that computer literacy is helping to reduce social isolation and is providing access to services (for example, **teleshopping,** home entertainment, and banking) for elders in Europe (James, Gibson, McAuley, & McAuley, 1995). Computerized technology increases older adults' independence and autonomy; it also helps people adapt behaviors, increase their options, and utilize multiple resources (Manheimer, Snodgrass, and Moskow-McKenzie, 1995; Moody, 1998). Other advantages of using com-

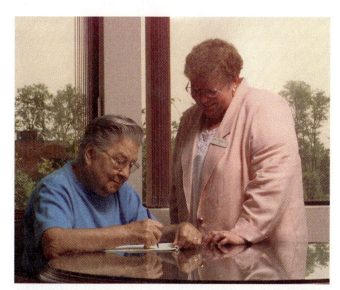

FIGURE 12-7 Providing encouragement will help the adult learner to succeed.

puters include the opportunity to participate in educational endeavors without restrictions such as physical impairments (for example, hearing deficits and arthritis) and travel to and from a course location.

Older adults are one of the two fastest growing age groups using the Internet. In 1995, 31% of Americans 55 and older owned personal computers; over 13 million older adults are currently on the Internet (Wrixon, 1998). In general, people use computer technology for a variety of educational purposes. Computer-assisted instruction can accommodate older learners' needs through self-pacing, individualization, privacy, learner active participation, immediate feedback, and the opportunity for repetition or practice (Manheimer, Snodgrass, and Moskow-McKenzie, 1995). Studies have shown that age, educational attainment, and previous experience with a keyboard are not related to effective older adult education using computer-assisted instruction (Manheimer et al., 1995).

A number of on-line training and information resources are available to older adults. Examples of Internet sites include SeniorNet at www.seniornet.org, ThirdAge at www.thirdage.com, Seniors in Cyberspace at www.intel.com, and numerous others. In addition, senior centers, community colleges, health programs, and a variety of other local resources are providing computer-assisted instruction for older adults.

Think About It

What are some of the advantages of the Internet for older adults? How can modern computer technology be made available to more older adults?

Evaluating Education for Older Adults

The evaluation process is perhaps the most important step in educational program planning and development. Program evaluation is defined as "a system of quality control to determine whether the process of education is effective, to identify its strengths and weaknesses, and to determine what changes should be made" (Holli & Calabrese, 1991, p. 208). It is important, especially when considering health outcomes, to know whether people are learning, instructors are teaching effectively, and goals and objectives are being accomplished. Whether the learning experience occurs in an individual or group setting and whether the instructional methods are formal or informal, program evaluation can ensure meaningful connections between knowledge, skills, experience, and health outcomes.

Kasworm and Marienau (1997) offered the following principles to guide the evaluation of education programs:

- Learning is derived from multiple sources.

- Learning engages the whole person and contributes to that person's development.

- Learning and the capacity for self-direction are promoted by feedback.

- Learning occurs in context; its significance relates, in part, to its impact on those contexts.

- Learning from experiences promotes meaning and creates diversity among adult learners.

As previously discussed, adult learners, and particularly older adult learners, bring rich and varied experiences to the learning environment. They learn by integrating new information with past and present understandings and then relating the newly acquired knowledge and skills to circumstances in their daily lives. They also "selectively learn, apply, synthesize, and critically reflect on new and old sources of knowledge from the world of their everyday life and the world of formal knowledge" (Kasworm & Marienau, 1997, p. 8). Thus, the evaluation process should:

- Reinforce learning from a variety of sources.

- Recognize cognitive, conative, and affective domains of learning.

- Focus on participant's active involvement in learning and assessment processes.

- Embrace the learner's participation in family and community responsibilities and activities.

- Accommodate differences and varied life experiences among learners.

Program evaluation should be designed to improve curriculum construction, teaching, and/or learning (Holli & Calabrese, 1991). Two types of evaluation, **formative** and **summative,** are used to assess these processes. Formative evaluation refers to assessments made during the course of education, with feedback used to modify the remaining educational endeavor. It involves a systematic appraisal for the purpose of improving teaching or learning during the course of instruction. Summative evaluation refers to a summary assessment of results at the conclusion of learning. Unlike formative appraisals, summative evaluation is performed to assess participants' progress or determine grades. Judgments are made about the effectiveness of learning, teaching, and/or curriculum and often result in anxiety or defensiveness about the evaluation process. Evaluations for adult education programs should be continuous and preplanned with suggestions from the learners (Holli & Calabrese, 1991). Formative methods provide a more positive learning experience.

At least three types of evaluation should be considered for group or individual health education programs: (a) knowledge and/or skills acquisition, (b) measures of behavioral change, and (c) attitudes or beliefs. It may also be necessary to evaluate other factors that could enhance or impede learning, such as the participants' reactions to the program, the instructor's attitudes or beliefs, health and social problems, and environmental issues. Program objectives, if written in terms of measurable performance, serve as the source of the evaluation. The objectives listed on the lesson plan in Box 12-7, for example, can be used to determine the degree to which learning was achieved, assuming that the lesson plan was followed. If facilitators find that participants are not able to perform the stated objectives, they should assume that instruction needs to be modified and repeated.

A number of methods can be used to collect evaluation data. Written examinations are probably the most common device for measuring learning (Holli & Calabrese, 1991) but are not always acceptable or effective with older adults. Multiple-choice, true-false, short-answer, completion, and essay questions are used to measure in the cognitive domain. In using any of these tools, the educator should take care not to evoke memories associated with authoritarian teachers or dependent students. The facilitator should also avoid assigning success or failure based on the outcome of the exam (Holli & Calabrese, 1991). Methods such as questionnaires, rating scales, checklists, interviews, visual observation, and simulations often provide more interactive and positive feedback in adult learning situations. All methods of evaluation have advantages and limitations. In assessing adult learning, the evaluator should always strive to protect the individual's self-concept and to treat errors as indicators for additional instruction (Holli & Calabrese, 1991).

Summary

Changes in the demographic characteristics of the U.S. population are dramatically affecting many elements of American culture. The graying of the population is producing trends that are beginning to reverse the effects of ageism and negative attitudes toward older adults and evaluate issues in all aspects of American life pertinent to the demographic shift (for example, work and retirement, family relationships, product design, advertising, political activity, financial security, and health). These trends will result in substantial increases in older adult education in the coming years.

The number of older adults participating in lifelong learning is growing in conjunction with the aging population. Despite the trends, American institutions, including health providers, community centers, colleges, universities, and technology suppliers, are slow to respond to the learning needs of older students. The demographic trends suggest that a comprehensive, age-integrated model of formal and informal education is needed that fosters diversity in intellectual, cultural, and social life by educating students of all ages about aging, aging issues, and ageism. Health educators have the responsibility of advancing the effective use of limited resources to meet society's needs. An aggressive response to this responsibility will help older adults create and shape change and obtain more control over their lives and the environment.

Review Questions and Activities

1. What is the role of the nurse in health education for older adults?

2. How do ageist myths affect the educational needs of older adults?

3. Where are major settings where older adults can learn information about health and wellness?

4. Find out whether universities and/or colleges in your area have special educational programs for older adults. Find out how well they are attended and what are the costs.

5. How can generational equity be built into health education programs?

6. What are the differences between behaviorist and cognitive learning principles?

7. What is meant by constructivist learning?

8. What are the most common barriers to learning for older adults?

9. Prepare a teaching guide to use with a group of older adults on the topic of osteoporosis. What teaching principles, methods, and materials will you use?

References

Adams, J. M., & Hoffman, L. (1994). Implications of issues in typographical design for readability and reading satisfaction in an aging population. *Experimental Aging Research, 20,*(1), 61–69.

Allen, M. E., & Belzer, J. A. (1997). The use of microteaching to facilitate teaching skills of practitioners who work with older adults. *Gerontology and Geriatrics Education, 18*(2), 77–86.

Battersby, D. (1990). From andragogy to geragogy. In F. Glendenning & K. Percy (Eds.), *Aging, education, and society: Readings in educational gerontology.* Keele, Staffordshire: AEG.

Bloom, B. (1956). *Taxonomy of educational objectives: Cognitive domain.* New York: McKay.

Cole, A. (1996, March–April). High-tech anxiety. *Modern Maturity.*

Cusack, S. (1998). What is the value of older adult education? *The older learner, 6*(4), 1, 7.

Czaja, S. J., Guerrier J. H., Nair, S. N., & Landauer, T. K. (1993). Computer communication as an aid to independence for older adults. *Behaviour and Information Technology, 12*(4), 197–207.

Eisen, M. J. (1998). Current practice and innovative programs in older adult learning. *New Directions for Adult and Continuing Education, 77,* 41–53.

Fischer, R. B., Blazey, M. L., & Lipman, H. T. (1992). *Students of the third age.* New York: Macmillan.

Furlong, M. S., & Lipson, S. B. (1996). *Young at heart: Computing for seniors.* Berkeley, CA: Osborne McGraw-Hill.

Gardner, H. (1983). *Frames of mind: A theory of multiple intelligences.* New York: Basic Books.

Gill, D. G., & Ingman, S. R. (Eds.). (1994). *Eldercare, distributive justice, and the welfare state: Retrenchment or expansion.* Albany, NY: State University of New York Press.

Glendenning, F. (1992). Educational gerontology and geragogy: A critical perspective. *Geragogics: European Research in Gerontological Education and Educational Gerontology, 13*(1&2), 5–21.

Holli, B. B., & Calabrese, R. J. (1991). *Communication and education skills: The dietitian's guide* (2nd ed.). Philadelphia: Lea & Febiger.

James, D., Gibson, F., McAuley, G., & McAuley, J. (1995). Adding new life to elders' lives. *Aging International, 22*(1), 34–35.

Johnson, R. J., & Wolinsky, F.D. (1994). Gender, race, and health: The structure of health status among older adults. *The Gerontologist 34*(1), 24–35.

Kasworm, C. E., & Marienau, C. A. (1997). Principles for assessment of adult learning. *New Directions for Adult and Continuing Education, 75,* 5–16.

Knowles, M. S. (1970). *The modern practice of adult education: Andragogy versus pedagogy.* New York: Association.

Lamdin, L., & Fugate, M. (1997). *Elderlearning: New frontier in an aging society.* Phoenix, AZ: Oryx.

Leon, J., & Lair, T. (1990). *Functional status of the noninstitutionalized elderly: Estimates of ADL and IADL difficulties.* DHHS Publication No. (PHS) 90-3462. National Medical Expenditure Survey Research Findings 4, Agency for Health Care Policy and Research. Rockville, MD: Public Health Service.

Mager, R. F. (1984). *Preparing instructional objectives.* Belmont, CA: Lake.

Manheimer, R. J., Snodgrass, D. D., & Moskow-McKenzie, D. (1995). *Older adult education: A guide to research, programs, and policies.* Westport, CT: Greenwood.

Moody, H. R. (1990). Education and the life cycle: A philosophy of aging. In R. H. Sherron & D.B. Lumsden (Eds.), *Introduction to educational gerontology* (pp. 23–39). New York: Hemisphere.

Moody, H. R. (1998). *Aging: Concepts and controversies* (2nd ed.). Thousand Oaks, CA: Pine Forge.

National Center for Health Statistics. (1990). Current estimates from the National Health Interview Survey, 1989. *Vital and Health Statistics,* Series 10, No. 176.

Nemshick, M. T. (1997). Designing educational interventions for patients and families. In K. F. Shepard & G. M. Jensen (Eds.), *Handbook of teaching for physical therapists.* Boston: Butterworth-Heinemann.

Rowe, J. W., & Kahn, R. L. (1998). *Successful aging.* New York: Pantheon Books.

U.S. Bureau of the Census. (1987). An aging world. *International Population Reports,* Series P-95, No. 78.

U.S. Bureau of the Census. (1990). Money income and poverty status in the United States: 1989. *Current Population Reports,* Series P-60, No. 168.

U.S. Department of Health and Human Services. (1985). *Report of the Secretary's Task Force on Black and Minority Health.* Washington, DC: Author.

U.S. Department of Health and Human Services. (1990). *Healthy people 2000: National health promotion and disease prevention objectives.* DHHS Publication No. (PHS) 91-50212. Washington, DC: U.S. Government Printing Office.

U.S. Department of Health and Human Services. (1991). *Aging America: Trends and projections.* DHHS Publication No. (FCoA) 91-28001. Washington, DC: Author.

U.S. Public Health Service. (1979). *Healthy people: Surgeon General's Report on Health Promotion and Disease Prevention.* Washington, DC: U.S. Department of Health and Human Services.

Resources

Senior Net: **www.seniornet.org**

Third Age: **www.thirdage.com**

Seniors in Cyberspace: **www.intel.com**

UNIT 4

Health Needs and Care

PERSPECTIVE...

A client and her daughter come to a comprehensive geriatric assessment program with complaints of falling, decreased appetite, decreased ability to care for herself, and mild memory problems. The daughter states that her mother has always been independent and active but now the daughter is having to assume many new roles to help her mother compensate for her declining abilities. The daughter is expressing a great deal of stress about her role as a caregiver for her mother and not knowing what resources are available or how to access those resources. The daughter has two children and a full-time job and is experiencing the sandwich generation syndrome. This African-American family is not interested in nursing home placement. Each member of the geriatric assessment team is critical in helping the daughter and her mother through this crisis.

The health care practitioner assesses the client for possible physical etiologies of the falls, decreased appetite, memory loss, and functional decline. This process includes physical examination, pertinent history, and testing that includes laboratory work-up and/or radiology screens. The social worker performs a social assessment and caregiver interview to assess the current psychosocial situation, including living arrangements, safety issues, current formal and informal support systems, financial resources, and caregiver knowledge and abilities to perform necessary care. Based on the findings of the health care practitioner, the daughter may require additional education and support. The social worker initiates referrals to appropriate community resources, such as adult day services, and home care. The pharmacist assists in a thorough medication evaluation to assess for the possibility of side effects that might be contributing to the falls, memory loss, decreased appetite, and functional decline. The dietitian can assist in assessing the client's nutritional needs and make recommendations to optimize her diet.

This family will need continued follow-up to ensure that the interdisciplinary plan of care is being implemented effectively and to reassess for any additional needs.

CHAPTER 13

Assessment, Diagnosis, and Planning

Katy Scherger, RN, MSN, CS

Barbara Harty, RN, MSN, CS

COMPETENCIES

After completing this chapter, the reader should be able to:

- *Describe techniques used in physical assessment of older adults.*
- *Describe physiological changes associated with aging and their clinical implications.*
- *Compare age-related laboratory values with normal laboratory values.*
- *Describe conditions with atypical presentations in the older adult.*
- *Discuss functional assessment in the older adult.*
- *Describe the basic components of a cognitive and affective assessment of the older adult.*
- *Discuss the importance of screening for both cognitive impairments and depression in the older adult.*
- *List objective tools that could be utilized in conducting a cognitive and affective assessment in the older adult.*
- *Describe the various components of a social assessment in the older adult.*
- *Discuss various tools that could be utilized in conducting a social assessment of older adults and their family members.*

MAKING THE CONNECTION

Refer to the following chapters to increase your understanding of assessment, diagnosis, and planning:

Techniques for Geriatric Assessment

The physical assessment of the older adult requires the health care team to consider and implement special considerations that are unique to the geriatric population. Adaptations are necessary to prepare the environment to compensate for the older adult's physiological and psychological changes.

Modifications to the physical environment start with a room that is comfortably warm and not exposing the client any more than is necessary. The room should be adequately bright but with indirect lighting to compensate for diminished visual acuity. Fluorescent lighting should be avoided, as should glare from windows. Straight-backed chairs with arms that are cushioned for comfort but that are not so low as to be difficult to rise from should be utilized. The examination table should be low and well padded to protect thin older adults from discomfort. The head of the examination table should be able to rise up, as some older adults may have difficulty lying flat for any amount of time. There should be adequate space in the examination room to accommodate mobility aides. The room should be free from distraction and background noises. It is important to take into consideration the energy level of the older adult and conduct the physical examination at the individual's own pace. This may mean conducting the examination over more than one session. It is helpful to organize the examination to minimize the change in body positions to conserve the client's energy.

Because the older adult may be disoriented in a different environment and/or have **sensory impairment**, various techniques need to be utilized to assess each individual adequately. At the start of the examination, it may be worthwhile for the examiner to spend some extra time establishing a nonthreatening relationship. As a sign of respect, older adults should be addressed by their last name and their first name not used unless invited to do so. Allow the older client enough time to respond to questions. Speak facing the client and use commonly accepted wording. Allow hearing-impaired clients to see your entire face and body so that they can detect lip reading and body language. If the client wears

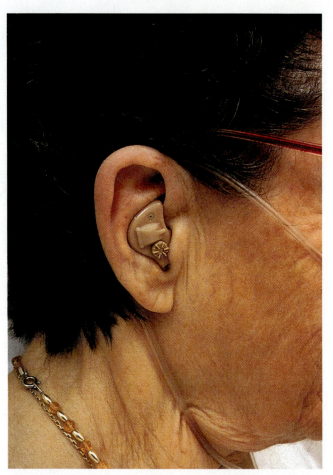

FIGURE 13-1   If a client relies on hearing aids, make sure they are functioning before beginning the assessment examination.

hearing aids, make sure they are on and functioning properly (Figure 13-1). For clients with visual deficits, be sure the clients have their glasses on and be prepared to use visual cues. Family members can provide important information, but the examiner needs to focus on the client.

Physical assessment on older adults requires a commitment of time and resources that is not always available in today's health care environment. An **interdisciplinary** team approach is required because of the **multidisciplinary** nature of the health problems expe-

Think About It

How would you prepare for a physical examination on an older adult with hearing impairment and severe chronic obstructive pulmonary disease (COPD)? What specialized equipment would you need in the room and what adaptations to the environment would need to be considered?

Nursing Tip

Because of time restraints and financial concerns in today's health care environment, it is essential to have an experienced geriatric team available for the initial assessment. One important member of the team should be a social worker who can evaluate the specific issues the client and family may have that require immediate attention.

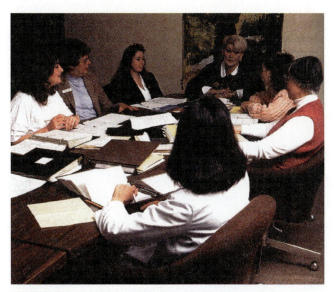

FIGURE 13-2 A multidisciplinary team meets to plan and communicate client care.

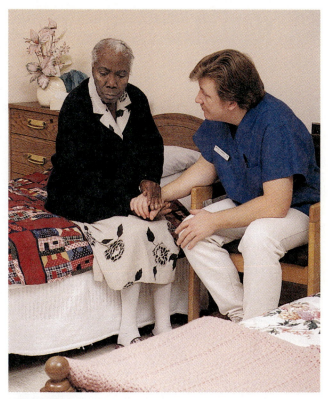

FIGURE 13-3 A client's cultural beliefs will have an impact on illness and recovery.

rienced by older adults. Operating within a managed care system, an interdisciplinary team with geriatric experience in several required disciplines will be able to communicate effectively and deliver a geriatric team approach (Figure 13-2). By using this approach, high quality and efficient geriatric care can be delivered at reduced costs (Fillit & Picariello, 1998). The nurse should include education about screening techniques for health promotion in the process of assessment (Goldberg & Chavin, 1997).

The relationship of the health care provider to the client requires recognition of and sensitivity to cultural differences (see Figure 13-3). The examiner must recognize that cultural groups have their own definitions of health and illness that may differ from the examiner's. These same cultural groups may also have their own health practices that attempt to promote health within the group and cure illness. All health care providers should be willing to attempt to modify health care in keeping with the client's cultural beliefs.

Ask Yourself

You are seeing a client from a culture that does not believe in traditional Western medicine. This client has a condition that would respond to antibiotics; however, the client refuses and informs you she has been using her culture's traditional herbs and roots. She is only seeing you because of her employer's insistence. She has missed work days because of her condition. How would you respond to her situation?

Physiological Changes Associated with Aging

In attempting to detect disease in the older adult, the health care provider must be able to compare physiological changes associated with aging with abnormal changes in the different organ systems and must also understand the clinical implications associated with these changes. Misidentifying an age-related change as induced by disease may lead to therapeutic attempts to reverse normal aging, which may result in **iatrogenic** harm. Incorrectly identifying changes induced by disease as age-related changes leads to therapeutic neglect of potentially or possibly treatable conditions (Beers & Besdine, 1987). For example, anemia is most likely caused by bleeding (Ania, Suman, Fairbanks, Rademacher, & Melton, 1997), so significantly lower hemoglobin and hematocrit blood counts are not a normal part of aging. Table 13-1 examines age-related changes and clinical implications or problems these changes may cause to older adults.

Table 13-2 gives a list of typical nursing diagnoses that could be utilized for the physical assessment of the older adult.

TABLE 13-1 Age Changes and Clinical Implications

Age-Related Change	Clinical Implication/Problem
General Overview	
Decreased lean body mass	Changes in pharmacokinetics
Decreased body water	
Increased body fat	
Decreased height	Osteoporosis
Skin	
Decreased subcutaneous fat	Increased chance for pressure ulcers
Decreased vascularity of dermis	Decreased body temperature regulation
Hair follicles produce less melanin	Greying of hair
Loss of collagen	Tendency to neoplasia
Flattening of dermoepidermal junction	Skin tears
Decreased sebaceous and sweat gland activity	Dry skin and less perspiration
Capillary fragility	Purpura
Diminished vascular supply to nailbed	Nails brittle, thick, and hard
Eyes	
Loss of elasticity of lens	Presbyopia, impaired adaptation to darkness, and glare
Rigidity of iris	Decreased size of pupils, sensitivity to light
Increased density of lens	Glaucoma
Accumulation of yellow substance in lens	Alteration of color perception
Lacrimal duct stenosis	Excessive tearing
Decreased strength of orbicular muscles	Ectropion, corneal drying, abrasion
Ears	
Loss of cochlear neurons	Hearing loss for higher frequencies
Decrease in activity of cerumen glands	Drier cerumen that may result in impactions
Degeneration of vestibular structures, loss of hair cells, and myelinated nerve fibers	Deficits in equilibrium and hearing
Nose	
Atrophy of olfactory bulbs	Diminished sense of smell
Mouth	
Resorption of gum and bony tissue	Loss of teeth and periodontal disease
Extrinsic stains and less translucent enamel	Darkened teeth
Tongue	
Papillae atrophy of lateral edges of tongue	Reduced taste sensation
Enlargement of tongue	Sign of hypothyroidism
Smooth, painful tongue	Vitamin B_{12} deficiency
Respiratory System	
Decreased vital capacity	Increased risk of pulmonary complications
Decreased maximum breathing capacity	

(continues)

TABLE 13-1 Age Changes and Clinical Implications *continued*

Age-Related Change	Clinical Implication/Problem
Respiratory System *continued*	
Increased residual volume	
Loss of interalveolar folds	Decreased alveolar surface available for gas exchange
Loss of muscle strength in thorax and diaphragm	Barrel chest
Cardiovascular System	
Increased peripheral vascular resistance	Hypertension
Fibrosis and sclerosis in heart valves	Aortic stenosis and mitral regurgitation
Decreased baroceptor reflex activity	Orthostatic hypotension
Loss of elasticity of aorta	Left ventricular hypertrophy
Heart rate slows with decrease in cardiac output	Response to stress and increased oxygen demand less efficient
Cellular alteration and fibrosis in the conduction system	ECG changes—first-degree atrioventricular block and atrial fibrillation
Renal System	
Decrease in creatinine clearance	Alteration in drug pharmacokinetics
Decreased tubular function	Tendency toward dehydration
Musculoskeletal System	
Loss of bone mineral density	Osteoporosis and fractures
Decreased intervertebral disk space	Increased curvature of spine
Decreased compliance of chest wall	Increased work of breathing
Loss of muscle mass	Decreased strength
Flattening of arch of feet	Gait impairment
Gastrointestinal System	
Diminished colonic motility	Constipation
Altered esophageal motility	Predisposition to aspiration
Decreased hepatic mass and blood flow	Altered pharmacokinetics
Decreased calcium absorption	Osteoporosis
Epithelial atrophy	Decreased secretion of digestive enzymes and protective mucosa
Less biologically active bacterial flora	Impaired digestive ability and tastes
Increase in biliary lipids	Gallstone formation
Nervous System	
Decreased brain weight (5%–7%) and blood flow	Increased risk of syncope
Deposition of the aging pigment lipofuscin in nerve cells and amyloid in blood vessels	Impairment in cognition, reasoning, judgment, and orientation
Altered sleep patterns	Increased sleep disturbances
Decreased vibratory sense	Altered gait
Increased postural instability	Accidents and falls
Decreased reaction time	Accidents, difficulty in operating machinery and driving

(continued)

TABLE 13-1 Age Changes and Clinical Implications *continued*

Age-Related Change	Clinical Implication/Problem
Nervous System *continued*	
Progressive loss of dendrites with progression to fragmentation and cell death	Failing short-term memory and learning ability
Endocrine System	
Moderate atrophy of thyroid gland	Hypothyroidism
Increased insulin resistance	Diabetes mellitus
Rise in bone resorption	Predisposition to osteoporosis
Decreased estrogen	Menopause

Adapted from Practical Guide to Health Assessment through the Lifespan (3rd ed.), by M. O. Hogstel and L. C. Curry, 2001, Philadelphia: Davis; Gerontological Nursing Certification Review Guide for the Generalist, Clinical Specialist, Nurse Practitioner, by C. Kopac and V. Millonig, 1996, Potomac, MD: Health Leadership Associates; Practical Guide to the Care of the Geriatric Patient, by F. Ferri and M. Fretwell, 1992, St. Louis, Mosby.

Think About It

A 65-year-old woman comes to your clinic complaining of low back pain and pain in her right wrist. You note that this client has listed her height as 5 feet, 4 inches; however, her height as measured today is 5 feet, 2 inches. Her weight is 95 pounds, she is Caucasian, and she has been a lifetime smoker. She also informs you her diet consists of frozen food and she is intolerant of milk products. What is a probable diagnosis for this client and what part of her complaints would need immediate attention?

Age-Related Laboratory Values

An important part of the comprehensive assessment of the older adult is evaluation of laboratory tests. The proper use of these laboratory tests in evaluating older adults requires knowledge of the normal ranges for age and the provider being aware of the client's health and medication history.

The blood urea nitrogen (BUN) or creatinine does not adequately reflect renal function in older adults. Because **lean body mass** declines with age, the total

TABLE 13-2 Typical Nursing Diagnoses for Older Adults

Altered body temperature	Sleep pattern disturbance
Risk for aspiration	Impaired swallowing
Decreased cardiac output	Impaired tissue integrity
Ineffective breathing patterns	Altered tissue perfusion
Fluid volume deficit	Altered urinary elimination
Risk for infection	Chronic pain
Altered nutrition	Altered health maintenance
Impaired skin integrity	Functional incontinence

Adapted from NANDA Nursing Diagnoses: Definitions and Classification, 1999–2001, by North American Nursing Diagnosis Association (NANDA), 1998, Philadelphia: Author.

production of creatinine declines. Creatinine clearance declines by almost 10% per decade after age 40, while the BUN is influenced by dietary protein intake.

Most liver function tests remain unchanged; however the alkaline phosphatase is frequently elevated in the older population. Total alkaline phosphatase may rise as a consequence of Paget's disease, minor bone trauma in osteoporotic patients, or fracture. In older adults, an elevation of total alkaline phosphatase is more likely to derive from bone than liver (Beers & Besdine, 1987).

Nursing Tip

When assessing the laboratory results of an older adult, be aware of concurrent medical conditions and what constitutes normal values in the older population.

Table 13-3 gives a list of laboratory values for the older adult with age-related changes described.

Atypical Presentation of Disease in the Older Adult

Altered presentation of illness is a common manifestation in the older population. Diseases may have unusual presentations with clinical signs and symptoms that can be confusing. Severe, acute illness will often present with nonspecific or vague symptoms. Typical signs and symptoms may be absent. At other times, diseases may present as merely failure to thrive, changes in mental status, falling, anorexia, or self-neglect. All health care providers need to be aware of these differences.

Table 13-4 contrasts classic presentations of illnesses and diseases in the younger population to presentations in the older population.

TABLE 13-3 Laboratory Values in Older Adults

Test	Age-Related Change	Geriatric Value
Hemoglobin	Slightly decreased, related to reduced hematopoiesis	M: 10–17 g/100 ml; F: 9–17 g/100 ml
Hematocrit	Slightly decreased, related to reduced hematopoiesis	M: 38%–54%; F: 35%–49%
Leukocytes	Decreased, related to decreased T and B lymphocytes	3,100–9,000 mm^3
Sedimentation rate	Slightly increased	Less than 22 mm/hr
Albumin	Decreased, related to reduced liver size and enzyme production	M: 2.3–4.7 g/100 ml; F: 2.6–5.0 g/100/ml
Alkaline phosphatase	Increased, related to decreased liver function	M: 21.3–80.8 units; F: 19.9–83.4 units
Blood urea nitrogen	Increased, related to compromised renal function	M: 8–35 mg/100 ml; F: 6–30 mg/100 ml
Creatinine	Increased	0.4–1.9 mg/100 ml
Calcium	Slightly decreased	9–10.9 mg/100 ml
Glucose	Increased	140 mg/100 ml
Potassium	Increased	3.0–5.9 mEq/liter
Creatinine clearance	Must be calculated to consider decreased glomerular filtration rate	M: $\dfrac{(140 - \text{age}) \times \text{kg body weight}}{72}$ F: $\dfrac{(140 - \text{age}) \times \text{kg body weight} \times 0.85}{72}$

Adapted from Primary Care Geriatrics: A Case-Based Approach *(2nd ed.), by R. Ham and P. Sloane, 1992, St. Louis: Mosby;* Practical Guide to Health Assessment through the Lifespan *(3rd ed.), by M. O. Hogstel and L. C. Curry, 2001, Philadelphia: Davis.*

TABLE 13-4   Comparison of Classical Presentation of Symptoms in Younger Adults and Older Adults

Illness	Presentation in Younger Adults	Presentation in Older Adults
Depression	Withdrawal, crying, and insomnia	Memory and concentration problems, increased sleep
Pneumonia	Productive cough, fever, chills	Nonproductive or absent cough, no fever or chills
Urinary tract infection	Frequency, urgency, nocturia	Incontinence, confusion, anorexia, weakness, normal temperature
Myocardial infarction	Severe chest pain, nausea	Atypical pain location, absent pain, tachypnea, confusion
Hyperthyroidism	Increased pulse, hyperactivity	Hypoactivity, depression, atrial fibrillation, weakness
Congestive heart failure	Dyspnea, fatigue, weight gain, rales	Same as in younger adults plus confusion, falls, agitation, and anorexia
Acute abdomen	Abdominal pain and tenderness	Acute confusion
Polymyalgia rheumatica	Headache, blindness	Mental changes or respiratory tract symptoms
Meningitis	Headache or nuchal rigidity	Fever, mental changes
Appendicitis	Right lower quadrant pain	Diffuse abdominal pain

Adapted from The Merck Manual of Geriatrics *(2nd ed.), by W. B. Abrams, M. H. Beers, and R. Berkow (Eds.), 1995, Rahway, NJ: Merck Research Laboratories;* Geriatrics, *by E. T. Lonergan (Ed.), 1996, Stamford, CT: Appleton & Lange.*

Functional Assessment

Older adults are often referred for a comprehensive geriatric assessment when functional status worsens. Functional ability is the combined effect of disease and disability on the person's ability to carry out a task associated with everyday living such as the ability to live alone independently, continue to drive, and to meet basic needs. Recommendations regarding type of housing and use of an automobile may depend on the results of the assessment. These recommendations could indicate minor changes rather than a complete change in lifestyle. For example, many older adults fear the loss of the ability to drive. However, assessment of functional ability may determine the cause of a problem (for example, vision or hearing) that could be corrected (Martolli, Richardson, Stowe, Miller, Brass, Cooney, & Tinetti, 1998). **Functional assessment** is a systematic attempt to measure objective performance in the areas of daily living, including physical activities of daily living (PADL) and instrumental activities of daily living (IADL). Assessing functional limitations in older adults can be important in detecting disease and dysfunction, selecting appropriate interventions, and evaluating the results of these interventions (Hogstel & Curry, 2001). Maintaining optimal function with the older adult being as independent as possible is the goal of the geriatric assessment

team. The team works toward promotion and maintenance of functional independence with the goal of assisting the older adult to live independently as long as possible and to prevent hospitalization and institutionalization. A functional geriatric assessment begins with a review of the major areas of functional ability—PADL and IADL.

Physical activities of daily living is the term used to describe basic self-care skills. The PADL are the activities that people must accomplish to survive without help. These include bathing, dressing, toileting, transferring, continence, and feeding. Older adults unable to perform these activities usually require caregiver assistance for at least 12 hours a day. Several reliable instruments have been developed to measure PADL. The Katz Index is "one of the best known and most carefully studied" tests to measure PADL (Kane & Kane, 1981, p. 45). It is a scale used to detect problems in performing PADL and to determine what kind of assistance may be needed (Katz, Ford, Moskowitz, Jackson, & Jaffee, 1963). The Katz scale records loss of independence in the six areas listed above and assigns a score based on the older adults' performance of those functions. This scale records loss of independence in the six skills in the order stated, because this is generally the order in which the skills are lost. They are regained, in the reverse order, during rehabilitation in the majority of people. A top

Research Focus

Citation:

Ania, B., Suman, V.J., Fairbanks, V.F., Rademacher, D.M., & Melton, L.J. (1997). Incidence of anemia in older people: An epidemiologic study in a well defined population. *Journal of the American Geriatrics Society, 45* (7), 825–831.

Purpose:

To assess the incidence and clinical spectrum of anemia among older adults.

Methods:

"Age- and sex-adjusted incidence rates, corrected for prevalent anemia, and survival estimates using the Kaplan-Meier method, with calculation of standardized mortality ratios for specific cause of death." (p. 825)

Findings:

The corrected annual incidence of anemia rose with age, and rates were higher in men (90.3 per 1,000) than women (69.1 per 1,000). In 465 cases (75%), anemia was detected in conjunction with a hospitalization, but admission was because of anemia in only 57 instances. Mortality attributable to malignancy, mental disorders, circulatory and respiratory diseases, ill-defined conditions, and injuries was significantly increased among those older clients with anemia.

Implications:

"The incidence of anemia among older people is 4 to 6 times greater than that suspected clinically, rises with age, and is higher in men than in women. The apparent cause in half the cases is blood loss. Even mild anemia is associated with reduced survival, especially during the first year, but this could relate to underlying comorbid conditions." (p. 825)

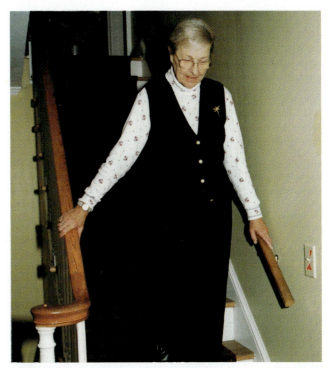

FIGURE 13-4 One of the IADL is the ability to use the stairs safely.

of patients to care for themselves" (Gallo, Reichel, & Anderson, 1995, p. 76) and to document improvement (Mahoney & Barthel, 1965).

Instrumental activities of daily living are used to describe the more complex activities a person needs for independent living. They include being able to shop, cook, manage finances, climb stairs, manage transportation, do housework and laundry, and manage medications (see Figure 13-4). Examples of IADL scales include the Rapid Disability Rating Scale and the Lawton IADL

Ask Yourself

Your widowed grandmother has been living alone in her own home in the town where she grew up. She has several life-long friends and is active in her church. You live 100 miles away and have children and a full-time job. Recently, you received a call from one of her church members telling you that your grandmother had been having difficulty with walking and that she had fallen three times in the last month. She also stated she had noticed your grandmother's legs were extremely swollen. Knowing that your grandmother has congestive heart failure and osteoarthritis, you are concerned with her ability to continue to function and live independently. You are also aware that she is extremely independent and has often stated that she "would never want to be a bother to her children." What actions would you take to ensure your grandmother's safety but also allow her to live according to her wishes?

score of 6 out of 6 will indicate that the person has full basic function, while lower scores indicate impairment in functional ability. A combined measure of all six PADL functions can be used to gauge changes over time. There are other PADL instruments that have been validated and been shown to be sensitive to change over time. Examples include the PULSES profile and the Barthel Index. PULSES is an acronym for physical condition, upper limbs (self-care), lower limbs (ambulation), sensory abilities, and social factors (Kane & Kane, 1981). The PULSES Index is similar to the Barthel Index. "The Barthel Index has been used to assess the ability

Scale. The Rapid Disability Rating Scale attempts to account for some of the functional disability related to the presence of confusion or depression. The scale rates what the individual actually does, not what the individual can potentially do. The Lawton IADL Scale asks nine questions related to IADL with three parts to each question. The first answer indicates independence; the second, capability with assistance; and the third, dependence (Adams, Beers, & Berkow, 1995; Lawton, 1988). Declining scores over time indicate decreased ability to function independently.

These tools assist the practitioner in objectively recording degrees of change over time and how fast functional change may be occurring. The practitioner who is aware of existing functional status will recognize changes that will enable earlier diagnosis of a possible emerging illness. Promotion and maintenance of functional independence to the highest possible degree is the primary goal of the geriatric health care team, and by utilizing assessment tools for PADL and IADL, these goals can be more adequately achieved.

Table 13-5 provides a list of nursing diagnoses that could be used in the functional assessment of the older adult.

Psychosociospiritual Assessment

Delivery of nursing care to the older adult requires a thorough understanding of the individual as a whole. A holistic assessment includes not only gathering data through the review of systems and physical examination, but also assessing the individual's psychosocial and spiritual background to gain a comprehensive view of individuals and how they are functioning within their social environment.

Psychosociospiritual assessment of the older adult can be a lengthy and complex process and is one that continues over the entire nurse-client relationship. It is important to remember that the data base is not static and that changes may occur in the individual's life situation. There must be ongoing assessment and alteration in the plan of care to optimize health and function of the older adult. There may be challenges faced in conducting the assessment, such as if the individual is confused, fatigued, or in pain. The nurse should be flexible in the assessment process and prioritize data to be gathered. Often additional information may be gathered at future meetings.

The depth of data gained will often depend upon the rapport that has been established between the nurse and client. The nurse should begin the interview with introductions and a general orientation to the nurses' role, the nature and purpose of the interview, and future plans for involvement with the individual. The nurse should make effective use of therapeutic communication skills and be sensitive at all times to the individual's feelings and for signs of anxiety or distress. The interview should generally proceed from less personal questions to those that might be considered more personal, such as questions regarding financial status. However, it is difficult at times to predict what topics might be sensitive for different individuals. For instance, when questioning a client about driving, the nurse may notice the client becoming increasingly agitated and may find out that this is an extremely sensitive subject for that person because the family has been repeatedly trying to convince the person to stop driving for safety reasons. In such situations, the nurse must be sensitive to the individual's feelings and utilize effective communication skills. The nurse should remember that the most important communication tool in conducting a psychosociospiritual assessment is the art of listening. It is not only important to gather as much quality information as possible through specific questioning, but it is critical to listen and observe carefully for nonverbal messages and feelings and caregiver-client interactions.

TABLE 13-5 Nursing Diagnoses in Functional Assessment	
Impaired adjustment	Altered role performance
Anxiety	Self-care deficit
Risk for loneliness	Social isolation
Powerlessness	Risk for injury
Impaired walking	Hopelessness

Adapted from NANDA Nursing Diagnoses: Definitions and Classification, 1999–2001, by NANDA, 1998, Philadelphia: Author.

Ask Yourself

How would you prepare to conduct a psychosociospiritual assessment of a cognitively impaired older adult? Would it be helpful to have the primary caregiver present? What would you do if the client started becoming anxious and agitated?

A comprehensive assessment should always involve family members and caregivers as appropriate. Frequently family members and direct caregivers can contribute information that might be overlooked if they are not included in the assessment process (Figure 13-5). Involving them not only gives the nurse the opportunity

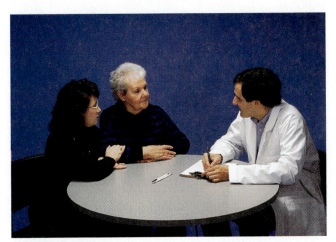

FIGURE 13-5 Family members and direct caregivers should be included in the assessment process.

to assess the status of their relationship with the individual, but also allows the nurse the opportunity to involve the caregivers in planning, education, and decision making. It is important to mention the potential mistakes health care providers often make in regards to family/caregiver involvement. One common mistake is to ignore the client and focus primarily on the caregiver to answer all the questions, receive information, and make decisions. Providers sometimes make certain ageist assumptions, underestimate clients' capabilities, and do not allow them to be active in their own care. On the other hand, sometimes they receive inaccurate information because they do not involve the family or caregivers when needed. Individuals with a dementing illness may still be quite socially skilled and may make the health care provider think that they are cognitively intact and that the information being given is accurate. Also, some older adults may overestimate their abilities out of fear that the health care provider might uncover certain information that could result in loss of independence or institutionalization.

The overall health and well-being of older adults is dependent not only upon their physical health but also on their psychosocial and spiritual health. All these components of an individual's being are interrelated. For example, an older adult may have severe urinary incontinence (physical issue) that causes low self-esteem and embarrassment (psychological issue), resulting in the older adult avoiding social outings with their friends (social issue). Relationships, social structures, and the environment are all important factors in psychosocial well-being, and older adults generally experience many role and life situation changes. It is important that the nurse remain aware of these factors when conducting an assessment of the older adult. Older individuals may have both positive and negative role and lifestyle changes that are impacting

their psychosocial health. Examples of some of these changes include retirement, loss of spouse or loved ones, increased time for leisure activities or volunteerism, and gaining new interests and hobbies. The nurse, along with other members of the health care team, can help the older adult identify and anticipate life changes and facilitate planning and implementation of adaptive strategies.

Psychological Assessment

Basic components of a psychological assessment include **cognitive** and **affective assessment**. The multiple physical, psychological, and environmental etiologies of cognitive impairment, as well as the common errorenous belief in our society that cognitive decline is simply a normal part of aging, often leads to inaccurate assessment of cognitive impairment in the older adult (Lueckenotte, 1994). Components of cognitive and affective assessment generally include memory, perception, language, attention, concentration, orientation, calculation, reasoning, judgment, insight, mood, and affect (Chenitz, Stone, & Salisbury, 1991). Many objective assessment tools are available for use in conducting cognitive and affective assessment of the older adult.

Cognitive Assessment

The Folstein Mini Mental State Examination (MMSE) (Folstein, Folstein, & McHugh, 1975) is a widely used cognitive assessment tool that does not require specialized training to administer and can be administered in approximately 10–20 minutes. It is a 30-point tool that measures orientation, registration, attention and calculation, recall, and language. However, the disadvantage to the Folstein MMSE is that it does not test the higher cognitive functions of judgment, problem solving, or abstract thinking (Chenitz, et al., 1991). Interpretation is as follows: If the individual scores 26 or greater out of a possible 30, there is probably no cognitive impairment; for scores between 20 and 25, the individual probably needs further testing, unless educational and language factors are thought to be playing a significant role; and scores less than 20 generally indicate cognitive impairment (Fillit & Picariello, 1998). Another relatively simple cognitive assessment tool includes the Short Portable Mental Status Questionnaire (SPMSQ) consisting of 10 items that test orientation, memory in relation to self-care ability, remote memory, and mathematical ability (Pfeiffer, 1975).

Affective Assessment

Depression is the most common mental health issue among older adults and is, unfortunately, often underdiagnosed and undertreated, which leads to loss of physical, cognitive, and social functioning (Ferri &

Fretwell, 1992; Fillit & Picariello, 1998). There are many risk factors for depression in older adults, including genetic predisposition, prior history of depressive episodes, sensory and social losses, certain chronic disease states (e.g., stroke, dementia, Parkinson's disease, alcoholism, hypothyroidism), and certain pharmacological agents (beta-blocker antihypertensives, analgesics, and sedatives) (Fillit & Picariello, 1998). Older adults frequently do not self-report feelings of depression, so it is often helpful to utilize objective tools to help screen for depression. The Geriatric Depression Scale (Yesavage, et al., 1983) is a 30-item tool that can be administered as a self-report or as an interview. Other examples of depression screening tools commonly used include the Beck Depression Inventory (Gallagher, 1986) and the Zung Self-Rating Depression Scale (Zung, 1965).

Sociospiritual Assessment

Social assessment involves attempting to gain a broad understanding of the individual's background, relationships, personal meaning of existence, environment, and how that person is functioning and interacting within the environment. Social factors can significantly impact a person's overall health, functional capacity, and well-being. Careful exploration of a person's social situation can provide answers about health problems they are having, and then interventions and treatments can be formulated. For example, identifying that a client with uncontrolled hypertension is not taking his medications because he has been unable to afford it would be very critical information. The nurse can then focus efforts on finding alternative ways to obtain the necessary medication or getting the medication changed to a more cost-effective alternative. Table 13-6 lists the essential components of a social assessment.

Support Systems

A **support system** is very often one of the most critical components of social well-being, which not only pro-

vides emotional support, but often is the determining factor of whether clients are able to remain living in the community. The general elements of social support include emotional support (e.g., affirmation and affection), assistance with task performance (e.g., bathing, shopping, transportation), financial assistance, and advice and guidance (Luggen, 1996). Support systems are comprised of both formal and informal supports. Examples of formal social supports include home health care, home-delivered meals, congregate meals, adult day services, nursing facilities, homemaker services, energy assistance, Medicaid, senior center activities, home repair services, and food stamps. Informal supports might include assistance from family, friends, neighbors, pets, and church group membership. In assessing support systems, the nurse can evaluate what supports are in place and help optimize and strengthen those and identify what additional support systems the individual might qualify for and benefit from.

It is important that the nurse also conduct a thorough assessment of the primary caregiver as appropriate, not only for quality of care and learning needs, but also for signs of stress and caregiver burden. Informal caregiving can involve many activities, including telephone calls, managing finances, visiting the individual, and providing direct physical care. More than 80% of care of older community-dwelling adults is delivered by family members (Fillit & Picariello, 1998). Caregiving responsibilities can potentially impact the caregivers' earning abilities or employment performance, other family obligations and relationships, and the caregiver's physical and emotional health. Providing care for an ill and/or cognitively impaired individual can be extremely stressful, and the nurse is in a good position to be able to identify signs of caregiver stress and provide assistance. A helpful tool for use in assessing for caregiver stress is the Burden Interview (Zarit & Zarit, 1983). It is critical for health care providers to be alert for signs of caregiver burnout and intervene to try and help relieve stress for the caregiver. Often caregivers are not even aware that they are experiencing burnout and stress or they do not know where to turn for information and support. Helping caregivers to optimize their caregiving knowledge and skills; assisting them in finding respite services, such as home care programs, short-term nursing home stays, and adult day services; and obtaining the help of volunteers to care for the client so the caregiver can get away are all valuable ways providers can assist caregivers.

Financial Resources

It is important to determine the individual's financial status so that health care providers are aware of any financial limitations and can adjust the care plan accordingly and facilitate getting the family assistance that they

TABLE 13-6 Components of a Social Assessment	
Support systems	Alcohol and tobacco use
Financial resources	Sleep hygiene
Occupational history	Sexuality
Education	Cultural background
Living arrangements	Signs of abuse/neglect
Interests/daily routine	End-of-life decisions
Nutrition	Spiritual values and beliefs

might need. Interview questions might include health insurance coverage, sources and amount of monthly income (to better assess status or eligibility for financial assistance programs), monthly expenses, and subjective opinion about adequacy of income to meet basic needs, for example, food, shelter, utilities, and health care needs. There may be special financial needs for assistance with the purchase of essential prescription medications for chronic health problems and dental care because of **periodontal disease**, which may eventually result in the need for the purchase of dentures.

Occupational and Educational History

Occupational history can include whether they are currently employed, what types of employment they have had, when they retired, and reasons for retirement. It is generally helpful also to clarify educational history and the highest level of education the individual completed.

Living Arrangements

Living arrangements and environmental assessment are important components of the social assessment. Some of the components of this assessment include marital status; where the individual lives and with whom; what type of living arrangement it is (e.g., home, family member's home, apartment, retirement community, or assisted-living facility); are they satisfied with their living arrangements; how accessible is the place of living to services and support systems; safety of the residence; accessibility to emergency assistance; and adaptive equipment.

CLINICAL ALERT

Be on the lookout for some of the following environmental safety hazards:

- *High crime area with poor locks/safety devices on the doors and windows*
- *Lack of running water, electricity, or telephone*
- *Lack of adequate heating/cooling system*
- *Use of space heater, wood stove, heating pads, or electric blankets for heating*
- *Inadequate lighting*
- *Stairs, railings, sidewalks in poor repair*
- *Lack of smoke alarms*
- *Cluttered walkways*
- *Durable medical equipment in poor working order*
- *Throw rugs, slippery floor surface, or loose carpet or linoleum*

Interests and Daily Routines

Finding out about the older adult's interests and daily routines provides the nurse with valuable information about the individual's level of activity and social health. It is good to question the individual about involvement in social groups, formal classes, recreational and leisure activities, exercise, hobbies, and a description of a typical day. It is important to ascertain whether clients have altered their activities or level of community involvement, and, if they have, what are the reasons for the change and how does the change in activity make them feel.

Nutrition

Nutrition is a very important part of any holistic assessment. **Malnutrition** in older adults is extremely serious and can predispose the individual to infection, skin problems, confusion, increased weakness, increased incidence of falls, and alterations in **pharmacokinetics** (Fillit & Picariello, 1998). Many factors can place an older adult at risk for poor nutritional health, including living alone, limited finances, transportation challenges, limited cooking facilities, decreased sensory function, poor dentition, polypharmacy, certain chronic illnesses (e.g., dementia, depression, dysphagia, arthritis, stroke, alcohol abuse, cancer, heart disease, and COPD), and limited understanding of nutrition (Fillit & Picariello, 1998). To assess nutritional health, the nurse should inquire about changes in weight and appetite, usual food and fluid intake, dietary preferences and restrictions, food intolerances, where and with whom meals are usually eaten, chronic use of laxatives, dental problems, difficulty chewing or swallowing, alcohol abuse, memory impairment, depression, and financial and functional issues as related to acquisition and preparation of the food (Fillit & Picariello, 1998). The nurse can then target interventions to optimize the individual's nutritional health, such as making community resource referrals (e.g., Meals-On-Wheels, senior centers, food stamps, transportation assistance), dietitian referral, adaptive equipment, occupational therapy referral, dental referral, dietary supplements, and nutritional education (Fillit & Picariello, 1998).

Alcohol, Drug, and Tobacco Use

A social assessment also includes questions related to alcohol, prescription or illicit drug use, and tobacco use. This information is usually most easily obtained by asking direct questions in a nonjudgmental manner. It is important to determine what substance(s) is used, the quantity that is used, and under what circumstances. It may also be beneficial to ask whether they have had any physical or social changes because of their substance use. Substance abuse is generally underreported and underdiagnosed in the older population, and nurses should look for signs of abuse.

Sleep Hygiene

It is also important to question older adults about their **sleep hygiene** or usual sleep patterns. Complaints about difficulty sleeping are extremely common in the older population. There are age-related changes in sleep patterns, including reduced time in the **rapid eye movement (REM)** stage of sleep and in deep (stage 4) sleep, increased wakefulness and fragmentation of sleep, and changes in circadian rhythms may occur, with increased wakefulness at night and fatigue in the daytime (Fillit & Picariello, 1998). Difficulty sleeping certainly can impact quality of life, and the nurse should try and identify any reversible causes and provide reassurance. It might be helpful to direct attention to the mattress and pillow the individual uses, potential environmental factors (e.g., noise, temperature, lighting), daytime napping, exercise and activity level, alcohol and caffeine intake, and fluid consumption in the evening (Fillit & Picariello, 1998).

Sexuality

Assessment of the older adult's sexual health is often overlooked, sometimes because of ageist assumptions that older adults are asexual beings, and sometimes because of a lack of comfort on the part of the nurse or the individual in discussing sexual matters. Healthy older adults often experience few changes in sexual interest or activity. Factors that might adversely impact libido or sexual activity in the older adult might include poor health, lack of a partner, lack of privacy (e.g., living in an institutional setting or in a three-generation household), or sexual dysfunction secondary to physical or psychological factors (e.g., diabetes, fear of failure, pain related to arthritis, change in body image). Other factors that might positively impact sexual function could include additional leisure time, no fear of pregnancy, and fewer family and work responsibilities (Roberts, 1989). Helpful questions to obtain sexual health information include sexual preferences, past and current sexual activity, number of partners, changes in sexual interest or activity, sexual difficulties, and methods used for protection against sexually transmitted diseases. The nurse can play an important role in providing education about sexual issues, such as safe sex practices, alternative methods or techniques for sexual expression, and available resources for help with sexual dysfunction.

Cultural and Ethnic Background

Cultural and ethnic history is an important component of the social assessment. The nurse should inquire about place of birth, native language, part of a special ethnic or cultural group, folk medicine practices, and practices that are unique to the ethnic or cultural group. It is important to identify and be sensitive to cultural and ethnic issues; however, the nurse should be cautious not to overgeneralize all individuals in a cultural group and miss the unique qualities of an individual (Hogstel, 1994).

Abuse and Neglect

Approximately one million cases of elder abuse occur annually, and this number is probably an underestimation as elder abuse is frequently not reported because of the victim's fear of retaliation, shame, or desire or need to protect the abuser (Fillit & Picariello, 1998) and lack of mandatory universal reporting laws. The nurse must try and remain nonjudgmental and begin with nonthreatening questions. It is important to interview the individual alone for this portion of the assessment and to be alert for any inconsistencies between history and physical findings. Types of abuse include physical, psychological, sexual, financial, and neglect. Physical abuse involves inflicting physical injury or pain, and psychological abuse involves the infliction of mental anguish, such as threats, insults, and purposeful social isolation (Fillit & Picariello, 1998). Financial abuse involves exploiting the older adult's funds, property, or assets, and neglect refers to failure to assist a vulnerable individual with basic or medical needs (Fillit & Picariello, 1998).

Some possible characteristics that might place an individual at risk of being a victim of abuse include being female, advanced age, functional dependence, intergenerational conflict, passive or stoic personality, social isolation, physical and/or cognitive deficits, and history of abuse (Fillit & Picariello, 1998). Characteristics that might place the caregiver at risk for abusing the older adult include substance abuse, mental illness, lack of knowledge or experience with caregiving, financial stressors, history of abuse as a child, lack of outside interests and involvement, extreme life stressors, aggressive and unsympathetic personality, and unrealistic expectations of the situation (Fillit & Picariello, 1998). The nurse should be suspicious of possible abuse if there are patterns of unexplained injuries; the older adult appears fearful of the caregiver; the caregiver appears indifferent or angry toward the individual; the caregiver appears overly concerned with the individual's assets; the presence of injuries or unexplained infections of the genital region; the presence of severe, unexplained dehydration or malnutrition; hypo- or hyperthermia related to environmental exposure; inadequate hygiene or inappropriate clothing; or unexplained medication mismanagement (Fillit & Picariello, 1998). If elder abuse or neglect is suspected, it is critical to report it immediately to the local Adult Protective Services so that an appropriate investigation can be conducted and intervention to ensure the older adult's safety can be initiated.

End-of-Life Decisions

Studies suggest that most individuals have inadequate information regarding **advance directives**, and discus-

TABLE 13-7	Examples of Psychosociospiritual-Related Nursing Diagnoses	
Impaired adjustment		Risk for injury
Anxiety		Altered nutrition
Caregiver role strain		Self-esteem disturbance
Ineffective individual coping		Sexual dysfunction/altered sexual patterns
Diversional activity deficit		Sleep pattern disturbance
Altered family processes		Social isolation
Dysfunctional grieving		Risk for spiritual distress
Impaired home maintenance		Altered thought processes
Hopelessness		Risk for violence
Relocation stress syndrome		Sensory/perceptual alterations

Adapted from NANDA Nursing Diagnoses: Definitions and Classification, 1999-2001, *by NANDA, 1998, Philadelphia: Author.*

sion and education regarding end-of-life decisions is best obtained when an individual is not acutely ill or under duress (Fillit & Picariello, 1998). The nurse should inquire whether the individual has executed a living will and a Medical Power of Attorney, document the client's wishes, and record where the formal documents are kept. As client advocate, the nurse should also educate the client and family, as appropriate, regarding these documents and facilitate completion of the documents if requested to do so. The living will helps document the individual's wishes regarding specific life-sustaining procedures if the person is in an irreversible or terminal condition, and the Medical Power of Attorney designates an individual as the decision-making proxy if the aging adult becomes unable to express personal health care choices.

Spirituality

Spirituality involves finding meaning and purposefulness in life and having a relationship with a higher being and does not necessarily have to be expressed through affil-

iation with a specific religion or church (Hogstel, 1994). The nurse can inquire about the individual's spiritual beliefs and practices, what spirituality means to that person, whether that person is affiliated with a specific religion, and if actively involved, whether spirituality is a source of support and strength, and whether the person has any special religious traditions, rituals, or practices. Table 13-7 lists examples of psychosociospiritual-related nursing diagnoses, and Box 13-1 gives a spirituality assessment guide.

Summary

Physical assessment of the older adult will require adaptations of the environment to compensate for physiological and psychological changes. Some of the changes would include modifications to the physical environment, such as a warm room, adequate lighting, age-appropriate chairs and examination tables, and adequate space to accommodate mobility aides. The client should be assessed for sensory impairment. The nurse should face the client, speak slowly to those who are hearing impaired, and use visual cues for the visually impaired. It is important to utilize an interdisciplinary team with geriatric experience to provide high-quality and efficient geriatric care in today's health care environment. The health care provider should also possess a knowledge of cultural beliefs and practices to deliver appropriate and sensitive care to different cultures.

Physiological changes associated with aging should be differentiated from abnormal changes in the aging body system. Each body system must be carefully assessed with the practitioner having a thorough knowledge of what constitutes normal aging and what are abnormal aging changes. The health care practitioner

BOX 13-1 Spirituality Assessment Guide

- Do you have a formal religious affiliation?

- If yes, how active is your involvement?

- Are there any specific spiritual practices that are important to you?

- How important is your spirituality or religion as a source of support to you?

- How important are your spiritual values and beliefs in your decisions about your health care?

CARE PLAN

CASE STUDY

Lucy Borgelli is an 89-year-old woman who lives alone in a one-bedroom independent living complex in the suburbs. She has "aged in place" there for the past 21 years, as have many of her friends. Mrs. Borgelli was once employed as a salesperson in a large department store. She enjoyed talking with customers and took great pride in her personal appearance and helpful manner. Her heritage is Italian American, second generation.

Mrs. Borgelli led a sedentary lifestyle. Although she remained busy and active around the house, she did not participate in regular sustained exercise. She never drove and relied on her husband to take her places until he died 22 years ago. She never smoked and drank red wine only at holidays. She is slightly overweight for her height.

Mrs. Borgelli's medical history comprises eye, vascular, and mobility problems. Her medical history includes glaucoma for 6 years (eye pressure has been consistently normal); history of cataracts with bilateral surgeries in 1994 and 1995, no complications; hypertension since 1984; and fall with bruising left leg and thigh in 1996 but no fracture. She is very cautious since the fall in 1996 and verbalized her fears. "Once old people fall, that's it. They go into a home [nursing facility] and never come out." This statement depicts her perception of her fall and her fear of loss of independence.

Medication: Timoptic, one drop to each eye twice a day; Zalatan, one drop to each eye at bedtime; Covera, one tablet after supper; Tylenol, one or two tablets for minor discomfort.

Mrs. Borgelli's ROM (range of motion) is becoming progressively limited and frustrating for her. She is unable as well as anxious and fearful of stepping into her tub-shower and thus sponge bathes daily. In addition, she can no longer hook her bra (hooks in the back). She still is able to wash major body parts and groin area. It is questionable whether she can reach her buttocks and rectum. At times, a mild odor has been noted. She denies urinary or fecal incontinence or "accidents."

Mrs. Borgelli has one daughter who lives 1 hour away and visits once weekly to buy groceries and assist with "odds and ends" and other errands. Mrs. Borgelli says she gets lonely, especially on Sundays, which was family day. But she is not ready for the nursing home until "my mind or my legs give out."

ASSESSMENT

Mrs. Borgelli may be at a turning point in her level of independence. Her advancing age and early deficits in mobility and self-care place her at high risk for home care services or assisted-living placement. In addition, she is afraid of falling and thus cautious of circumstances surrounding going out to social and other functions. She is unable to leave her home and is at risk for social isolation, although she has neighbors and friends close by. Three positive aspects of Mrs. Borgelli's health are (1) minimal use of medications, (2) cognitive ability (no signs and symptoms of dementia or memory loss), and (3) she never smoked.

It is critical that the nurse establishes with Mrs. Borgelli a care plan aimed at maximizing her strengths and minimizing her deficits to maintain and extend her level of independence and overall well-being. This care plan identifies some key nursing diagnoses and interventions to support positive life-enhancing outcomes.

NURSING DIAGNOSIS

Self-care deficit, bathing related to inability to wash body parts and get in and out of tub-type shower.

Outcomes:

Mrs. Borgelli will:
- *Shower once/weekly (goal accomplishment: within 4 weeks).*
- *Use shower seat safely and effectively; demonstration and return demonstrations (goal accomplishment: within 4 weeks).*
- *Express and overcome fears about shower transfer (within 4 weeks).*

(continues)

CARE PLAN *continued*

Planning/Interventions:

The nurse will:

- *Assess shower area and environment for conduciveness to self-care.*
- *Observe and assess muscle strength, balance, and upper and lower body movements associated with bathing activities.*
- *Observe effectiveness of sponge bath.*
- *Consult with physical therapy to arrange a full physical therapy evaluation.*
- *Consult with a home care agency for follow-up teaching.*
- *Facilitate discussion on fear of falling and loss of independence.*
- *Encourage daughter's involvement with Mrs. Borgelli's showering once weekly.*

EVALUATION:

Mrs. Borgelli will shower once weekly with her daughter's assistance. The home health aide will visit her home once weekly to assist her. Physical therapy will perform an assessment and establish a plan of care to support mobility, safety, and fall prevention. A shower safety chair seat will be ordered by the home care agency. The home care nurse will successfully teach by demonstration and return demonstrations on how to get in and out of the tub-shower. Mrs. Borgelli will begin to verbalize her fears about losing her independence and being institutionalized as a first step in learning how to cope with changes in meeting her self-care needs.

NURSING DIAGNOSIS

Risk for injury related to history of falls, affective orientation (fear of falling), and altered mobility.

Outcomes:

Mrs. Borgelli will:

- *Experience zero falls.*
- *Describe environmental hazards related to falls and methods of fall prevention.*
- *Express fear of falling and identify ways to combat the fear.*

Planning/Interventions:

The nurse will:

- *Assess fall risk status, including orthostatic hypotension, balance, gait, and medications (refer to a fall risk assessment instrument such as the Tinnetti Scale).*
- *Consult with physical therapy on fall risk interventions.*
- *Explain/list environmental hazards pertaining to fall prevention.*
- *Discuss fall prevention with Mrs. Borgelli's daughter so that teaching may be reinforced.*

EVALUATION:

Mrs. Borgelli will have no further falls. She will express and cope with her fear of falling so that her fears do not compromise independence. In addition, environmental hazards will be screened for and eliminated from her house. The safety plan will be presented to her daughter so that both can work together to attain a hazard-free, low-fall-risk environment.

NURSING DIAGNOSIS

Impaired physical mobility related to postural instability during activities of daily living, limited range of motion, and anxiety.

(continues)

CARE PLAN *continued*

Outcomes:

Mrs. Borgelli will:

- *Walk 50 feet three times daily within 4 weeks.*
- *Perform physical therapy recommended upper and lower body exercises within 2 weeks.*
- *Verbalize feelings of increased confidence in walking and moving within 4 weeks.*
- *Consider a front-hooking bra.*

Planning/Interventions:

The nurse will:

- *Assess range of motion.*
- *Assess shower area for safety; recommend shower mat and shower seat.*
- *Discuss anxiety about falling.*
- *Consult with physical therapy for muscle strengthening, stretching, and coordination exercises/activities.*
- *Consult with psychiatric nurse specialist and social worker on approaches for building Mrs. Borgelli's confidence and reducing fear.*

EVALUATION:

Mrs. Borgelli will be able to walk extended distances and improve range of motion. She will carry out prescribed exercises and recognize the importance of safety without allowing fear of falling to consume her. By involving the interdisciplinary team, Mrs. Borgelli will meet the psychosocial as well as physiological challenges of impaired mobility from advanced age. Increased confidence and physical strength will be achieved and are realistic for Mrs. Borgelli, who is somewhat weak physically but has many positive aspects of health to her benefit.

---

must also be aware of age-related laboratory values and how clients' health history will affect their laboratory work. Finally, the older adult will often present with atypical presentation of illness. Diseases and illnesses may present with vague or confusing signs and symptoms. A practitioner educated in geriatric medicine and gerontological nursing will be able to understand physiological changes, laboratory values, and atypical disease presentations in the older adult as compared to a younger person.

One of the most important tasks of the geriatric practitioner is assessing functional status of the older adult. Functional ability is the combined effect of disability and disease on the older adult's ability to carry out the tasks associated with daily living. Functional assessment is a systematic attempt to measure performance objectively in physical activities of daily living (PADL), which include basic self-care skills such as bathing, dressing, toileting, transferring, continence, and feeding. Instrumental activities of daily living (IADL) describe the more complex tasks a person needs for independent living, such as shopping, cooking, and managing finances, transportation, and medications. There are multiple tools available to the practitioner to assess both PADL and IADL. These tools assist the provider in assessing change over time and how fast the

changes are occurring. The primary goal of the practitioner is promotion and maintenance of functional independence to the highest degree possible for the older adult.

The comprehensive assessment of the older adult should also focus on psychosocial and spiritual health. This holistic view of the individual will enable the health care professional to understand better how older adults are functioning in their total environment. Components of a psychological assessment include cognitive and affective assessment, which consists of memory, perception, language, attention, concentration, orientation, calculation, reasoning, judgment, insight, mood, and affect. Social assessment is composed of many different components. Support systems need to be assessed, as this may be the determining factor of whether the older adult will be able to remain independent in the community. Financial resources should be discussed to assist individuals to receive any benefits they may be entitled. Other components include occupational and educational history; living arrangements; interests and daily routines; nutrition; alcohol, drug, and tobacco use; sleep hygiene; sexuality; cultural and ethnic background; abuse and neglect; and spirituality. End-of-life decisions are best discussed when the individual is not acutely ill or undergoing life changes.

Review Questions and Activities

1. Describe five techniques used in the physical assessment of older adults.

2. Why is it important to understand physiological changes associated with aging?

3. List six nursing diagnoses common in the older adult.

4. What are the major differences in laboratory values for older adults?

5. Contrast classic presentations of illnesses and diseases in the older population to those in the younger population.

6. What are four tools used in the functional assessment of older adults?

7. Name the most important communication tool for conducting a psychosocial assessment.

8. What are the two basic components of a psychosocial assessment?

9. What are four types of elder abuse?

10. What is the name of the legal document that designates a decision-making proxy for an individual who does not have the mental or physical ability to make health care decisions?

References

Abrams, W. B., Beers, M. H., & Berkow, R. (Eds.). (1995). *The Merck manual of geriatrics* (2nd ed.). Rahway, NJ: Merck Research Laboratories.

Ania, B. J., Suman, V. J., Fairbanks, V. F., Rademacher, D. M., & Melton, L. J. (1997). Incidence of anemia in older people: An epidemiologic study in a well defined population. *Journal of the American Geriatrics Society, 45*(7), 825–831.

Beers, M., & Besdine, R. (1987). Medical assessment of the elderly patient. *Clinics in Geriatric Medicine, 3*(1), 17–27.

Chenitz, W. C., Stone, J., & Salisbury, S. (1991). *Clinical gerontological nursing: A guide to advanced practice.* Philadelphia: Saunders.

Ferri, F., & Fretwell, M. (1992). *Practical guide to the care of the geriatric patient.* St. Louis: Mosby.

Fillit, H., & Picariello, G. (1998). *Practical geriatric assessment.* London: Oxford University Press.

Folstein, M., Folstein, S., & McHugh, P. R. (1975). Mini-mental state: A practical method for grading the cognitive state of patients for the clinician. *Journal of Psychiatric Research, 12,* 189–198.

Gallagher, D. (1986). The Beck Depression Inventory and older adults: Review of its development and utility. *Clinical Gerontology, 5,* 149–161.

Gallo, J. J., Reichel, W., & Andersen, L. M. (1995). *Handbook of geriatric assessment.* Gaithersburg, MD: Aspen.

Goldberg, T. H., & Chavin, S. I. (1997). Preventive medicine and screening in older adults. *Journal of the American Geriatrics Society, 45*(3), 344–354.

Ham, R., & Sloane, P. (1992). *Primary care geriatrics: A case-based approach* (2nd ed.). St. Louis: Mosby.

Hogstel, M. O. (1994). *Nursing care of the older adult* (3rd ed.). Albany, NY: Delmar.

Hogstel, M. O., & Curry, L. C. (2001). *Practical guide to health assessment through the lifespan* (3rd ed.). Philadelphia: Davis.

Kane, R. A., & Kane, R. L. (1981). *Assessing the elderly.* Lexington, MA: Lexington Books.

Katz, S., Ford, A. B., Moscowitz, R. W., Jackson, B. A., & Jaffee, M. W. (1963). Studies of illness in the aged. The Index of ADL: A standardized measure of biological and psychosocial function. *Journal of the American Medical Association, 185*(12), 914–919.

Kopac, C., & Millonig, V. (1996). *Gerontological nursing certification review guide for the generalist, clinical specialist, nurse practitioner.* Potomac, MD: Health Leadership Associates.

Lawton, M. P. (1988). Scales to measure competence in everyday activities. *Psychopharmacological Bulletin, 24*(4), 609–614.

Lonergan, E. T. (Ed.). (1996). *Geriatrics.* Stamford, CT: Appleton & Lange.

Lueckenotte, A. (1994). *Pocket guide to gerontologic assessment.* St. Louis: Mosby.

Luggen, A. (1996). *NGNA core curriculum for gerontological nursing.* St. Louis: Mosby.

Mahoney, F. I., & Barthel, D. W. (1965). Functional evaluation: The Barthel Index. *Maryland State Medical Journal, 14,* 61–65.

Marottoli, R. A., Richardson, E. D., Stowe, M. H., Miller, E. G., Brass, L. M., Cooney, L. M., & Tinetti, M. E. (1998). Development of a test battery to identify older drivers at risk for self-reported adverse driving events. *Journal of the American Geriatrics Society, 46*(5), 562–568.

Pfeiffer, E. (1975). A short portable mental status questionnaire for the assessment of organic brain deficit in elderly patients. *Journal of the American Geriatric Society, 23*, 433–441.

Roberts, A. (1989). Sexuality in later life. *Nursing Times, 85*(24), 65–68.

Yesavage, J. A., Brink, T. L., Rose, T. L., Lum, O., Huang, V., Adey, M., & Leirer, V. O. (1983). Development and validation of a geriatric depression screening scale: A preliminary report. *Journal of Psychiatric Research, 17*, 37–49.

Zarit, S., & Zarit, J. (1983). *Working with families of dementia victims: A treatment manual.* Los Angeles, CA: Andrew Older Adult Center.

Zung, W. (1965). A self-rating depression scale. *Archives of General Psychiatry, 12*, 63–70.

Resources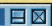

Sigma Theta Tau International Honor Society of Nursing: **www:nursingsociety.org**

Geriatrics: **www.geri.com**

AJN, American Journal of Nursing: **www.nursingcenter.com**

CHAPTER 14

Major Diseases: An Overview

Carol A. Stephenson, EdD, RN, C, CRNH

COMPETENCIES

After completing this chapter, the reader should be able to:

- *Relate cardiovascular risk factors to older adults.*
- *Discuss older adult-specific signs, symptoms, and nursing manage-ment of the following conditions: hypertension, congestive heart fail-ure, cerebral vascular accident, obstructive airway diseases, Parkinson's disease, cancer, pneumonia, urinary tract infections, sex-ually transmitted diseases, and Lyme disease.*
- *Discuss a variety of specific interventions, observations, and cautions related to medications commonly used by older adults.*
- *Discuss the impact of common diseases on older adults.*
- *Identify interactions between common comorbidities in older adults.*
- *Evaluate safety needs of older adults with selected conditions and drug therapy.*
- *Discuss selected issues with relation to morbidity and mortality in older adults.*

MAKING THE CONNECTION

Refer to the following chapters to increase your understanding of major diseases affecting older adults:

- **Chapter 5** *Biological and Physiological Aspects of Aging*
- **Chapter 11** *Wellness and Health Promotion*
- **Chapter 15** *Acute Care Issues*
- **Chapter 16** *Chronic Illness*

General Indicators of Disease in Older Adults

The rapidly rising numbers of older adults are contributing to increasing numbers of people with health problems and to increasing economic costs of diseases in that age group. This chapter will highlight some of the major physical health problems of older adults: cardiovascular (CV) disease, pulmonary disease, cancer, Parkinson's disease (PD), and some of the infectious diseases. The risk factors for disease in older adults are the same as those for disease in anyone of any age. However, older adults are often at higher risk related to the same risk factors or have higher rates of severity and mortality. In general, given any condition, older adults who have a specific disease will not fare as well as younger adults. This is coupled with the fact that older adults are more likely to have one or more coexisting conditions, may have a less healthy lifestyle, and often have less economic ability to cope with major illness.

It is important to consider health long before one becomes an older adult: Build a healthy **lifestyle**, correct **risk factors** and potential problems, strive for adequate financial status and health care funding, and build a personal network of friends and relatives.

When older adults become ill, their symptoms are often less specific to the body system that is involved than is true in younger adults. As a result, the health care provider must be alert to subtle or nonspecific condition changes and seek the cause. For example, urinary incontinence is a nonspecific finding that may occur at the onset of many pathological conditions in older adults, whether or not the pathology is related to the urinary system. A decreased level of consciousness is another common, nonspecific finding of disease in older adults. A sudden change in level of consciousness should not automatically be assumed to be the result of neurological pathology. Older adults may not have fevers in situations where this finding would ordinarily be expected. The usual body temperature of older adults is often less than 98°F, so a temperature of 99°F or 99.5°F may be regarded as a fever for them. Other atypical findings in older adults are described throughout this chapter.

Research Focus

Citation:
Lantz, P. M., House, J. S., Lepkowski, J. M., Williams, D. R., Mero, R. P., & Chen, J. (1998). Socioeconomic factors, health behaviors, and mortality. *Journal of the American Medical Association, 279*(21), 1703–1708.

Purpose:
This study was designed to test the widely held assumption that the elevated risk for disease and death in the poor is related to lower levels of education and income and behaviors that put their health at risk.

Methods:
The behavioral risk factors of cigarette smoking, drinking alcohol, sedentary lifestyle, and obesity were studied in relation to socioeconomic factors and morbidity rates in 3,617 adult men and women over a period of 7.5 years.

Findings:
The study found a strong correlation between income and educational levels. More important, even considering all related factors, the risk of dying was significantly elevated for the lowest income group.

Implications:
The researchers concluded that even if risky behaviors or lifestyle were changed, the very poor would still be at a higher risk of dying than those who are not poor.

Cardiovascular Diseases in Older Adults

Cardiovascular diseases are currently the leading overall cause of death in the United States, although their rank varies by age. Although the percentage of deaths from CV disease as opposed to total deaths from all causes has declined about 28% since 1985 [see American Heart Association (AHA) web site], the increasing numbers of aging persons will continue to result in rising numbers and economic costs of CV disease (Halm, 1997). Cardiovascular disease can be quite severe in older adults. About 85% of all CV deaths occur in those age 65 years or older. In 1995, about 56% of **coronary artery bypass graft (CABG)** procedures, 48% of **percutaneous transluminal coronary angioplasties) (PTCAs)**, and 59% of heart transplants were performed on persons age 65 years or older (AHA Website).

Nonmodifiable Risk Factors for Cardiovascular Disease

It has long been known that many lifestyle factors contribute to disease morbidity and mortality, in addition to **nonmodifiable risk factors** such as age, race, gender, and ethnicity. In addition, without significant changes in the many factors related to poverty, the poor will continue to die at higher rates than others.

Age

Although CV disease can occur in any age group, the vast majority of cases occur in those who are age 65 or over, in which case it is the first ranked cause of death.

Gender

The gender differences in risk, symptoms, and treatment of CV disease between men and women have been largely overlooked. Prior to menopause, the CV risk of men is far higher than that of women. In women, CV disease generally occurs about 20 years behind men, unless women have diabetes mellitus or renal disease, which can cause CV disease at about the same age as men (Jadin & Margolis, 1998). After age 65, the incidence of coronary heart disease in women is about one in three, compared with one in eight for breast cancer, a number that has been far more widely publicized (Halm, 1997). Heart disease and stroke in women cause about 500,000 deaths per year, which far exceeds the combined total for breast, uterine, ovarian, and cervical cancers with obstetrical mortality rates also factored in. Women who smoke are five times more likely to have sudden cardiac death than those who do not (Halm, 1997).

In general, CV disease is more difficult to diagnose in women. Women's symptoms may be atypical, and some of the usual tests may be unreliable. The most reliable tests in women appear to be the resting electrocardiogram (EKG), thallium scan, resting echocardiogram, and cardiac catheterization (Halm, 1997).

Race and Ethnicity

Racial and ethnic differences related to CV diseases, while publicized more than gender differences, have generally been underappreciated. All types of CV disease occur at a higher rate in blacks than nonblacks and the conditions are more severe. For example, black women have a 33% higher heart disease rate than white women. They have a heart attack death rate twice that of white women and three times that of women of other races (Halm, 1997).

Modifiable Risk Factors

Tobacco Use

One of the most important lifestyle causes of morbidity and mortality is the use of all kinds of tobacco. Tobacco is the most important contributor to CV disease. Stopping smoking is the one most important thing that anyone, including older adults, can do to promote optimal health. Studies show that women who currently smoke more than 24 cigarettes a day have 10 times the CV risk of nonsmoking women. However, this risk declines rapidly when women stop smoking. Within 3–4 years, CV disease risk is at the same level as for women who have never smoked (Halm, 1997). Smoking cessation may also help to slow the risk of osteoporosis and fractures (Lueckenotte, 1996).

Elevated Cholesterol and Triglycerides

Elevated cholesterol and triglycerides have been recognized for many years as major risk factors for CV disease. Three major studies, the Framingham Heart Study, the Pooling project, and another study done in Israel all showed that cholesterol levels over 200 mg/100 ml were associated with increased coronary risk. Above 200 mg/100 ml, coronary risk essentially doubled for every 50 mg/100 ml increase in cholesterol level (Ernst, Mullis, Sootey-Bochenek, & Van Horn, 1988; Frick et al., 1987; Kris-Etherton et al., 1988; Lueckenotte, 1996; Murray, Kurth, Mullis, & Jeffery, 1990). Triglycerides are the most common type of fat in the body. High triglycerides often accompany high total cholesterol and **LDL (low-density lipoprotein)** levels. **High-density lipoprotein (HDL)**, known as the good cholesterol, helps to transport lipids away from the arteries, preventing lipid accumulation within the arterial walls. High triglyceride levels are an associated risk for CV disease, perhaps more for women than for men (AHA web site). Although the association between cholesterol and triglyceride levels and coronary risk is less well defined in older adults than those who are younger, a low-fat diet continues to be a good health practice. However, it is more critical to ensure that the older adult has a balanced and adequately nutritious diet than to limit fat (Lueckenotte, 1996).

Diabetes

Diabetes is an associated risk factor in that it alters the metabolism and levels of cholesterol and triglycerides in the body. More than 80% of diabetics die of heart or blood vessel disease. Type II diabetes affects more women than men after age 45, partly because there are many more older women than men. Compared to nondiabetics of the same age, diabetics have twice the risk of heart attack and a much higher risk of stroke. The risk of a second heart attack is much higher in diabetic women than men, although it has not yet discovered why this is so (AHA web site). It is critical that diabetics not smoke. Smoking drastically increases the risk of CV disease in diabetics. When diabetics stop smoking, the risk of coronary artery disease drops quickly in only 2–3 years, reaching the baseline for diabetics in 10 years. Cutting down to even a few cigarettes per day, however, results in a continued high CV risk (Kawachi et al., 1994).

Sedentary Lifestyle

Older adults are not the only age group who may have a sedentary lifestyle. However, older adults are more at risk for the hazards of immobility and the development of disease because of lack of exercise. Overall, studies have shown that CV disease is nearly twice as likely to develop in sedentary people than in those who continue to be active (AHA Web site). Even moderate exercise levels have been shown to be associated with a reduced risk of CV disease and death. Lack of activity has been clearly identified as dangerous for health. Older adults may have difficulty exercising because of pain and reduced joint function from arthritis or other musculoskeletal problems, decreased coordination and muscle function, and limitations from such problems as dyspnea, reduced cardiac output, angina, adverse effects from drugs, and intermittent claudication (poor blood supply to the leg muscles) (Lueckenotte, 1996). Diabetics may have reduced mobility caused by peripheral neuropathy and inability to feel their feet, peripheral vascular disease, or reduced vision.

Nursing Tip

Exercise for Cardiopulmonary Clients
Many cardiopulmonary clients are extremely sedentary, which increases their debilitation. One of the most important therapies for them is exercise, beginning very gradually at the level of their current activity.
Why exercise? Exercise . . .
- Strengthens the heart
- Normalizes blood pressure
- Improves deep breathing
- Is an outlet for stress and tension
- Reduces bone demineralization and osteoporosis
- Improves mobility
- Improves outlook on life
- Aids in weight loss
- Reduces CV disease risk
- Reduces cardiopulmonary work load
- Improves muscle conditioning
- Reduces the amount of oxygen needed for any activity

Adapted from "Exercise: Wellness Maintenance for the Elderly Client," by E. J. Forbes, 1992, Holistic Nursing Practice, *6(2), pp. 14–22.*

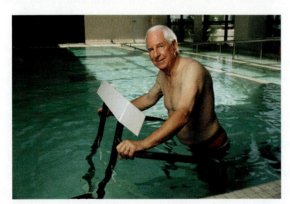

FIGURE 14-1 Using an underwater treadmill is a safe and effective workout for an older adult.

It is never too late to start an exercise program. This process should be done very gradually with the advice of a physician, nurse practitioner, exercise physiologist, or other appropriate health care provider. The goal is moderate levels of aerobic activity: continuous, rhythmic activity at least three times weekly for a minimum of 15–30 minutes at a time. The exercise should be one that is safe and enjoyable for the older adult. The program should include realistic goals. There should be a slow increase in activity levels and adequate warm-up and cool-down periods (Forbes, 1992). The exercise should be safe and noninjurious to joints, which excludes activities such as jogging for most older adults or bending exercises such as touching the toes, which could pull muscles or dislocate the hip joints. Walking is an excellent activity for older adults, as is swimming and cycling if balance or danger of falls is not a problem (see Figure 14-1). Strategies such as exercising with a friend, group exercise such as low-impact aerobics, line dancing, and the like can encourage staying with the exercise program. High-intensity, competitive activities and isometrics such as weight lifting not only do not build cardiopulmonary fitness but also may be hazardous. Isometrics, in particular, tend to raise blood pressure and generally should be avoided.

It is critical that older adults strive for achievable goals during exercise. If they overexercise to the point where they need one or more days to recover, they have jeopardized their exercise program and potentially reduced their fitness level. Sometimes, cardiopulmonary patients complain that they cannot exercise because they become dyspneic. They should be taught that everyone becomes somewhat dyspneic on exercise. **Dyspnea** should not be cause for concern, but rather for consultation with the health care professional as to what level is acceptable and how to manage it. The dyspnea should not become so severe that the older adult cannot recover from it relatively quickly. Older adults should be taught to monitor their pulse and stop to rest when the **target pulse rate** is exceeded; pulmonary patients can be taught to rest when dyspneic and to use **pursed-lip breathing** in order to maintain breathing control during exercise. Often, exercise programs are carried out in a supervised setting, with or without EKG and oxygen saturation level monitoring.

Obesity

Many studies confirm that obesity is a risk factor for CV disease, diabetes, and degenerative joint disease (osteoarthritis). The criteria for obesity are changing, however. Guidelines for weight-to-height ratio are generally being revised downward from those that have been long-standing. The reader is encouraged to consult a current chart for the most recent guidelines. While older adults should be encouraged to maintain a healthy weight, they should avoid dieting to the point of becoming malnourished.

Stress

The role of stress in CV disease and in the tendency to use other unhealthy lifestyle behaviors has not been clearly defined, although research is underway. It is postulated that responses to stress vary between individuals: Many are at higher CV risk because of stress. Older adults may have high stress levels caused by a variety of factors: loss of job, lifestyle, home, friends, roles, or pets, economic stressors, and many other factors. Any program or support system that reduces stress can promote a better outlook on life and potentially reduce problematic lifestyle behaviors and disease risks.

Estrogen Loss

After menopause, the risks of heart attack and stroke rise. Until recently, the studies of CV disease risk as related to estrogen have included few women over 65 (Lueckenotte, 1996) and have been limited to healthy women. As a result of the findings of these studies, the American Heart Association guidelines related to hormone replacement therapy (HRT) recommended that women who take estrogen after menopause may reduce their heart attack risk, although the stroke risk relationship was less consistent. This recommendation is currently controversial as a result of the Heart and Estrogen/Progestin Replacement Study (HERS) which was conducted over a 4-year period and published in 1998 (Hulley et al., 1998). The study involved 2,700 women from 44 to 79 with a mean age of 66.7 years. All of the women had a positive CV history. The results of the study were neutral, producing no data that HRT does or does not prevent heart and CV disease. The study also found that the risk of cardiac incidents was increased in the first year of the study; some reviewers have speculated this was because of starting the HRT when the client was unstable, but this is not a proven fact. In contrast, the cardiac risk was lower in the last 2 years of the study. Additionally, the study found that the risk of deep vein thrombosis (DVT) was increased in participants who took HRT. As a result, more studies are recommended. The impact of this study does not include other known facts regarding HRT. For example, HRT reduces the risk of osteoporosis and fractures and may reduce the risk of **Alzheimer's disease**. Although HRT does increase the risk of breast, endometrial, and uterine cancer, the risk of heart and CV disease is far higher. The result is that women and their health care providers should jointly decide if HRT is appropriate therapy for them (AHA Web site).

Selected Cardiovascular Diseases in Older Adults

Cardiovascular diseases that are prevalent in older adults include, but are not limited, to coronary artery disease, CAD, [angina, myocardial infarct (MI)], hypertension (HTN), congestive heart failure (CHF), peripheral vascular disease (PVD), and cerebral vascular accident/ stroke (CVA).

Hypertension

Hypertension fits into a unique category: It can result from the risk factors and lifestyle behaviors mentioned previously. It, in turn, becomes a serious risk factor for many types of CV and renal diseases. Therefore, the prevention and treatment of HTN in older adults is critical to continued good health and function. Hypertension, which has been labeled a **silent killer**, is so-called because at least one-third of people with it do not know that they have it. Of those who are aware, at least half are not on therapy while about 27% more are on inadequate therapy (AHA Web site), possibly because of cost of the medication or undesired side effects. Only one in four hypertensive persons has their blood pressure under control (Hurley, 1998). Although the percentage death rate for HTN is stable, the actual number of deaths is rising because of the higher number of persons at risk. In 1995, HTN killed nearly 40,000 people and contributed to the deaths of nearly 200,000 more (AHA Web site). It is estimated that about half of the 65-and-older population is hypertensive (Lueckenotte, 1996). More than 60% of women age 65 and older are hypertensive; over 75, women are far more likely than men to be hypertensive (AHA Web site)

The Framingham Heart Study found that systolic blood pressure was superior to either diastolic or **mean arterial pressure (MAP)** as a predictor of coronary heart disease in people over 45. Hypertensive persons had twice the risk of death not only from coronary heart disease, but from other diseases as well. Hypertensives had a sevenfold increase in strokes. Among the 159,000 subjects in the study, the death rate for treated hypertensives was 7.7% compared to a rate of 17.6% for untreated hypertensive persons (Kannam & Levy, 1993).

There are occasions when hypertension may be overestimated because the blood vessels in older adults may become rigid, which gives a blood pressure reading higher than it actually is. This is because the blood pressure cuff cannot compress the vessel. This phenomenon, **pseudohypertension**, can be identified by the fact that the radial pulse fails to disappear when the blood pressure cuff is inflated to high levels.

As previously described, the risk factors for hypertension are the same as those for other CV diseases. The combination of diabetes and smoking is more dangerous than either factor alone because smoking reduces blood flow and increases the likelihood of atherosclerosis (ADA, 1999). Therefore, the 1997 Hypertension Guidelines include risk factor identification as critical decision-making data for hypertension treatment. The guidelines define hypertension as a blood pressure 140/90 or above measured on three separate readings. It is critical that older adults undergo regular blood pressure screening and, if they are hypertensive, that they follow the directions of their physicians.

Hypertension treatment guidelines vary somewhat. Regardless, treatment of hypertension has been shown to reduce morbidity and mortality in all ages, genders, and races (Kannam & Levy, 1993). Risk stratification is often used to make decisions regarding treatment for hypertension. In clients with low CV risk factors, even a blood pressure as high as 160/100 mm Hg may be treated with lifestyle modifications alone. In contrast, in clients at high risk, such as those with diabetes, antihypertensive drug therapy may be recommended even when the blood pressure is ≤140/90 mm Hg. The treatment target is a blood pressure of ≤130/85 mm Hg (Kaplan, 1998).

The current guidelines for staging and treating hypertension are listed in Table 14-1. Treatment of hypertension is generally started with diet and lifestyle modification and once-daily dosing of drugs if needed using a gradual approach. Drugs are increased very gradually until optimal control is attained. In general, first-line therapy consists of diuretics and beta blockers. Angiotensin-converting enzymes (ACE inhibitors), calcium antagonists, alpha blockers, and alpha-beta blockers are used for first-line therapy only when the diuretics and beta blockers are contraindicated.

Problems with Antihypertensive Drugs

Many adverse effects can result from antihypertensive therapy. Older adults who are beginning therapy should be warned that adverse effects may occur and be urged to consult their physician or gerontological nurse practitioner for a modification of therapy when the adverse effects are not tolerable or acceptable. It is important to start antihypertensive therapy very slowly and with careful monitoring in older adults because there is great danger of lowering the blood pressure so quickly that symptoms such as dizziness, weakness, falling, and impotence can be induced. Long-acting drugs should be used in order to enhance compliance with once-daily dosing and reduce early morning surges of blood pressure with resulting catastrophic events. Therapy can also be enhanced by combining drugs from different classes to keep doses and adverse effects low (Kaplan, 1998).

Beta blockers have been proven to reduce the rate of complications in hypertensive clients. They may reduce the risk of a second heart attack and may decrease the frequency of migraine headaches or angina (Kuncl & Nelson, 1997). Despite this effectiveness, beta blockers can cause problems. While they lower heart rate, which is helpful, the lower rates can be problematic, especially in those with preexisting heart failure. Lowering the rate and contractile force can relieve angina but can hinder attempts to exercise since the heart rate will not increase to meet the increased metabolic need. Clients might complain of increased fatigue and shortness of breath when exercising. Nonselective beta blockers such as propranolol (Inderal) also affect the beta-2 receptors that cause bronchodilation. The result may be shortness of breath and bronchospasm (wheezing), especially if the patient has asthma or chronic obstructive pulmonary dis-

TABLE 14-1   Guidelines for Treatment of Hypertension

	Blood Pressure Stages		
Risk Group	**High–normal:** 130–139 85–89	**Stage 1:** 140–159 90–99	**Stages 2 and 3:** 160+ 100+
A. No risk factors	Lifestyle changes	Lifestyle changes for up to 12 months before treating	Drug therapy, lifestyle changes
B. At least one risk factor (e.g., smoking), but excluding diabetes, organ damage, or heart disease	Lifestyle changes	Lifestyle changes for up to 6 months; several risk factors may warrant drug therapy	Drug therapy, lifestyle changes
C. Organ damage or heart disease	Lifestyle changes; also drug therapy for clients with heart failure, renal insufficiency, or diabetes	Drug therapy, lifestyle changes	Drug therapy, lifestyle changes

Adapted from the Sixth Report of the Joint National Committee on Prevention, Detection, Evaluation, and Treatment of High Blood Pressure, *1997, Bethesda, MD: National Institutes of Health.*

ease (COPD). An alternative might be the administration of a cardioselective beta blocker, reducing the dose, or discontinuing the drug (Kuncl & Nelson, 1997). In asthmatics, beta blockers tend to increase bronchospasm. In addition, the beta₂ antagonist drugs (bronchodilators) interact adversely with the beta blockers. In diabetics, beta blockers can lengthen an episode of hypoglycemia or mask its signs. They also increase the risk of hypoglycemia (Kuncl & Nelson, 1997). Persons on beta blockers will not be able to raise the heart rate when needed, such as in the case of acute blood loss.

Diuretic administration reduces blood pressure and cardiac workload but can also reduce potassium levels. It is essential to monitor and replace potassium as needed. Usually, added dietary potassium is insufficient for this purpose; supplements must be administered.

Angiotensin-converting enzyme inhibitors may help control renal hypertension and decrease the risk of kidney failure in clients with proteinuria. They can reduce the complications that are associated with heart failure in diabetics or reduce risk of heart failure after MI. However, they can also cause a cough that may be mistaken for asthma. The cough should subside if the ACE inhibitor is discontinued. The ACE inhibitors can also elevate serum creatinine potassium if the client has decreased renal function. These levels should be monitored and the drug discontinued if necessary (Kuncl & Nelson, 1997).

Many antihypertensive agents can cause constipation: a frequent cause is the calcium antagonist verapamil (Calan). Diltiazem (Cardizem) causes it less frequently. The constipation should be managed with the usual measures: fiber, fluids, and activity. Other symptoms that may result from verapamil and diltiazem include pedal edema and headache. Calcium antagonists reduce heart rate, which can precipitate heart failure, but clients with atrial fibrillation or supraventricular tachycardia (SVT) can benefit from the reduced rate. Those with angina benefit from the resulting improved cardiac blood flow and reduced workload (Kuncl & Nelson, 1997)

Alpha-adrenergic blockers such as terazosin (Hytrin) may be used to manage hypertension, but they may cause dizziness and weakness, especially with the first dose. Therefore, it is helpful to administer the first dose at bedtime (Kuncl & Nelson, 1997).

Treatment guidelines emphasize four conditions in which more vigorous, specific drug therapy is indicated as first-line therapy to prevent life-threatening complications. These include the following: diabetes with **proteinuria**, myocardial infarct, heart failure, and **isolated systolic hypertension** in older adults. Isolated systolic hypertension, in which systolic blood pressure rises disproportionately to diastolic pressure, is the most common type of hypertension in older adults. Although there is no consensus of what numbers constitute iso-

lated systolic hypertension, it is generally assumed to involve a systolic blood pressure over 160 mm Hg with a diastolic blood pressure of less than 90. Isolated systolic hypertension may be underrecognized and undertreated because of the common focus on diastolic rather than systolic blood pressure numbers. Studies have shown that those with isolated systolic hypertension have an increased incidence of **left ventricular hypertrophy (LVF)**, or congestive heart failure.

Lifestyle modification includes weight loss for the obese, regular aerobic exercise, maintenance of adequate calcium, potassium, and magnesium levels, and reducing sodium intake to 2–4 g/day. The **DASH (dietary approaches to stop hypertension) diet** is low in saturated and total fat and rich in fruits, vegetables, and low-fat dairy foods (Appel et al., 1997). This diet has been found effective not only for hypertensive persons and those at CV risk, but for everyone. Older adults should stop smoking and limit alcohol intake to one glass of wine or beer per day.

Congestive Heart Failure

Congestive heart failure is the single most frequent cause of hospitalization for those age 65 and older. Four and seven-tenths (4.7) million people in the United States have CHF, with about 400,000 new cases each year (Kellerman, 1990). Both the incidence and prevalence of CHF increase with age. Its presentation and outcome are often influenced by the presence of comorbidity. About 80% of all clients with CHF are age 65 and older.

The term congestive heart failure may be used to refer to left ventricular failure or right ventricular failure (RVF). The pathology in most older adults is left ventricular dysfunction. Right ventricular failure may result from LVF (fluid backs up through the lungs, overwhelms the right ventricle, and causes it to fail.) Once congestive heart failure develops, the 6-year mortality rate approaches 80% in men and 65% in women (Kannel, 1989). A variety of factors can precipitate CHF, the most common of which are MI and CAD (Freed & Grines, 1994). Other causes of CHF include valvular dysfunction, arrhythmias, infections, MI, rheumatic heart disease, hyperthyroidism, anemia, excess salt and fluid intake, steroid administration, and stopping medications related to the heart (Cheitlin, 1999). The focus of this discussion is the care and maintenance of older adults with chronic CHF. It is critical to maintain these clients at the highest possible level of wellness and avoid the development of frank failure, pulmonary edema, or cardiogenic shock.

The major cause of transition from chronic failure to acute failure and/or **pulmonary edema** in the older adult is often infection, **exacerbation** of other **comorbidities**, surgery, trauma, or other severe stress.

The classic clinical presentation of CHF is the insidious development of shortness of breath, which is often exertional at first and then progresses to dypsnea at rest, **orthopnea**, and **paroxysmal nocturnal dyspnea (PND)** or dyspnea when lying down, which is relieved by sitting up (see Figure 14-2). Chronic nonproductive cough may be another finding, along with fatigue, weakness, memory loss, confusion, diaphoresis, tachycardia, palpitations, anorexia, and insomnia (Mancia, 1990). Many older adults may not develop dyspnea on exertion during acute episodes of CHF because their normal lifestyle may habitually include little or no exertion. They may complain of chest pain or tightness, fatigue, general weakness, a nonproductive cough, insomnia, and other vague symptoms. Their orthopnea may be hidden by the fact that they usually sleep in a chair or with the head and chest elevated because of **gastroesophageal reflux disease (GERD)**, COPD, or obesity. The usual **crackles** resulting from the client's COPD may mask those that develop caused by CHF. The pedal edema or weight gain of CHF may be masked by the client's level of **cor pulmonale** (right-sided heart failure caused by COPD) or the effects of drugs such as steroids. The **hemodynamic** abnormalities of CHF may also be masked by the body's adaptive changes to CHF.

When the client develops right-sided heart failure, the result may be weight gain, pedal edema, possible liver enlargement and abdominal distention, gastric distress, or anorexia and nausea (Mancia, 1990).

The usual cornerstones of treatment for chronic CHF are weight loss for obese clients, sodium restriction, alternating periods of activity and rest with avoidance of activity levels that exacerbate symptoms, and appropriate drug therapy. Although intense physical exercise should be avoided, moderate exercise to tolerance should be encouraged. Too much activity restriction can result in severe muscle and cardiac deconditioning, which can cause the older adult to become a **cardiac cripple**, that is, severely disabled and unable to tolerate normal levels of activity because of severe deconditioning. Clients should alternate aerobic activity and rest and avoid isometric exercises such as push-ups or weightlifting because these raise the cardiac workload (Figure 14-3).

Drug therapy for chronic CHF usually includes a combination of ACE inhibitors, digoxin, and diuretics. An anticoagulant, warfarin (Coumadin) is added if there is a history of thrombi or emboli. At times, vasodilators (nitrates) are also necessary (Freed & Grines, 1994). Angiotensin-converting enzyme inhibitors reduce mortality and symptoms and improve exercise tolerance, but they must be used cautiously in clients with an elevated serum creatinine clearance or renal impairment. In these clients, any condition that depletes intravascular volume, such as diarrhea, high-dose diuresis, or marked sodium or water restriction can exacerbate renal insufficiency or increase its risk as a result of ACE inhibitor therapy (Weinberg, 1993). If ACE inhibitors are not tolerated, then isosorbide and hydralazine may be used instead.

Diuretics are often used for CHF clients; however, it is critical to restrict sodium intake to ≤2 g/day rather than attempting to treat edema with diuretic therapy alone. In this way, it may be possible to reduce diuretic doses. Potassium supplements are used along with the diuretics as needed. However, **hyperkalemia** should be avoided. Dangerous hyperkalemia may occur if ACE inhibitors are used with potassium-sparing diuretics or large doses of potassium supplements, so potassium-sparing diuretics are avoided and the older adult is monitored carefully. In general, nonsteroidal anti-inflammatory drugs (NSAIDs) interact with potassium-sparing diuretics and can result in hyperkalemia and hypernatremia in the client with

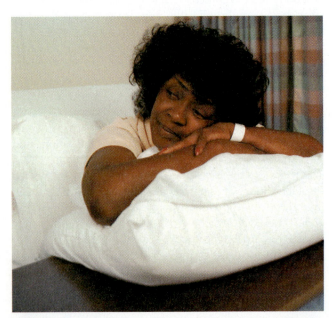

FIGURE 14-2 The orthopneic position shown here aids ventilation for the client with CHF.

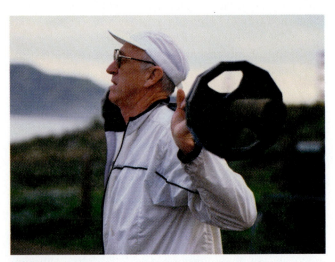

FIGURE 14-3 The client with CHF should avoid isometric exercise such as weightlifting because it increases the cardiac workload.

severe heart disease. As a result, NSAIDs should be avoided in these clients (Williams, et al., 1995). Digoxin remains controversial for clients on ACE inhibitors who are in sinus rhythm, but it is commonly used. Clients who are stable on digoxin may deteriorate if it is withdrawn (Williams et al., 1995).

Other drugs used for CHF depend on symptoms and on the mechanism of failure (systolic or diastolic). Beta blockers are commonly used. However, beta blockers can be problematic for older adults, as previously discussed.

When an older adult with chronic CHF develops mild to moderate symptoms of **decompensation**, the treatment is often the administration of intravenous diuretics and optimization of the client's long-term treatment for CHF. If there are no complicating factors, such as a recent MI or concurrent threatening conditions such as symptomatic **arrhythmias** or marked **hypokalemia**, the client may be treated or observed for several hours in the emergency department or outpatient facility and then sent home. Moderate to severe symptoms usually require hospital admission (Sonneblick & LeJemtel, 1993).

Angina and Myocardial Infarction: Mens' Diseases?

Women may have any of the various types of angina as a first manifestation of coronary heart disease. Often, women's pain is somewhere other than the chest: the arm, neck, jaw, or back. Women's pain is often less likely to be taken seriously (see Figure 14-4). Women tend to

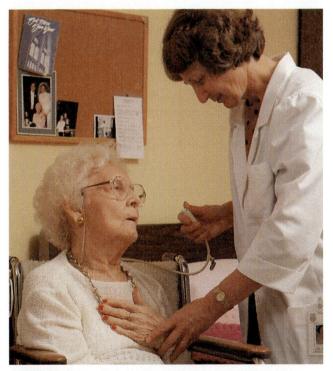

FIGURE 14-4   Never discount a female client's complaint of arm, neck, jaw, or back pain. Know all the signs and symptoms that can lead to a heart attack.

remain on medical management without extensive diagnostic testing or surgical intervention longer than men. This may be because both clients and their physicians view heart disease as a man's disease. Other reasons may be the atypical presentation or that women might delay seeking treatment longer than do men (Halm, 1997).

Regardless of sex, the pain and dysrhythmias of MI may be more serious in older adults than in younger persons due to older adults' poor tolerance of reduced cardiac output. Additionally, older adults may not display the so-called *normal* presentation of MI: crushing, radiating chest pain, gray or cyanotic skin, diaphoresis, severe anxiety, nausea and vomiting, and hiccough. In older adults, there may be no symptoms of MI (silent

Think About It

Mrs. S. is an 85-year-old woman who has had several MIs over the past 5 years. A retired bank vice-president, she lives with her 67-year-old niece, who also has serious CV disease, in a one-story house, which she owns in a family neighborhood. Her only other relatives are the niece's two adopted daughters, both in their early 20s, who live about 1,500 miles away and are unavailable except for an occasional telephone call.

Mrs. S. is nearly 6 feet tall but weighs less than 100 pounds. She does cook at least one balanced meal of meat, potatoes, and vegetables daily, although the amounts of each food she eats are small. Otherwise, she snacks occasionally during the day. She does not like the foods her niece cooks. She and her niece both describe her as much less flexible than she used to be and "very set in her ways."

Mrs. S. is up and about in the house and occasionally goes to church or the store with her niece driving. Otherwise, her outings are restricted to visits to the physician. She has given up golf and volunteer work, in which she was very active. She has weekly hired help for housekeeping and yard work. A lifelong heavy smoker, she is still smoking and considers this practice essential to her state of mind. Her husband died many years ago. Her longtime male friend died about two years ago.

Two weeks ago, after attending a funeral, she collapsed with crushing chest pain and was rushed to the hospital by the paramedics. An MI was confirmed, but after 2 days of rest and medication adjustment, she was sent home because she was not felt to be a candidate for any surgical intervention, including a percutaneous coronary angioplasty (PTCA). After she was hospitalized, she told her niece that she had experienced severe anginal pain for 2 days prior to the funeral. She was taking her sublingual nitroglycerin during this time.

What nursing problems can be identified here? What outcomes would be realistic for her? What interventions, teaching, and support might be appropriate to assist this woman?

heart attack); older adults may not experience chest pain but instead may complain about any combination of pain in the back, shoulder, jaw, or abdomen, diminished level of consciousness or acute confusion, nausea and vomiting, hiccoughs, **hypotension**, dizziness or **syncope**, acute confusion, **transient ischemic attack (TIA)**, CVA, weakness, fatigue, falls, restlessness, or incontinence.

Cerebral Vascular Accident

Stroke is the leading cause of serious long-term disability in the United States, accounting for about half of all neurological diagnoses. The risk of stroke more than doubles for each decade after age 55. About 75% of new strokes and 88% of stroke deaths occur in those age 65 and older. About one-third of all initial stroke clients die within a year, with the percentage being higher in older adults. About two-thirds of surviving stroke clients die within 12 years poststroke, although women tend to outlive men (AHA Web site).

The risk factors for stroke are the same as those for other CV diseases. The incidence of occurrence and death are higher for blacks than for white persons. There are three types of stroke: hemorrhage, usually caused by hypertension, emboli from distant areas, such as the heart or carotid artery, and plaque actually forming in the cerebral vasculature.

Many persons have "little strokes" or warning strokes called transient ischemic attacks for up to 2 years prior to a major stroke. Symptoms of TIAs are the same as those of stroke, but they last only 20 minutes to 24 hours. When a person has a TIA, it is critical to seek a cause and treat it if possible to prevent a major stroke. This may include measures such as carotid **endarterectomy** (cleaning plaque from the carotid artery), which will enhance blood flow to the brain and reduce the chance of emboli breaking off from the plaque and moving to the cerebral vasculature. Auscultating the carotid arteries for **bruits** (the sound of turbulent blood flow) enables the nurse to refer the client for treatment prior to the occurrence of a TIA or a stroke. Preventive measures for strokes caused by both plaque and emboli include anticoagulants, such as one aspirin per day, ticlopidine (Ticlid), or warfarin (Coumadin), and management of hypertension.

Symptoms

The symptoms of stroke vary widely; sometimes a stroke may progress for as much as a week. The classic symptoms include sudden weakness or numbness in the face, leg, or arm on one side of the body, a sudden dimness or visual loss in one eye, difficulty in speaking or understanding, a sudden, extremely severe headache, unexplained dizziness, unsteadiness, or falling, or a lowered level of consciousness.

First Aid for Stroke

Time is critical in the treatment of a stroke, yet the delay in presenting at the emergency department (ED) may be up to 24 hours (Whitney, 1994). The client who may be having a stroke needs to go to the ED as quickly as possible. Treatment decisions must be made quickly. While waiting for an ambulance, the client should be turned on the side and a clear airway maintained, tight clothing loosened, and reassurance given.

Treatment of Stroke

At the hospital, a patent airway is maintained and oxygen is administered. Vital signs and neurological signs are monitored often. Diagnostic tests may include a **lumbar puncture** to detect blood in the spinal fluid, a sign that the stroke is caused by hemorrhage. Other diagnostic studies might include a **computed tomography (CT) scan**, or **carotid** or **cerebral angiography**. If a stroke due to clot or thrombus has occurred within 3 hours prior to treatment, and the client has no contraindications, **tissue plasminogen activator (tPA)**, a clot-dissolving drug, may be administered. The tPA has the potential to dissolve the clot that caused the stroke and potentially quickly restore cerebral blood flow. After the tPA, the client is started on intravenous heparin and other treatment is administered according to the client's symptoms (Apple, 1996).

Nursing Care of the Client with Stroke

In general, the nursing care plan for a stroke client is developed according to the individual client's condition and needs. Some common problems are communication, urinary incontinence, and the behavioral manifestations of strokes of various locations. Clients with strokes may have no communication alterations (rare), problems with understanding (**receptive aphasia**), problems with speaking and communicating (**expressive aphasia**), or problems with both speaking and understanding (**global aphasia**). If the client cannot speak intelligible syllables, understanding can be checked by ability to follow simple commands. If the client can speak, cognitive ability can be assessed by requesting a count of a few simple objects placed on the overbed table. The nurse should not ask the client to count to 10 or say the alphabet, because those can be done automatically, without active thought processes. When speaking to the stroke client, the nurse should use short sentences, express one thought at a time, and give the client time to respond (Figure 14-5). Client education may be limited because of functional disabilities.

Urinary incontinence is often a rationale for the insertion of an indwelling catheter. This procedure, however, is a nearly guaranteed method of acquiring a urinary tract infection. Instead, the nurse could initiate a record of voiding times for 24 hours and then plan to

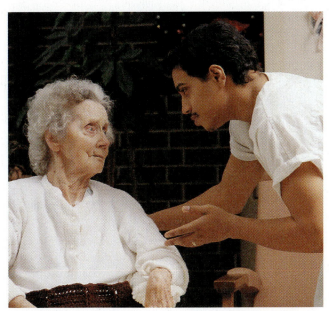

FIGURE 14-5 When speaking to a client who has had a stroke, speak slowly, in short sentences, and give the client time to respond.

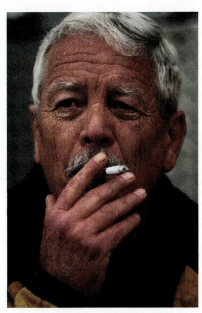

FIGURE 14-6 A direct link has been established between older adults who continue to smoke and COPD mortality.

offer the opportunity to void about 30 minutes prior to usual voiding times if the client is able to void at all.

The behavioral manifestations of stroke vary somewhat by whether the lesion is on the right or the left side of the brain. Those with left-sided lesions tend to be cautious, plodding, and very careful. They often need some encouragement to cooperate with rehabilitation activities. Those with right-sided lesions, on the other hand, tend to be impulsive, with poor judgment, and need supervision to prevent injury (Ignatavlcius, Workman, & Mishler, 1999). Emotional lability is also a common behavioral manifestation of stroke. The long-term consequences of stroke vary widely; usually the lives of the older adult and his or her family is changed forever as a result of the stroke.

Obstructive Airway Diseases

Although there are many obstructive airway diseases, the three major ones that affect older adults are chronic bronchitis and emphysema, which are generally grouped together under the heading of COPD, chronic obstructive pulmonary disease, or COLD, chronic obstructive lung disease, and asthma. Chronic bronchitis, which is caused by airway inflammation, involves airway mucosa edema and copious sputum production, with a tendency to airway closure on expiration. Emphysema is damage to the alveolar structures, causing them to enlarge and be damaged, resulting in reduction of the alveolar-capillary diffusion interface and airway closure caused by the loss of support for the airway structures.

Scope of the Problem

Although COPD can be the result of other factors or combinations, such as air pollution, smoking continues to be the most important cause. While there is no specific number of cigarettes at which COPD occurs, it is known that small airway changes begin early, perhaps at about a 20-pack-year history (packs per day times years smoked). Persons who have COPD tend to ignore their symptoms for a long time, which means that clients may be admitted to the hospital, treated for other problems, or go to surgery without a clear diagnosis of COPD, even though it is present. As a result, they may develop unforeseen pulmonary problems along with whatever treatment is being given. It is critical to elicit a history of smoking or prolonged exposure to second-hand smoke and history of COPD symptoms whenever health professionals are caring for a client. When a COPD diagnosis or risk is recognized, appropriate pulmonary hygiene may be utilized prior to surgery, or appropriate pulmonary treatment provided along with treatment of the presenting problem. In this way, pulmonary complications may be minimized or avoided.

Obstructive airway diseases are ranked as the fourth leading cause of death in the United States. Unlike CV disease, whose percentage rate is declining, the mortality rate for COPD continues to rise steeply, with the rates for women rising considerably more than for men. The rise in COPD mortality is especially striking among older people who continue to smoke (Speizer, 1989). See Figure 14-6.

Although smoking does not cause it, asthma is a common comorbidity and must also be recognized and treated appropriately. Asthma is a reversible or potentially reversible expiratory airway obstruction, with exacerbations and remissions, which is characterized by bronchospasm, mucosa edema, and copious sputum production by the airway mucosa. This process results in air trapping, diaphragmatic flattening, wheezing, and severe respiratory distress. Asthma is on the rise, with incidence and mortality increasing yearly in all age groups. Older adults can and do have asthma, some longstanding from their youth, and some having developed it as adults (Lueckenotte, 1996). In older adults, the clinical course of asthma tends to be more severe; complete remission of symptoms is rare (Bramann, 1993). The rate of asthma deaths is climbing in all age groups. Most asthmatics who die are over 50 years of age (Friebele, 1996). Urban residence and minority status are critical risk factors, although the asthmatic is at risk for dying. As with other diseases, poverty seems to be a more important risk factor than race or residence. The highest numbers of asthma deaths in the United States occur in poor, urban areas (Lantz, et al., 1998).

Comparing and Staging Obstructive Airway Diseases

The three major obstructive airway diseases have many commonalities and even overlapping of pathologies, although their etiologies and treatment are different. Those who have COPD often have a combination of emphysema and chronic bronchitis, although one or the other may predominate. Many develop a combination of chronic bronchitis and asthma, which is referred to as asthmatic bronchitis. In most people, the basis of asthma is now thought to be a major allergic or inflammatory reaction, although this is less likely to be true of older adults, especially if the asthma is of new onset.

It can be difficult to distinguish between diagnoses of COPD and asthma because the features of the diseases are not as clear-cut in a particular individual as they seem to be in the texts. Commonly believed to have little or no reversibility with drug therapy, COPD may often look a lot like asthma, which is commonly believed to have a great deal of reversibility with treatment. Often, COPD may include a significant reversible component while clients with asthma may go on to develop irreversible airflow obstruction indistinguishable from COPD (Celli et al., 1995). Age-related changes in the respiratory system and smoking history can also blur the diagnosis. Both COPD and asthma can exist on any of several levels, from mild and clearly episodic to chronic, with constant or nearly constant symptoms, though exacerbations may make symptoms much more severe. The diagnosis should include a detailed history as well as pulmonary function testing and possibly testing for an allergic component (Brown, Evans, &

Ferdman, 1997). Standard allergy testing is of little value in older adults because their skin sensitivity is poor related to airway reactivity. Neither is desensitization therapy particularly helpful for most older adults. One important method of determining an allergic basis for adult asthma and differentiating it from COPD as a diagnosis is a very detailed history. A laboratory finding of serum eosinophilia can further validate allergies but may be absent in older adults because of reduced immune responses or steroid therapy.

Problems That Can Complicate the Diagnosis

It is not uncommon for other pathologies to be mistaken for COPD or asthma. One important condition in older adults is chronic aspiration, which may be the result of GERD, in which the person chronically aspirates gastric acid. Chronic aspiration may also be related to neurological deficits: impaired cognitive status or level of consciousness, impaired swallowing ability or reflexes due to conditions such as strokes (CVA) or chronic neurological diseases such as Parkinson's disease. Referral to a **speech/language pathologist** for a swallowing evaluation and plan of treatment is essential for neurological clients; treatment of the GERD should be initiated when indicated.

Sometimes, a person has a long-term isolated wheeze in one area of the chest. This is not usually caused by asthma but may be related to foreign-body aspiration (foreign bodies may or may not be radio-opaque) or to obstruction or pressure on a bronchus or bronchiole from such pathology as tumors or **aneurysms**. Other occasional causes of wheezing include **pulmonary emboli**, respiratory infections, and the pulmonary edema of left ventricular cardiac failure. Asthma may be confused with CV disease when the client with left-sided heart failure develops nocturnal dyspnea or wheezing caused by wet lungs. One diagnostic clue is that distress caused by heart failure typically occurs an hour or two after going to bed, while asthmatics tend to worsen in the early morning hours (Brown et al. 1997). As previously mentioned, ACE inhibitors can cause a cough that can be confused with asthma.

Management of Obstructive Lung Diseases

Although specific interventions vary by disease, the goals of COPD and asthma therapy and management are similar (Box 14-1). Classification of severity, diagnosis, and treatment of COPD and asthma have changed a great deal in the 1990s. Many of the problems encountered and treatments used are similar for all of the obstructive airway diseases. The National Institutes of

Health, American Lung Association, and American Thoracic Society are excellent sources of information regarding current COPD and asthma treatment.

Drug Therapy for Obstructive Airway Diseases

The drugs that are used for asthma and COPD are similar, even though they are used according to different guidelines. The mainstay drugs of asthma are now considered to be steroids, with bronchodilators as back-up drugs, while, in contrast, the mainstay drugs for COPD are bronchodilators, with steroids used only for exacerbations or ongoing problems that cannot be adequately managed without steroids.

Steroids are the drugs of choice for the management of asthma. Although inhaled steroids are commonly believed to be safe, it is now known that both inhaled and oral steroids can lead to skin thinning, easy bruising, and adrenal suppression in older adults. Because the oral drugs (prednisone, prednisolone) are more prone than the inhaled drugs to cause these problems, the focus of long-term management is on inhaled steroids as much as possible. Another reason to avoid the oral drugs is that the systemic steroids are cleared more slowly from the bodies of older adults than they are in younger people. Other problems with long-term steroid use are reduction of bone density, which worsens osteoporosis, increased difficulty in regulating blood sugar, a predisposition to developing cataracts, and a much higher risk of gastrointestinal bleeding.

A commonly used category of bronchodilators is the beta agonists. These are especially problematic in older adults because those who are on beta blockers for CV disease or glaucoma are placed at a higher risk for arrhythmias and hypertension. The use of beta blockers, as previously mentioned, should be avoided in clients with asthma or COPD because they can cause bronchospasm. The beta agonists also have potential interactions with antidepressants, especially the tricyclics, and some of the anti-Parkinson drugs.

Theophyllines, another common bronchodilator class, can be problematic for older adults. Many practitioners are now avoiding these drugs or using them only in very small doses for older adults. Theophylline is poorly cleared from the bloodstream of older adults, so toxicity is a constant hazard. They may develop signs of toxicity long before they reach the top of the stated theophylline therapeutic level range of 10–20 μg level. Extreme nervousness and arrhythmias also are common theophylline-induced problems.

Anticholinergics may be used to reduce bronchospasm and decrease mucus production. However, they should be avoided if glaucoma or benign prostatic hyperplasia (BPH) are present, as they can exacerbate both of these conditions. Anticholinergics are contraindi-

---

BOX 14-1 Goals for the Management of Obstructive Lung Diseases

- Optimal ventilation and secretion clearance.

- Optimal pharmacotherapy with minimal adverse effects.

- Prevention of chronic troublesome symptoms, symptom progression, recurrent exacerbation, and complications; minimal ED visits and hospitalizations.

- Maximal quality of life: maximal comfort, maximal ability to participate in normal activities and ADL, positive outlook on life.

- The client and family have an adequate knowledge base and are able to participate in self-management and self-monitoring.

- The client and family expectations of care are met.

---

cated in clients who are taking antidepressants or who have seizure disorders or diabetes mellitus.

Combination drugs for pulmonary symptoms should be avoided in pulmonary clients. Many of these combinations include drugs that have serious adverse effects and which then require more drugs to counteract those adverse effects. Ephedrine is one of the most serious offenders in the combination drugs, causing both cardiac stimulation and worsening BPH. Over-the-counter bronchodilators should also be avoided. Most of these are either adrenalin alone or in combination, which, while they do provide quick, short-term ventilatory relief, also cause dangerous stimulation of the heart.

Clients who have asthma and COPD should avoid antihistamines, which dry secretions and make clearing the chest difficult. In addition, the nonsedating antihistamines, if combined with diuretics or B₂ agonists, can cause arrhythmias or hypertension. Clients who have pulmonary diseases should generally avoid sedatives, which can depress respiratory drive and cause hypoventilation. Cough suppressants are often avoided as they can impair the ability to clear one's airway. However, in situations of severe, nonproductive cough, measures to suppress cough can greatly aid client comfort and improve sleep. There are exceptions to these rules, in which certain selected medications can safely be used to aid sleep and in terminal situations, in which opioids have been proven safe and effective to reduce terminal dyspnea and respiratory distress. These should be administered only by those who are experienced in their use.

Antibiotics are indicated for pulmonary clients who have documented respiratory infections. For all older adults with obstructive airway disease, respiratory infection is an especially important precipitator of crises and should be avoided. Older adults should receive influenza vaccine yearly. Pneumococcal vaccine should be administered every 5–7 years for older adults aged 60–75, and every 3–4 years if >age 75 (Lueckenotte, 1996).

Besides drug management, the management of obstructive lung diseases focuses on maintaining optimum health (exercise, nutrition, rest, stopping smoking), avoiding activities or settings that exacerbate symptoms, monitoring one's own condition, and early awareness of and treatment for condition changes and problems. Along with drugs, other measures such as oxygen therapy may be used. Oxygen therapy is generally indicated for a po_2 of <55 mm Hg or a **pulse oximetry** reading of <85 mm. Pulmonary rehabilitation programs are an effective method of improving general health and ventilatory status. Older adults should be encouraged to participate in them.

Drug administration and self-monitoring may be problematic for older adults. Common problems in older adults can include arthritis and/or impaired strength and coordination, which may affect their ability to use metered-dose inhalers (MDIs) or peak flowmeters, which are commonly used by asthmatics to monitor ventilatory status. A spacer can be added to the MDI or a nebulizer may be used to reduce the amount of coordination needed for drug delivery. Some clients never learn to use peak flowmeters effectively and must be taught to carefully monitor symptoms instead as a method of recognizing changing ventilatory status. Some key indicators of changing status are listed in Box 14-2.

Parkinson's Disease

Although Parkinson's disease (PD) can occur at any age, the vast majority of cases occur after age 60. With about 50,000 cases being newly diagnosed each year, the number of older adults with PD remains at about 1% of the population (Goldsmith, 1998; Hopfenspenger & Koller, 1991). At any time, more than one million Americans have PD—more than the total who have multiple sclerosis, muscular dystrophy, and amyotrophic lateral sclerosis (ALS) combined. Anyone is at risk, but PD affects males more than females and whites more than those who are black or Asian. For the population as a whole, the incidence of PD is about 100/100,000, or 1 in 1,000 persons. However, after age 65, the incidence is 1,000–2,000/100,000, or 1–2 in 100 persons (Rakel, 1997). Besides being debilitating and progressive and shortening life, PD is expensive. It is estimated that PD costs the nation about $5.6 billion annually. Of that, the medication cost alone for each client is about $2,500/year.

Although the causes of PD have not been clearly identified, there are several theories. A genetic component recently has been identified by research, although the magnitude is yet to be determined. Other causes that have been implicated include environmental toxins, poisons, viruses, and medications. Drug-induced PD is usually reversible when the cause is removed. Some drugs that have been implicated as potential causes of PD symptoms include prolonged use of the following: tranquilizers such as chlorpromazine (Thorazine) and haloperidol (Haldol), the antihypertensives reserpine

---

BOX 14-2   Monitoring Pulmonary Status

1. Use the peak flowmeter daily (especially for asthma). Follow an established plan for the results:

   - Good ≥80% personal best. No intervention needed.

   - Moderate impairment: 51%–79% personal best. Implement predetermined action plan.

   - Severe impairment: ≤50% personal best. Call physician. Get treatment immediately.

2. The following symptoms indicate worsening of pulmonary status and are reasons to notify the health care provider:

   - Early morning or nocturnal wakening with wheezing, coughing, shortness of breath

   - Increased orthopnea, cough

   - Increased use of bronchodilator inhalers

   - Biweekly weight check shows gain of >3 pounds

   - Development of or increase in dependent edema

   - Change in color, amount, consistency of sputum

   - Less able to eat and drink

   - Reduced level of consciousness or increased irritability and uncooperativeness

   - Development of fever or chills

   - Reduced exercise and activity tolerance— unable to tolerate the same amount of exercise

   - Increased dyspnea

(Serpasil) and methyldopa (Aldomet), and the GI stimulant metachlorpramide (Reglan).

Diagnosing Parkinson's Disease

There are no specific diagnostic tests for PD. Instead, the physician must observe the often vague and variable client symptoms and then rule out other causes of those symptoms in order to diagnose PD. The disease is one of slow, insidious onset; about 70%–80% of the dopamine-producing neurons in the brain are destroyed by the time symptoms are obvious. As a result, the diagnosis may be missed for a long time or an inaccurate diagnosis may be made. Often, the diagnosis is confirmed by observing the client's response to levodopa (L-dopa), the most common drug therapy for the disease. If the client does not respond to L-dopa, another cause for the symptoms should be sought (Lang & Lozano, 1998).

Pathology

Although the pathology of PD is complex, it can be briefly summarized as resulting from the death of dopamine-producing neurons in the brain. Dopamine is a critical chemical messenger that controls body movement and balance. In the brain, it exists in balance with another chemical transmitter, acetylcholine, which is not destroyed by the disease, so as dopamine decreases, the balance is not maintained and acetylcholine dominates, which aggravates the disease symptoms. There are enzymes in the brain that break down dopamine and further reduce the supply. It is theorized that the breakdown of dopamine by these enzymes releases free radicals which are highly toxic to nerve cells and which can further reduce the dopamine supply. Drug therapy is directed at any or all of these processes.

Signs and Symptoms

There are four major or classic symptoms of PD. However, the range is wide and symptom combinations are extremely variable. The classic symptoms include the following:

- *Tremor.* Surprisingly, **tremor** is absent in up to 25% of PD clients. When present, it predominates in the hands and arms but may also occur in the feet and legs. Tremors commonly occur at rest, when stressed, or when the arms are stretched in front of the body and disappear during sleep or activity; are often unilateral or asymmetrical; and include pill rolling motions. A few clients exhibit tremors on activity rather than rest; these are less likely to respond to the current PD drugs (Varon & Jacobs, 1990).

- *Muscle rigidity and weakness.* Increased muscle weakness and rigidity are present when the limbs are still and are thought to be caused by the constant tension of opposing muscle groups. This is different from the spasticity that can follow paralysis. Early symptoms of rigidity include jerky, cogwheel movements. As the disease progresses, the client may develop a masklike face and dysphagia. Loss of eyelid control can result in inability to blink or even to open the eyes or keep them open. The voice often becomes a soft, difficult-to-understand monotone. In the late stages, chest muscle rigidity can reduce the ability to breathe and cough (Varon & Jacobs, 1990).

- *Bradykinesia.* This problem can be quite disabling. **Bradykinesia** is manifested as slow movement and a delay in starting movement (impaired ability to initiate or modify a movement once begun). As a result, it may take hours to do physical activities of daily living (PADL) such as bathing, dressing, and eating. The client may take tiny, fast steps (fenestation) and be unable to stop walking (Varon & Jacobs, 1990).

- *Postural instability.* The client has impaired balance and coordination, develops a shuffling gait, and leans backward or forward when walking (see Figure 14-7). The combination of motion disorders can cause the client to freeze during

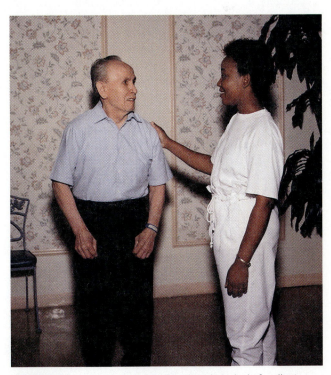

FIGURE 14-7 This man's stooped posture is typical of a client with PD.

motion or fall if bumped (Goldsmith, 1998). Eventually, the client may lose the ability to ambulate (Varon & Jacobs, 1990).

The secondary symptoms of PD appear in many combinations and cause a variety of client care problems. They may include cognitive and emotional problems (depression, memory loss, slow thinking, and emotional instability, although intelligence is unimpaired); dementia of varying severity in some clients—a problem that can occur in addition to Alzheimer's disease (AD) or can be mistaken for AD when AD is not present; sleep abnormalities; **autonomic dysfunction** (constipation, excess salivation and consequent drooling, and **orthostatic hypotension**, oily skin and scalp); and *sexual dysfunction* (impotence or loss of interest) (Varon & Jacobs, 1990).

Treatment

Treatment for PD includes symptomatic care, health promotion, drug therapy, and sometimes surgery. Often, drugs are not begun until symptoms interfere with ADL because many of the drugs tend to lose their effectiveness over time. There can also be great fluctuations in symptoms throughout a single day. Both because of this phenomenon and the commonality of adverse effects, drug doses are kept as low as possible. Table 14-2 summarizes the major drugs for PD, their actions, and drug information that is particularly related to older adults.

Surgery is usually reserved for clients whose disease has progressed to later stages, although the surgeries available and indications for use are changing rapidly. Currently, the surgeries which are available are the **thalamotomy** (destruction of part of the thalamus) and the **pallidotomy**, which is performed on the globus pallidus, or motor communications center of the brain. The symptom relief provided by the surgeries may not be long-lasting but may last 2 or more years. Brain pacemaker-type implants are being researched and will probably soon be available. The electrical pulsations block the malfunctioning brain signals that cause the tremors. Its settings can be adjusted with a magnet.

Comorbidities and Cautions

Clients who have PD are not immune from the comorbidities common to older adults. Many conditions and their treatments can cause significant problems if health care providers are unaware of them or their interactions with the Parkinson's drugs. These conditions include the following:

- *Glaucoma.* **Glaucoma** can be exacerbated by the use of anticholinergic drugs. It is not essential to discontinue the anticholinergics if they are

relieving Parkinson's symptoms, but the client should be closely monitored by an opthalmologist. L-Dopa and Sinemet also cause serious problems for glaucoma clients and should be avoided (Aminoff, 1997).

- *Hypertension.* Rarely, antihypertensive drugs may worsen PD symptoms. Clonidine (Catapres) can do this, but the effects will be relieved when the Catapres is tapered and discontinued. Another antihypertensive agent, Aldomet, may compete with carbidopa (in Sinemet) for the enzyme that changes L-dopa into dopamine. This problem can decrease the beneficial effects of Sinemet. Although Aldomet need not be discontinued in PD clients, health care providers should be aware of potential drug interactions. Diuretics, which are often used for the treatment of hypertension, can decrease the amount of fluid in the body and worsen the body dryness resulting from PD and its drug therapy, as well as worsen postural hypotension and increase the risk of dizziness, syncope, and falls. This effect can be a particular problem in those who take Sinemet. Other antihypertensives that may interact with PD drugs include reserpine (Serpasil) and rauwolfia (Raudixin).

- *Gastrointestinal disorders.* Parkinson's disease has a direct effect on the GI tract: Swallowing is difficult and prolonged, the stomach takes longer to empty, and food passes through the intestinal tract more slowly. Although no direct effects of Sinemet and the dopamine agonists have been proven, there have been some reports of bleeding ulcers. These drugs can also relax the cardiac sphincter of the stomach, resulting in gastroesophageal reflux, which can cause discomfort, esophageal inflammation, and even aspiration of stomach contents. This condition can be accompanied by nausea and vomiting, which is a common adverse effect of many PD drugs, further increasing the risk of aspiration. The reflux situation is even more problematic in clients who have hiatal hernia. They may require antacids, elevation of the head of the bed, and other measures to prevent aspiration. Those who have a history of liver disease are at particular risk when taking PD drugs and should have their liver function monitored periodically. Antiemetics and GI stimulants that may interact with PD drugs include prochlorperazine (Compazine), metoclopramide (Reglan), and thiethylperazine (Torecan).

- *Use of antidepressants and antipsychotics.* Depression is often an important symptom in PD clients and should be treated when necessary. In

TABLE 14-2 Overview of Drug Therapy for Parkinson's Disease

Drug	Major Action	Comments, Special Information for Older Adults
Primary Drugs: Assist with Production, Release, or Prolongation of Dopamine Action		
Levo-dopa (L-dopa)	Provides raw material to be converted to dopamine.	Extremely variable blood levels, symptom relief. Avoid in those with glaucoma, melanoma, hypertension, heart disease, or taking certain antipsychotic drugs (Aminoff, 1997).
Sinemet, Atamet Madopar, CD/LD (combinations of L-dopa and carbidopa)	More effective than L-dopa alone but does not slow neuron loss.	Over time, action is less predictable; larger doses are needed.
Deprenyl, Eldepryl seligiline	Block the enzymes responsible for the chemical breakdown of dopamine so it remains in the brain longer. May slow neuron destruction and death.	Concurrent use with Sinemet allows lower doses and fewer adverse effects of Sinemet as well as significantly improved functional ability (Brunt, 1994). May be used alone early in the disease to slow its progress.
Tolcapone (Tasmar)	Blocks a major enzyme that breaks down L-dopa.	When given with Sinemet, smoother and more sustained levels of L-dopa are available to the brain (Center Watch, 1998).
Bromocriptone (Parlodel), pergolide (Permax), ropinirole (Requip), pramipexole (Mirapex), Lisuril	Dopamine agonists (mimic effect of dopamine).	Effectiveness does not decrease as the number of neurons decrease. Requip and Mirapex have lower side-effect profiles.
Amantadine (Symmetrel)	Increases amount of dopamine released with each nerve impulse. May also block acetylcholine.	Can be a first-line medication. Less effective over time in some clients. Improves all symptoms.
Secondary Drugs: Anticholinergic; Block Influence of Acetylcholine		
Trihexyphenidyl (Artane), Akineone, benztropine, Pagitate	Improve symptoms in spite of reduced available dopamine.	Artane reduces rigidity but has little effect on tremors. Cogentin can reduce tremors and rigidity, increase mobility.

fact, the treatment of depression may lessen the PD symptoms. However, the health care provider should be aware of potential interactions when using the following antidepressants: amoxapine (Asendin), phenelzine (Nardil), and tranylcypromine (Parnate, Triavil). The following antipsychotics might cause interactions: haloperidol (Haldol), loxapine (Loxitane), thioridazine (Mellaril, which may be used in low dosages), molindone (Moban), thiothixene (Navane), pimozide (Orap), fluphenazine (Prolixin, Permitil), mesoridazine (Serentil), trifluoper-

azine (Stelazine), chlorprothixene (Taractan, Thorazine), acetophenazine (Tindal), perphenazine (Trilafon), and triflupromazine (Vesprin). The tricyclic antidepressants Elavil and Tofranil are safe for use with PD clients (Bonander, 1995).

- *Bladder conditions.* The anticholinergic Symmetrel and some of the antidepressants used for PD clients may cause an inability to void. This problem is especially true in those who have BPH. The clients should be monitored and the drugs used very carefully.

- *Orthopedic problems.* Clients with PD are at high risk for falls. Many older adults have concurrent osteoporosis and are at special risk of fracture if they fall. If a PD client with severe tremors or dyskinesias needs treatment for a fracture, these symptoms must be relieved to treat the fracture.

- *Cancer.* There have been some reports in which the use of L-dopa has been associated with the growth or exacerbation of melanoma. This may be caused by the fact that L-dopa participates in melanin formation. Although this relationship is not proven, and there are reports of melanoma clients taking L-dopa with no exacerbation, it is important to use a great deal of caution. If the client's PD worsens to the point where it is a much more serious problem than melanoma, then the drugs should be used cautiously and with careful monitoring.

CLINICAL ALERT

It is critical that PD clients who are to undergo surgery inform the anesthesiologist, the surgeon, and the neurologist so that potential interactions between PD drugs and anesthetics and narcotics can be avoided. Fatal interactions have occurred, particularly with the commonly used narcotic analgesic meperidine (Demerol) (Bonander, 1995).

Think About It

Mr. Jenson is a 70-year-old man who has advanced PD. He and his wife live in a spacious home on a busy street in a developing neighborhood, so there are no sidewalks. Over the past 2 years, the disease has progressed. Mr. Jenson has severe dementia. He sleeps extremely poorly, often wandering at night. He has been found in the street by the police several times. During the day, he has a paid caregiver, who assists Mrs. Jenson with his personal care and feeding. He sits on the couch most of the time but can walk to the table or bathroom when encouraged and assisted to do so. He does not interact verbally. He is occasionally combative. The house is designed with a bedroom at the back of the house that opens onto a screened porch. The porch also opens into the living room. There is a large fenced back yard. Mrs. Jenson wants to keep him at home but is exhausted from being up all night to keep him safe.

What suggestions can be given to Mrs. Jenson to attempt to keep Mr. Jenson safe and allow her to get some sleep? What other interventions would be appropriate for this couple?

Nursing Care

There are a number of common nursing problems for clients with PD. Some of these are discussed in Table 14-3. Along with these specific client problems are the problems of coping and caregiving. These must be evaluated on an individual basis and support provided as needed. Often, support groups can be extremely helpful as well as support and assistance with day-to-day care.

Cancer

Although cancer can and does occur in all age groups, over half of all malignancies in the United States occur in those age 65 and older, who, at present, constitute only about 13% of the population. The rate for cancer occurrence in those age 65–69 is approximately double that for those age 55–59. Age is also an important predictor of cancer stage; those of advanced age often have their cancers diagnosed at later stages than do younger persons. Therefore, the outcomes of cancer treatment appear to diminish as age increases (Ruger, 1997).

For all age groups, lung cancer is still the number-one cancer killer. For older men, the other major cancer killers in order are prostate, colon/rectum, and pancreas. The standard screening laboratory test for prostate cancer, the prostate-specific antigen (PSA), may not be helpful for older men, because it can also be elevated by the common condition BPH.

For older women, colon/rectum cancer is the highest killer, followed by cancers of the lung, breast, pancreas, and ovary. In older women, breast cancer has been related to estrogen deficiencies and imbalance. There may be other reasons for breast cancer to become advanced prior to detection; older adults may have visual, tactile, motor, and cognitive deficits that interfere with their ability to perform breast self-examination. Many avoid self-exam and mammograms because of attitudes that one does not touch oneself or expose one's breasts to others. This may be cultural or a holdover from the teachings of their mothers and grandmothers.

Differences between Older Adults and Younger Adults

Historically, older adults have not been targeted for educational programs regarding risk awareness or prevention, detection, and screening activities. There are many reasons for this. Only recently have third-party payers begun to pay for some of the necessary screening activities. Older adults tend to have more difficulty in attending cancer prevention, awareness, and screening activities because of lack of funds or transportation.

TABLE 14-3 Client Problems and Nursing Interventions for Parkinson's Disease

Problem	Related Causes	Suggested Interventions
Altered nutrition	Dysphagia, anorexia, nausea, vomiting, increased metabolic need, high risk for aspiration.	Eat small frequent meals. Balanced diet with adequate fiber, fluids, and calcium; liquid supplements, multivitamins, antioxidant vitamins (A, C, E) (Carter, 1992).
Altered fluid balance	Thirst diminished by aging, anti-Parkinson drugs; ability to ingest fluids diminished by dysphagia, motor abilities.	Make adequate fluid intake a priority. Schedule fluid intake.
Altered mobility	PD pathology; comorbidities.	Daily gentle exercise is extremely beneficial. Stretching, walking, swimming, formal programs are all good.
Potential for falls	Altered balance and mobility; postural hypotension.	Use safety aids such as canes and walkers as needed; change position slowly; keep environment clear of obstacles. Never carry objects in both hands.
Depression	More common in PD clients than others of same age group; sometimes drug induced.	Need care and medication program by component psychiatrist. Treatment of depression may reduce PD symptoms.
Dementia	Can be severe, associated with confusion, disorientation. PD drugs may be cause.	Care by qualified professional. Keep client safe and calm. Monitor. Adjust drug therapy as needed. See case study.
Sleep disturbances	Commonly have trouble falling asleep, staying asleep, leading to daytime exhaustion. They may reverse day and night sleeping patterns or have vivid dreams, nightmares, or talk in their sleep. They may have restless leg syndrome or difficulty changing position in bed.	Some are wakeful because of L-dopa; it makes others sleepy. Some need it at night so they are not too rigid to turn in bed. Time doses accordingly. Have a regular sleep-wake cycle. Avoid going to bed too early. Use standard relaxation and presleep routines. Hypnotic drugs may help but must be used with caution.
Impaired verbal communication	Caused by PD pathology. Intelligence unimpaired. Leads to frustration of both client and caregiver.	Seek new communication methods. Voice training, including singing, can be very helpful. A speech/language pathologist can assist. Take time to listen respectfully.
Dysphagia, drooling reflux	Caused by PD pathology. At risk for aspiration, weight loss.	Feed slowly and frequently; use easy-to-swallow foods, liquid supplements. Position upright for feeding. Provide tissues or other appropriate means to keep skin dry and appearance acceptable.
Constipation	Caused by PD pathology, reduced fiber and fluid intake, comorbidities, and drugs.	Monitor stools. Use standard methods to prevent and treat constipation.
Difficulty voiding	Caused by PD pathology, drugs, reduced mobility, and intake.	Monitor voiding patterns. Seek medical intervention as needed.
Pedal edema	PD pathology, drugs, benign prostatic hypertrophy. PD drugs, poor circulation.	Elevate legs when seated; do not cross legs; usual foot and leg care for those with poor circulation.

(continues)

TABLE 14-3   Client Problems and Nursing Interventions for Parkinson's Disease   *continued*

Problem	Related Causes	Suggested Interventions
Sexual dysfunction	PD pathology, loss of energy and mobility, loss of interest.	Plan intimacy for times of maximal energy, alter drug therapy when necessary and possible, and use alternate means for satisfaction.
Dyspnea, difficulty in breathing	Reduced chest wall strength and mobility.	Alternate exercise and rest; elevate head and chest when dypsneic; oxygen as needed; maximize fluid intake to thin secretions; influenza and pneumonia immunization; avoid respiratory infection.

Sensory and cognitive deficits may prevent them from understanding or utilizing the information that is given. Fatalistic attitudes that cancer treatment for older adults is hopeless also contribute to the problem.

Until recently, age was considered a major factor in treatment choices for cancer. A newer trend, however, considers physiological age and comorbidities when estimating the probability of success rather than utilizing chronological age alone as the determining factor in anticipating treatment success or failure. Older adults as a group tend not to be as assertive as younger adults in becoming informed once a cancer diagnosis is made. While younger persons may be searching the libraries and the Internet, older adults may be more likely to use their previous health care strategies, which is to do whatever the doctor says to do. As a result, they are less able to help decide what treatment would be best for them. Once treatment is begun, they may be less able to cope with multiple drug therapy routines and to tolerate the adverse effects of the cancer treatment.

Psychosocial Impact

The diagnosis of cancer in an older adult should be considered as much of a crisis as it is in a younger person. Although the older adult may appear more fatalistic, Houldin and Wasserbauer (1996) demonstrated that the older cancer clients reported feeling dependent, having problems with memory, and feeling out of control and helpless, upset, tense, and angry. They did not cope any better than younger persons and were just as much in need of spiritual and psychological assistance. Often, they lived far from family and had lost many friends so that they had less support systems to help them cope. Health care providers should be sensitive to these needs and seek to obtain or provide the support and encouragement that is needed for older adults to cope with a cancer diagnosis.

Infectious Diseases

Older adults can be predisposed to a variety of infectious diseases due to aging. Some of the most prevalent are pneumonia, urinary tract infection (UTI), sexually transmitted diseases, HIV/AIDS, and Lyme disease.

Pneumonia

Although it affects all age groups, pneumonia is a particular problem in older adults. Community-acquired pneumonia (CAP) is the leading cause of death from infectious disease and the overall sixth leading cause of death in the United States (Institute, 2000). Pneumonia is the second leading nosocomial infection in the United States in both hospitals and nursing homes, trailing only UTIs. Mortality is high, especially in older adults who have had surgery or mechanical ventilation (Mick, 1997). Its economic and social impact is substantial. Pneumonia rates will probably increase because of the growing numbers of older adults and those who are immunocompromised (Rubins & Janoff, 1997).

In general, aging tends to predispose older adults to pneumonia as the result of lowered immune status and less efficient ventilation, gas exchange, and airway clearance. In addition, the upper airways of older adults tend to be colonized with gram-negative bacilli that can cause pneumonia if they enter the lower respiratory tract (Caruthers, 1990). Those who are compromised by diseases such as COPD or CHF, who are malnourished, or who have a low albumin are at high risk for pneumonia. Other risk factors include exposure to children and those with influenza and infections; reflux, impaired swallowing, or tube feeding; immobility; atelectasis; lung cancer; collagen vascular disease; radiation therapy of the chest; or treatment with drugs such as methotrexate or amiodarone (Rubins & Janoff, 1997).

Older adults are at particular risk for delayed diagnosis and treatment of pneumonia, which in turn can lead to increased mortality. This is because pneumonia has a wide variety of presentations in older adults. Rather than the classic cluster of symptoms—cough, fever, and dyspnea, purulent sputum, and pleuritic chest pain—a high percentage of older adults have an atypical pneumonia presentation—confusion or delirium, altered functional abilities, and/or decompensation of underlying illnesses. One or more of the classic cluster is often present along with the atypical symptom or symptoms, but not in all cases. The most common of the classic symptoms to be present in all age groups is the pleuritic chest pain. Other common presenting symptoms of pneumonia in older adults may include falls, incontinence, failure to thrive, sepsis, tachypnea, tachycardia, or congestive heart failure (Mick, 1997). A 1997 study found that for a high percentage of older adults, the atypical presentation caused a diagnosis of pneumonia to be missed at the first clinic visit for the symptoms; for many, the diagnosis was delayed as long as 3 days (Riquelme et al., 1997).

The Riquelme study confirmed that delirium at the first clinic visit or admission was significantly more common for older adults with pneumonia than for the nonpneumonia control group. When an older adult presents with acute confusion or delirium, a careful history should be taken to differentiate it from other causes such as chronic dementia, depression, or psychosis. If the client has chronic confusion or dementia, pneumonia can cause deterioration of the baseline cognitive and functional status. As a result, standard diagnostic testing for all acutely confused older adults should include a chest x-ray and white blood count (Riquelme et al., 1997). However, the chest x-ray may not provide a definitive diagnosis in the early stages if the client is dehydrated. The infiltrates may not show up until the client is adequately rehydrated (Buehrens, 1995). Serologic testing and blood cultures are generally not recommended for outpatients with pneumonia (Institute, 2000).

Treatment of pneumonia is based on identification of the cause, which often includes more than one pathogen (Institute, 2000). There does not seem to be a relationship between the etiology and whether the client presents with typical or atypical symptoms (Riquelme et al., 1997). Although most clients who have pneumonia can be treated at home, it is important to identify those who are at high risk for complications or who should be hospitalized. A model for identifying whether the client has a high or low risk of serious complications has been developed. It assigns points for age, whether the person is institutionalized or not, symptoms, laboratory results, and the presence or absence of comorbidity. The points are then summed to establish a complication risk score, although clinical judgment must also be utilized in the decision-making process (Fine et al., 1997). A treatment algorithm has also been established and may be found at www.icsi.org (Institute, 2000).

In general, the treatment of pneumonia includes medicating for the causative organism or virus, proper diet, high fluid intake, acetaminophen or NSAIDs for discomfort, rest, and assisting the client to clear the chest if necessary utilizing such techniques as postural drainage and percussion. Clients who are being treated at home should be contacted in 24–48 hours to assess progress. The client should be monitored for signs of complications that require follow-up and/or further therapy: dyspnea, worsening cough, the onset or worsening of chills, fever occurring more than 48 hours after drug therapy is begun, or intolerance of the medications. Older adults' recovery period from pneumonia varies. In many cases, it is weeks before the client feels normal again. At 6–8 weeks, a follow-up chest x-ray should be obtained for anyone over 40 years old or who is a smoker. If the infiltrate has not resolved, cancer should be suspected (Institute, 2000).

Although an excellent fluid intake is necessary to thin secretions enough to clear them from the chest, caution should be the rule with older adults. It is possible to overhydrate the client enough to cause congestive heart failure. Cough suppressants are usually avoided unless they are needed to help promote sleep at night. Both cough suppressants and antihistamines can impair the individual's ability to clear the chest of the products of the pneumonia.

The prevention of pneumonia in older adults is essential. Those under 80 years of age should have the pneumonia vaccine once. After age 80, the vaccine should be repeated every 5–7 years (Mick, 1997), although the current Medicare policy is to pay for only one dose of pneumonia vaccine in a lifetime. Influenza vaccine should be administered yearly. Older adults should avoid persons with respiratory infections, practice excellent handwashing, and maintain optimal nutritional and health practices.

Urinary Tract Infection

Urinary tract infection is the most common cause of fever-producing illness in older adults (Duffield, 1997). However, not all **bacteriuria** equals a UTI. Bacteria in the urine is a common finding in older adults, especially the very old and those residing in institutions. More common in women than men at all ages, it is less common in community-dwelling older adults than in those who reside in institutions. Bacteriuria is usually asymptomatic and does not appear to cause renal damage or to affect long-term survival (Nicolle, 1993). Cranberry juice has been long used prophylactically. However, studies to support this practice are just now occurring. The use of cranberry juice has been supported, but the protective effects seem to take several weeks to occur (Avorn, Monane, Gurwitz, Glynn, Choodnovskly, & Lipsitz, 1994). One gram of vitamin C daily in four divided doses may be used instead.

When a symptomatic UTI does occur, the symptoms may not be those that are typical: urinary frequency, dysuria, suprapubic discomfort, fever, and/or costovertebral tenderness. An atypical presentation is common in older adults: any combination of confusion, delirium, apathy, nocturia, and incontinence (Haus, 1998; McCue, 1993).

Bacteriuria is always present in persons with long-term indwelling catheters (Gleckman, 1992). The annual cost of catheter-related UTIs is high, resulting in more than seven million physician visits and one million hospitalizations annually (Hardyck & Petrinovich, 1998).

When a UTI is suspected, collecting usable urine specimens from older adults is often problematic. If a clean catch midstream specimen is necessary, the client needs clear instructions and sometimes assistance. If the client is confined to the bed, the specimen collection is even more challenging. It is not recommended that men use pediatric collection bags because of the high contamination rate (Nicolle, 1993). Obtaining a catheterized specimen should be avoided if possible because of the high infection rate from any bladder instrumentation. If a catheter is already in place, the old one should be removed and a new one inserted to collect the specimen (Brechtelsbauer, 1992).

Even if sediment develops, routine cultures are not done on asymptomatic clients with indwelling catheters. All catheterized clients develop bacteriuria. Treatment is unnecessary unless a symptomatic UTI develops.

Regardless of whether the older adult has an indwelling catheter or not, treatment of UTIs should be instituted only if the client is symptomatic or is at risk for developing serious complications (Duffield, 1997; Nicolle, 1993). One indication for prophylactic treatment is anticipated urinary tract procedures. This is particularly important for diabetics, those who are immunocompromised, and those with new urinary incontinence (Melillo, 1995). To prevent medication-related complications, the treatment goal should be symptom relief, not total eradication of microorganisms (Nicolle, 1993).

Although current guidelines for treating uncomplicated symptomatic UTIs in younger adults is a short course of about 3 days of antibiotics, older adults are less likely to respond. They are commonly treated with 7–14 days of antibiotic therapy after verification of the UTI via urine culture.

Although indwelling catheters should be avoided if possible, long-term catheterization may be the only option for clients who have intractable incontinence or urinary retention. When this occurs, special care is necessary to prevent infections and complications. Some guidelines include:

- Use small silicone or silicone coated catheters to reduce irritation.

- Attach the tubing to the thigh or abdomen without tension and rotate the attachment site daily.

- Empty the drainage bag about three times daily.

- Make sure the urine flow is unobstructed and that the drainage bag remains below the bladder.

- If changing between a leg bag and a large bag, use sterile technique, cleanse the tubing ends with alcohol, and cover the end of the unused tubing.

- Reduce manipulation to a minimum.

- Encourage an oral intake of at least 2000 ml/day.

- To reduce sediment, use cranberry juice or vitamin C as described above. If sediment is a severe problem, irrigations with a solution of one part vinegar to four parts water may be necessary (Brechtelsbauer, 1992).

- Cleanse the perineum twice daily and apply an antibiotic ointment at the insertion site to improve comfort and reduce the chance of ascending infection. If infections are particularly chronic or troublesome, a suprapubic catheter may be considered (Reznicek, 2000).

- Change the catheter and drainage bag every 2 weeks (Stamm & Hooten, 1998). Consider using disposable drainage bags. Hardyck and Petrinovich (1998) conducted a study in which catheters were changed every 2 weeks and which compared the use of the usual drainable bags versus disposable nondrainable collecting bags that were changed once daily using sterile technique. The cost of treatment of clients with the nondrainable bags was half that of those using the more conventional bags.

Sexually Transmitted Diseases (STDs) and HIV/AIDS

Of the many negative myths regarding aging, none is more pervasive than that desirability, erotic capacity, and sexual worth peaked long ago and are now diminished (Billhorn, 1994). As a result, health care providers tend not to include sexual practices in their history taking or to consider the common STDs, HIV, or hepatitis in diagnosing problems of older adults. In fact, older adults still have sexual needs and drives (Figure 14-8). The most common reason for lack of sexual activity is

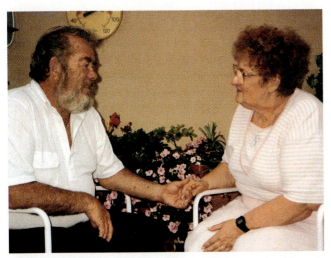

FIGURE 14-8 Because older adults still desire companionship and intimacy, it is very important that the health care provider include this information when taking a complete health history.

no acceptable partner. Because there are so many more older women than men and because men often prefer younger women, a higher percentage of older men continue to have sexual activity. This is heightened by the availability of Viagra. Men often have more than one sexual partner, including both older women and prostitutes. Because older adults no longer fear pregnancy and safe-sex education is lacking, the percentage of older adults who use condoms is low. The presence of sexual abuse, both in the community and in the institutionalized older adult, must also be considered in diagnosing and treating older adults (Letvak & Schoder, 1996). A STD may be present in an older adult who is no longer sexually active (Letvak & Schoder, 1996).

Health care providers must include a history of sexual practices in their screening of older adults. This may be a difficult discussion for the older adult, who has learned or has cultural biases against discussing such information. Some may be hesitant to verbalize their feelings for fear of being considered as lecherous or depraved (Billhorn, 1994). Privacy for the discussion and the establishment of a trusting relationship are essential. Respect for the older adult's sexual beliefs and practices should be communicated along with acknowledging the sensitive nature of the topic. The nurse should be attentive to nonverbal clues from the client during the discussion and proceed accordingly. Asking open-ended questions is more helpful than those that can be answered "yes" or "no." The history should include information regarding partners, practices, physical signs and symptoms, problems or satisfaction with sex life, and the use of protection and precautions (Letvak & Schoder, 1996). Education for both individuals and groups should include the hazards of STDs, HIV, and hepatitis, along with safe-sex practices and condom use.

In general, STDs are more easily transmitted from males to females than vice versa (Emmert & Kirchner, 2000; Letvak & Schoder, 1996). This is true in all age groups, but older women may experience vaginal dryness and have tissues that are more easily traumatized and broken, which increases their risk of disease transmission during sexual encounters (Wooten-Bielski, 1999). In addition, some older adults have STDs continuing from earlier years. Some examples include **genital herpes**, HIV, and hepatitis. Blood transfusion is the most common cause of HIV in older adults, but if the HIV was acquired recently, the most common cause is sexual activity (Letvak & Schoder, 1996).

Current statistics show that about 10% of HIV/AIDS cases occur in adults over 50 years of age. This number is probably low because of misdiagnosis and will continue to rise as the population of older adults rises (Wooten-Bielski, 1999). The number of cases of other STDs and hepatitis will also rise accordingly. In older adults, the symptoms of HIV may be confused with commonly perceived problems of aging: fatigue and decreased endurance or altered cognitive status. Some of the major manifestations of HIV/AIDS in older adults include *Pneumocystis carinii* pneumonia, herpes zoster, tuberculosis, cytomegalovirus, oral thrush, *Mycobacterium avium* complex, and HIV dementia. Women who are HIV positive are at high risk for cervical cancer. A common problem in HIV-positive older adults is that HIV dementia may develop more rapidly than in older adults who are not HIV positive. Because HIV is not suspected, the HIV dementia is often mistaken for AD or PD. In general, HIV dementia has a relatively sudden onset over a few months and may be accompanied by tremors, seizures, peripheral neuropathy, and/or ataxia. Occasionally, the dementia is the only presenting symptom of HIV in the older adult (Wooten-Bielski, 1999). Because HIV can be transmitted simultaneously with other STDs, the health care provider should encourage anyone who is diagnosed with an STD to be tested for HIV (Kirchner & Emmert, 2000).

With regard to STDs such as chlamydia, gonorrhea, syphilis, and other diseases, women often have few or no symptoms. As a result, the diagnosis is missed more often than in men, and female patients are more at risk for complications (Kirchner & Emmert, 2000). Gonorrhea is a common cause of pelvic inflammatory disease (PID), which may present with minimal symptoms. If the following are present with no other cause, PID should be considered in the woman of any age: adnexal tenderness, cervical motion tenderness, and lower abdominal tenderness. There may or may not be a cervical or vaginal discharge or fever (Emmert & Kirchner, 2000). The diagnosis of syphilis may also be complicated by the fact that there are many factors that can cause false positives on the serologic testing: advanced age, other bacterial infections, Lyme disease, chronic liver disease, malignances, and viral infections (Emmert & Kirchner, 2000).

The goals for treatment of STDs, HIV, and hepatitis are the same in older adults as they are for those of other age groups. Appropriate drug therapy is administered with care monitoring for adverse effects and interactions. Opportunistic infections and complications should be avoided as much as possible and treated when they occur (Wooten-Bielski, 1999). Follow-up testing should be done after the treatment of STDs along with the identification, testing, and treatment of sexual partners.

Lyme Disease

Lyme disease is now the most common tick-borne infection in the United States. It is caused by *Borrelia burgdorferi*, a spirochete, which the ticks acquire by feeding on small animals such as mice. The bite is usually painless and the tick eventually falls off, so most people are unaware of being bitten. Although children and adults under 50 years old are more likely to be exposed to and develop Lyme disease, those 70 and older have been shown to be in great danger of acquiring the disease and its complications. Although Lyme disease is most commonly acquired in rural coastal or wooded areas, it is not limited to them (Simon et al., 1999).

The symptoms of Lyme disease are diverse, which complicates the diagnosis. Some of the possible symptoms of early Lyme disease are a distinctive skin rash that burns rather than itches, followed days to weeks later by symptoms involving the joints, nervous system, or the heart. Expert opinions vary as to what percentage of clients develop the skin rash. If it occurs, it may be transient. It usually begins as a pimplelike spot that expands over a few days to a purple circle up to 6 inches in diameter and with a red rim. Sometimes, it becomes as large as 20 inches in diameter. The center of the rash may clear or turn bluish. Concentric rings may develop within the original ring, creating the impression of a bull's eye. A person may have more than one ring or may have a partial ring that looks more like an arc. The ring usually fades completely in about a month. The rash is often accompanied by flulike symptoms, muscle and joint aches, swollen glands, headache, nausea, vomiting, and/or sore throat. These symptoms may occur with or without the rash. Some clients develop Bell's palsy (facial paralysis). A year or more later, symptoms such as skin disorders, prolonged bouts of arthritis, and neurological problems may occur. Fatigue is a significant symptom in both early and late Lyme disease (Simon et al., 1999).

Prevention, early detection, and prompt treatment are critical to improve the prognosis for persons with exposure to Lyme disease. The longer the disease is present before treatment, the more persistent the symptoms will become. Protective, long-sleeved clothing should be worn when there is a possibility of tick exposure. The skin of both persons and pets should be inspected for ticks after being in tick-prone areas. If a tick is found, it should be carefully pulled out with tweezers, without crushing, twisting, or handling it with bare fingers. None of the folk methods of removal, such as matches, petroleum jelly, or nail polish should be used since this prolongs exposure and may cause the tick to eject more noxious substances into the skin. Clothing should be run through a dryer at high temperatures for 30 minutes, because washing does not kill ticks. Insect repellents should be used, but they do not confer predictable protection. There is a vaccine, but it is not very predictable (Simon et al., 1999).

Diagnosis of Lyme disease can be difficult if the symptoms are unclear. The diagnostic tests that are available are expensive and not very precise. False negatives and positives may be caused by a wide variety of factors. Commonly used antibody tests are the enzyme-linked immunosorbent assay (ELISA), indirect immunofluorescence assay (IFA), the PreVue Burgdorferi Antibody Detection Assay, and the polymerase chain reaction (PCR). If one of these is positive, it is followed by the Western blot test (Simon et al., 1999).

The treatment for Lyme disease usually consists of antibiotics such as doxycycline (Vibramycin), amoxicillin, or azithromycin (Zithromax) for a course of 21–30 days. A second course of antibiotics may be given if symptoms recur. If the disease is severe or widespread, intravenous antibiotics such as ceftriaxone or cefotaximine are given. Pain-relief medications may include acetaminophen or NSAIDs (Simon et al., 1999).

Summary

Older adults are more likely than other age groups to have serious chronic conditions. The possibilities are not limited to those listed in this chapter, although some of the more common cardiovascular, pulmonary, endocrine, neurological, and infectious conditions have been discussed. When managing any older adult with medication or other treatment, it is critical to consider the interactions of drugs for different pathologies and with the pathophysiology of unrelated conditions. Many older adults manage a high functional ability and quality of life even when chronic conditions are present. They should be supported toward this goal in any appropriate manner.

CARE PLAN

CASE STUDY

Mr. and Mrs. Zenkowski are in their late sixties. Mr. Zenkowski is a retired railroad worker. Mrs. Zenkowski is a retired elementary school teacher. They visit the senior center on Tuesdays and Thursdays for aerobic exercise classes and also to socialize with a group of friends. In addition, they participate in health screening and teaching sessions offered at the center. They have four grandchildren and are expecting one more. They also take advantage of discounted senior bus trips.

Recently, Mr. Z. has been diagnosed with hypertension and a hypothyroid condition. After four blood pressure readings of 160–172/85–95, Mr. Z.'s physician confirmed the diagnosis of hypertension (HTN) and prescribed a medication, dietary, and exercise regimen. He is on Vasotec (enalapril) and Synthroid (levothyroxine) along with a 1 gm. low-sodium diet. Mr. Z. enjoys cold cuts and salty foods, according to his wife. He says he "feels perfectly fine." In addition to exercising at the senior center, they take turns every other day walking their dog.

Mrs. Zenkowski has been recently diagnosed with osteoporosis, based on results from bone mineral density studies showing loss of bone mass (osteopenia). In addition, she is borderline overweight (>20% over ideal body weight) and admits she eats when under stress. She is on an adequate calcium supplement. Hormone replacement therapy (HRT) is under consideration. After the exercise class, Mrs. Z. sets up an appointment with the gerontological nurse practitioner, who has regular hours at the senior center for consultation on health-related issues. She privately tells the nurse she is concerned about her husband. He has been acting different and "snapping" at her since he has been diagnosed with HTN. She states that "he doesn't take his high blood pressure seriously enough." Mr. Z. is ambivalent about the meeting but goes along with his wife. The nurse finds out three important pieces of data: (1) Mr. Z. denies his illness and hates his diet, (2) the couple's sexual patterns have changed (decreased frequency), and (3) Mrs. Z. is afraid that her husband might have a stroke.

ASSESSMENT

It is not unusual that individuals first diagnosed with HTN are asymptomatic and thus "feel just fine." However, HTN is a precursor to stroke, which can cause devastating paralysis, aphasia, and cognitive deficits requiring months of rehabilitation, dramatic potential lifestyle changes, and undue financial burden on our health care system. Stroke is preventable. By controlling his HTN, Mr. Z. can reduce his risk of having a stroke. But without acceptance of his diagnosis of HTN, Mr. Z.'s adherence to a disease management program is unlikely. Mrs. Z. recognizes this and is very concerned, as evidenced by her initiating the meeting with the nurse. Her current level of stress over her husband's condition could prompt increased weight gain. Medication teaching and evaluation of progress are warranted. The decreased sexual activity may be caused by the anti-HTN medication. Three key nursing diagnoses have been selected for the care plan, although certainly not comprehensive of this situation.

NURSING DIAGNOSIS

Ineffective denial related to not perceiving personal relevance of symptoms or danger; unable to admit impact or the disease on life pattern.

Outcomes:

Mr. Z. will:

- *Verbalize feelings about his diagnosis.*
- *Comprehend facts about high blood pressure.*
- *List all aspects of his therapeutic regimen, including medications, side effects, diet, and exercise regimen.*
- *Continue with follow-up visits with his physician/gerontological nurse practitioner.*

(continues)

CARE PLAN *continued*

Planning/Interventions:

The nurse will:

- *Encourage verbalization of Mr. Z.'s feelings.*
- *Explain/clarify facts on high blood pressure.*
- *Review Mr. Z.'s plan of care: medications, diet, and exercise program.*
- *Encourage and support continued physician/nurse practitioner visits.*

EVALUATION:

Mr. Z. will accept his diagnosis of hypertension and understand facts of the disease and its prevention. He will express any fears, concerns, anger, and other feelings which may be associated with his perception of the disease. He will find value in follow-up physician/nurse practitioner visits.

In approaching individuals about preventive care, it is easy for clinicians to be paternalistic. Additionally, a nurse might unintentionally become threatening or punitive. This approach is unacceptable and usually ineffective in the long run, although some clients respond initially out of fear for their health.

NURSING DIAGNOSIS

Altered sexuality patterns related to changes in sexual behaviors/activities as expressed by Mrs. Z.

Outcomes:

Mr. and Mrs. Z. will:

- *Verbalize feelings of stress, tension, and concern to one another.*
- *Discuss with one another any changes in sexual behaviors that they have noticed.*
- *Discuss with physician/nurse practitioner possible alterations in Mr. Z.'s blood pressure medication.*
- *Examine the need for obtaining counseling.*

Planning/Interventions:

The nurse will:

- *Encourage Mrs. Z. to open up discussion with her husband about her concerns.*
- *Offer to facilitate subsequent discussions; assess sexual patterns and Mr. and Mrs. Z.'s perceived level of satisfaction.*
- *Encourage them to contact the physician/nurse practitioner regarding consideration of a medication change.*

EVALUATION:

Mr. and Mrs. Zenkowski will talk with one another about the change in sexual activity and behaviors. Anti-HTN medication will be scrutinized as a possible contributor along with Mr. Z.'s inner fears and concerns about his disease. Continued husband-wife interpersonal communication is essential, as opposed to avoidance, to promote quality of life.

NURSING DIAGNOSIS

Anxiety, as evidenced by expressed concerns related to change in health status of spouse.

Outcomes:

Mrs. Z. will:

- *Express her feelings about her husband's illness.*
- *Discuss her concerns directly with him.*

(continues)

CARE PLAN *continued*

- *Identify nonpharmacological methods of relaxation.*
- *Practice the selected relaxation method (i.e., meditation, prayer, exercise, deep breathing) at least twice daily for a 1-month trial.*
- *Work for her health improvement.*

Planning/Interventions:
The nurse will:
- *Facilitate Mrs. Z.'s expression of her concerns while helping to put feelings into perspective.*
- *Explain different relaxation methods; instruct on Mrs. Z.'s method of choice.*
- *Explain the hazards of over-the-counter antianxiety agents; inform about herbal remedies, benefits, and risks.*
- *Recommend an appropriate reading list and self-help guides.*
- *Offer information on HRT, osteoporosis, and healthy eating styles.*

EVALUATION:
Mrs. Z. will channel and control her anxiety by using relaxation techniques, which she will perform at least twice daily over the next month. She will verbalize benefit and reduced anxiety at the end of the month. Her husband will become aware of her concern for his health and keep open communication flowing. In addition, Mrs. Z. will not forget to focus on improving her own health.

NURSING DIAGNOSIS

Lack of adherence to dietary plan.

Outcomes:
Mr. Z. will:
- *Identify reasons for noncompliance of the low-sodium diet.*
- *Become knowledgeable in high- and low-sodium foods.*
- *Identify preferred alternatives to the high-sodium foods.*

Planning/Interventions:
The nurse will:
- *Assess nutritional status and Mr. Z.'s food likes and dislikes.*
- *Explore reasons for failure to adhere to dietary plan.*
- *Provide a list of foods with the sodium content in milligrams.*
- *List alternative foods low in sodium.*
- *Involve Mrs. Z. in food preparation classes offered by the community dietitian.*

EVALUATION:
Mr. Z. will select appealing foods low in sodium. To make this life-long change in eating patterns, he will express and cope with feelings about his new diet. Mrs. Z. will participate in food preparation classes relating to low-sodium and heart-healthy meals. As both become increasingly knowledgeable and aware, they will integrate this lifestyle change into their everyday routine.

Review Questions and Activities

1. Overall, which factor is probably the most important predictor of morbidity and mortality?

   a. Number of chronic diseases present

   b. Lifestyle: smoking, drinking, sedentary lifestyle

   c. Poverty

   d. Presence of factors that cause immunosuppression

2. The disease that kills the most older adults is:

   a. Pulmonary disease: COPD.

   b. Cardiovascular diseases

   c. Cancers: lung, colon, breast, prostate

   d. Accidents

3. The most important thing that people of any age can do to improve their health and lower their risk of dying is to:

   a. Wear seat belts.

   b. Exercise regularly.

   c. Avoid alcohol and drug use.

   d. Stop smoking.

4. A client with cardiac or respiratory disease asks why the physician has suggested an exercise program. The best answer is that:

   a. "It will help you lose weight."

   b. "It will condition your muscles so that they need less oxygen for any activity."

   c. "It will make you feel better."

   d. "It will enable you to sleep better at night."

5. When hypertension is diagnosed, treatment is usually begun in which of these ways?

   a. All clients are counseled on losing weight, salt reduction, and exercise. This is tried for several weeks or months prior to prescribing drugs.

   b. All clients with a blood pressure of 160/90 or higher must begin drugs immediately.

   c. Choice of treatment depends on whether the hypertension is causing any symptoms.

   d. Treatment choice is based on a variety of individual factors.

6. Beta blockers are a popular class of drugs for older adults with cardiovascular disease. The nurse knows that:

   a. These are relatively safe with few adverse effects.

   b. They cause the client to be at risk for potassium loss.

   c. They reduce the ability to raise the heart rate when needed.

   d. They may cause constipation.

7. A patient who is taking ACE inhibitors may be mistakenly believed to have:

   a. Emphysema

   b. Asthma

   c. Angina

   d. A CVA

8. Symptoms of congestive heart failure, such as reduced exercise tolerance, may go unnoticed because the client:

   a. Is often sedentary

   b. Has COPD

   c. Has a good attitude and denies the problem

   d. Both a and b

9. Match the primary drug treatment to the disease categories:

   a. COPD: bronchodilators; asthma: steroids

   b. COPD and asthma: bronchodilators and steroids

   c. COPD and asthma: bronchodilators

   d. COPD and asthma: avoid drug use as much as possible

10. Which are included in the major or most common symptoms of Parkinson's disease?

    a. Dementia, immunosuppression, and reduced activity tolerance.

    b. Severe muscle rigidity and inability to speak coherently.

    c. Tremors, rigidity, weakness, slow movement, and tendency to fall.

    d. Difficulty and tremor when starting movement, but once begun it is effective, smooth, and well controlled.

11. Which of the following may cause constipation in older adults?

    a. Parkinson's disease, sedentary lifestyle, and some CV drugs.

    b. Low-fiber diet, many respiratory drugs, and inability to get to the bathroom quickly.

    c. The disease is severe and the client is confined to bed.

    d. Nausea, poor food intake, and inability to take medications.

12. Which of these statements are true about gastric reflux?

    a. It is not a common problem in older adults.

    b. It can result from the administration of some drugs such as Sinemet.

    c. It is a common cause of pneumonia in older adults.

    d. All but a.

13. When administering drugs such as Sinemet to older adults with Parkinson's disease, the nurse knows that:

    a. It should be given with meals.

    b. Its onset and effects are unpredictable.

    c. It should not be taken by anyone less than 60 years of age.

    d. There are many drugs that interact with it; use caution when administering.

References

American Diabetes Association (ADA). (1999). *Standards of Medical Care for Patients with Diabetes Mellitus* [On-line]. Available: www.diabetes.org.

Aminoff, M. J. (1997). *Nervous system in current medical diagnosis and treatment: 1997 at-large medical book* (pp. 919–921). Stamford, CT: Appleton and Lange.

Appel, L. J., Moore, T. J., et al. (1997). A clinical trial of the effects of dietary patterns on blood pressure. *New England Journal of Medicine, 336*(16), 1117–1124.

Apple, S. (1996). New trends in thrombolytic therapy. *RN, 59*(1), 30–34.

Avorn, J., Monane, M., Gurwitz, J., Glynn, R., Choodnovskly, I., & Lipsitz, L. (1994). Reduction of bacteriuria and pyuria after ingestion of cranberry juice. *Journal of the American Medical Association, 271*(10), 751–754.

Billhorn, D. R. (1994). Sexuality and the chronically ill older adult. *Geriatric Nursing, 15*(2), 106–108.

Bonander, A. (1995). *Problem drugs in PD* [On-line]. Available: http:iipdweb.mgh.harvard.edu.

Bramann, S. S. (1993). Asthma in the elderly patient. *Clinics in Chest Medicine, 14*, 413–422.

Brechtelsbauer, D. A. (1992). Care with an indwelling urinary catheter. *Postgraduate Medicine, 92*(1), 127–132.

Brown, E., Evans, M., & Ferdman, R. (1997, November). Asthma in the older patient. Treatment updates—a clinical series for physicians [On-line]. Asthma Information Center, *Journal of the American Medical Association*. Available: http://www.ama-assn.org/special/asthma/treatment/updates/older.htm

Brunt, E. (1994, Summer). *Deprenyl, a 1994 update.* Staten Island, NY: American Parkinson's Disease Foundation.

Buehrens, P. E. (1995). Effectiveness of oral antibiotic treatment in nursing-home acquired pneumonia (letter). *Journal of the American Geriatrics Society, 1995*(43), 1443.

Carter, J. H. (1992). *A special diet for Parkinson's disease.* Staten Island, NY: American Parkinson's Disease Association.

Caruthers, D. D. (1990). Infectious pneumonia in the elderly. *American Journal of Nursing, 90*(2), 56–60.

Celli, B. R., Snider, G. L., Heffner, J., Tiep, B., Ziment, I., Make, B., Braman, S., Olsen, G., & Phillips, Y. (1995). Standards for the diagnosis and care of patients with chronic obstructive pulmonary disease. *American Journal of Respiratory Critical Care Medicine, 152*, S77–S120.

Center Watch. (1998). *Newly approved drug therapies* [On-line]. Available: Centerwatch.com.

Cheitlin, M., (1999). *Clinical cardiology* (7th ed.). Norwalk, VA: Appleton and Lange.

Duffield, P. (1997). Urinary tract infections in the elderly: A common complication of aging. *Advances for Nurse Practitioners, 5*, 30–32.

Emmert, D. H., & Kirchner, J. T. (2000). Sexually transmitted diseases in women: Gonorrhea and syphilis. *Postgraduate Medicine, 107*(2), 181–97.

Ernst, N. D., Mullis, R., Sootey-Bochenek, J., & Van Horn, L. (1988). The national cholesterol education program: Implications for dietetic practitioners from the adult treatment panel recommendations. *Journal of the American Dietetic Association, 88*(11), 1401–1411.

Fine, M. J., Auble, T. E., Yearly, D. M., et al. (1997). A prediction rule to identify low-risk patients with community-acquired pneumonia. *New England Journal of Medicine, 336*(4), 243–250.

Forbes, E. J. (1992). Exercise: Wellness maintenance for the elderly client. *Holistic Nursing Practice, 6*(2), 14–22.

Freed, M., & Grines, C. (1994). *Essentials of cardiovascular medicine.* Birmingham, MI: Physicians Press.

Frick, M. et al. (1987). Helsinki heart study: Primary prevention trial with gemfibrozil in middle-aged men with dyslipidemia. *New England Journal of Medicine, 317*(20), 1237–1245.

Friebele, E. (1996). The attack of asthma. *Focus, 104*(1), 1–9.

Gleckman, R. A. (1992). Urinary tract infection. *Clinics in Geriatric Medicine, 8*(4), 793–803.

Goldsmith, C. (1998, March 2). Advances in treatments for Parkinson's disease. *Healthweek*, pp. 24–25.

Halm, M. A. (1997). *Women and heart disease. Type I continuing education for Texas nurses* (pp. 17–45). Sacramento, CA: CME Resource.

Hardyck, C., & Petrinovich, L. (1998). Reducing urinary tract infections in catheterized patients. *Ostomy/Wound Management, 44*(12), 36–43.

Haus, E. (1998). Urinary tract infections in the homebound elderly. *Home Healthcare Nurse, 16*(5), 323–327.

Hopfensperger, K., & Koller, W. C. (1991). Recognizing early Parkinson's disease. *Postgraduate Medicine, 90*(1), 49–59.

Houldin, A. D., & Wasserbauer, N. (1996). Psychosocial needs of older cancer patients: A pilot study abstract. *MEDSURG Nursing, 5*(4), 253–256.

Hulley, S., Grady, D., Bush, T., Furberg, C., Herrington, D., Riggs, B., & Vittinghoff, E. (1998). Randomized trial of estrogen plus progestin for secondary prevention of coronary heart disease in postmenopausal women. *Journal of the American Medical Association, 280*(7), 605–613.

Hurley, M. L. (1998, March). New hypertension guidelines. *RN*, pp. 25–28.

Hutton, J. T., & Hutton, T. (1998). *Young Parkinson's handbook* [On-line]. Available: http:iipdweb.mgh.harvard.edu (site no longer available).

Ignatavlcius, D. D., Workman, M. L., & Mishler, M. A. (1999). *Medical-surgical nursing across the health care continuum* (3rd ed.). Philadelphia: Saunders.

Institute for Clinical Systems Improvement (ICSI). (2000). Community-acquired pneumonia: Outpatient treatment of patients 16 years and older. *Postgraduate Medicine, 107*(2), 246–253.

Jadin, R. L., & Margolis, K. (1998). Coronary artery disease in women. *Postgraduate Medicine, 103*(3), 71–84.

Joint National Committee on Prevention, Detection, Evaluation, and Treatment of High Blood Pressure. (1997). *The Sixth Report of the Joint National Committee on Prevention, Detection, Evaluation, and Treatment of High Blood Pressure.* Bethesda, MD: National Institutes of Health.

Kannam, J. P., & Levy, D. (1993, September 15). Isolated systolic hypertension in the elderly. *Hospital Practice*, pp. 57–74.

Kannel, W. B. (1989). Epidemiological aspects of heart failure. *Cardiology Clinics, 1989*(7), 1–9.

Kaplan, N. M. (1998). Treatment of hypertension: Insights from the JNC-VI report. *American Family Physician, 6*(58), 1323–1330.

Kawachi, I., Colditz, G. A., Stampfer, M. J., Willett, W. C., Manson, J. E., Rosner, B., Speizer, F. E., & Hennekens, C. H. (1994). Smoking cessation and time course of decreased risks of coronary heart disease in middle-aged women. *Archives of Internal Medicine, 154*(2), 169–175.

Kellerman, J. (1990). Introduction. *American Heart Journal, 120*(6), 1529–1531.

Kirchner, J. T., & Emmert, D. H. (2000). Sexually transmitted diseases in women: *Chlamydia trachomatis* and herpes simplex infections. *Postgraduate Medicine, 107*(1), 55–65.

Kris-Etherton, P., Krummel, D., Russell, M. E., Dreon, D., Mackey, S., Borchers, J., & Wood, P. D. (1988). The effect of diet on plasma lipids, lipoproteins, and coronary heart disease. *Journal of the American Dietetic Association, 88*(11), 1373–1400.

Kuncl, N., & Nelson, K. M. (1997, August). Antihypertensive drugs: Balancing risks and benefits. *Nursing*, pp. 46–49.

Lang, A. E., & Lozano, A. M. (1998). Parkinson's disease. *New England Journal of Medicine, 339*(15), 1044–1053.

Lantz, P. M., House, J. S., Lepkowski, J. M., Williams, D. R., Mero, R. P., & Chen, J. (1998). Socioeconomic factors, health behaviors and mortality. *Journal of the American Medical Association, 279*(21), 1703–1708.

Letvak, S., & Schoder, D. (1996). Sexually transmitted diseases in the elderly: What you need to know. *Geriatric Nursing, 17*(4), 156–160.

Lueckenotte, A. G. (1996). *Gerontologic nursing.* St. Louis: Mosby.

Mancia, G. (1990). Neurohumoral activation in congestive heart failure. *American Heart Journal, 120*(6), 1532–1537.

McCue, J. (1993). Urinary tract infections in the elderly. *Pharmacotherapy, 13*(2, Pt. 2), 51S–53S.

Melillo, K. D. (1995). Asymptomatic bacteria in older adults: When is it necessary to screen and treat? *Nurse Practitioner, 20*(8), 50–66.

Mick, D. J. (1997). Pneumonia in elders. *Geriatric Nursing, 98*(3), 99–102.

Murray, D. M., Kurth, C., Mullis, R., & Jeffery, R. W. (1990). Cholesterol reduction through low-intensity interventions: Results from the Minnesota Heart Health Program. *Preventive Medicine, 19*(2), 181–189.

Nicolle, L. E. (1993). Urinary tract infections in long-term care facilities. *Infection Control and Hospital Epiemiology, 14*, 220–225.

Rakel, R. E. (Ed.). (1997). *Conn's current therapy* (pp. 963–972). Philadelphia: Saunders.

Reznicek, S. G. B. (2000). Common urologic problems in the elderly. *Postgraduate Medicine, 107*(1), 163–178.

Riquelme, R., Torres, A., El-Ebiary, M., Mensa, J., Estruch, R., Ruiz, M., Angrill, J., & Soler, N. (1997). Community-acquired pneumonia in the elderly: Clinical and nutritional aspects. *American Journal of Respiratory and Critical Care Medicine, 156*(6), 1908–1914.

Rubins, J. B., & Janoff, E. N. (1997). Community-acquired pneumonia. *Postgraduate Medicine, 102*(6), 45–62.

Ruger, T. (1997). *Nursing oncology 2000.* Paper presented at M. D. Anderson Cancer Center, Houston, TX.

Simon, H., Etkin, M. J., Godine, J. E., Heller, D., Juter, I., Shellito, P. C., & Stern, T. A. (1999). *Lyme disease and ehrlichiosis* [On-line]. Available: http://www.well-connected.com.

Sonneblick, E. D., & LeJemtel, T. H. (1993, September 15). Heart failure: Its progression and therapy. *Hospital Practice*, pp. 121–130.

Speizer, F. E. (1989). The rise in chronic obstructive pulmonary disease mortality: Overview and commentary. *American Review of Respiratory Disease, 140*, S106–S107.

Stamm, W. E., & Hooten, T. M. (1993). Management of urinary tract infections in adults. *New England Journal of Medicine, 329*, 1328–1334.

Varon, J., & Jacobs, M. B. (1990). Treating the progressive stages of Parkinson's disease. *Postgraduate Medicine, 90*(1), 63–71.

Weinberg, J. (1993). Renal effects of angiotensin converting enzyme inhibitors in heart failure: A clinician's guide to minimizing azotemia and diuretic-induced electrolyte imbalances. *Clinical Therapeutics, 1993*(15), 3–15.

Whitney, F. (1994). Drug therapy for acute stroke. *Journal of Neuroscience Nursing, 26*(2), 110–113.

Williams, J. F., Bristow, M. R., Fowler, M. B., Francis, G. S., Garson, A., Jr., Gersh, B. J., Hammer, D. F., Hlatky, M. A., Leier, C. V., Packer, M., Pitt, B, Ullyot, D., J., Wexler, L. F., & Winters, W. L, Jr. (1995). *Guidelines for the evaluation and management of heart failure.* Dallas, TX: American Heart Association.

Wooten-Bielski, K. (1999). HIV and AIDS in older adults. *Geriatric Nursing, 20*(5), 268–272.

Resources

Alzheimer's Disease Education and Referral Center (ADEAR): `www.alzheimers.org`

American Cancer Society: `www.cancer.org`

American Diabetes Association (ADA): `www.diabetes.org`

American Heart Association (AHA): `www.heartsource.org`

Institute for Clinical Systems Improvement: `www.ICSI.org`

Parkinson's Disease Foundation (PDF): `www.pdf.org`

Answers to Review Questions

1. c
2. b
3. d
4. b
5. d
6. c
7. b

8. d
9. a
10. c
11. a
12. d
13. b

CHAPTER 15

Acute Care Issues

Carol A. Stephenson, EdD, RN, C, CRNH

COMPETENCIES

After completing this chapter, the reader should be able to:

- Discuss the concerns and needs of older adults who become hospitalized.
- Discuss the need for balance between autonomy and safety in the hospitalized older client.
- Identify some of the major nursing problems of older hospitalized clients and appropriate interventions related to each.
- Explain some possible causes of concern and stress for older hospitalized clients and their families.
- Discuss some major issues and techniques in the management of acute pain in the older adult.

MAKING THE CONNECTION

Refer to the following chapters to increase your understanding of acute care issues:

Older Adults as Health Care Consumers

Older adults are the largest consumers of health care in the United States. This trend will continue as the number of older adults rises dramatically in the coming years. Not only is the American population aging, but the numbers of older old adults will continue to rise as well. Although many older adults continue to be relatively healthy into old age, a large percentage of them have one or more chronic health problems—often they have several. They are also at higher risk for acute and recurring health problems than are younger adults.

Models of Caring for Older Adults

The largest, although not the only, third-party payer for older adult health care is the government (Medicare, Medicaid, state, and local programs). The astronomical costs of health care for older adults are fueling a national debate on how to reduce those costs. To reduce total costs may require extensive cuts in the services provided to each older adult, given the fact that there are so many more older adults in the system each year and that the cost of goods and services is constantly rising. To date, one of the results of efforts to reduce health care expenditures is limiting hospitalizations to those with major injury or illness and/or who cannot be cared for in other settings. Therefore, hospital inpatients are much more acutely ill than they were in the past. Other outcomes of the changing health care environment include the development and/or expansion of wellness education programs; outpatient and gerontological clinics; outpatient and ambulatory surgery centers; subacute, transitional care, and rehabilitation units; and adult day services programs. Nursing facilities are in transition as other options are becoming available. There is a need for home care, although its availability has been greatly reduced by funding cuts.

Health care providers must be well prepared to meet the needs of the rapidly expanding group of gerontological clients. Acute care of older adult clients is increasingly complex, and no more so than when they are acutely ill and hospitalized. From the time of the client's admission to the health care system until discharge, nurses have closer contact with the client than does any other member of the health care team. Nurses must understand not only the normal aging process but also the common deviations from normal, individual differences among older adults, and the many issues and problems that confront these clients and their families.

The ideal model for providing comprehensive care to older adults is an interdisciplinary care team whose members have special preparation in gerontology: physicians, nurses, pharmacists, dietitians, therapists, social workers, or case managers. Besides providing direct care and problem solving, the gerontological health care team should be proactive rather than reactive with regard to polices and protocols related to older adult care. They should be client advocates in the legislative and policymaking arenas as well as advocating for quality rather than cost as the driving force in client care.

The entire team works together to provide appropriate individualized support and intervention to older adults. For example, a pharmacist might recognize that a particular drug ordered by the physician or gerontological nurse practitioner interacts with other drugs being taken by the older adult or that the drug might be metabolized differently than in the younger adult. The pharmacist then uses this knowledge to alert the physician and nurse to prevent the client from receiving a drug that could possibly have adverse effects. The use of specially prepared gerontological nurses, gerontological resource nurses, gerontological clinical nurse specialists, and gerontological nurse practitioners (GNPs) is extremely helpful in the acute care setting, where the client mix commonly includes a high proportion of older clients. Not only do nurses with gerontological preparation relate better to aging persons, but also they are more alert to problems of aging often missed by others and provide more comprehensive, individualized care for older adults; they are more prepared to discuss issues such as role change and losses, autonomy, right to life, and other related issues with clients, families, health care providers, and the public. Gerontological nurses are aware of the potentially overwhelming nature of the health care system, the payment system, and the magnitude and implications of what is happening to older clients. Gerontological nurses have a responsibility to challenge stereotypes and inappropriate care or behaviors as they assist other team members to examine their own knowledge of and attitudes toward older adults. Gerontological nurse practitioners and clinical specialists lead the nursing team, serve as a liaison with other providers and as a resource for health care team members as well as provide direct client care. The GNPs often act as primary care providers for gerontological clients in settings such as clinics, private or group medical practices, and independent settings. The gerontological resource nurse is usually a staff member who has completed formal or informal course work and perhaps an apprenticeship to become knowledgeable regarding the common problems experienced by older clients. This nurse, while usually remaining a part of the nursing staff of the unit, also is able to serve as a resource and teacher to other staff members, families, and clients.

Case management is a useful approach to improving the care of older clients before, during, and after hospitalization. Case management terminology, however, lacks a clear definition. The term *case management* is used in many ways: in some cases, the primary nurse is called the case manager; in others, the discharge planner holds the title of case manager. However, the larger definition of case management includes not only coordination of care within the agency but also referral to the most appropriate resources or settings after hospitalization, coordination of support services, and prevention of future hospitalizations by the coordination of education, support services and personnel, and community services. Many insurance companies and third-party payers employ case managers who work with the client long term because good case management is cost effective. Gerontological clients often require a variety of resources and services, which, without the coordination of the case manager, might not be identified or accessed, might be overlapping, or with gaps, or be over- or underutilized. An excellent case manager can not only maximize care for a particular client and maximize the outcomes of that care but also can enable the care to be provided in the most cost-effective manner, which is a critically important factor for third-party payers.

The Admission Process

Admission to a hospital is most often a stressful event for anyone. It can be even more stressful to an older adult for a variety of reasons. Older adults may be in pain; perceive the illness or injury as possibly ending a lifestyle as they know it; be worried about how to pay for the hospitalization; have few or no support persons available to them; or be confused because of the illness, pain, or drug therapy, or because of the different environment. The nursing staff should be alert to signs of anxiety, discomfort, confusion, and other problems during the admission process. The admission can become a time for calming the client and establishing trust that excellent care will be given, or it can serve to further confuse or cause anxiety regarding what will happen during the hospitalization.

Establish Rapport and Trust

Even if the hospital admission of an older adult is a crisis situation, the admitting nurse should make a serious effort to establish rapport and trust. In serious illness or injury, the admission process may involve a great deal of urgent activity. If there is no opportunity for extensive discussion during the admission, the nurse, by kindness and courtesy while performing necessary procedures or treatments in an efficient and comfortable manner, can establish a sense of confidence and expectation of competent, quality care throughout the hospitalization. Any procedures that are not absolutely essential should be

delayed: nonessential portions of the history, physical exam, and diagnostic procedures. Clients should be allowed to wear their own clothing or pajamas and to keep a few personal possessions at the bedside, including glasses, hearing aids, dentures, prostheses, walkers, and other items that enhance adjustment and independence. Both comfort and dignity are preserved as much as possible. The client is informed about what is going to happen and given support and encouragement while procedures are carried out. Physical exposure is kept to an absolute minimum. There is no excuse for unnecessary exposure, even if the client is unresponsive. Lying on a hard table for diagnostic and therapeutic procedures for long periods in areas such as the emergency department is extremely uncomfortable and may even damage skin and subcutaneous tissue. Such discomfort should be minimized as much as possible and skin prominences padded if the procedure will take extended time (beyond 2 hours). Clients may be asked to assume positions that are uncomfortable or even impossible for them. The staff must listen to clients and adapt the procedures and positions as much as possible.

All staff members are expected to clearly identify themselves to clients and families by name and title. Older adults are often confused by the wide variety of uniforms and have no idea who is a nurse and who is not. They may believe they never saw a "real nurse" during the entire hospitalization. They may believe that the people in street clothes or other non-uniform-appearing clothes with missing nametags do not belong in their rooms and they are right. Many clients cannot read the names and titles on the nametags when staff do wear them, so verbal identification of name and title is important.

Common Client Concerns

Even if the situation for which the client is being admitted is not considered to be a crisis by the staff, it is often a crisis to the older adult and the family. Anyone who is being admitted to a hospital is usually anxious. Older adults are often more vulnerable than younger clients to such anxiety. This is not solely because they may personally be less resilient. Older adults often have a variety of other fears and concerns, which are very realistic and well founded. Some people reach their later years without ever being hospitalized, resulting in significant fear of the unknown when it finally happens. Others have had unpleasant and even frightening previous experiences in hospitals, which contribute to their expectation of more traumatic experiences. There may be many other concerns swirling through their minds: "Will this be the end of my independence?" "Will I be able to live at home on my own?" "What will happen to my spouse or my pets?" "Will I die?" "Can I tolerate the pain?" "Can I afford this?" "I don't want to lose my privacy and my dignity." "If I tell them I don't understand what they are saying to me, they will think I'm ignorant." "Will I have to leave the hospital before I am able or ready to care for myself?" "I don't want to be a burden to my family." "I don't even know what questions to ask." Nurses must be alert to comments about fears or other verbal and nonverbal indicators that the client is anxious. For example, some older adults become ill within a few months after the death of a spouse. Nurses should notice when older adults are confused and/or distressed, not only at the time of admission, but throughout their stay in the health care system. It is important to clearly and frequently ask them about their feelings, to listen attentively to their replies, to ask questions as often as necessary for clarification, and then to address their concerns in every way possible. The staff should tell older adults and their families what steps are being taken to address their concerns so that they are aware that attempts on their behalf are being made even if actual resolution takes time.

Older adults may be anxious about their diagnoses, the tests and treatments to be performed, their consequences and outcomes, and/or their ability to understand and cope with what the health care providers are telling them. They may request that a family member or a close friend be with them when the health team members speak with them. This request is respected and encouraged, even if waiting for the requested person causes inconvenience. Others are very private and want to be alone when health care providers speak with them or give news of test results or surgical outcomes. They may not convey this information to the physician or nurse if others are in the room when care providers visit. Clients are asked if they want to talk with the doctor or nurse *alone* and that request is respected.

Older clients often have many financial concerns related to the hospitalization. Medicare does not pay all of the bills. There are often deductibles and copays, even with Medicare, insurance supplements, and health maintenance organizations (HMOs). Older adults may have already incurred extremely high bills for outpatient care and medications prior to entering the hospital. Each time a different health care provider visits, they may wonder or even ask how much it will cost. They may tell nurses and other providers that they "just have Medicare," hoping to convey the information that they cannot afford costly treatment that is not covered by standard Medicare benefits. On the other hand, older adults may fear that their treatment will be inadequate or inappropriate because they are just on Medicare or are being cared for in a public hospital.

Most older clients and their families are familiar enough with the payment system to realistically dread its complexities. It takes a great deal of time and energy to cope with treatments, bills, and regulations and requirements. Even a healthy younger person can be overwhelmed. Social workers are of great assistance in helping older adults to understand and cope with the health care and the payment system. Some communities have volunteers who help clients make and keep appointments, manage finances, and understand and cope with bills as well as handle other complexities of day-to-day life.

It is important to ask the client and family about their chief concerns regarding the illness or hospitalization. The health care team gives excellent care and solves many problems during the hospitalization, but if clients do not feel that their major personal concerns have been addressed, they are likely to perceive the experience as a failure. It is also important to determine their goals for treatment (short and long term) and to inquire about personal schedules and preferences. Perhaps they are used to sleeping late and staying up late or eating many snacks throughout the day rather than three meals daily or have devised ingenious ways to cope with their ongoing medical problems. As much as possible, treatments should continue in the same manner in which the client is doing them at home. Listening to the client about what works and what does not prevents many problems. Nurses also should listen to what clients say they have been taught by physicians, GNPs, office staff, and home care nurses. This can prevent situations such as the cancer client whose **peripherally inserted central catheter (PICC)** was lost during a week-long hospitalization for severe nausea. "I told them exactly how you irrigate it, but they wouldn't listen. My roommate lost his line too!" When asked what he told the nurses, his description was accurate in every detail. The wife of another client was quite verbal to the home care nurse who was administering intravenous antibiotics after the client's implanted port became both infected and occluded during a hospitalization. "I told them they weren't doing it right, but they wouldn't listen!" Besides being dangerous, not listening to clients and families is disrespectful and destroys trust and rapport. The staff should also make an attempt to identify particular fears or concerns and then make every effort to prevent problems from occurring.

For example, Mrs. J. is a 78-year-old woman who lived on a farm without electricity in the early days of raising her family. She was overcome by fumes from her gasoline washing machine and survived only because her husband returned from the fields unexpectedly on that day. The most important long-term result was chronic dysphagia. Over the years, she developed an unpredictable and serious esophageal spasm problem as well. She became a licensed vocational nurse and worked in nursing facilities for several years. As a result of all of the above, she is terrified that she will die of choking when being fed by a staff member in a hospital or an older adult care facility. So far, she and her husband continue to be independent and live on their own, but she is concerned about the future. If she is admitted to a hospital or nursing facility, special efforts must be made to acknowledge her fears as valid *and* to make sure that all feeding is done in an extremely slow and careful manner.

Think About It

Mrs. P., age 68, has been admitted for the treatment of unstable angina. She is now a client in the step-down coronary care unit. Mrs. P. has had renal failure for several years and has been managing her own continuous ambulatory peritoneal dialysis (CAPD). She is now comfortable, alert, oriented, and stable with regard to her cardiac status. She states that she wishes to manage her own dialysis while in the hospital rather than allowing the nursing staff to do it for her. Her rationale is that she knows how to do it and would be more comfortable that sterile technique is maintained if she did it herself.

Do you think Mrs. P. should be allowed to manage her own dialysis?

The Need for Respect and to Avoid Labeling

The nursing staff conveys respect by both word and deed. Older clients may not be treated as respected adults for a variety of reasons. Even if they are articulate and independent, illness and ageism may skew staff perception. Older adults who cannot recall instructions or information, who cannot follow instructions, or who appear to be overwhelmed are more likely than younger people to be stereotyped as incapacitated, confused, dependent, helpless, or unable to make decisions. Often, older adults are inappropriately labeled because of an isolated incident related to the disease, problem, or treatment, such as becoming confused or combative after the administration of drugs or anesthesia. Even more frightening is the tendency to consider such problems to be those of normal aging. Once older adults are stereotyped, staff tend to treat them as though the stereotype is true and expected. Staff members then make less effort to identify and overcome the problems that may have contributed to the confusion. For example, nurses were receiving shift change report on a particular day when the client being discussed was an 81-year-old priest who was 24 hours postoperative. The nurse reported his confusion and lack of cooperation along with a comment that "after all, he's quite old." This would probably have been accepted as his norm by the staff except for the fact that one nurse spoke up: "He's my marriage counselor; his mind is very sharp despite

his age!" This brought a new expectation to the situation and a search for the cause, which was found to be medication.

The personalities of some older adults change with illness and medications. Most simply continue with their usual personalities and reactions, whether these were flexible and easy-going or somewhat difficult and uncooperative. Reactions to illness and stress vary widely. The nurse should be alert for verbal and behavioral clues that the client needs a different approach than the one being taken or that priorities need to be adjusted (Figure 15-1). For example, a nurse is attempting to take a history at the time of admission of a man who has just come from the physician's office after being told that he has inoperable cancer and probably will die soon. He is rather quiet and stoic, but his wife is quite upset, agitated, and teary. She is throwing out many nonverbal clues regarding her extreme distress, but the nurse calmly goes on with the admission—"when was this originally diagnosed . . . what were the symptoms . . . what medicines is he on . . . is he allergic to any medicines?" Unless the history taking is extremely urgent, and usually it would not be in this situation, the nurse needs to stop and either listen to the wife and give support or, if the workload is too heavy, call the chaplain or counselor to assist her.

Part of the admission process includes asking what the older adult wants to be called. Many are distressed when they are called by their first names or by terms of endearment such as "dearie" or "sweetie." Until given permission to do otherwise, older adults should be addressed by respectful, proper names, such as Mr. Smith. One retired minister and missionary was appalled

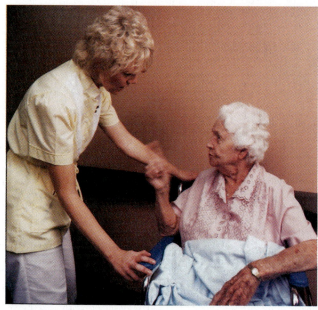

FIGURE 15-1 A client may express anger and frustration as a result of illness, stress, or medication.

when his nurse addressed him as John. His response: "You may call me Dr. Smith; you may call me Mr. Smith; you may call me Reverend Smith; you may call me Sir. Don't call me John. What will people think?" Most older adults are not willing to be this blunt about their displeasure; staff members must ask rather than making assumptions. The exceptions to this rule are those clients who have had disease or injury that renders them unconscious or semiconscious. In attempting to elicit a response, the nurse uses the name or nickname that the person has used throughout life. The reason for this is that clients are likely to respond to their lifelong name or nickname that has been used from birth, rather than to a name that was acquired later, such as Mr. Jones. Information regarding how the client is usually addressed by friends and family is elicited from these friends and family members.

Room Accommodations

Room accommodations may be problematic for older clients. It is still common for double rooms to be the norm because third-party payers cover them (Figure 15-2). However, sick older adults may be unable to cope with the noise or loss of privacy that is common in double accommodations. Sometimes, one roommate makes life unpleasant for the other person by refusing to share control of the television or the telephone or with numbers of visitors. Sometimes roommates, by virtue of their illness or personality, make so much noise that older adults are unable to get enough sleep. Sometimes, the person in the back bed is too far from the bathroom to get there safely. Many older adults, because of their own physical or mental condition, or because of their personalities, do much better in a private room. This is especially true for confused older adults, because of the more limited number of distractions and/or the ability for a significant other to be in the room with them all or most of the time.

The sick older adult may not want to share a room with a total stranger or be where family members cannot visit freely. Privacy is important when the physician or nurse is giving critical or personal information. Discussion of personal information begins with the admission nursing assessment and continues throughout the hospital stay. Many adults are often uncomfortable discussing private information when strangers are present in the room. Others may prefer a double room because they feel they will be lonely or they like company. Some accept a double room that they do not really want because they believe that is all that is covered by their third-party payer.

Room assignments are often made by admitting office personnel who are aware only of the client's sex and admission diagnosis. Clients are often assigned by the medical service with which the client's physician works with little regard for individual needs. Not only might clients be placed with an incompatible roommate; they might be placed in dangerous situations. For example, a client in her nineties might be placed in the room with a client who has pneumonia. It is almost certain that, before long, the client in her nineties may also have pneumonia if she remains in that room. Once clients are assigned to rooms, staff members should be alert to problems, because reassignment may be necessary for health, safety, or comfort.

Intensive care units (ICUs) are often extremely noisy, with the lights on for 24 hours daily. Clients become disoriented not only because of the noise and the medications being administered but also from disruption of sleep and confusion resulting from loss of the normal light-dark cycle. The limited visiting time, discomfort, strange procedures, and monitors are disorienting and contribute to confusion, fear, and anxiety. If older clients are in a private ICU room with a door that closes and have a significant other in the room most of the time, they are more likely to remain oriented and comfortable.

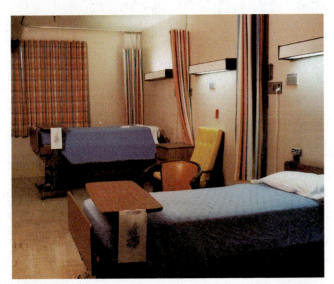

FIGURE 15-2 Double-occupancy rooms like this one are the norm in most acute care settings.

The Need for Consistent Caregivers

When possible, the client is cared for by the same staff members, even if this violates their usual assignment policy. For example, a client might be transferred to a room at the opposite end of a nursing unit that is traditionally covered by a different care team. It is helpful for the original staff to continue to care for the client during the remainder of the hospital stay, even if they must walk to the other end of the hall to do so. If this is impossible, perhaps some transition time could be effected by creative staffing with both teams.

The hospital is not the only place where consistent caregiving can be a problem because of usual policies for staffing patterns. An older woman with multiple myeloma has been in a nursing facility. Even though the nursing facility staff provides 24-hour care, the same hospice nurse and hospice aide have visited several times weekly, provided her care and case management, and bonded with her. She had a crisis and was admitted to a hospital. The hospice nurse visited her there but the aide did not. The client requested to go to a different nursing facility on release because she did not feel the quality of care at the first home was good. Her eventual goal: to become strong enough to live with her son for the remainder of her life. A different hospice team is assigned to clients in the second nursing facility, so the move would require a new nurse and aide. To complicate the situation, the regular hospice nurse for the new nursing facility is on vacation while a substitute nurse provides care. According to agency protocol, the substitute nurse would care for the client until the regular nurse returns from vacation. When and if the client is discharged to her son's home, a hospice home care team will be assigned to her care—all new personnel again. The original hospice nurse is talking with the other teams involved in an effort to continue to visit this client in the interest of continuity of care and continuing her trust and bonding—not the usual agency protocol, but good for the client.

Teaching and Discharge Planning

As the reader is aware, everyone is now discharged from the hospital "sicker and quicker" than was formerly the case. Older adults are often not able to care for themselves at home when ill or injured. Many older adults live alone or with other ill older adults. There may be no family members who live nearby or they may have outlived their family and friends. A case manager should begin discussing **discharge planning** with the older adult and any potential caregivers as early as possible into the admission so that the older adult will be discharged to a location and situation that will maximize safety and recovery.

When teaching older adults, the usual principles of client teaching apply. Teaching should not be attempted when the client is exhausted, distracted, hypoxic, in pain, or distressed about factors such as prognosis, outcomes, or test results. If the client usually wears glasses and hearing aids, these should be used during the teaching process. Teaching should be done in extremely short segments and reinforced often. An excellent way to structure teaching is to begin with a discussion of what the client knows, believes, and practices about the topic as well as eliciting concerns and then structure teaching from there. Instructions should be written in

clear, simple language, with the major points emphasized and nonessential material omitted or deemphasized. Written instructions should be given to aid retention. These written materials should be in large, bold type on nonglare paper and should be read with the client, rather than assuming that the client can or will read them independently.

When teaching older adults, it is important to teach strategies that can and will be used by the client (see Figure 15-3). Often, merely taking all of the prescribed drugs on time and in the proper manner can be overwhelming. Written materials regarding each drug may not be enough to help the client get them all straight, although they can be helpful to those who can read them. One strategy that may help is to highlight the written descriptions, the dose schedule, the medication bottles, and a chart for filling a medication box or taking medications from the original bottles with color-coded dots or labels. Sometimes, it is more effective for the nurse to visit weekly to monitor the client's condition and fill the medication box. At other times, a friend or relative may be able to fill the medication box and call for drug refills when necessary.

Sometimes, the problem is that the client simply cannot read the label well enough to use the right drug in the right manner at the right time. One home care nurse arrived at a client's home the day following eye surgery. Her bottles of eye drops had been picked up at the pharmacy and dropped off at her house, but she had not used any in the 24 hours since surgery. Why? The print on the label of the bottle was small (standard 10-point type) and the printer ribbon was so faded that it was barely visible to the nurse. The client could not tell which eye drop was which, much less when and how to use each. The problem was solved quickly and easily when the nurse placed each bottle individually in a zip-lock plastic bag. The nurse wrote the label information for each drug on wide adhesive tape with a bold black marker and placed it on the outside of each appropriate bag. The client was now able to manage her medications independently.

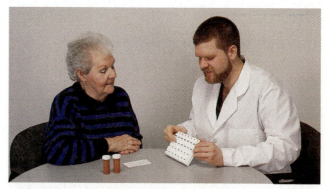

FIGURE 15-3 This client is learning to manage her medication regimen by using a pillbox correlated to the days of the month.

If the client is discharged to another health care facility, to home care, or to home before teaching is completed and understanding can be demonstrated, the teaching plan should be communicated to the receiving nurses: in the new facility, the home care agency, or the clinic, physician's, or GNP's office. All too often, little or nothing is communicated. Either no follow-up is done or the client is retaught what has already been learned. For example, a 70-year-old woman had a Stokes-Adams attack, lost consciousness, and fell, fracturing her shoulder. At the hospital, her cardiac arrhythmia was documented. A **pacemaker** was inserted, her shoulder was set, and she was discharged to a rehabilitation hospital all within the space of three days. The communication from the referring hospital included the date when her pacer stitches should be removed but not the information that NO pacer teaching had been completed because of the client's pain and sedation during hospitalization. Only when a nursing student assigned to her care was questioned by her instructor regarding the client's knowledge about the pacer and related long-term care was it discovered that no teaching had been done.

Current reimbursement policies for client teaching are, for the most part, miserly. Payers appear to assume that all clients are willing, able, and motivated to learn everything they need to know in very short order. Teaching in the hospital must begin earlier than ever before and the client will still be discharged before it is completed. Giving clients a written list of what they need to know as they are being discharged is NOT adequate client teaching. Nurses must be assertive in proving the need for further teaching and monitoring visits when these are needed and indicated. In any setting, complete and accurate documentation of what is taught, client response, written materials given, and strategies devised is critical. It is important to remember that even though clients may respond appropriately to the teaching in the hospital, there is no guarantee that they will use the information at home or even remember it if they were tired, anxious, in pain, or on medication at the time of the teaching. Teaching family caregivers is essential in many cases.

Appreciate Cultural Differences

Understanding and appreciation of the client's culture are critical throughout the client's hospital stay and are always considered when teaching, although people are individuals within their cultures and should not be stereotyped. Instead, pertinent questions are asked to gain cultural information and individualize care. The client's culture should always be valued and respected. However, if a cultural practice seems truly unsafe in view of the client's condition, this should be discussed with the client and family.

There are some cultures in which it is considered protective of the client to be relieved of the burden of information and decision making. In these cultures, conferences are usually held with family leaders, such as the oldest or most educated child or the family as a whole. The client and family are asked their preferences. It is good nursing practice to have regular discussions with clients when they are alone, if at all possible, so that if they have an opinion or want to give information that is not acceptable to the family, they are able to do so. For example, the family may believe that pain and suffering are important in order to atone for sins or to gain entrance into heaven, while the client may not agree.

Sometimes, nurses who have not had cultural discussions with clients and families are frustrated in their attempts to teach or provide care. For example, nurses caring for an older Hispanic woman were frustrated when attempting to teach her the skills she would need to care for herself after discharge. She seemed totally disinterested and did not pay attention. What they learned, after discussion with a Hispanic nurse, was that the woman's daughters and daughters-in-law were expected

Think About It

My grandmother developed a lump on her right breast in 1994. She was 68 and had never been sick enough to ever go to the doctor! It is amazing to find that a woman who has never had any health problems could develop such a deadly disease. The whole ordeal was a very strange and scary process. She does not speak English and she has never been to the doctor, so after her second visit to the internist, her diagnosis was made and she was instructed to go have an MRI, CT, more x-rays, and blood work. This was exhausting and scary for her. Thank God that we could be here to support her through this. She had a mastectomy and they also tried to insert a port, but when she was younger, she had a broken collar bone that healed incorrectly, because she never went to the doctor for it. Since the port was not feasible, the doctor decided to wait and see how she was progressing before talking to us again about chemotherapy. Throughout all of this, my grandmother prayed and asked us a lot of questions about the procedures and what was next. She came through fine and did not have to have chemotherapy or radiation. She is on oral medications and is doing great. She has a whole new outlook on her life and her health, and so does the rest of the family. The doctor said she would probably end up outliving him (and he was a fairly young doctor!) It seems to amaze me every time I think about it, that she went through all of these procedures and surgery when she had never even gone to the doctor for anything in her life. She has a lot of courage and a great will to live. She has taught me a lot about the human spirit.
Written by Dipa Triveti, a junior nursing student in a gerontology class.

to be responsible for her care and intended to do so. As a result, the client did not feel a need for any knowledge about self-care.

In some cultures, adults believe that their duty to parents supercedes duty to spouse and children. Although that is not usually the case, they may leave a spouse or child in need to care for an ill parent. Discussing this issue with cultural or religious leaders is helpful. They can discuss the situation with the family and help to ensure safe care of all family members.

Care During Hospitalization

The staff strives to provide high-quality, individualized care, which, when many of the current staffing levels are analyzed, seems to be impossible. Nurses and other health care providers need to be articulate and informed so that they can justify adequate staffing levels in a context that administration and HMO providers can understand. Older adults have special needs to consider. One frequently encountered problem resulting from low staffing is long waits for call lights to be answered. For older adults, as well as for other clients, the failure to answer call lights in a timely manner is one of the most distressing aspects of the hospitalization and can lead to unnecessary problems, particularly falls and incontinence. Nurses should be advocates for staffing patterns that are adequate to meet the needs of their clients and to ensure that the attitudes and work patterns of the staff also meet those needs.

Commonly Encountered Problems

Regardless of diagnosis, there are problems that are common to older adults in the hospital setting. These include the following:

- Altered mental status: orientation, cognition, confusion

- Anxiety

- Safety: oxygen precautions, falls, **restraints**, swallowing difficulties

- Potential **hazards of immobility**

- Potential **dehydration** or fluid and electrolyte imbalance

- Potential drug interactions and adverse effects

- Absence or masking of standard symptoms of complications

- Potential for infection

- Possible drug and alcohol **withdrawal**

- Altered comfort

Altered Mental Status: Orientation, Cognition, and Confusion

When the environment changes, older adults are vulnerable to **delirium** (confusion). When factors such as pain, disease, stress, drug therapies and interactions, dehydration, electrolyte imbalance, altered light-dark cycle, and near-constant noxious stimuli are added, confusion increases during hospitalization. Antipsychotic drugs often are used to treat confusion and behaviorial changes in the older adult. This may result in further cognitive deficits. A clear cause for the behavior should always be sought, rather than simply administering another drug (Semia, Beizer, & Higbee, 1997).

Many nonpharmacological interventions can be effective for the prevention or management of confusion or disorientation. Older adults should be placed in a quiet, private room with a window when possible. This minimizes the effect of a roommate who is awake and noisy all night, constant alarms and equipment noises, the lack of a normal light-dark cycle, and misinterpretation of environmental stimuli. Contrary to popular practice, the TV should NOT be left on all the time in the name of stimulation. Actually, many older adults dislike TV or consider it an annoyance; in this case, the TV would add to the person's stress. Confused clients may believe that whatever is happening on the TV is happening in their environment and that they are in danger. Others have a few favorite programs, which should be provided when possible. Some like soft music from a favorite radio station. Some gain comfort from a tape recorder and favorite tapes or tapes of family members' voices. Many clients are far more comfortable when a family member or friend is in the room with them (Figure 15-4). As much as possible, this should be encouraged rather than discouraged by restrictive visiting rules. Both the client and the family member will be more comfortable when they are together. The family members or friends should be encouraged to touch and talk to the client and to participate in care if they wish to do so.

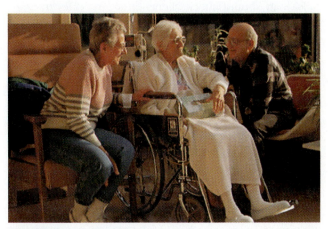

FIGURE 15-4 Family members should be encouraged to spend time with clients during an acute care hospitalization.

A clock and a calendar that is current and large enough for clients to read also are helpful. However, it is unrealistic to expect anyone always to be oriented to day and time after a few days of hospitalization. They should, however, remain oriented to the larger environment, such as month, year, city, and who is president, if they were oriented prior to the hospitalization. Disoriented clients should be reoriented frequently, with a gentle rather than an argumentative manner: "Mr. Jones, you are in Germ-Free Memorial Hospital after a bicycle accident. You can't move because your leg is in traction. I'm your nurse, Juan Gonzales. Your wife, Mary, is sitting right here beside you. Today is Tuesday. It's a beautiful fall day." Unless the client has a hearing deficit, it is not necessary to speak loudly to communicate with a confused or unresponsive client because this may cause aggressive behaviors.

Safety

Safety is a critical concern for older hospital clients. There are many ways for them to be unsafe. Clients may need to get up to go to the bathroom and climb out of bed, either because their need is urgent, their call light is not answered promptly, they forgot how to use the call light or dropped it or it was not left within reach, they forgot they were not at home, or they are embarrassed to ask for assistance for such personal needs.

Falls and Restraints

If the side rails are up, the client may climb over them or the end of the bed and fall or become lodged between the side rails and the mattress. If the older client is extremely confused, climbing out of bed, wandering, and at extremely high risk for injury, hospital personnel often restrain them. Restraints should be avoided whenever possible. Beds should be kept in low position (although this is still too high for very short people) and only the top side rails raised whenever possible, so that if clients do get up, they will not fall further because of the high rails. Staff should check clients often and offer to assist them to the bathroom when needed. If night safety is a chronic problem, a sitter or family member may need to stay with the client to prevent falls. Some units have video monitors for clients who may be unsafe, but this is not much help in the middle of the night if no one is at the desk watching the monitors. Bed alarms can be very useful in alerting the staff if the client attempts to get up. There are also chair alarms that may be used during the day when the client is up in a chair or wheelchair. Bed and chair alarms are pads that are placed under the client and which set off an audible alarm if the client's weight is removed. Auditing charts and tracking the time of day and/or causes of attempting to get out of bed without assistance can be useful. One client in a nursing home fell and broke his hip at 3 AM. A chart audit showed that on four different occasions in the three weeks prior to the fall, he had been found caught in the side rails or climbing out of bed between 2:30 and 4 AM. This should have been occasion for intensive observation and a fall prevention protocol. In reality, safety was not even included as a problem on his care plan and no precautions or special observations were documented. His family was never advised of the problem either.

When there is constant or severe wandering or the client is so confused as to be unsafe when left alone, the Vail Bed is quite useful. This looks like an adult crib, the sides and top of which are covered with sturdy netting (Figure 15-5). It is said that from the inside, the netting tends to fade out and not be perceived as a barrier. Clients can move about as much as they want to in this bed, but they cannot climb out, fall out, or become entangled. Though the Vail Bed can be useful to provide safety and establish boundaries for confused and disoriented clients, it should not be used for those who are oriented.

Wheelchair safety is another problem. There are trays, bars, and lap buddies that can be placed across the arm rests to prevent the client from sliding forward or getting out of the chair. Sometimes, seat belts are used. As mentioned earlier, seat alarms may be helpful. Vest restraints, though commonly used, are dangerous, whether used in a bed or wheelchair. Clients can and do get out of them; those who try but do not succeed can become entangled and choke to death in the restraint. They can slump to the side and remain in uncomfortable positions for long periods of time. Clients can get their hands and feet caught in wheelchair spokes, especially if they lack sensation or proprioception. Pads and bolsters can be used to sup-

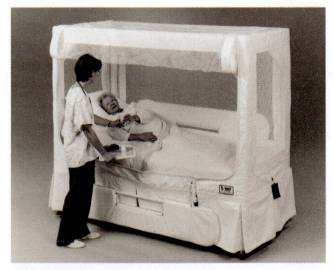

FIGURE 15-5 The Vail Bed is a safety strategy for a very confused client. *(Photo courtesy of Vail Products, Inc.)*

port them in proper alignment. Appropriate measures should be utilized to keep hands and feet safe.

The need for any mechanical or chemical restraint (sedating with drugs specifically to control movement or behavior) must be well documented and a physician's order secured. There should be a protocol for reevaluating the need for the restraint at frequent intervals and securing new orders or discontinuing the restraints at that time. Restraints are used much too routinely, especially in the ICU as a precaution against pulling out tubes and lines. Even clients who are sedated and/or paralyzed are often restrained. Many clients have enough self-control to leave tubes and lines alone without restraints. Others can be kept just as safe with the application of commercial mitts filled with batting or soft elbow restraints. The use of either of these allows the client freedom of movement, which promotes comfort and more sense of self-control and is much more conducive to frequent turning and repositioning of the client. Some clients who have been restrained have spoken not only about how confined and victimized they felt but also of how embarrassed they were for visitors to see them "tied down to the bed." American hospitals need to commit to a restraint-free environment.

Another safety precaution is the use of shoes when older adults get up while in the hospital. Slippers that fit loosely or may shift or fall off or which have slick soles can lead to falls. The older adult should wear well-fitting shoes with nonskid soles and with socks whenever getting up in order to help prevent accidental falls. Shoe soles should also be of a nonstick variety to prevent falls. Rails on the walls of the bathroom and corridors are of great assistance in fall prevention. A client's fall risk should be assessed on admission and updated as necessary with this information as well as precautions to be taken and the information clearly noted in the care plan.

Oxygen Precautions

Many older adults use oxygen, either continuously or on an as-needed basis. Safety precautions should be emphasized. Clients should not smoke while using oxygen and should be monitored to ensure that this precaution is being followed. In addition, tubing should not be so long that they become entangled in it and fall. Staff must monitor whether oxygen tanks are full or not.

Swallowing Precautions

In acute care settings, the most frequent diagnosis of clients referred for speech pathology evaluation is dysphagia. Generally, it is thought that dysphagia exists in about 12% of the overall hospitalized population and is twice that in stroke clients (Horner & Massey, 1991). Gordon, Hewer, and Wade (1987) further demonstrated that older stroke clients are at particularly high risk

for dysphagia and consequent **aspiration** and pneumonia. A particular older adult may have more than one problem that contributes to dysphagia and resulting aspiration.

The threshold for the cough reflex is much higher for older adults than for younger ones. This decreased cough sensitivity could help explain the high occurrence of aspiration in the neurologically impaired or sedated older adults, although it has not been shown to occur in healthy older adults (Matteson, McConnell, & Linton, 1997; Pontoppidan & Beecher, 1960). Unfortunately, dysphagia may not be recognized until the client aspirates and develops a subsequent pneumonia. Although no statistics are available, a casual review of weak and neurological clients in rehabilitation facilities shows that a high percentage of them aspirated prior to arriving in rehabilitation. Often, no effort is made to evaluate swallowing in the hospital setting; rather it is left for the rehabilitation facility. Box 15-1 details signs of swallowing disorders for which the nurse should be alert.

Some of the causes of dysphagia in older adults include:

- *Physical changes:* dentures (having them, needing them, or having some that fit poorly); even if dentures fit well, it takes much longer to chew with them than with teeth, which slows the eating process (Hogstel & Robinson, 1989); inability to see the food or fluid; inability to hold cups, glasses, silverware or to place the food or fluid in the mouth properly because of arthritis, pain, weakness, and other problems with the hands and arms.

- *Neurological conditions:* stroke, **Parkinson's disease**, amyotrophic lateral sclerosis (ALS), multiple sclerosis, brain tumors, head trauma, and other neurological disorders (Horner & Massey, 1991); altered **gag reflex**, altered taste, sensation, or ability to manipulate the mouth and tongue; diminished level of consciousness or cognitive changes that reduce the ability to understand and follow directions to chew and swallow; the client is too weak to use a straw or to chew and swallow; impairment from alcohol or drug use; from medications, anesthesia, or local anesthesia to mouth and throat.

- *Other causes:* overfilling of the stomach because of constipation or reduced intestinal peristalsis; neoplasms of any area of the gastrointestinal (GI) tract that may lead to food intolerance, early satiety, or esophageal strictures; diminished secretion of saliva or general dehydration; dilated esophagus, decreased esophageal peristalsis, or **hiatal hernia**, which is most common in older

BOX 15-1   Signs of Possible Swallowing Disorders

Subjective and/or objective difficulty in swallowing:
- Not being able to swallow or having difficulty with certain types of food or fluid

- Choking or coughing after meals that is often accompanied by watering eyes

- Difficulty initiating a swallow

- Multiple swallows—must swallow foods or pills repeatedly

- Complaints of pain or discomfort when swallowing

Excessive secretions:
- Significant drooling during mealtime or even when not eating

- Hoarse, wet, breathy, or weak voice quality

Signs of actual or potential difficulty manipulating mouth and/or tongue:
- Slurred speech or difficulty in speaking

- Solid material remaining on the tongue or palate after swallowing

- Clears throat frequently

- Decreased tongue mobility

- Facial weakness

- Decreased gag reflex (do not check the gag reflex if client cannot swallow or cough spontaneously; if he vomits, he may aspirate)

- Impaired sensitivity in mouth or face

- Chronic respiratory distress

Miscellaneous:
- Clients who have a functional cough can still aspirate.

- Self-report of dysphagia or the lack of it may not be accurate: studies show a lack of relationship between complaints of food caught in the throat and residue found on videofluoroscopy. When in doubt, the video fluoroscopy should be done.

- Many clients aspirate silently, without symptoms; two-thirds of stroke clients in one study were found to have silent aspiration.

- Lack of interest in or refusal to eat and drink.

- Signs that aspiration may have occurred: respiratory distress, pneumonia, wheezing, stridor, and coughing, dehydration or malnutrition of unknown cause, fever of unknown origin.

Adapted from Rapp (1997); Cole-Arvin, Notich, & Underhill (1994); Horner & Massey (1988); and Lugger (1994).

obese females (Hogstel & Robinson, 1989); adverse effects of many drugs (Rapp, 1997); poor positioning (eating and drinking while lying down or in a semireclining position is a prescription for choking); fatigue; pain; weakness; and diminished cognitive status or coordination related to medication.

When admitting a client, a mini–nutrition assessment should be completed. If the client has lost a great deal of weight or is chronically very thin, a discussion of possible reasons for this problem should be instituted. The client or family may describe particular eating or swallowing problems. The nurse should be alert to the presence of conditions that could cause dysphagia and aspiration **[cerebral vascular accident (CVA, stroke)**, Parkinson's disease, **Guillain-Barré syndrome]**, or drug therapy (Table 15-1). Any client who is at high risk for dysphagia should be evaluated by a speech language pathologist prior to feeding.

No single plan for managing all dysphagia is possible or appropriate (Lugger, 1994). However, the general guidelines in Boxes 15-2 and 15-3 can be helpful.

The speech language pathologist can recommend specific techniques to enhance the ability to swallow and prevent aspiration in individual clients. These recommendations should be followed meticulously. One technique often used to control the consistency of food and fluids is presented. Semisoft foods, such as applesauce, scrambled eggs, oatmeal, and pudding, are much easier to chew and swallow than either liquids such as water or solids such as meat, bread, and vegetables. The therapist can recommend the best consistency for a particular client. There is a product called Thick-It that when added to any fluid—such as water or juice—causes the consistency to become thicker so that the client can swallow it more easily. The usual terminology for specification of fluid consistency includes *nectar* (as thick as commercially prepared fruit nectars), *honey* (as thick as honey), and *pudding* (as thick as pudding). Thick-It must be added to the liquid and stirred in well immediately prior to drinking and should be used for all fluids consumed, including those used to take medications. If Thick-It is unavailable, instant potatoes, tapioca, or baby cereal may be used as a substitute thickener (Killen, 1996).

TABLE 15-1 Drugs That May Affect Swallowing and Their Effects

Symptoms	Drugs Which May Cause the Symptoms
Dry mouth	Anticholinergics (Bentyl, Donnatal)
	Antihistamines (Benadryl, Antivert, Phenergan, Sominex)
	Tricyclic antidepressants (Elavil, Sinequan, Pamelor)
	Minor tranquilizers (Valium, Atarax, Librium)
	Antihypertensives (Catapres)
Increased salivation	Cholinergics (Pilocarpine, Miotics for glaucoma)
Anorexia	Antineoplastic agents (chemotherapy)
	Sympathomimetic agents (nasal decongestants)
	Antibiotics; digitalis or theophylline toxicity
Heartburn, gastric distress	Antiemetics (Vontrol, Tigan)
	Aspirin
	Antidiabetic drugs (Dymelor, Diabeta, Glucatrol)
	Taking theophyllines or steroids on an empty stomach
	Possible systemic effects of steroid therapy
Nausea and vomiting	Antineoplastic agents (chemotherapy)
	Oral iron or potassium preparations
	Estrogens
	Sulfonamides
	Antibiotics
	Toxicity: digitalis, theophyllines
Dyspepsia (uncomfortable feeling of fullness)	Nonsteroidal anti-inflammatory drugs
	Diuretics
	Antihypertensives
Stomatitis (mouth pain and ulcers) or thrush (candidiasis of the mouth)	Antineoplastic drugs (chemotherapy)
	Sulfonamides
	Aspirin
	Dilantin (phenytoin)
	Penicillin allergic reaction
	Steroids, especially if inhaled without rinsing mouth afterward
Gum and mouth bleeding	Anticoagulants (Coumadin, Heparin, Lovenox)
	Aspirin
	Antineoplastic agents (chemotherapy)
Gum swelling	Dilantin (phenytoin)
Abnormal taste	Antineoplastic agents (chemotherapy)
	Antithyroid preparations
	Catapres (clonidine)
	Proventil (albuterol) and many other inhaled drugs

Adapted from Rapp (1997).

BOX 15-2   Foods to Avoid When Clients Have Difficulty Swallowing

- Food with skin (corn, tomatoes, grapes)
- Stringy foods (greens, okra)
- Fibrous foods (cabbage, lettuce)
- Gelatin (jello)
- Grainy foods (rice, uncooked oats)
- Foods with seeds (tomatoes, squash, cucumbers)
- Breads (dry, crackers, toast)
- Crunchy, textured foods (bacon, jerky, popcorn, crackers, pickles, relish, dry cereals, pizza)
- Hard candy, raisins, onions, broccoli, nuts, coconut, M & M's, olives
- Chewing gum
- Some fruits (raw or fresh, oranges, apples)
- Sticky foods (peanut butter)
- Eggs
- Foods that may liquify in the mouth and choke client (ice cream, other frozen treats)

Adapted from Rapp (1997) and Killen (1996).

BOX 15-3   General Rules for Safe Feeding of Clients at High Risk for Choking or Aspirating

- Sit the client up (preferably in a chair) for eating and drinking and for 1–2 hours afterward.
- Always follow the directions of the speech language pathologist.
- Many can swallow more easily if the head is supported at midline and flexed slightly forward while eating.
- Be sure the client is as awake and rested as much as possible prior to eating and drinking.
- Provide oral hygiene before and after eating.
- Be sure dentures are in place and stable prior to feeding.
- Avoid using straws for liquids unless specifically ordered by the speech language pathologist.
- If the client is self-feeding, supervise eating and drinking when an aspiration risk or diminished cognitive status exists.
- Choose foods of suitable consistency.
- Feed slowly. Provide very small bites, consistencies that the client can chew and swallow, and finger foods if the client can handle them.
- Encourage thorough chewing before swallowing.
- Do not force-feed clients.
- Do not feed with a syringe.
- Use liquid oral medications rather than tablets or capsules as much as possible.
- Be certain the client is able to swallow pills if they are ordered. If pills are to be crushed and placed in pudding, applesauce, or ice cream, check to be certain that it is safe to crush the pill or open the capsule. Never crush or open sustained-release or enteric coated medications.
- Choose foods the client likes.
- Avoid distractions while eating to allow the client to concentrate on chewing and swallowing.
- Avoid milk products if the client has thick secretions; milk thickens secretions.

When clients are simply too weak to eat and drink, they may be enabled to do so by using other techniques instead of or in addition to those mentioned in Box 15-3. One technique is using a spoon to place very small amounts of liquid or pureed foods in the mouth. The nurse or aide should be certain that each bite is swallowed before placing more food in the mouth. Those with extreme cognitive impairment sometimes retain their sucking reflex and can be given an adequate diet per spoon without resorting to tube feedings. Sucking on a straw requires some coordination and effort: Extremely weak clients can often take fluids more easily if fluid is placed in a small spouted or sipper cup and held to their lips. Above all, the nurse must be prepared to spend time with the client.

Potential Hazards of Immobility

Older adults are especially prone to the hazards of immobility. It does not take very long, when the client is ill, in bed, medicated, and nutritionally depleted, for the client to decondition and develop any or all of the following problems: skin breakdown or pressure ulcers, constipation, thrombi, **atelectasis** and even hypostatic pneumonia, and **contractures**. Nurses should utilize all of the skills that they learned in basic nursing classes to prevent these complications in a manner that is individualized to the client (see Table 15-2).

Potential Dehydration and Fluid and Electrolyte Imbalance

As people age, body composition changes, though it cannot be specified exactly how much it changes for each individual. Regardless, older adults are at higher risk for complications related to dehydration.

Many factors during hospitalization contribute to dehydration in older adults. Clients may be unable to ingest an adequate amount of fluids for many reasons, the most obvious of which is problems related to the gastrointestinal tract: surgery, trauma, and nausea after anesthesia. Another problem that contributes to dehydration in older adults is the diagnostic tests they are undergoing and the necessary related protocols. For example, a client may be scheduled for diagnostic tests over a period of several days. The client is NPO (allowed no oral intake) for the first test. Upon returning to bed, the client is exhausted or food and fluid are not provided so the client misses a meal or two and does not drink very much. For the next day, a clean intestinal tract is required, so the client receives laxatives or enemas. The NPO status is resumed, the test is done, and the client is again exhausted and eats and drinks very little. This may go on for several days, until the client is extremely dehydrated, laboratory values are skewed [increased sodium and blood-urea-nitrogen (BUN); increased hematocrit], **postural hypotension** develops, and cognitive status becomes impaired. One outcome is that the client faints, falls, and breaks a hip. Nurses must pay close attention to the hydration status of older clients and not assume that because food and fluid are available, they are being ingested. Besides monitoring intake and urinary output, cognitive status, and signs of dizziness upon arising, laboratory values are helpful. When a client is becoming overhydrated, sodium and hematocrit decrease.

TABLE 15-2	Hazards of Immobility
Problem	**Preventive Measures That Should be Individualized to the Client**
Skin breakdown	Complete a skin risk assessment scale at admission and according to protocols thereafter; sheets dry and tight; appropriate mattress for skin condition; no crumbs or particles in bed; turn and move client often; move carefully; avoid skin shearing; check pressure points often; keep heels supported and off bed; place pillows between knees, ankles, other bony prominences; apply appropriate strengthening or cushioning products to reddened, intact skin or protocols for other stages of breakdown; mobilize as soon as possible (ASAP).
Atelectasis	Turn and move client often; mobilize ASAP; cough and deep breathe often, especially after general anesthesia; encourage fluids; discourage smoking; frequent respiratory assessment.
Constipation	Mobilize ASAP; check and record stools; regular abdominal assessments and monitoring of food intake; seeking reasons for nausea, reflux, or complaints of feeling extremely full; institute bowel protocols if client goes more than 3 days without a stool or if taking drugs that promote constipation, such as opioids, antidepressants, or iron; encourage fluids to tolerance; encourage bulk and natural laxative foods to tolerance; obtain orders for GI stimulants as indicated (Reglan, Propulsid).
Contractures	Gentle ROM (range-of-motion) exercises several times daily: passive when necessary and active when possible. Encourage generalized active movement of all extremities. Self-care activities such as brushing the hair can encourage arm and shoulder motion. Use measures to promote extremities always being in a position of function (hand and wrist splints, foam boots or high-top tennis shoes on feet, hand rolls), use of passive-motion devices as ordered after joint replacement surgeries or similar problems.
Thrombi	Position to prevent pressure on extremities; monitor legs for signs/symptoms of deep vein thrombosis (DVT) or thrombi; elastic hose that fit (remove for 1 hour 2–3 times daily), sequential foot or leg massage devices.
Deconditioning	Mobilize ASAP; exercise with light weights or whatever activity can be done to improve cardiopulmonary fitness and muscle conditioning.

Potential Drug Interactions and Adverse Effects

Older clients develop physiological changes that alter drug absorption, distribution, metabolism, excretion, sensitivity, and response. An acute illness may exacerbate these changes: for instance, liver trauma or disease would magnify already existing drug detoxification problems in an older client. Many older adults are protein depleted and have low albumin levels. Because many of the drugs they might receive are lipid soluble and protein bound, increased sensitivity and a prolonged response to the drugs would be expected (Lee & Burnett, 1998). If these problems were not enough, older adults are often excellent candidates for polypharmacy—the administration of many drugs concurrently. The metabolism, actions, and interactions of the drugs may cause further problems. Drug administration should be kept to essential drugs. A high percentage of drug orders for hospitalized clients are PRN (as needed) orders. Therefore, the nurse has a major responsibility with regard to what drugs are administered. The nurse should check interactions and compatibilities and note contraindications because the older adult may have some contraindicating condition to a drug that would otherwise be an excellent drug for another problem or condition. There are some drug texts available that discuss drug therapy for the older adults specifically, but most still do not. The physician, nurse, and pharmacist are required to learn as much as possible about the known effects of a particular drug in older adults *before* it is ordered and administered. A general rule of thumb is to start low and go slow. Drug doses may need to be lower than for younger adults or intervals between administration longer. Because older adults are often more sensitive to the effects of drugs, they may develop symptoms of toxic effects before the highest therapeutic drugs levels are reached. It is essential to monitor responses to drugs and associated laboratory values, such as liver and renal function, as well as therapeutic drug levels in order to prevent toxicities from occurring.

Absence or Masking of Standard Symptoms of Problems or Complications

Older adults often do not display the same signs and symptoms of disease, injury, or complications as younger people do. It is therefore essential for those caring for older adults to be familiar with common differences in presentation. For example, the middle-aged person with pneumonia might display a cough, sputum production, and chest discomfort caused by the excessive coughing. It is not uncommon for an older client to have none of these pneumonia symptoms, although a chest x-ray would show pneumonia just as severe as that of the younger person. The first symptom of pneumonia in an older adult may be altered cognitive status, confusion, or even loss of consciousness resulting from hypoxia. As a result, the person may be subjected to a variety of neurological tests prior to a chest x-ray. This increases the cost of care, the discomfort, and the length of time before definitive diagnosis is available and proper treatment begun.

Older adults may show atypical signs of myocardial infarcts. This is especially true if they are women or members of some ethnic groups. Myocardial infarcts may cause no symptoms (silent heart attack) or atypical symptoms, a few of which might be pain only in the back, shoulder, arm, jaw, abdomen, or diminished level of consciousness caused by cerebral **hypoxemia** (Hawkins, Kwentus, & Price, 1990) or severe gastrointestinal symptoms such as nausea and vomiting.

It is widely believed that the classic sign of appendicitis is rebound tenderness at **McBurney's point** in the right lower quadrant of the abdomen. However, the very old and the very young often do not have this sign. Rather, their appendicitis symptoms may be those of diffuse, nonspecific gastrointestinal distress. This phenomenon is a major factor in subsequent rupture of the appendix of the very old and the very young.

The normal body temperature of older adults is often low compared to that of younger persons. It is extremely helpful to know the client's norm. Older adults often develop only subtle temperature elevations, if any, when ill. An oral temperature of 99°F or 100°F in an older adult whose normal is between 96°F and 97°F or who is immunosuppressed should be cause for serious appraisal of possible sources of infection.

The fact that someone is older complicates any diagnosis. Regardless of the diagnosis or number of comorbidities, the older client is more likely to develop complications, heal more slowly, or even die from a given acute event.

> ### Nursing Tip
>
> Many older adults do not present typical symptoms of disease; as a result, they are often undiagnosed until the problem is well advanced. For example, since older adults often have a subnormal temperature, a temperature of 99°F may constitute a fever. However, if the temperature is not being monitored, the skin is cool, and any other symptoms are nonspecific and mild or vague, the illness may be unrecognized. Even subtle symptoms in older adults should alert health care providers to the possible presence of illness. Many problems mimic what is commonly believed to be normal aging.

Potential for Infection

One result of aging is lowered general immunity. Along with that, the person may be taking drugs, such as steroids, or have chronic conditions, such as diabetes, that reduce immunity. Older adults are more likely to develop skin tears and other breaks in the body's protective mechanisms. As a result, the potential for infection is magnified. Caregivers should always be aware of the risks and strive to prevent infection by such methods as the use of strict aseptic technique; avoiding the use of products that may damage the tissues; taking great care to avoid skin tears from tape or other products; protecting skin tears promptly with products such as gel patches; using commercial pads and protective products on reddened skin as well as effective but gentle commercial products for perineal care; avoiding the use of harsh soaps; and using appropriate overlays and mattresses on beds. If the person has reduced perfusion or sensation of the legs and feet, as many older adults do, it is critical to avoid injury by avoiding heating pads, testing water temperatures prior to bathing, using only well-fitting shoes with socks, having a qualified person carefully cut toenails, and preventing injury such as dangling extremities in wheelchairs. The skin should be thoroughly inspected on a daily basis to recognize an actual or potential injury as early as possible and treat it before it becomes a more complicated problem or focus of injury and/or infection.

One of the most common causes of infection in older adults is the indwelling urinary catheter. In the hospital, catheters are typically inserted at the first sign of problems without a thorough analysis of why a problem is occurring or if the catheter can be avoided. A nonsymptomatic finding of bacteria on a culture probably should not be treated with antibiotics. If older adults have documented, symptomatic urinary tract infections, the infection should be treated rather than a catheter inserted because of incontinence. Males who are incontinent can often wear external catheters and avoid indwelling ones. Even before that, a urinal should be offered to men and the women offered a bedpan or preferably be assisted to the commode on a regular basis (every 2–3 hours). These measures alone may be enough to keep them dry. If not, the nursing staff can maintain records of the times the client is found wet for 24–48 hours. People void on predictable schedules. The nurse can avoid incontinence by offering the opportunity to urinate about one-half hour prior to usual voiding times. If a catheter is absolutely necessary, it should be in place for as short a time as possible. The insertion site should be washed well with soap and water at least twice daily.

Potential Drug and Alcohol Withdrawal

The number of older adults who use alcohol (and perhaps illegal or prescription drugs to excess) is higher than is generally believed. Often, the family is unaware of how much alcohol, tranquilizers, antidepressants, pain relief

medications, or illegal drugs are being consumed by the older adult. Sometimes, the client has been medicating with alternative or over-the-counter drugs or drugs obtained in another country, the discontinuation of which can cause withdrawal symptoms. All drugs that cause withdrawal symptoms are not harmful drugs in themselves. For example, if a person who is steroid dependent (on steroids regularly for several weeks or months) is not continued on the drugs and/or given a bolus of steroids in a time of physiological crisis, the client can develop a steroid crisis and die. Clients who chronically take drugs that must not be stopped abruptly should wear **medical alert bracelets** or necklaces for their own protection in case they cannot give health information to a caregiver. Wallet cards are not as effective because they may not be found until too late, if they are found at all.

A person whose body is dependent on alcohol or certain drugs can develop troublesome or even critical symptoms. Any development of new symptoms after a day or two in the hospital should not automatically be assumed to be the result of the client's acute condition or its treatment. The possibility of drug or alcohol withdrawal should always be considered, investigated, and treated appropriately.

Some antihypertensive drugs should not be discontinued abruptly. When certain antihypertensive drugs are abruptly withdrawn, the client can develop serious symptoms of withdrawal, which include but are not limited to extremely high blood pressure, altered level of consciousness or behavior, **delirium tremens (DTs)**, cardiac arrhythmias, or even death. One client on clonidine (Catapres) was advised by his rural physician to stop all of his drugs prior to going to the large city hospital for cardiac surgery. No one told the surgeon. After the surgery, the client's blood pressure rose rapidly and was extremely difficult to control for many days. Fortunately, the client survived, but he could have ruptured his coronary grafts due to the extremely high blood pressure or had a myocardial infarct because of the increased work load.

Alcoholics who are abruptly discontinued from alcohol tend to develop serious psychological hyperactivity (DTs) within a few days. If the staff is unaware of the alcoholism, the first sign may be when the client does something injurious to himself (such as pulling out intravenous lines or dismantling balanced traction). To prevent DTs, alcohol can be given to many seriously ill clients. It can even be given intravenously if there is no way to give it orally or by feeding tube. However, for many clients, the administration of alcohol is contraindicated by their condition. In this case, intramuscular chlordiazepoxide (Librium) is the drug of choice to prevent or lessen the possibility of DTs. For some reason, oral Librium does not seem to work as well. Librium is also available as an intravenous preparation.

Altered Comfort

One of the common adverse outcomes of hospitalization of older adults is discomfort or pain. Ignoring or undertreating pain in older adults is not unusual. The most frequently reported causes of chronic pain in older adults are arthritis and neuralgias (Helme, Katz, Gibson, & Corran, 1989). Although everyone should have a right to adequate pain relief (Box 15-4), there is significant evidence that pain in older adults is inadequately managed or not managed at all. At least 40%–80% of community-dwelling and 15%–30% of institutionalized individuals have been reported to receive no treatment for pain, although more than 70% of the nursing home residents report having significant pain, while 33% report constant pain (Ferrell, 1991; Ferrell, Ferrell, & Osterwell 1990). One-fourth to one-half of the noninstitutionalized persons over 60 who were surveyed reported pain (Ferrell et al., 1990).

Barriers to Pain Management

There are many possible reasons for undertreatment of pain in older adults. When they have pain, they may not report it for many reasons: They may fear that the disease process is progressing or that pain is a normal part of aging. They may fear expensive or painful diagnostic tests to evaluate the cause of the pain. They may desire to be "good" clients and not bother caregivers or to avoid distracting their physicians from treating the causative problem. They may believe that everything possible has been done or that nothing can be done for the pain. They may be unaware that control of their pain is possible. Often, they fear **addiction, dependence**, or the side effects of pain medications. They may be unable to use the pain questionnaires that are provided, or they may fear that the medication will be ineffective

later, when it is needed more. Some do not use the term *pain* but may use other terms such as hurt, pressure, twinge, tiring, exhausting, nagging, annoying, or worrisome. Thus, when they are asked about pain, they deny it (Pitorak, 1998) and nurses do not probe further.

Older adults also are at risk for undertreatment because of a lack of knowledge and experience of the clinicians that are managing their pain. Most pain research has been conducted on young adults, so clear data on pain in older adults is minimal at best. Many clinicians use their own beliefs about pain in older adults as fact when managing pain (Wallace, 1994). Some professionals believe that older adults are less sensitive to pain, that they are adversely affected by pain medications, or that complaints of pain reflect emotional disorders. Age-associated changes in pain sensation have not been documented (Ferrell, 1991). Some believe that previous experience with pain makes it easier to bear; actually the opposite is true. Health professionals often have an inadequate appreciation of the possibility of relieving pain in older adults and may even criticize the protocols or dosages that are used appropriately to relieve severe pain. Some believe that all pain has a clear, identifiable, documentable cause. This is not the case. Sometimes, the cause of the pain is never clearly identified. The search for and identification of the cause of pain should not delay its treatment.

Issues and Terminology Related to Pain Management

Addiction, tolerance, and withdrawal are commonly cited rationales for failure to attempt to relieve pain adequately. These phenomena are generally misunderstood and inappropriately used. Addiction refers to drug-seeking behaviors. There are two paths for pain medications in the body. One is the pleasure path, which applies to those who are using drugs for pleasure in the absence of pain. Seeking the drug and its resulting "high" becomes the consuming activity of their lives—they forego food and care of themselves and their children and are willing to prostitute themselves, commit crimes, and do just about anything else to obtain drugs. When people who are in pain take pain relief medications, the drugs act on the pain path. Instead of demonstrating pain behaviors such as irritability, inability to work or care for children, or inability to move, the pain medication gives them their personality and lifestyle back. They are now able to work, provide child care, and have their usual personality. The drug does not give them a high or cause them to commit crime to obtain it. **Pseudoaddiction** is the term for the person whose pain is inadequately relieved and who is actively seeking relief, either by requesting medication frequently or by changing physicians and pharmacies. They may display decreased socialization, sleep disturbance, increased

---

BOX 15-4 Bill of Rights for Persons with Pain

- I have the right to have my pain believed by health professionals, family, friends, and others around me.

- I have the right to have my pain controlled, no matter what its cause or how severe it may be.

- I have the right to be treated with respect at all times. When I need medication for pain, I should not be treated like a drug abuser.

- I have the right to have pain resulting from treatments and procedures prevented or at least minimized.

Adapted from the Wisconsin Pain Initiative (undated).

health care utilization, deconditioning, gait disturbances, falls, slow rehabilitation, polypharmacy, cognitive dysfunction, malnutrition, and poor quality of life (Ferrell, 1991). When relief is obtained, these behaviors cease.

Physical dependence to many drugs develops when the drugs are administered on a long-term basis to relieve pain. This is no different from the dependence that results when steroids or certain antihypertensives are administered as described in the drug withdrawal section earlier in this chapter. Having a withdrawal response to analgesics does *not* mean that the person is addicted. It is an expected physiological phenomenon. Tapering drug doses when pain has been relieved can prevent withdrawal reactions. In any case, dependence will not develop unless the pain and the need for pain medication are prolonged. It will not occur in short-term situations.

Tolerance may occur if a pain medication is needed for a long time—perhaps after a major trauma that takes many months to heal. Tolerance does not develop quickly. If it does develop, the dose of the drug may be increased safely. It is important to recognize that the most common reasons for needing increased drug doses are undertreatment of pain and progression of or complications of the disease—not tolerance or dependence. The fear of developing tolerance or dependence should not be a rationale for withholding adequate pain relief (Woodin, 1993).

Consequences of Poor Pain Management

There are many consequences of poor pain management: Clients whose pain is not adequately relieved may refuse to or be unable to turn, move, and ambulate, thus slowing their recovery. They may be irritable and uncooperative, exhausted from lack of rest, depressed, or even suicidal. They may demonstrate signs of pseudo-addiction and "hop" from doctor to doctor or use whatever drugs they can obtain appropriately. The relationship between pain and depression is circular. Either may cause or increase the other. A significant amount of depression has been demonstrated in older adults who are experiencing pain. The suspicion of depression should not reduce the appreciation of the severity of the older adult's pain or reduce the need for a comprehensive pain assessment (Gagliese & Melzack, 1997). A client should not be treated for depression until pain has been adequately relieved.

A person should not have to demonstrate expected pain behaviors or state "I have pain" in order to receive treatment for pain. Unfortunately, this is often not the case. Parmelee, Smith, and Katz (1993) found no evidence of pain masking by cognitively impaired older adults (Alzheimer's and dementia) in more than 700 clients in a nursing facility. They suggested that although cognitively impaired older adults may slightly underreport and may not recall previous episodes of pain, their reports are no less valid than those of older adults who are cognitively intact.

Lack of recognition of or inadequate treatment of pain is even more common in persons who are nonverbal, mentally retarded, cognitively impaired, or emotionally disturbed or whose cultural, racial, or socioeconomic backgrounds, lifestyle, or language differ from that of the caretakers (Shapiro & Ferrell, 1992). Those who communicate their discomfort in some way (preferably verbally) are the most likely to be treated, whether or not this treatment is sufficient to adequately relieve the pain. Commonly, this means that the client must either be able to say "I have pain" or behave in a manner that communicates pain—moaning, crying, or writhing. Without such communication, there is great danger that the pain will not be identified or treated unless there is a clear anticipatory cause such as recent surgery or trauma (Shapiro & Ferrell, 1992). One study of older adults with dementia showed that 84% of those with potentially very painful comorbidities received no medication for pain (Marzinski, 1991). In another study, physicians identified pain in 43% of verbal clients, but in only 17% of the nonverbal. Worse, only 21% of the communicative clients and 4% of the nonverbal were receiving analgesia (Sengstaken & King, 1993). Even if the pain is identified and orders received, studies show that nurses actually administer only a very small percentage of the ordered analgesics. Some nonverbal signs of pain in older adults might include refusal to turn or move, increased confusion, agitation, combativeness, moaning, rapid blinking, or rocking (Pitorak, 1998). Cognitively impaired clients' symptom reports should be taken seriously. They can often provide clear information about their symptoms, if the staff will take them seriously.

One type of pain often overlooked in the hospital but that can be significant is the pain from brief diagnostic or therapeutic procedures. For example, the insertion and removal of chest tubes and major drains and other diagnostic and therapeutic procedures may last for only a few minutes, but they can be intolerable to the client during that length of time. Local or topical anesthesia is not enough for these types of procedures. The health care team should make every effort to premedicate the client adequately and with safe drugs for that person for the procedure so the pain can be avoided. Even when local anesthesia will be adequate, a topical anesthetic product should be applied to reduce the pain of injecting the local anesthetic.

Pain: The Fifth Vital Sign

It is critical for nurses to become advocates for the optimal treatment of pain. The most important activity related to pain relief, and one of the most overlooked, is assessment and documentation of pain. Pain assessment should be viewed as of equal importance with the vital signs. In fact, it could be called the *fifth vital sign.* Unless the client is unable to communicate verbally or nonverbally, the nurse should use the client's report of pain as fact. According to McCaffrey and Beebe (1989), pain is

Research Focus

Citation:

Ferrell, B. A., Ferrell, B. R., & Osterwell, D. (1990). Pain in the nursing home. *Journal of the American Geriatrics Society, 38*(4), 409–414.

Purpose:

To describe the scope of the problem of pain in a long-term care facility.

Methods:

Ninety-seven residents in a long-term care facility were interviewed; charts were reviewed for pain problems and management strategies, and functional status, depression, and cognitive impairment were evaluated.

Findings:

Seventy-one percent of the residents had at least one pain complaint. Of those with pain, 34% described constant or continuous pain; 66% described intermittent pain. Of those with intermittent pain, 51% reported pain occurring on a daily basis. The major sources of pain identified were low back pain (40%), arthritis of the joints (24%), pain at previous fracture sites (14%), and neuropathies (11%). Other sources of pain reported included leg cramps, intermittent claudication, headaches, generalized pain, cancer pain, cardiac pain, and eye pain. Moderately strong correlations were found between pain and infrequent participation in social and recreational activities. Although little correlation was observed between pain and the Yesavage Depression Scale, the Folstein Mini-mental State Scale, or basic activities of daily living (ADL) measured by the Katz Scale, many clients did report depression, anxiety, sleep disturbances, impaired bowel or bladder function, and impaired memory or ability to carry out dressing and grooming activities. Pain management strategies included analgesic drugs, physical therapy, and heating pools. Only 15% of the residents who reported pain had received pain medication in the previous 24 hours.

Implications:

The findings suggest that pain is a major problem in nursing home residents. Strategies for pain management appear to be limited in scope and application in this setting.

what the client says it is and exists when the client says it does. Clients are authorities regarding their own pain. Only the person who is experiencing the pain knows what it feels like and what relieves it. Neither vital signs nor behavior should be used in lieu of a client's self-report of pain (Palos, 1997). The client's pain level should be assessed and documented before surgery, routinely after surgery with the onset of each new or unexpected pain, and after administering analgesia—1 hour later for oral drugs other than those labeled as short acting and 30 minutes after parenteral or short-acting oral drugs (Agency for Health, 1994). Analgesia should not be administered without inquiring about the location and character of the pain as well as its intensity. If the need for pain medication is increasing, a careful analysis is necessary to discover why the increase is needed.

Most pain assessment tools are either unidimensional estimates of pain intensity or multidimensional measures of the pain experience (Melzack & Katz, 1992). Both are important to a comprehensive pain assessment.

A comprehensive pain assessment should include the characteristics of the pain, precipitating and relieving factors, and the effects of the pain on the client and family's quality of life. The most commonly used multidimensional assessment tools are the short and long forms of the McGill Pain Questionnaire (MPQ) (Melzack, 1975). Unfortunately, these scales may be too complex for older adults or the illiterate to use. Even cognitively intact older adults may be unable to use the scales in the way that they were intended or to understand them.

Ferrell, Ferrell, and Rivera (1995) studied the ability of nursing facility residents to use the various pain scales and found that 83% of the subjects could complete at least one scale. The Pain Intensity Scale of the McGill Pain Questionnaire had the highest completion rate—65%—while 59% of the older subjects completed the Memorial Pain card subscale. Clients had more difficulty with the verbal scale; 32% were unable to complete the visual analogue scale, either because of inability to follow commands or to hold a pencil; and 17% were unable to complete any of the scales despite having appropriately answered yes or no questions about the presence of pain during an interview. The nurse should collaborate with clients to choose a pain-reporting method that works for them. This method should then be used consistently to rate the client's pain.

Physical and behavioral manifestations are different for acute and chronic pain. As has been previously stated, the hospitalized older adult may have both types of pain simultaneously and may or may not display typical pain manifestations. Some may be stoic or try to ignore the pain as much as possible. Typical behaviors of clients who are experiencing acute pain may include such findings as elevated blood pressure, pulse, and respiration; dilated pupils; **diaphoresis**; reduced concentration; manifestations of anxiety, apprehension, distress, and restlessness; crying, moaning, grimacing, furrowed brows, clenched fists or teeth, lying rigidly in bed; and resisting turning, moving, or ambulating. Even though their pain may be just as severe, those with chronic pain may not display these signs. Their vital signs and pupils are usually normal and the skin is dry. They may be irritable, depressed, withdrawn, fatigued, and even suicidal. They may be generally inactive or combative, confused, rubbing at painful body areas, or quiet and stoic. They may sleep a great deal more or less than usual. It is critical that the nurse not expect clients to behave in a particular way to "prove" that they are in pain. Nurses should also consider the differences between acute and chronic manifestations when assessing cognitively impaired or nonverbal clients (Forrest, 1995).

It is not enough to assume that hospitalized clients have pain related only to their surgery, trauma, or admitting diagnosis. New pain can always arise. The client could develop appendicitis, a myocardial infarct, a pulmonary embolus, or a pathological fracture, for example. Others have ongoing chronic problems in addition to their admitting diagnosis: arthritis, migraine headaches, and other sources of long-standing pain. The location and characteristics should be investigated for every pain complaint. Charting that a specific drug and dose were administered for pain is inadequate.

Interventions for Pain Relief

In providing pain relief, it is important to choose the intervention that will provide maximum pain relief with the fewest adverse effects. Often, this is a combination of pharmacological and nonpharmacological interventions. Nonpharmacological methods of pain relief should be used whenever possible. These are often not enough to completely relieve pain but can significantly reduce the amount of pain medication needed. These techniques include massage, backrubs, relaxation, imagery, the use of heat and cold (avoid using heat on persons with vascular impairments), the use of **transcutaneous electrical stimulation (TENS units)**, changing position, **acupuncture, biofeedback, hypnosis**, the use of humorous or musical videotapes and audiotapes, acupressure, foot massage, art therapy, meditation, prayer, and talking and playing games with friends.

Older adults are often not given the same level of relief for acute pain that might be given to a younger person. One study of older hospitalized clients showed that acetaminophen was the most commonly prescribed analgesic, while naproxen, aspirin, and codeine were the only other drugs prescribed to study clients. Most had only PRN therapy ordered. The only nonpharmacological pain management method prescribed was physical therapy, despite the fact that there is growing evidence that multimodal therapy can be very useful. In the same study, difficulty in evaluating pain management was found. Clients expressed satisfaction with their pain management despite the continuation of pain, making statements such as "They're doing all they can", "I know the pain can't get any better", and "I'm not one who complains." Health care providers reinforce these attitudes with comments such as "you'll have to live with it" (Grymonpre & Kirshen, 1993), which further reinforces the norm of undertreatment.

Ask Yourself

A 58-year-old woman remained in the ICU of a small hospital 1 month after she had had coronary bypasses, which she did not want but was talked into by her husband and physician. She had experienced nearly every complication imaginable. On the day described here, she was awake and agitated and had tears in her eyes. She was on a ventilator with an endotracheal tube in place. Although her nasogastric tube was still in place, her tube feedings had been stopped on the day before. She was receiving intravenous fluids via a central line, but the antibiotics had also been discontinued the day before when her husband signed a do-not-resuscitate form. Her chest and leg wounds had become infected; they were open and being packed with wet-to-dry dressings twice daily. She had NO pain medication orders. Her many physicians visited throughout the day for a few seconds each. Her husband's visit did not last much longer. When asked about pain medication by the nurses, the various physicians' comments included "I'm not the primary—I can't do those orders" or "we're trying to wean her off the vent." No one was willing to concede that the situation was inhumane.

What ethical issues are involved in this case? Does this situation warrant the use of opioid analgesics? What do you think the nurse should/could do now?

At times, the mixed agonist-antagonists pentazocine (Talwin), nalbuphine (Nubain), butorphanol (Stadol), and buprenorphine (Buprenex) may be used to achieve pain relief. These are antagonists to the **opioids** and so should not be used in addition to them. Only clients who are not on opioids should receive these drugs. They do have a dose-related ceiling effect, so doses cannot be continually increased if pain levels increase (Agency for Health Care, 1994). The mixed agonist-antagonists tend to have a high level of adverse effects when used long term, so they should be used only for short periods. Their major adverse effects are drowsiness, occasional nausea, and psychotic reactions. Talwin, in particular, tends to cause delirium and agitation in older adults and should be avoided.

A myth regarding administration of intravenous or intramuscular opioids is that administering the drugs promethazine (Phenergan) or hydroxyzine (Vistaril) along with the opioid will enhance the pain relief. In actuality, these drugs tend to detract from pain relief and should not be routinely administered as part of the analgesia prescription (McCaffrey & Beebe, 1989).

Meperidine (Demerol) is a commonly used analgesic in the hospital, although it has been shown to be a poor choice, especially for older adults. Although its pain relief lasts only about 3 hours, its metabolites last about 15 hours. Hence, the second dose for pain relief adds to the existing normeperidine metabolite, and the third dose does the same. This accumulation is particularly severe in older adults and in those with impaired excretion capabilities. The normeperidine accumulation can cause central nervous system (CNS) excitation and toxicity: tremors, shakiness, irritability, **myoclonus** (jerking), seizures, altered level of consciousness, and confusion. The effects of normeperidine *cannot* be reversed by naloxone (Narcan), the administration of which could actually worsen or precipitate a seizure. In short, Demerol is best avoided in older adults. Table 15-3 further discusses pain management in older adults (McCaffrey & Beebe, 1989).

When it is time to change from intravenous to oral administration of narcotics, the order is often written for the same dose of oral medication that was given intravenously or intramuscularly. Clients then complain that they prefer the intravenous route or the shot rather than the oral drug. Nurses then state that the client "really likes the shots." Actually, the client really likes pain relief. A review of the **equianalgesic** dose concept reveals that the pass-through effect of drug metabolism in the intestines causes a loss of much of the drug's potency. Therefore, a much higher dose must be used when a drug is given orally than when it is given parenterally. For morphine, the pain relief capability of a parenteral dose of 10 mg requires an oral dose of 30 mg. For Demerol, a 300-mg oral dose is required to equal the pain relief capability of 75 mg administered parenterally. For Dilaudid, a 7.5-mg oral dose equals a 1.5-mg parenteral dose. A review of equianalgesic concepts will also enable the health care providers to convert client orders from one drug to another. For example, a parenteral dose of 10 mg of morphine is equal to the pain relief capability of 200 mg hydrocodone (Vicodin, Lortab) (Texas Cancer Pain Initiative, undated). Equianalgesic charts may be obtained from the major pharmaceutical companies or found in the AHCPR guidelines *Management of Cancer Pain: Adults* (Agency for Health Care, 1994), which can be obtained from pharmaceutical representatives or pain management clinics or by calling 1-800-4CANCER.

Constipation as an Adverse Effect

One adverse effect of pain medications in general and opioids in particular, to which tolerance does not develop, is constipation. This can be a serious problem in hospitalized older adults, who may be immobile, not eating well, on other constipating drugs, and receiving pain medications other than nonsteroidal anti-inflammatory drugs (NSAIDs.) Bowel management should be a standard part of care for clients on opioid analgesics: Monitor and record stools, institute a bowel program early to prevent constipation or impaction, and listen to client symptoms and complaints. Even when not eating, most people should have a bowel movement every 2–3 days at minimum. Some commonly used bowel protocols include the use of intestinal stimulants such as Reglan (metoclopramide) and Propulsid (cisapride). Other commonly used drugs include stool softeners such as Colace (ducosate) or a combination of softener and stimulant such as Senokot-S (senna and ducosate). Other products may be added as necessary: magnesium citrate, lactulose (cephulac), suppositories, and enemas. The fiber laxatives should never be used unless adequate fluid intake can be ensured—at least 1.5–2 liters of fluid. Whatever combination and amount of drug is necessary to accomplish the task may be used. However, it is important to assess carefully for signs of paralytic ileus, which is not uncommon postoperatively and requires much more invasive treatment.

> ### Nursing Tip
>
> Any time pain management medications stronger than NSAIDs are begun, the older adult should be instructed that constipation is a probable adverse effect and that the risk increases with increases in the dose of pain medication. It is wise for the person to start on a stool softener or a combination drug containing a stool softener and gentle stimulant when the pain medication is begun. More or stronger medications can be added or substituted if necessary. A record of bowel movements should be kept to ensure that the person has a bowel movement at least every 3 days. If this does not happen, suppository administration is the usual next step.

Summary

The care of hospitalized older adults is a complex and challenging aspect of nursing. The nurse must be aware of the special needs of this age group along with the general pathophysiology of whatever their diagnoses may be. Nurses must be alert to special psychosocial and communication needs as well as physiological needs that are unique to the older individual. Discharge planning should consider special teaching needs and the fact that they might not be returning to a safe environment without case management intervention. Some of the many problems that call for special consideration include altered mental status, anxiety, safety, potential hazards of immobility, potential dehydration and fluid and electrolyte imbalances, potential drug interactions and adverse effects, absence or masking of standard symptoms of complications, potential for infection, possible drug and alcohol withdrawal, and altered comfort.

TABLE 15-3 Acute Pain Management in Older Adults

Drugs	General Considerations
Morphine—has no ceiling dose	The gold standard for pain relief. Available for intravenous (IV), intramuscular (IM), subcutaneous (SC), epidural, and intrathecal and oral administration.
Hydromorphone (Dilaudid)—has no ceiling dose	Available for IV, PO, and rectal administration. There are two parenteral preparations. Dilaudid HP is a high-potency concentrated solution, intended for diluted use only in opioid-tolerant clients. Dilaudid is a good choice for those few who are truly allergic to morphine.

Oxycodone
   With acetaminophen: Percocet, Roxicet, Tylox
   With aspirin (ASA): Percodan, Roxiprin
   Alone: Roxicodone
	All preparations are by mouth (PO). For moderate pain levels. Any preparation mixed with an NSAID is limited by the safe daily dose of the NSAID. Generally, acetaminophen doses >4 g should not be administered to healthy adults; the amount should be lower in older adults and those with hepatic compromise. The ceiling for NSAIDs is the standard dose of each. Beyond that, adverse effects rise but pain relief does not.

Hydrocodone
   With acetaminophen: Vicodin
   With ASA: Lortab tabs or liquid
   With ibuprofen: Vicoprofen
	All preparations are PO. For moderate, short-term pain. Dose limited by NSAID content.

Acetaminophen with codeine, Fiorinal with codeine	These are not safe for long-term use, particularly in older adults. Any dose of Fiorinal or Tylenol #3 over 65 mg (2 tablets) will not increase relief but will increase adverse effects. At doses >1.5 mg/kg/day of codeine, there is increased danger of gastrointestinal effects. If clients are deficient in certain enzymes or taking Tagamet (cimetadine) or quinidine, they may not be able to convert codeine to morphine in the body and thus will not receive pain relief.
Level 1 NSAIDs: Anaprox, ASA, Dolobid, Advil, Disalcid, Motrin, Naprosen, Orudia, Rimadyl, Indocin, Lodine, Toradol, Ultram, Trilisate; acetaminophen (not anti-inflammatory)	These drugs may be given alone for mild pain or with opioids to potentiate their action. They are the drugs of choice for bone pain; they may need to be administered along with opioids for the bone pain of cancer or for an acutely ill client who also has severe arthritis. The ceiling for NSAIDs is the standard dose of each. Beyond that, pain relief does not increase, but adverse effects do. Of the NSAIDs, Indocin generally has the most central nervous system (CNS) adverse effects and should be avoided in older adults. In general, the NSAIDs other than acetaminophen have more adverse effects in older adults: platelet dysfunction, impaired clotting, bleeding, and severe gastrointestinal distress. All but acetaminophen are contraindicated in clients with bleeding disorders. Acetaminophen has the potential for severe hepatic toxicity with overdosage. *Note:* Toradol is labeled for 5 days only. It is often given on a regular schedule to reduce the need for opioids.
Darvon (propoxyphene), Darvocet	These are no more effective than NSAIDs (and perhaps not as effective) but have significantly more adverse effects, especially in older adults. They can be habit forming and have the side effects of the stronger narcotics. They may cause constipation, sedation, confusion, and slowed respiration. They should be avoided in older adults.

CARE PLAN

CASE STUDY

Mrs. Lu Chang was admitted to the hospital with a fractured hip. She is 90 years old and lives with her family in a large city. With her husband as owner, they all work together to run an Asian grocery store. Mrs. Chang speaks very little English and is unable to read or write in the language. She is the "matriarch" of the household and is respected by all family members.

While sweeping snow from the steps outside the market, Mrs. Chang slipped and fell. She was taken to the hospital unwillingly but with urging from other family members. Mrs. Chang has never been hospitalized.

Mrs. Chang has seven children, two of whom work in the store along with her 85-year-old sister and several cousins and grandchildren. Her medical history is somewhat vague as one of her grandsons interprets for the admission nurse in the emergency department. She is on a variety of Chinese herbs for headaches, weak bones, and pain, according to her grandson. Herbal teas have been used more frequently lately for gastric distress. Her vital signs are 101.0 PO temperature, 110 regular pulse, 36 respirations, and blood pressure 144/90. She has no allergies that her grandson is aware of. Her right hip is tender to the touch and swollen. An x-ray confirms a right-hip fracture.

Mrs. Chang speaks rapidly and is very upset about the hospitalization. As she is brought to her room, she tries to get up, intending to leave, against her family's wishes. She flails her arms and pushes away the nurse. The grandson attempts to explain to her what is occurring. Mrs. Chang appears to be out of control, a harm to herself and others, and the decision is made to restrain her, both chemically with 0.5 mg Haldol IM and physically with a waist restraint jacket. As she falls asleep, the nurse, physician, and nurse's aide gather with the family to establish a strategy for Mrs. Chang's safety during the night and postsurgery.

ASSESSMENT

The challenge is to establish a care plan for Mrs. Chang that is culturally and medically acceptable. There are individuals who have never been hospitalized and who will find the hospital a very restrictive and unsettling environment. Yet hospital personnel will require them to conform to the rules and routine typical of an institutional setting. In addition, language and cultural diversity are challenges to all involved. Patterns of behavior and coping mechanisms need to be considered given this crisis. Besides high risk for further injury, several nursing diagnoses are appropriate to this situation.

NURSING DIAGNOSIS

Impaired verbal communication related to cultural differences, emotional condition, and environment changes.

Outcomes:

Mrs. Lu Chang will:
- *Express ideas, questions, feelings, needs, and thoughts in her native language.*
- *Understand/comprehend what has transpired as well as the care anticipated in her rehabilitation*

Planning/Interventions:

The nurse will:
- *Assess facial expressions and body language given Mrs. Lu Chang's cultural background.*
- *Arrange for a 24-hour interpreter, that is, her grandson and family members.*
- *Involve Mrs. Lu Chang directly in her care planning with help from an interpreter.*
- *Collaborate and consult with resources on Chinese culture and medicine.*
- *Use pictures to express basic ideas, requests, and actions.*
- *Consult with occupational therapy.*

EVALUATION:

Mrs. Lu Chang will effectively communicate her thoughts and needs to staff and staff to her. With assistance from an interpreter, the language and cultural barrier will not become a hindrance to health and recovery. Sociocultural norms will be respected.

(continues)

NURSING DIAGNOSIS

Powerlessness perceived as and related to the health care environment, perceived lack of control over the entire situation.

Outcomes:

Mrs. Lu Chang will:
- *Express and confirm an understanding of what has happened to her.*
- *Express feelings of control.*
- *Verbalize ways she can participate in her own care.*

Planning/Interventions:

The nurse will:
- *Elicit expression of Mrs. Lu Chang's feelings.*
- *Explain to her what has happened.*
- *Describe usual hospital routine.*
- *Orient her to her surroundings.*
- *List ways she can participate in her care and rehabilitation.*

EVALUATION:

Mrs. Lu Chang will be involved in her own care. She will comprehend what has and will happen to her. She will begin to understand the environment and use it to facilitate her recovery.

NURSING DIAGNOSIS

Risk for altered body temperature related to illness/trauma and advanced age.

Outcomes:

Mrs. Lu Chang will:
- *Show no signs and symptoms of infection.*
- *Reduce temperature to 97°F–98°F orally.*
- *Demonstrate no change in mental status and no signs and symptoms of delirium.*
- *Ingest adequate (1500–2500 cc) fluids daily.*

Planning/Interventions:

The nurse will:
- *Assess vital signs every shift.*
- *Assess mental status every shift.*
- *Check labwork for infection and abnormalities: urine for culture and sensitivity, electrolytes, BUN, creatinine, chest x-ray, white blood count, leukocytes, and neutrophils.*
- *Investigate Chinese herbs for diuretic effect and adverse interactions.*

EVALUATION:

Mrs. Lu Chang will maintain normal vital signs. Her temperature will return to normal limits after she has taken adequate fluids. Mental status, a very good barometer of infection in older adults, will remain at baseline status. Related labwork will remain normal. Chinese herbs will be continued unless contraindicated.

Review Questions and Activities

Sample Test Items

1. Which drug is unsafe for administration to older adults?

   a. Morphine

   b. Meperidine (Demerol)

   c. Hydromorphone (Dilaudid)

   d. Acetaminophen (Tylenol)

2. Pain should be defined in which of the following manners?

   a. It is an unpleasant sensation, the result of which can be observed in client behaviors.

   b. It is a sensation that can be relieved by analgesic drugs.

   c. It is what the client says it is.

   d. Pain occurs as a predictable result of illness, surgery, or trauma.

3. Drug and alcohol withdrawal:

   a. Are rarely a problem in acutely ill older adults.

   b. Can usually be prevented; the older adult will advise the nurse of ongoing alcohol use.

   c. Are a problem only if older adults are seriously ill.

   d. Occur more frequently than is often anticipated.

4. If a client with alcohol withdrawal is having symptoms and it is inappropriate to administer alcohol, the drug of choice is:

   a. Morphine, administered intravenously

   b. Chlordiazepoxide (Librium) administered intramuscularly

   c. Naloxone (Narcan), administered intravenously

   d. Chlorodiazepoxide (Librium), administered orally

5. What are four potential hazards of immobility? Identify at least two nursing actions to prevent each.

6. What are three methods by which the nurse can safely feed someone with a swallowing difficulty?

7. Discuss three strategies the nurse can use to establish trust and rapport with the older adult who is being admitted to the hospital.

Activities

1. From an acute, long-term, outpatient, or home care setting, identify an older adult who takes five or more medications on a routine, long-term basis.

   a. Prepare a chart showing the therapeutic effects, interactions, and possible adverse effects of these drugs.

   b. Telephone or visit at least two neighborhood pharmacies to determine the approximate cost of these drugs per month.

2. Agency visits:

   a. Visit a rehabilitation facility to observe the speech language pathologist and/or other staff members evaluating and managing clients with actual or potential swallowing problems.

   b. Visit a rehabilitation, acute care, or long-term care facility to explore restraint policies, methods available for managing safety, and methods utilized. Compare your finding with those of students who visited other types of facilities. What are your suggestions for policies and equipment to keep older adults safe?

   c. Visit a gerontological nurse practitioner and observe his or her interactions with assessment and management of older clients for several hours. How does the practice of this health professional compare with others you have observed? Discuss your findings with your instructor and peers.

References

Agency for Health Care Policy and Research. (1994). *Clinical practice guidelines: Management of cancer pain: Adults.* AHCPR Pub. No. 94-0593. Rockville, MD: U.S. Department of Health and Human Services.

Cole-Arvin, C., Notich, L., & Underhill, A. (1994). Identifying and managing dysphagia. *Nursing, 24*(1), 48–49.

Ferrell, B. A. (1991). Pain management in elderly people. *Journal of the American Geriatrics Society, 39*(1), 64–73.

Ferrell, B. A., Ferrell, B. R., & Osterwell, D. (1990). Pain in the nursing home. *Journal of the American Geriatrics Society, 38*(4), 409–414.

Ferrell, B. A., Ferrell, B. R, & Rivera, L. (1995). Pain in cognitively impaired nursing home patients. *Journal of Pain and Symptom Management, 10*(8), 591–598.

Forrest, J. (1995). Assessment of acute and chronic pain in older adults. *Journal of Gerontological Nursing, 21*(10), 15–20.

Gagliese, L., & Melzack, R. (1997). Chronic pain in elderly people. *Pain, 70*(1), 3–14.

Gordon, C., Hewer, R. L., & Wade, D. T. (1987). Dysphagia in acute stroke. *British Medical Journal, 295*(6595), 411–414.

Grymonpre, R. E., & Kirshen, A. J. (1993). The management of pain in the hospitalized elderly. *American Journal of Pain Management, 3*(4), 191–195.

Harkins, S. W., Kwentus, J., & Price, D. D. (1990). Pain and suffering in the elderly. In J. J. Bonica (Ed.), *The management of pain* (2nd ed., pp. 552–559). Philadelphia: Lea and Febiger.

Helme, R. D., Katz, B., Gibson, S., & Corran, T. (1989). Can psychometric tools be used to analyze pain in a geriatric population? *Clinical Experiences in Neurology, 26*, 113–117.

Hewer, R. L., & Wade, D. T. (1987). Motor loss and swallowing difficulty after stroke: Frequency, recovery, and prognosis. *Acta Neurologica. Scandinavica, 76*(1), 50–54.

Hogstel, M., & Robinson, N. B. (1989). Feeding the frail elderly. *Journal of Gerontological Nursing, 15*(3),16–20.

Horner, J., & Massey, E. W. (1988). Silent aspiration following stroke. *Neurology, 38*(2), 317–319.

Horner, J., & Massey, E. W. (1991). Managing dysphagia. *Postgraduate Medicine, 89*(5), 203.

Killen, J. M. (1996). Understanding dysphagia: Interventions for care. *MEDSURG Nursing, 5*(2), 99–105.

Lee, V. K., & Burnett, E. (1998). A case report: Special needs of hospitalized elders. *Geriatric Nursing, 19*(4), 185–191.

Lugger, K. E. (1994). Dysphagia in the elderly stroke patient. *Journal of Neuroscience Nursing, 26*(2), 78–84.

Marzinski, L. R. (1991). The tragedy of dementia: Clinically assessing pain in the confused, nonverbal elderly. *Journal of Gerontological Nursing,17*(16), 25–28.

Matteson, M. A., McConnell, E. S., & Linton, A. D. (Eds.). (1997). *Gerontological nursing.* Philadelphia: Saunders.

McCaffrey, M., & Beebe, A. (1989). *Pain: Clinical manual for nursing practice.* St. Louis: Mosby.

Melzack, R. (1975). The McGill Pain Questionnaire: Major properties and scoring methods. *Pain, 1*(1975), 277–299.

Melzack, R., & Katz, J. (1992). The McGill Pain Questionnaire: Appraisal and current status. In D. C. Turk & R. Melzak (Eds.), *Handbook of pain assessment* (pp. 152–168). New York: Guildford.

Palos, G. (1997). The influence and assessment of culture on cancer pain. *Nursing Interventions in Oncology, 9*, 8–12.

Parmelee, P. A., Smith, B., & Katz, I. R. (1993). Pain complaints and cognitive status among elderly institution residents. *Journal of the American Geriatrics Society, 41*(5), 517–522.

Pitorak, E. F. (1998). *The challenge of pain management in the elderly hospice patient.* Unpublished presentation, Hospice and Palliative Care Nurses Association, San Diego, CA.

Pontoppidan, H., & Beecher, H. K. (1960). Progressive loss of protective reflexes in the airway with the advance of age. *Journal of the American Medical Association, 174*(18), 2209–2213.

Rapp, D. (1997). *Dysphagia education series.* Unpublished, Health South Rehabilitation Hospital, Fort Worth, TX.

Semia, T. P., Beizer, J. L., & Higbee, M. D. (1997). *Geriatric dosage handbook.* Cleveland: Lexi-Comp.

Sengstaken, E. A., & King, S. A. (1993). The problems of pain and its detection among geriatric nursing home residents. *Journal of the American Geriatrics Society, 41*(5), 541–544.

Shapiro, B. S., & Ferrell, B. R. (1992, October/November). Pain in children and the frail elderly: Similarities and implications. *APS Bulletin*, pp. 11–13.

Texas Cancer Pain Initiative. (Undated). *Oral and parenteral opioid analgesic equivalencies and relative potency of drugs as compared with morphine.* Austin, TX: Texas Cancer Council.

Wallace, M. (1994). Assessment and management of pain in the elderly. *MEDSURG Nursing, 3*(4), 293–298.

Wisconsin Pain Initiative. (Undated). A bill of rights for persons with cancer pain. *The pain relief papers.* Titusville, NJ: Janssen Pharmaceuticals.1:5.

Woodin, L. M. (1993). Cutting post-op pain. *RN, 56*(8), 26–33.

Resources

National Foundation for the Treatment of Pain: **www.paincare.org**

Pain.com. "A World of Information about Pain": **www.pain.com**

CHAPTER 16

Chronic Illness

Gail C. Davis, EdD, RN

Barbara M. Raudonis, PhD, RN, CS

COMPETENCIES

After completing this chapter, the reader should be able to:

- *Explain the prevalence of chronic illnesses in the older adult population.*
- *Discuss the impact of chronic illnesses on the U.S. health care delivery system.*
- *Identify the major chronic illnesses affecting older adults.*
- *Describe the possible effects of chronic illness on health status and quality of life.*
- *Describe approaches to assessing the impact of chronic illness on the older adult.*
- *Identify methods and techniques to assess and measure pain intensity.*
- *Discuss approaches for meeting the needs of older adults experiencing chronic pain.*
- *Relate the problem of depression to diagnoses of arthritis and cancer in older adults.*
- *Describe the purposes and functions of the Arthritis Foundation and the American Cancer Society.*
- *Design new approaches that will meet the needs of older adults with chronic illnesses within a changing health care delivery system.*

MAKING THE CONNECTION

Refer to the following chapters to increase your understanding of chronic illness:

Demographics of Chronic Illness

The major purpose of this chapter is to increase the reader's awareness of the special needs of older adults who experience chronic illnesses and ways in which their optimum health status can be maintained or improved and **quality of life** promoted.

Because terminology related to chronic conditions varies, the terms as they are used here are identified for consistency of discussion. The definitions developed by the Robert Wood Johnson Foundation (1996) have been selected and are noted in Table 16-1. Discussion will focus primarily on selected chronic illnesses (**arthritis** and **cancer**), as well as on the **secondary conditions** such as **pain** and **depression** that frequently occur in association with them.

Estimates related to the growing percentage of people age 65 and older, along with projections of increasing chronic illness, underscore the importance of planning effective health care services for older adults experiencing chronic illness. In 1991, it was predicted that people age 65 and over would account for 13% of the U.S. population by the year 2000 and 22% by 2030 (Public Health, 1991, p. 23). Worldwide, the percentage of the older population will increase from 6.2% in 1990 to 9.7% in 2025 (Preston & Martin, 1994). As the proportion of older adults increases, so will the number of persons with chronic illness. By 2030, approximately 150 million persons will have a chronic condition as compared with 99 million in 1995 (Robert Wood Johnson, 1996). Currently, the three major chronic conditions in the older population are arthritis, hypertension, and hearing impairment (Verbrugge & Patrick, 1994). **Osteoarthritis (OA)** is the most common type of arthritis, having almost universal prevalence in those age 80 and over (Downe-Wamboldt, 1991).

A high percentage (86%) of older adults have at least one chronic disease (McConnell, 1997). Up to 70% of those over age 80 who live in the community have at least two chronic conditions (Agency for Health Care, 1998). Almost 40% of community-dwelling older adults experience some limitations related to chronic conditions. Of these, about 10% were unable to perform some activities associated with independence, such as shopping, dressing, bathing, or eating (Robert Wood Johnson, 1996). Requirements for assistance with daily activities increase with age, sharply increasing in the age 85 and older group. These numbers have strong implications for the planning of health care services and considering options that will address the needs of those who may require only minimal assistance to maintain independence (see Figure 16-1). Such services may be offered by professionals, skilled workers, family members, and volunteers who often need some specific training and available support.

Even if the necessary kinds of services are offered, how these will be accessed—both physically and financially—is also an important consideration. Health care considerations for older adults must be viewed within a social, political, and economic context (Diamond, Catanzaro, & Lorensen, 1997). The **functional limitations** associated with many chronic illnesses, in combination with such **financial limitations** and **social limitations** as transportation and **social support,** may limit the older adult's ability to take advantage of services that might be offered within a community.

Financial Issues

Financial issues can severely limit the person's access to care. Low income is an important risk factor for "virtually all of the chronic diseases that lead the Nation's

TABLE 16-1 Terminology Related to Chronic Illness	
Term	**Definition**
Chronic conditions	A general term that includes chronic illnesses and impairments.
Chronic illness	The presence of a long-term (i.e., 3 or more months) disease or symptoms. Examples: arthritis, diabetes, cancer, and heart disease.
Impairment	A physiological, psychological, or anatomical abnormality of bodily structure or function; includes all losses or abnormalities, not just those attributable to active pathology. Examples: blindness, hearing impairment, head injury, and spinal injury.
Secondary condition	Conditions related to the main illness or impairment that further diminish the person's quality of life, threaten his or health, or increase vulnerability to further disability. Examples: pain, depression, and pressure ulcers.

From the Robert Wood Johnson Foundation, 1996.

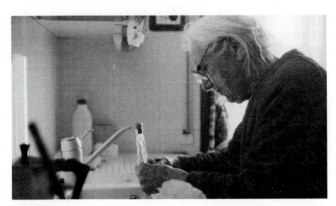

FIGURE 16-1 Chronic illness can severely limit the ability to live independently.

list of killers," including heart disease and cancer (Public Health Service, 1991, p. 29). Groups who are especially vulnerable include persons age 80 and older, women, and ethnic minorities. Data show, for example, that older African-Americans are two times less likely than whites age 65 and over to have health insurance coverage, including Medicare, Medicaid, or assistance from the Department of Veterans' Affairs (Ries, 1987). Women in the young-old group (65–74 years) experience more chronic illnesses such as **rheumatoid arthritis (RA),** hypertension, and/or osteoporosis than do men; thus, they are more likely to have greater out-of-pocket expenses. This is of special concern considering the fact that their economic level is less than that of men (Sofaer & Abel, 1990). Twenty-four percent of an age 80 and older study population reported financial difficulties, and 25% reported activities of daily living (ADL) limitations. They were eight times more likely to delay health care because of the costs and twice as likely to encounter structural barriers to care as those without financial problems (Agency for Health Care, 1998).

The costs associated with arthritis provide one example of how a long-term chronic illness becomes a financial issue for older adults. The direct costs across all age groups, approximately $15.2 billion in 1992, included hospital and physician inpatient costs, outpatient costs, nursing facility care, medications, and nonphysician health care visits (Callahan, 1996). While Medicare coverage helps in providing those services that are acute in nature, it does not provide for many of these direct costs that are long term, such as rehabilitation services, outpatient physician or nurse practitioner visits, outpatient medicines, and mobility aids. Because so many older adults are financially unable to purchase Medicare supplemental health insurance **(Medigap)** coverage or to pay for these items or services, it is important that public policy address these financial issues that are so important to the overall health status and quality of life of the older adult.

Cost data at the patient level of cancer care have been difficult to obtain (Riley, Potosky, Lubitz, & Kessler, 1995). However, Riley and associates were able to estimate the Medicare costs of care from the time of diagnosis through to death using tumor registry data (1995). There were variations in the cost of care based on the phase and site of the cancer. Persons with bladder cancer had the highest total cost of care ($57,629) and those with lung cancer ($29,184) the lowest cost. Lower costs were related to shorter survival rates. Initially, early detection and treatment may seem to incur greater cost. However, when cancer was detected early, the Medicare payments per year of survival were lower (Riley et al., 1995).

Ask Yourself

Imagine that all the women on your maternal side of the family were diagnosed and died from breast cancer during their late fifties. As a female, would you request genetic testing for breast cancer at an early age (for example, 30)?

Major Chronic Illnesses

Persons age 85 and older now represent the fastest growing group of older adults, and women constitute 72% of this group (Roberto, 1994). Because people are more vulnerable to chronic conditions as they age (Robert Wood Johnson, 1996), the incidence of chronic illness is expected to rise. Those that often affect older adults include essential hypertension, arthritis, musculoskeletal impairments, cancer, heart disease, diabetes, chronic airway obstruction, and peripheral vascular disease. Any of these may occur in combination. In the case of comorbidity, or when the individual experiences more than one chronic condition, treatment becomes complex and treatment-related complications are more likely to occur. Numerous complications are related to the side effects of single or multiple medications, a point that deserves the attention of health care professionals.

Regardless of the body system affected (for example, musculoskeletal, cardiovascular, or endocrine), the adaptive issues of any chronic illness are very much the same. Functional status and pain are major issues associated with many chronic conditions. Of persons age 65 and older in 1987, about 13% had difficulty performing one or more physical activities of daily living (PADL) such as bathing, dressing, toileting, and eating. About 17.5% had difficulty performing one or more instrumental activities of daily living (IADL), such as telephoning, managing money, and preparing meals (Haber, 1994). While the reported percentage of older adults who experience pain varies across studies, it ranges from 70% to 86% (Davis, Cortez, & Rubin, 1990). One group of older adults, when asked to describe a physical or mental problem that had occurred within the previous 24 hours, identified pain as the most frequent symptom. They also noted pain as having the greatest interference with activities such as walking, performing household chores, and leisure and social activities (Brody & Kleban, 1983).

Individuals with a cancer diagnosis experience many other symptoms in addition to pain. Cancer pain cannot be treated in isolation from problems such as nausea and vomiting, anorexia, constipation, **fatigue,** skin breakdown, **sleep disturbances,** and sexual dysfunction (Hogan, 1997). Poorly controlled symptoms compromise both survivors of cancer (decreased energy, despair, impaired quality of life) and the bereaved family members of deceased cancer clients (complicated bereavement based on memories of the cancer client's ordeals) (Hogan, 1997).

Functional limitations are associated with most chronic conditions, and comorbidities only exaggerate these. Specific medical diagnoses such as arthritis, cardiovascular disease, diabetes, and cancer each affect function in specific ways. Guccione et al. (1994) found that the conditions having the greatest effect on the function of older adults include knee osteoarthritis (OA), stroke, heart disease, and depressive symptoms.

For the competencies to be addressed as part of this chapter, arthritis and cancer were selected to provide the basis for further discussing chronic illness. The prevalence of these illnesses increases with age; the major difference is in terms of their prognosis. Arthritis is not considered to be a life-threatening illness; rather, it is one that can be tremendously *wearing* and requires a great deal of self-management and adaptation over time. These two conditions provide a way of conceptualizing two different ways of thinking about symptom and disease management. Cancer is generally associated with a poorer prognosis, and therefore, the focus of management is more likely to be on the relief of symptoms using pharmacological methods, as opposed to learning and using nonpharmacological techniques to manage symptoms over a long period of time.

Arthritis and musculoskeletal diseases affect approximately 49% of persons age 65 and older in the United States (Callahan, 1995). Arthritis is a general term that encompasses more than 100 different conditions, with the most common being osteoarthritis (OA) and rheumatoid arthritis (RA); others commonly occurring in older adults include tendinitis, intervertebral disc disorders, gout, and osteoporosis. Osteoarthritis alone affects more than 80% of persons age 75 and older, and the majority of persons at age 65 show radiographic evidence of OA in one or more joints (Brandt & Slemenda, 1993). Age is definitely a risk factor for OA, as it is for osteoporosis. As an age-related condition, osteoporosis affects both women and men (Hamdy, 1992), although it occurs in men about 10 years later than women (Kleerekoper, 1999). While osteo-

porosis is most often described in terms of decreased bone mass, a major consideration is also bone fragility. More than 1.5 million osteoporotic fractures occur annually at an estimated cost of $14 billion for hospital and nursing facility care (Kleerekoper, 1999). Vertebral fractures are the most common (700,000), followed in frequency by fractures of the hip (300,000) (Kleerekoper, 1999). More than 30% of women will have osteoporosis by age 60–70 and 70% will by age 80 (Taxel, 1998).

Cancer also represents a group of diseases; these are characterized by uncontrolled growth and spread of abnormal cells that disrupt any body system. Although cancer can potentially be a terminal illness, it is now considered a chronic disease. Factors contributing to its change from acute to chronic illness include advances in technology and research that have made the long-term treatment in outpatient settings and ongoing care in the home by family caregivers possible (Given & Given, 1998). An average 5-year survival rate of 58% is currently expected for all types of cancer. Survival rates include individuals living 5 years after diagnosis whether disease free, under treatment, or in remission (American Cancer Society, 1998).

Despite the change in the classification of cancer to a chronic illness, it continues to be a leading cause of death in individuals age 65 and older. Age is considered the single most significant risk factor for the development of cancer (Baird, McCorkle, & Grant, 1991). In 1998, it is estimated that 564,000 new cases of cancer will be diagnosed in the United States. Currently, the leading sites of cancer death in men are lung (32%) and prostate (13%). The leading site in women is lung (25%), followed by breast (16%) (Landis, Murray, Bolden, & Wingo, 1998).

Individuals control their own lifestyle behaviors; thus risks for developing cancer can be changed by altering environmental and lifestyle behaviors. These changes alone can significantly impact the prevention, detection, and early treatment of cancer. Cancer screening guidelines by the **American Cancer Society (ACS)** have positively impacted the early detection and treatment of cancer in older adults. The guidelines suggest who should be targeted, what type of examination should be done, and how frequently the screening should be performed.

Effects of Chronic Illness on Health Status and Quality of Life

The effects of chronic illness have major implications for the individual's quality of life. These effects include those conditions that are secondary to the illness, such as pain, decreased functional status, depression, fatigue, sleep disturbance, hopelessness, and decreased socialization. Researchers are attempting to measure quality of life using scales, interview guidelines, and questions. It is difficult to define the concept. If it can be measured, efforts can be made to enhance components of it. Whereas the treatment of an acute illness is closely supervised by a health care professional, it is important that the individual assume a major role in the self-management of a chronic illness when possible. This self-management focus requires that the individual develop certain skills and coping strategies, such as how to balance activities to avoid worsening the condition or its symptoms, managing self-medication and other required therapies, adapting the performance of daily activities and using mobility aids such as a cane or walker as necessary, and adjusting to changing patterns of socialization. Accomplishing these things may be highly dependent on the person's **self-efficacy,** or the confidence in one's own ability to manage the effects of the illness and make the necessary adaptations.

Pain

Chronic pain is a major symptom associated with such chronic illnesses as arthritis, cancer, postherpetic neuralgia, and peripheral vascular disease. Population studies have estimated that the prevalence of pain is two times greater in those age 60 and older than in those who are younger (Crook, Rideout, & Brown, 1984). Arthritis-related pain alone affects approximately 80% of people age 65 and older (Davis, 1988), and the incidence of pain related to conditions such as OA and osteoporosis can be expected to increase with age.

The pain itself has major effects on the individual's quality of life. Davis (1998a) found that the response to living with persistent nonmalignant pain was essentially the same for all adult age groups. Dimensions underlying this experience are (1) perceived effects on **functional ability,** (2) affect, and (3) helplessness. A study conducted in a multilevel long-term care facility found that 54% of residents acknowledged that their pain interfered with their enjoyment of activities available in the facility and 53% related it to impaired ambulation (Ferrell, Ferrell, & Osterweil, 1990).

While little is known about the prevalence of pain in the older adult during the terminal phase of life, several retrospective studies of hospice patients with a diagnosis of cancer have confirmed that their pain was a major issue toward the end of life (Mor, 1987; Morris, Suissa, Sherwood, Wright, & Greer, 1986). Moss, Lawton, and Glicksman (1991) conducted interviews with the closest available survivors of 200 older persons approximately 6 months after their death. Pain was reported to have increased during the last year of the person's life. While

37% had pain at the beginning of the year preceding death, 66% reported pain 1 month before death. More specifically, 27% had increased pain during the last 30 days of life. Such findings suggest an approach to **pain management** that is aimed at relief, primarily pharmacological. Involving persons in their own management by self-monitoring and reporting **pain intensity** and pain relief levels is an important part of this approach. Commonly used measures of pain intensity are shown in Figure 16-2.

The research-based Agency for Health Care Policy and Research (AHCPR) guidelines on the *Management of Cancer Pain* (Management of Cancer Pain Guideline Panel, 1994) state that pain can be controlled in 90% of cancer patients. However, their pain continues to be undertreated and pain management remains generally ineffective. The AHCPR panel believed that cancer clients and their families should be involved in the process of effective pain management; therefore, a Patient Guide to the management of cancer pain also was published.

> ### Nursing Tip
>
> Functional limitations related to chronic illness can impact the individual's quality of life. Be aware and assess for these limitations.

Functional Limitations

The nature of arthritis and other musculoskeletal conditions affects functional ability. Community-residing older

Visual Analogue Scale:

Instructions ask individuals to rate their current level of pain by marking a line across the line provided. (This is a 10-cm, or 100-mm, line, and the person's score is determined by measuring the point at which the line is drawn. The given line can be horizontal—as shown—or vertical.)

No pain	Worst possible pain

Verbal Descriptive Rating:

This example of the Present Pain Intensity (PPI) rating from the McGill Pain Questionnaire asks individuals to check the word that best describes current pain.

0	No pain	_____
1	Mild	_____
2	Discomforting	_____
3	Distressing	_____
4	Horrible	_____
5	Excruciating	_____

FIGURE 16-2 Frequently used measures of pain intensity. *(Adapted from* The McGill Pain Questionnaire, *by R. Melzack, 1975. Copyright 1975 by Ronald Melzack. Adapted with permission.)*

adults with arthritis and joint pain have indicated problems with mobility, upper extremity function, household management, and **self-care** activities of daily living (Fried & Guralnik, 1997). Self-reported arthritis also has been identified as a risk factor for falls among older adults (King & Tinetti, 1995). Osteoarthritis-associated factors such as muscle weakness of lower extremities and balance deficits, along with other factors such as impaired vision, medications, and comorbidity have been identified as possible causes of falls (Ling & Bathon, 1998).

In cancer, functional limitations may result directly from the disease process or interventions such as surgery and chemotherapy. However, cancer therapy also produces symptoms such as nausea, diarrhea, and fatigue. These symptoms can directly cause functional limitations. Cancer-related fatigue is an excellent example of an indirect cause of functional limitations.

Depression

Like pain, reports of depression among older adults have been varied. The incidence of depression may be small, but dysphoria or depressed mood may be greater. Anthony and Aboraya (1992) suggested that, despite the diagnostic criteria used, the incidence of depression in older adults is too great to be ignored. Its measurement may also be confounded by factors such as sleep abnormalities, functional limitations, somatic complaints, and fatigue (Bolla-Wilson & Blecker, 1989; Casey, 1994; Turk, Rudy, & Stieg, 1987). These associations suggest that depression has a close tie to chronic illness.

The close alliance between pain and functional ability in older adults has already been noted. Likewise, depression has also demonstrated an association with functional impairment (Guccione et al., 1994; Husaini & Moore, 1990; Katz & Yelin, 1993) and pain (Williamson & Schulz, 1992). Parmelee, Katz, and Lawton (1991) discovered a significant relationship between depression and functional ability in older residents of skilled nursing facilities. Also, when they controlled for functional disability, the correlation between pain and depression remained strong. This finding suggests that the pain-depression relationship is at least partially independent of the association with functional ability (Figure 16-3). More likely, the relationship between pain and depressed mood is mediated by functional ability (Williamson & Schulz, 1992).

Fatigue, Sleep Disturbance, and Social Support

Other factors that may affect the quality of life of persons with a chronic illness include fatigue, sleep disturbance, and the availability of social support. Fatigue may be largely caused by the inactivity and resulting decon-

ditioning that often occurs in the case of chronic illness. As one's activity level diminishes, conditioning is affected and tiring occurs more easily. In the case of inflammatory conditions such as RA, components of the inflammatory process may contribute to fatigue (Belza, 1996). A study of older adult RA clients revealed that 60% of the variance of fatigue was explained by pain, sleep disturbance, inactivity, comorbidities, poorer functional status, and newly diagnosed disease (Belza, Henke, Yelin, Epstein, & Gilliss, 1993).

> ### Nursing Tip
>
> Nurses need to assess for fatigue in all clients with a chronic condition. Fatigue may be associated with the disease process or may be a result of deconditioning. Fatigue should become the sixth vital sign. Pain is the fifth.

Cancer-related fatigue can produce lingering, chronic effects on the quality of life of cancer survivors (Haberman, 1998). This symptom has been rated as the most underassessed and undertreated symptom of cancer (Haberman, 1998). However, this situation is currently changing. The Fatigue Initiative through Research and Education (FIRE) project jointly sponsored by the Oncology Nursing Foundation and the Oncology Nursing Society, is a three-phase project initiated in 1995 and funded through 2000. Phase 1 focused on providing professional education for oncology nurses about the need to assess and treat

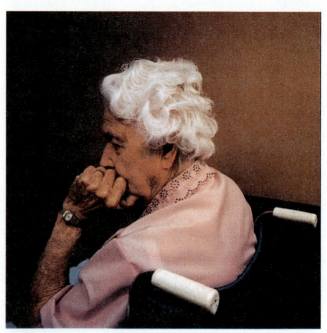

FIGURE 16-3 Older adults may experience depression secondary to pain and functional disability.

cancer-related fatigue throughout the trajectory of the disease and across cancer care settings (Haberman, 1998). The second phase continued through 1998 and focused on public education regarding the symptom of cancer-related fatigue. The focus of the third phase was on multifaceted, multi-institutional research. The project closed with a state-of-the-knowledge conference in 1999 (Haberman, 1998).

Because sleep disturbances are usually associated with pain, they are commonly found in painful chronic illnesses. Sleep issues represent an important concern within the older population (Roy, 1986). Some of this is due to the changing sleep patterns with age. While older adults have more midsleep awakening periods, they often maintain the amount of needed sleep through daytime naps (Wegener, 1996). Sleep disturbance has been documented in persons with OA (Moldofsky, Jue, & Saskin, 1987).

Social support, as used here, broadly refers to the social support that is beneficial to the individual's health promotion and well-being (Figure 16-4). There are many interpretations of social support, and the findings related to its importance vary. Much of this variation is probably related to the individual cultural, social, and physical needs of the person and how social support is conceptualized. In a study examining the role of social support in modifying the effects of pain and functional limitations on depression, Roberts, Matecjyck, and Anthony (1996) examined the effects of four types of social support: tangible, emotional, informational, and integrative. The sample included 59 persons (mean age 65) with end-stage joint disease just prior to joint arthroplasty of the hip or knee. The sample indicated moderately high emotional and integrative social support but received

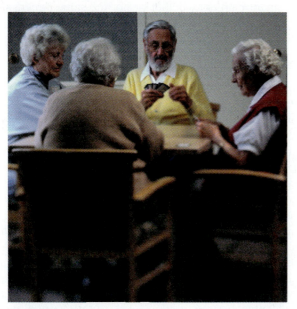

FIGURE 16-4 Social support is beneficial to the older adults' well being, but the effect on chronic illness is still being studied.

little tangible or informational support. Findings suggested that not all types of social support reduced the effects of pain and functional impairment on depression; rather, findings were mixed. Functional mobility (i.e., mobility, physical activity, and performing household activities) and depression were moderated by emotional and tangible support. Functional coordination (for example, dexterity and ADL) and depression were moderated by tangible support. These findings, along with others that have even suggested that there might be some adverse effects of social support, emphasize the importance of continuing to study its role in chronic illness.

Approaches to Assessment

In considering approaches to assessment with older adults there are a number of factors that may play a role. They should be remembered when selecting an instrument or an approach to assessment, because they will certainly affect the accuracy of the assessment. These factors include (a) visual impairments such as presbyopia, decreased visual acuity, cataracts, and glaucoma; (b) hearing impairments; (c) fatigue and discomfort related to such problems as muscle atrophy, decreased circulation to coronary arteries, and decreased fat cells; (d) decreased abstract thinking abilities; and (e) cognitive impairments (Shaw, 1992).

The relationships among chronic illness and pain, decreased functional ability, depression, and other associated variables vary with the individual person; therefore, they should be clinically evaluated for each individual. There are numerous assessment tools available for this purpose. Relevant and accurate assessment is necessary to intervene appropriately. Following is a discussion of some selected valid and reliable instruments that might be considered by nurses and other health professionals for the ongoing clinical assessment of older adults with a chronic illness. It should be noted that all of these require self-report.

Health Status

The measures used most often for assessing the health status of persons with arthritis include the Health Assessment Questionnaire (HAQ) (Fries, Spitz, & Kraines, 1980) and the Arthritis Impact Measurement Scales (AIMS) (Meenan, Gertman, & Mason, 1980) or their shorter versions, the Modified Health Assessment Questionnaire (MHAQ) (Pincus, Summey, Soraci, Wallston, & Hummon, 1983; Wolfe, 1995) and the AIMS2 (Meenan, Mason, Anderson, Guccione, & Kazis, 1992). These self-report instruments include components addressing ability to perform IADL and PADL, pain level, and emotions/mood. The shorter versions are more applicable for use in the clinical setting. These instruments have been successfully used with a variety of rheumatic diseases and with different age groups in community settings. Their sensitivity to measuring change in the person's condition contributes to their usefulness as clinical measures, as well as measures in outcome studies. They would be useful as part of a routine clinical measurement protocol for persons with arthritis in a variety of settings, such as offices of primary care providers, clinics, and rehabilitation settings.

The Medical Outcome Study Short Form 36 (SF-36) (McHorney, Ware, Lu, & Sherbourne, 1994; Stewart & Ware, 1992) is a health status instrument that has been used across a wide variety of client populations, including those with rheumatic disease. Its widespread use in outcomes studies contributes to its usefulness as a clinical measure in primary care settings, because there is a great deal of normative data available. Like the MHAQ, it can be completed quickly. Unlike the arthritis-specific tools, though, it does not yield some of the functional assessment information (Hawley, 1996).

Pain Intensity

A common approach to measuring pain intensity has simply been to ask persons to rate their current level of pain using a single-item measure such as a visual analogue scale (VAS) or a present pain intensity (PPI) rating, a verbal descriptor scale (VDS) that asks the individual to rate pain on a six-point scale from 0 (none) to 5 (excruciating) (Melzack & Katz, 1992). The VAS and VDS have demonstrated high correlations (Ekblom & Hansson, 1988; Kremer & Atkinson, 1983). This subjective rating of the single dimension of intensity most likely reflects the sensory/discriminant aspect of pain. When measuring pain intensity with persons who have chronic illness, the clinician should consider the number of comorbid conditions the person has and which of these have a pain component. Such considerations have important implications for planning and evaluating interventions.

The most commonly used unidimensional measure has been the VAS, though it has been suggested that there is a higher incidence of incorrect responses as age increases (Jensen, Karoly, & Braver, 1986). When six different one-item scales were compared, the correlations were high but the average scores varied. There seemed to be a greater problem in using the horizontal than the vertical VAS; thus, the vertical presentation of the scale may be more appropriate for older adults.

Pain Experience

The McGill Pain Questionnaire (MPQ) introduced by Melzack (1975) has been extremely valuable in differentiating the various dimensions of pain and their measurement. It gives persons an opportunity to describe their pain on the following dimensions: sensory, affective, or evaluative. Additionally, there is a miscellaneous category. The total pain rating index (PRI) score is the total of the ranked values selected by the individual. An alternative scoring method using weighted rank values has also been developed to provide increased sensitivity (Melzack, Katz, & Jeans, 1985).

A shorter version, the SF-MPQ, is especially useful for clinical applications. It provides 15-word descriptors representing the sensory and affective dimensions, and each is ranked on a scale of 0 (none) to 3 (severe). The resulting total PRI score has demonstrated high correlations with the PRI from the original MPQ (Melzack, 1987).

Herr and Mobily (1991) have suggested that the MPQ word choices may be too complex and overwhelming and the length of time required to complete it too long for some older adults. While information is not available related to its specific use with older clients, it has been widely used with this age group. Clinicians might consider using the short form with older clients and administering it verbally so that directions and word choices can be clarified if there are questions.

Davis (1991) has developed an instrument intended to measure the chronic **pain experience,** or response to persistent nonmalignant pain. The Chronic Pain Experience Instrument (CPEI) has been used with older clients, primarily with arthritis, and has demonstrated high estimates of validity and reliability with this age group (Davis, 1998a). The underlying dimensions of the CPEI provide direction for planning and evaluating ongoing pain management; these include perceived effects on functional ability, distress, and helplessness. The CPEI has not been tested with those experiencing malignant pain, so whether or not the same dimensions compose this experience is unknown.

Depression

Even though depression, or depressed mood, has been identified as a major problem in older adults who have chronic illness, health care professionals have not generally considered its assessment to be important. Primary care physicians' screening for and treatment of depression among community-dwelling older adults seldom occurs (Diamond et al., 1997). Perhaps the fact that it can be masked by a physical illness is one explanation for this oversight. Several instruments that serve as common screening tests for older adults include the Geriatric Depression Scale (GDS) (Yesavage et al., 1983), the Center for Epidemiological Studies-Depression Scale (CES-D) (Radloff, 1977), and the Beck Depression Inventory (BDI) (Gallagher, 1986). Short forms of both the GDS (Yesavage, 1986) and the BDI (Beck & Beck, 1972) are also available for use as screening measures. The CES-D was initially tested with persons living in the community, instead of persons in a psychiatric treatment setting. This contributes to its usefulness with the chronic illness population where depressed mood may be secondary to the illness itself. Not surprisingly, disability has been identified as the most important predictor of depression in persons with rheumatoid arthritis (Newman, Fitzpatrick, Lamb, & Shipley, 1989). The CES-D has been successfully used with older adults and with individuals with chronic pain (Davis, 1998a).

Fatigue

Development of measures to describe the type and occurrence of fatigue has been pioneered by Piper and her research team (Piper, Dibble, Dodd, Weiss, Slaughter, & Paul, 1998). The revised Piper Fatigue Scale (PFS) consists of 22 numerical scales providing choices from 0 to 10 that measure four dimensions of subjective fatigue: the affective dimension related to the emotional meaning attributed to fatigue; the behavioral dimension related to the severity, distress, and degree of disruption in ADL; the cognitive dimension related to mental and mood states; and the sensory dimension related to the physical symptoms of fatigue (Figure 16-5). Subscale scores can be determined separately for each dimension. A total fatigue score can also be calculated (Woo, Dibble, Piper, Keating, & Weiss, 1998).

As described earlier, the FIRE project continues to conduct multi-institutional research on the symptom of cancer-related fatigue. Examples of this research include the development of studies to test an exercise intervention for cancer-related fatigue (Mock et al., 1998). Another research team is investigating fatigue and quality of life (Grant et al., 1998).

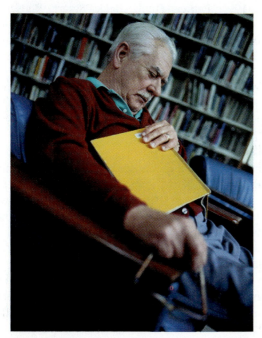

FIGURE 16-5 Fatigue is a common side effect of chronic illness.

Approaches and Services Addressing Chronic Illnesses and Their Effects

A variety of services are available to older adults experiencing chronic illnesses, though locating and accessing them may present a challenge. Nurses and other health professionals, especially those in primary care, can serve as catalysts in helping people locate resources that are a fit for them. In addition to the type of service (for example, informational, exercise, support group, counseling, and medical treatment), consideration of the setting where it is offered is important. Realistically, will the individual be able to access it? Will supportive arrangements such as assistance with transportation or mobility aids and learning to use the Internet be necessary?

When helping people access resources, professionals need to keep in mind that a major goal of using these resources is that of assisting individuals to maintain, or increase, their level of independence and quality of life. To do this, a thorough assessment of physical and cognitive abilities, as well as motivation, is necessary. Such assessment should include the person's current level of function, as well as its potential level. Stevenson (1997) noted that, in some cases, older adults may not have stretched their cognitive abilities for a long time, may have negative attitudes about a specific type of intervention, or may have a very low level of fitness. These issues need to be acknowledged in selecting the appropriate services and approaches and in allowing the time for the intervention to make a difference. When people are functioning below their potential, extra time will be necessary to see the benefits of participation in a new activity.

Health care services that address the issues of the client with chronic illness may involve a variety of approaches, many of which are interdisciplinary and focus on assisting the individual with self-management. The **cognitive-behavioral perspective** provides a way of addressing these important elements.

Cognitive-Behavioral Perspective

Approaches that use a cognitive-behavioral perspective assist the individual to recognize the connections among cognition, affect, and behavior, together with their joint consequences (Turk, Meichenbaum, & Genest, 1983). Cognitive-behavioral strategies have been used successfully for a variety of chronic conditions, for example, rheumatoid arthritis (Keefe & Van Horn, 1993; O'Leary, Shoor, Lorig, & Holman, 1988; Sinclair, Wallston, Dwyer, Blackburn, & Fuchs, 1998), cardiac rehabilitation (Taylor, Bandura, Ewart, Miller, & Debusk, 1985), tension headache (Mosley, Grothues, & Meeks, 1995), and unexplained physical symptoms (Speckens & van Hemert, 1995). The following research example demonstrates the importance of focusing on both cognitive and behavioral outcomes as part of an exercise treatment program for older adults with OA of the knee (Rejeski, Ettinger, Martin, & Morgan, 1998).

Research Focus

Citation:

Rejeski, W. J., Ettinger, Jr., W. H., Martin, K., & Morgan, T. (1998). Treating disability in knee osteoarthritis with exercise therapy. A central role for self-efficacy and pain. *Arthritis Care and Research, 11,* 94–101.

Purposes:

(a) To describe the effects of aerobic and resistance exercise on the self-efficacy beliefs of older adults with knee osteoarthritis (OA) and (b) to determine whether self-efficacy and knee pain mediate the effects of exercise therapy on stair-climbing performance and health perceptions.

Methods:

Three hundred fifty-seven older adults (age 60 and over) with knee OA were randomly assigned to one of three treatment groups: aerobic exercise, resistance training, or health education control. Data collection measures of self-efficacy, knee pain, stair-climbing performance, and health perceptions were collected prior to randomization and 18 months following implementation of the exercise programs.

Findings:

The two exercise treatments increased self-efficacy for stair climbing in comparison with the health education control group. The effect of each of the exercise treatments on self-efficacy was consistent with improvement in stair climbing. Both knee pain and self-efficacy mediated the effect of the treatment on stair-climbing time, while only knee pain mediated health perception.

Implications:

The findings suggest that both self-efficacy beliefs and changes in physical symptoms such as pain are important outcomes, along with physical performance and health perception, of an exercise intervention. The promotion of self-efficacy beliefs in combination with either of the exercise programs was superior to health education alone; thus it seems important to link physical activity and performance improvement with information.

A cognitive-behavioral perspective recognizes the importance of cognitive and affective factors on behavior and the importance of various behavioral techniques, especially positive reinforcement for adaptive behaviors. The following goals are supported: (a) positive reconceptualization of a helpless and hopeless view; (b) monitoring thoughts, feelings, and behaviors during activities and identifying the relationships between these, the environment, and symptoms experienced; (c) dealing effectively with problems by using necessary behaviors; and (d) developing and using increasingly more effective and adaptive ways of thinking, feeling, and responding (Holzman, Turk, & Kerns, 1986). These cognitive-behavioral goals, as specifically applied to the successful handling of chronic illness, are an integral part of self-management.

Self-efficacy, defined as "beliefs in one's capabilities to organize and execute the courses of action required to produce given attainments" (Bandura, 1997, p. 3), is a concept important within this perspective. Strengthening one's self-efficacy expectations should enhance self-management behaviors and health status (Taal, Rasker, & Wiegman, 1996). One's self-efficacy beliefs can influence behavior, motivation, thoughts, and emotions (Buckelew et al., 1994). People are more likely to perform behaviors if they view these as being within their capabilities and resulting in positive consequences. Success should then reinforce the behavior.

Even though the cognitive-behavioral approach has been well recognized within the pain management literature, it has been used very infrequently for that purpose with older adults. The studies testing this approach with the older population have been few in number (Cook, 1998; Fry & Wong, 1991; Hamm & King, 1984; Mosley et al., 1995; Parker, Frank, Beck, Smarr, Buescher, & Phillips, 1988; Puder, 1988). Results have demonstrated that older adults can successfully use such interventions as stress inoculation training (SIT) that combines cognitive restructuring, imagery-based pain control, and progressive muscle relaxation (Puder, 1988) and an attention/support intervention that provides minimally structured and supportive group therapy (Cook, 1998).

Education

Education has been recognized as an important method of learning to cope with chronic illnesses such as arthritis. It is an approach that, when properly implemented, can incorporate the four components of cognitive-behavioral therapy: (a) education, (b) skills acquisition, (c) cognitive and behavioral rehearsal, and (d) generalization and maintenance (Bradley, 1996).

A well-established Arthritis Self-Help Course exemplifying this approach is offered through local chapters of the **Arthritis Foundation (AF).** This course was developed and tested by Lorig and Fries (1995) at the

Stanford Arthritis Center; *The Arthritis Helpbook* (Lorig & Fries, 1996) has been prepared to accompany this program. Lorig and Associates (1996) have prepared a book for health care providers who would like to provide client education that supports self-management, sharing information that has undoubtedly been used for and learned from offering the arthritis self-help course. Three primary features of the self-management model are identified as (a) dealing with the consequences of the disease; (b) concern with problem solving, decision making, and client confidence, as opposed to prescription and adherence; and (c) placing clients and health professionals in partnership relationships.

Davis and White (2000) used an educational approach to promote osteoporosis self-management activities with older adult residents in a retirement home setting. The development of the osteoporosis educational program (OEP) was based on a cognitive-behavioral perspective with the belief that behavioral practices such as using specific strategies, taking calcium supplements, and performing simple exercises for maintaining bone health and preventing falls are influenced by one's understanding of the associated condition (e.g., osteoporosis). Experimenting with strategies such as goal setting and games to actively involve individuals in the process were questions important to the pilot testing. Although the sample ($n = 10$) for this pilot study was small, the results supported further development of this group education approach that extended over a 4-week period. The participants' knowledge about osteoporosis and its management increased, and their participation was marked by interest and enthusiasm. Such programs are suggested for older adult groups across a variety of settings.

Support Groups

Approaches that actively involve the person may also include support groups. Because many older adults with a chronic illness have limited activity that has restricted their socialization, it may be important to involve them outside the home when possible. When community social workers in Canada offered home-based counseling to persons with arthritis, for example, they found that social isolation was a common experience. As a result, they planned and implemented a successful group intervention (Kowarsky & Glazier, 1997).

Cronan, Groessl, and Kaplan (1997) found that both social support and educational interventions and a combined social support/educational intervention provided cost-effective approaches to helping older adult participants learn self-management strategies by interacting with and learning from each other. In this case, using volunteers rather than professionals for implementing the interventions demonstrated a cost-saving technique. Participants' quality of life showed some improvement, though not significantly different from a control group.

In the study conducted by Cook (1998) cited above, a combination support group/educational intervention also was used. Combining these approaches provides a way of incorporating the components of the cognitive-behavioral perspective. Even though social support has not demonstrated consistently positive effects in past studies, the way in which social support is interpreted may be an issue. These studies suggested that when it is structured in a well-defined manner, a support group provides a method by which individuals can learn from each other. As a method that has been used rarely with older adults, further testing seems merited.

> ### Nursing Tip
>
> Be knowledgeable about assistive devices, organizational supports, and informational and community resources. Clients and families may ask or you may need to make referrals for them.

Organizational Resources

Numerous organizations that are disease-specific exist primarily for education and research. The AF and the ACS represent the major organizations focusing on arthritis and cancer, respectively. Additional **organizational resources** are presented in Table 16-2. [For a more comprehensive list that includes a variety of chronic conditions, see Davis and Raudonis (1998).] The AF offers numerous educational resources through its approximately 70 local AF chapters throughout the United States and its national office. Published materials include a wide variety of pamphlets, some of which are specific to such rheumatic diseases as OA, RA, lupus, and gout. A magazine, *Arthritis Today,* that is published by the AF six times annually also provides information that is very practical in nature. In addition to the AF, there are other arthritis-related organizations that provide education and support for their members. These include The American Lupus Society (TALS), Spondylitis Association, and National Osteoporosis Foundation (NOF).

The ACS is dedicated to eliminating cancer as a major health problem. The programs and services offered are categorized as research, education, and client services. The ACS organizational structure provides a national, community-based network, with state or division offices and local units throughout the 50 states. Materials and information about client services are available online through the ACS web site. In addition to the ACS, there are other cancer-related organizations that provide support and informational resources for specific types of cancer. These include the American Brain Tumor Association, Breast Cancer Information Clearinghouse, and National Coalition for Cancer Survivorship.

TABLE 16-2 Organizational Resources

Organization	Resources
American Cancer Society (ACS) 1599 Clifton Road, NE Atlanta, GA 30329 1-800-ACS-2345	Provides information on a wide variety of cancer-related topics and, in addition, the opportunity to do added searches. These may be related to specific types of cancer. Gives up-to-date statistics for clients and families and guidelines for prevention and detection. Links to information about activity in one's state.
American Fibromyalgia Association (AFSA) 6380 E. Tangue Verde, Suite D Tucson, AZ 85715	Nonprofit organization dedicated to research, education, and client advocacy for fibromyalgia (FMS) and chronic fatigue syndrome (CFS). Web site provides basic information about FMS and information about how to contact support groups.
American College of Rheumatology (ACR)/ Association of Rheumatology Health Professionals (ARHP) 1800 Century Place, Suite 250 Atlanta, GA 30345	Provides information for clients and practice standards for health professionals. Fact sheets on numerous rheumatic disease conditions are available in print and on-line.
Arthritis Foundation (AF) P.O. Box 7669 1330 W. Peachtree Street Atlanta, GA 30357-0669 1-800-283-7800	Provides up-to-date information about arthritis that includes facts, figures, and tips. Some of this is selected from resources and brochures that are available from AF. Provides information about how to contact local AF offices and other resources.
Fibromyalgia Network P.O. Box 31750 Tucson, AZ 85751 1-800-853-2929	Provides educational material on FMS and CFS. Discusses the basics of FMS, including diagnostic criteria and commonly associated symptoms. Provides coping tips from prior issues of its printed publication, *Fibromyalgia Network*.
National Cancer Institute (NCI) Office of Cancer Communications Bldg. 31, Room 10A18 Bethesda, MD 20205 1-800-4CANCER	The NCI coordinates the government's cancer research and is part of the National Institutes of Health (NIH). The web site provides information for cancer clients, the public, and mass media. This includes research information, latest research developments, information about a variety of therapies, and help for clients related to such issues as how to manage treatment side effects and talk with health care providers about pain.
National Osteoporosis Foundation (NOF) 1150 17th Street NW, Suite 500 Washington, DC 20036 1-202-223-2226	Provides professional education and client advocacy information. Web site provides a list of client brochures and other publications and ordering instructions.
Osteoporosis and Related Bone Diseases-National Resource Center 1150 17th Street NW, Suite 500 Washington, DC 20036	Provides information about a number of conditions, including Paget's disease and osteoporosis. Web site is linked to related sites such as National Institute of Arthritis and Musculoskeletal Diseases (NAIMS), another excellent resource for arthritis.
Spondylitis Association of America P.O. Box 5872 Sherman Oaks, CA 91413 1-800-777-8189	Provides information about ankylosing spondylitis and associated diseases such as Reiter's syndrome and psoriatic arthritis.

Planning for the Future

Little attention has been given to the nonpharmacological management of chronic illness in older adults, a consideration that is especially important when comorbidity is a potentially complicating factor. Treatment is often limited to the use of medicine, with older adults taking two to three times more drugs than those who are younger (Bressler, 1993). If attention from the traditional curative model is shifted to one of health promotion that focuses on the individual's quality of life and sense of well-being, nonpharmacological methods will need to be better integrated with the use of medicine. Additionally, more attention can be given to involving the individual in self-monitoring the effects of medicines taken.

Cognitive-behavioral strategies that provide a way for people to avoid this reliance on medication management deserve more recognition as feasible approaches to managing chronic illness. Even though such strategies have long been recognized in enhancing the self-management of pain, they have had very limited use with older adults. Because older individuals may be more sensitive to the effects of medications and be more likely to take multiple medications because of comorbidity, nonpharmacological approaches could be especially helpful.

Examples of **nonpharmacological pain management** approaches that are sometimes used by older adults for modulating chronic musculoskeletal pain include the following (Davis, 1998a): (a) distracting techniques; (b) relaxation methods such as meditation or guided imagery; (c) heated pool, tub, or shower; (d) stress control methods; (e) positive self-talk; and (f) pacing activities, or performing activities in a balanced way to avoid overexertion. The strategies aimed at cognitive restructuring are not used as often by older adults as by middle-aged and younger adults, perhaps indicating that older adults had not been exposed to these methods as often. Such methods provide an example of approaches that might be incorporated into an educational program using a cognitive-behavioral framework for assisting older adults to self-manage chronic illness. How to use complementary methods and alternative therapies such as exercise, music, light, and massage should also be considered (see Figure 16-6). Since functional ability, pain intensity, fatigue levels, and mood are commonly affected by chronic illness, their presence should be acknowledged in implementing new therapies and changes in them monitored to determine effectiveness.

There are many possibilities for developing and implementing innovative approaches for promoting the health status of the older adult with a chronic illness. As previously noted, it is important that such methods (a) actively involve the individual, (b) have an interdisciplinary approach, (c) address health as being multidimensional in nature, (d) be goal oriented, (e) allow persons to experience and acknowledge success, (f) build on where the person is, and (g) provide physical and emotional support as needed.

As opposed to acute illness, the emphasis of future services provided will be on maintaining or improving health status and promoting health rather than on curing the condition. When considering the care of the older adult, specifically, much emphasis needs to be given to assisting the individual to remain independent. Such a goal is important to increasing the quality of life.

Because the enhancement of quality of life is difficult to translate into financial data, outcomes will need to be documented in several ways. Including a combination of clinical and sociodemographic data, along with cost analysis, will be vital to influencing public policy changes. As Haber (1994, p. 1) notes, "Moving from this costly emphasis on disease and medical treatment to one of disease prevention and health promotion in the United States . . . will require creative and cost-effective strategies." A positive reorientation of health care practices is overdue. Getzen (1992) cautions that the aging population is not responsible for the increasing costs; rather, growing problems and concerns are inherent within the present system (or nonsystem) as it has been constructed.

Summary

As the percentage of the age 65 and older population increases, so will the incidence of chronic illness. Over 80% of this age group have at least one chronic condition, with most having more than one. The fact that assistance with the performance of many daily activities increases with age is not surprising. The increasing functional, social, and financial limitations associated with chronic conditions call for a variety of resources to be offered within the community.

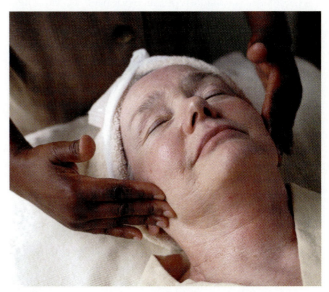

FIGURE 16-6 A facial massage can be relaxing as well as therapeutic.

CARE PLAN

CASE STUDY

Mr. Horace Edmunds, an 80-year-old man, has been diagnosed with congestive heart failure, hypertension, and arthritis for 20 years. He lives in retirement housing with his wife, Emily, and youngest son, who is 35 years old. It is thought that his son is a drug dealer in the neighborhood. Mr. and Mrs. Edmunds do not condone their son's actions, but they are ambivalent about asking him to leave. Mr. Edmunds is a retired assembly-line worker for a car manufacturer. He has adequate health care benefits and is retired with an adequate pension. His Social Security is also adequate. Emily worked part-time in the town library. They both are concerned about their youngest son.

Mr. Edmunds has been hospitalized three times with CHF (congestive heart failure) over the 20-year course of his disease. He has a history of smoking since 12 years old and has no intention of stopping: "I got this far. Why should I change." He is 6 feet 2 inches tall and weighs 275 pounds. His blood pressure ranges from 158/80 to 180/95. His ejection fraction is <40%. His medications include Coreg (carvedilol), Monopril (fosinopril), digoxin, and Lasix (furosemide).

Lately, Mr. Edmunds has been complaining of a cough, insomnia, and dyspnea. His wife says he seems confused sometimes, forgetting his phone number and appointments he has made with friends and family. He climbs steps and becomes out of breath at the second flight. Fatigue and tiredness warrant his napping during the daytime. He feels like he has been gaining weight and states, "My shoes are tight." His favorite foods include fried chicken and ice cream, which he eats two to three times weekly.

ASSESSMENT

Mr. Edmunds has classic signs and symptoms of congestive heart failure. He has not controlled many of the risk factors such as smoking, increased weight, diet, and high blood pressure. Symptom control and risk factor management are key to successful treatment of this chronic illness. Here is the essential content of his care plan and pathway for congestive heart failure. In the pathway, note the terms "PCG" (primary care giver) and "POC" (plan of care). Three aspects of the pathway are illustrated: session/visit 1, a portion of session/visit 2, and an outcome sheet. Compare the pathway with the care plan and note the similarities in the content of care. Practice filling in the pathway using the care plan as a guide.

NURSING DIAGNOSIS

Decreased cardiac output as evidenced by variable blood pressure readings, altered mental state (forgetfulness), fatigue, edema, and weight gain related to left-sided heart failure.

Outcomes:

Mr. Edmunds will:
- *Have decreased and consistent blood pressures.*
- *Exhibit no crackles, no S_3 or S_4 heart sounds.*
- *Manifest no edema, shortness of breath, insomnia, fatigue, or other signs and symptoms of CHF.*
- *Adhere to low-sodium dietary guidelines.*
- *Commit to stop smoking.*
- *Stop smoking.*
- *Decrease weight.*

Planning/Interventions:

The nurse will:
- *Assess cardiovascular and respiratory status.*
- *Assess for jugular vein distention (JVD) and peripheral pulses.*
- *Monitor weight and vital signs.*

(continues)

CARE PLAN *continued*

- *Assess for edema.*
- *Examine most recent labwork: electrocardiogram, cardiac enzymes, chest x-ray, pulse oximeter readings.*
- *Collaborate with physician on medication regimen with consideration to increasing diuretic and carvedilol or angiotensin-converting enzyme (ACE) inhibitor.*
- *Encourage and facilitate smoking cessation program.*
- *Teach about CHF control and risk factors.*
- *Teach Mr. or Mrs. Edmunds how to monitor daily weights, pulse, and blood pressure.*

EVALUATION:

Mr. Edmunds will remain free of signs and symptoms of CHF. He will take charge of managing his illness by monitoring weight, pulse, and blood pressure. He will maintain consistent blood pressure readings within normal limits (WNL). Heart and lung sounds will range WNL. He will adhere to dietary and smoking cessation—no easy task. His wife will play a critical role as his immediate social support network.

NURSING DIAGNOSIS

Decisional conflict related to family values and beliefs regarding son's activities, as evidenced by verbalized uncertainty about asking him to move out.

Outcomes:

Mr. and Mrs. Edmunds will:
- *Express their values and feelings to their son.*
- *Make a decision consistent with their beliefs and feelings.*

Planning/Interventions:

The nurse will:
- *Encourage the Edmunds to talk with their son and express their concerns and beliefs.*
- *Explore and evaluate all feasible options related to the son's situation.*
- *Facilitate a resolution acceptable to the Edmunds.*

EVALUATION:

Mr. and Mrs. Edmunds will resolve their conflict surrounding their son's actions inconsistent with the current living arrangement. After exploring all options, they will commit to a plan that promotes a healthy home and healthy community while supporting a positive change in their son's (and their) life.

Chronic illnesses that are the most common among older adults include hypertension, arthritis, musculoskeletal impairments, cancer, heart disease, diabetes, chronic airway obstruction, and peripheral vascular disease. Often these exist in combination. The issues associated with most conditions are the same, with pain and functional limitations being the most common. Overall, the individual's quality of life is affected.

Because of the nature of chronic illness and the need for developing coping and adaptation skills, it is important that the individual be involved in self-care to the greatest degree possible. This involvement is highly dependent on other factors such as cultural background, age, and the person's confidence in being able to manage the effects of the illness and make the necessary adaptations.

Assessment of the individual should be comprehensive, including such areas as pain, functional ability, and depression. Likewise, treatment approaches are complex and interdisciplinary in nature. Cognitive-behavioral approaches are applicable, because they assist the person to recognize connections among knowledge and beliefs, feelings, and behavior. Nonpharmacological interventions are also important in reducing some of the issues associated with medications and polypharmacy. Managing chronic illness also requires a variety of organizational and community resources of which the client and the nurse should be aware.

CONGESTIVE HEART FAILURE
SKILLED NURSING PATHWAY

PATIENT NAME	PATIENT ID#
DATE OPENED:	DATE CLOSED:

STANDARD:

The physical assessment standard and standard for nursing interventions are based on Agency for Health Care Policy and Research (AHCPR) guidelines for nursing care of the patient experiencing Congestive Heart Failure.

DISCHARGE CRITERIA:

1. Client/caregiver will demonstrate understanding of CHF and self-care management.
2. Client will integrate diet modifications, medications, and any prescribed exercise regimens into daily living plan.
3. Client's vital signs, weight and cardiovascular status are normal for client range.
4. Other: _____

NURSING DIAGNOSES: (Choose appropriate diagnoses)

1. ☐ Knowledge deficit regarding disease process and home care management.
2. ☐ Alteration in cardiac output related to mechanical factors.
3. ☐ Alteration in fluid volume; excess, related to increased systemic venous congestion and/or left ventricular failure.
4. ☐ Potential for alteration in skin integrity related to edema.
5. ☐ Ineffective coping related to diagnosis and prognosis.
6. ☐ Activity intolerance related to decreased cardiac output.
7. Other: _____

TEACHING TOOLS:

Medication Teaching Sheets
CHF Management Packet
_____
_____

SN VISIT FREQUENCY:

Recommended: 6-8 visits
Other Disciplines Active in Care Plan: ☐ PT   ☐ OT   ☐ ST   ☐ MSW   ☐ HHA   ☐ Other:

VARIANCE CODES:

A: Patient too physically impaired/ill
B: Co-morbid interference
C: Psychosocial issues interfering
D: Caregiver limitations/difficulties

E: Equipment problems
F: Pt/CG learning difficulties
G: Pt/CG decision
H: Does not apply (explain)

Nursing pathway for congestive heart failure, including first and second visits. *(Courtesy of Connecticut VNA, Inc.)*

CONGESTIVE HEART FAILURE
PATIENT OUTCOME LOG: SKILLED NURSING

For each visit made, enter date of visit and place a check-mark (√) next to any outcomes achieved during the visit. If an outcome can not be achieved during this plan of care due to some interfering factor, enter a variance code from the list at the bottom of the page. Explain the use of a variance code in the "Explanation of Variances" area.

DATE OF VISIT:								
VISIT #	**1**	**2**	**3**	**4**	**5**	**6**	**7**	**8**
Verbalizes s/s requiring emergency action; has emergency procedures in place.								
Explains correct medication schedule/demonstrates effective medication management.								
Verbalizes primary concern and personal goals of care; verbalizes projected length of services and plan for discharge.								
Demonstrates adherence to keeping weight and symptom log.								
Demonstrates radial pulse taking.								
Demonstrates safety awareness during position changes.								
Demonstrates effective skin care techniques/management of edema.								
Verbalizes s/s of electrolyte imbalance and action to take if noted.								
Verbalizes s/s of CHF and action to take if noted.								
Verbalizes s/s of fluid retention/advancing edema and action to take if noted.								
Verbalizes role of medication, diet and activity/rest balance in treatment of disease.								
Patient exhibits freedom from s/s of exacerbation of CHF.								
Demonstrates adequate self care capacity and identifies family/social supports needed to manage disease at home.								
Other:								
Other:								
TOTAL GOALS MET THIS VISIT								
INITIALS OF RN								

EXPLANATION OF VARIANCES:

SIGNATURE BLOCK:
NAME/TITLE _____ INITIALS _____
NAME/TITLE _____ INITIALS _____
NAME/TITLE _____ INITIALS _____
NAME/TITLE _____ INITIALS _____

TOTAL OUTCOMES MET:
_____
TOTAL POSSIBLE: _____
% ACHIEVED (ACHIEVED/POSSIBLE): _____

VARIANCE CODES:
A: Patient too physically impaired/ill
B: Co-morbid interference
C: Psychosocial issues interfering
D: Caregiver limitations/difficulties
E: Equipment problems
F: Pt/CG learning difficulties
G: Pt/CG decision
H: Does not apply (explain)

PATIENT NAME:		PATIENT ID#	
PATIENT SIGNATURE:	INSURANCE TYPE/ PAYER:	DATE	VISIT #1

FIRST EPISODE CHF? ☐ Yes ☐ No

☐ Systolic CHF ☐ Diastolic CHF
EJECTION FRACTION: %   Date

CONFINED TO HOME DUE TO:	NOT CONFINED TO HOME:
Unable to leave home w/o use of device/another person due to:	Attends SOCIAL adult day care program
Trips out of home are medically contraindicated due to:	Leaves home frequently without assistance
Experiencing extreme weakness/pain related to illness/surgery:	Leaves home for long periods of time without asst.
Cardio/respiratory tolerance to ambulate only _____ ft. due to:	Other:
Unsafe to leave home due to psychiatric illness:	
Other (specify):	

SUBJECTIVE DATA/PRIMARY COMPLAINT PER PATIENT:

VITAL SIGNS/ASSESSMENT STATISTICS/LAB VALUES

Temp	BP: lying/sitting/standing	PEDAL EDEMA:		LAB VALUES:	
Resp	Right	Left ankle	Right ankle	O_2 sat	
Radial Pulse	Left	Left instep	Right instep	Protime	INR
Apical Pulse	Abd Girth (cm)	Left calf	Right calf	FBS/RBS	
Weight (Actual)	Other:			Other:	

SUBJECTIVE SYMPTOMS/PRIMARY COMPLAINT PER PATIENT:

☐ Exercise tolerance/weakness   ☐ Paroxysmal Nocturnal Dyspnea: ☐ Other: _____
Comments:

RESPIRATORY	CARDIOVASCULAR
WNL	WNL
lungs clear to auscultation	ascites:
lung sounds diminished:	chest pain (describe/specify location):
lung sounds absent:	pleuritic pain (describe/specify location):
dyspnea/SOB	neck vein distention: cms
orthopnea	(+) peripheral pulses Left/Right
crackles/location by lung field:	abnormal heart sounds:
rhonchi/location by lung field:	Other pulses:
wheeze/location by lung field:	cyanosis
cough: productive/non-prod.	Rhythm: regular/irregular
sputum:	
O_2 @ liters/minute	

PAIN MANAGEMENT

No pain per client	■ Per patient, pain affects:

Location of Pain:
Per patient, rate level of pain: LEAST 0 1 2 3 4 5 6 7 8 9 10 WORST

OTHER OBJECTIVE FINDINGS/NARRATIVE COMMENTS:

ANALYSIS OF FINDINGS:

VISIT #1

MEDICATION MANAGEMENT:

☐ Written medication information given to patient ☐ Adheres to medication regimen ☐ Verbalized dose/schedule
☐ Medications re-ordered: ☐ Med box prefill from (date) to (date)
☐ Medications assessed for side effects/contraindications/effectiveness. Medications instructed (specify):

TREATMENT/PROCEDURES

TEACHING/TRAINING

Instructions given to: ☐ Pt. ☐ PCG. ☐ Other:	Teaching/training regarding:	☐ Instructed ☐ Reinstructed	Retention verified via: ☐ demonstration ☐ verbal response	Level of understanding: ☐ Complete ☐ Partial ☐ None
Instructions given to: ☐ Pt. ☐ PCG. ☐ Other:	Teaching/training regarding:	☐ Instructed ☐ Reinstructed	Retention verified via: ☐ demonstration ☐ verbal response	Level of understanding: ☐ Complete ☐ Partial ☐ None

CLIENT RESPONSE TO CARE
Document response to treatments and interventions, progress toward discharge goals, and understanding of and compliance with treatments/interventions.

Notified MD of following: ☐ Weight gain greater than 2 lbs. in 24 hours or 4 lbs. in one week; ☐ O_2 Sat <90%; ☐ chest pain ☐ BP <90 systolic

PLAN FOR NEXT VISIT: (include follow-up to treatments, interventions, and demonstrations) **Approx. Next Visit Date:**

COORDINATION OF CARE: Document case conference content on Conference Form ☐ CC WITH (NAME):
☐ TELEPHONE CALL TO:

Next MD appt:

Care Plan Management/Discharge Planning: Care Plan [ ] Reviewed and/or [ ] revised with patient/cg involvement;
Discharge plan [ ] formulated with patient/PCG [ ] Reviewed with patient/PCG

Home Health Aide Orientation/Supervision   Name of HHAide _____

Yes	No	Orientation/Supervision/Activity	Yes	No	Orientation/Supervision/Activity
		Patient care plan revised/updated			Care given as per the Plan of Care
		Patient care needs assessed by HHA prior to starting care			Universal Standards practiced by HHA
		Pt/PCG participated in POC changes prior to implementation			Continued need for HHA services
		Rapport between HHA and Pt/cg satisfactory			Follow up required (specify)
Activities requiring specific instruction and return demonstration:			Other activities performed/observed		

DISCHARGE CRITERIA:

1. Client/caregiver will demonstrate understanding of CHF and self-care management.
2. Client will integrate diet modifications, medications, and any prescribed exercise regimens into daily living plan.
3. Client's vital signs, weight and cardiovascular status at baseline for client.

SIGNATURE/TITLE

PATIENT NAME:		PATIENT ID#	
PATIENT SIGNATURE:	INSURANCE TYPE/ PAYOR:	DATE	VISIT #2

NURSING ASSESSMENT/OBSERVATION: MARK ALL APPLICABLE WITH AN "X"; CIRCLE APPROPRIATE ITEM(S) SEPARATED BY "/".

CONFINED TO HOME DUE TO:	NOT CONFINED TO HOME:
Unable to leave home w/o use of device/another person due to:	Attends SOCIAL adult day care program
Trips out of home are medically contraindicated due to:	Leaves home frequently without assistance
Experiencing extreme weakness/pain related to illness/surgery:	Leaves home for long periods of time without asst.
Cardio/respiratory tolerance to ambulate only _____ ft. due to:	Other:
Unsafe to leave home due to psychiatric illness:	
Other (specify):	

VITAL SIGNS/ASSESSMENT STATISTICS/LAB VALUES

		PEDAL EDEMA:		LAB VALUES:	
Temp	BP: lying/sitting/standing				
Resp	Right	Left ankle	Right ankle	O₂ sat	
Radial Pulse	Left	Left instep	Right instep	Protime	INR
Apical Pulse	Abd Girth (cm)	Left calf	Right calf	FBS/RBS	
Weight (Actual)	Other:			Other:	

SUBJECTIVE SYMPTOMS/PRIMARY COMPLAINT PER PATIENT:

☐ Exercise tolerance/weakness   ☐ Paroxysmal Nocturnal Dyspnea: ☐ Other: _____
Comments:

RESPIRATORY	CARDIOVASCULAR
WNL	WNL
lungs clear to auscultation	ascites:
lung sounds diminished:	chest pain (describe/specify location):
lung sounds absent:	pleuritic pain (describe/specify location):
dyspnea/SOB	neck vein distention: cms
orthopnea	Pulses:
crackles/location by lung field:	abnormal heart sounds:
rhonchi/location by lung field:	S1/S2
wheeze/location by lung field:	cyanosis
cough: productive/non-prod.	Rhythm: regular/irregular
sputum:	
egophony	Other:
O₂ @ liters/minute	
Other:	

PAIN MANAGEMENT	
No pain per client	Per patient, pain affects:
Location of Pain:	
Per patient, rate level of pain: LEAST 0 1 2 3 .4 5 6 7 8 9 10 WORST	

OTHER OBJECTIVE FINDINGS:

ANALYSIS OF FINDINGS:

MEDICATION MANAGEMENT:

☐ Adheres to medication regimen ☐ Verbalized dose/schedule ☐ Med box prefill from (date)   to (date)
☐ Medication administered by nurse (specify med, dose, route, site, response):

TREATMENTS/PROCEDURES

Pathway continued

VISIT #2

√	NURSING INTERVENTIONS	√	NURSING INTERVENTIONS
	Teach definition/causes of disease process		Teach fluid/dietary restrictions; have patient keep a diet log and assess understanding and compliance
	Instruct daily weights and use of weight/symptom log; assess understanding and compliance		Instruct in medication effects/side effects/contra-indications; leave medication list in patient's home
	Teach s/s of CHF and action to take if noted		Teach slow position changes/rationale for this; assess management of ADLs/IADLs; teach activity pacing
	Instruct on radial pulse taking and parameters for use of digitalis; assess skill level		Teach patient to avoid temperature extremes and other environmental hazards which may exacerbate CHF
	Teach s/s of electrolyte imbalance and symptoms to report		Teach patient to elevate feet when resting; assess tolerance of gradually increased activities
	Teach s/s of fluid retention and action to take if noted		Establish an emergency plan; teach emergency procedures
	Instruct on skin care and risk of skin breakdown due to edema		Other (specify):

CLIENT RESPONSE TO CARE Document response to treatments and interventions, progress toward discharge goals, and understanding of and adherence to treatments/interventions.

☐ Notified MD of following: Weight gain greater than 2 lbs. in 24 hours or 4 lbs. in one week; O_2 Sat <90%; chest pain

PLAN FOR NEXT VISIT: (include follow-up to treatments, interventions, and demonstrations) **Approx. Next Visit Date:**

COORDINATION OF CARE: Document case conference content on Conference Form ☐ CC WITH (NAME):
☐ TELEPHONE CALL TO:

Next MD appt:

Care Plan Management/Discharge Planning: Care Plan [ ] Reviewed and/or [ ] revised with patient/cg involvement;
Discharge plan [ ] formulated with patient/PCG [ ] Reviewed with patient/PCG

Home Health Aide (circle one) Orientation/Supervision Name of HHAide _____

Yes	No	Orientation/Supervision/Activity	Yes	No	Orientation/Supervision/Activity
		Patient care plan revised/updated			Care given as per the Plan of Care
		Patient care needs assessed by HHA prior to starting care			Universal Standards practiced by HHA
		Pt/PCG participated in POC changes prior to implementation			Continued need for HHA services
		Rapport between HHA and Pt/cg satisfactory			Follow up required (specify)
Activities requiring specific instruction and return demonstration:			Other activities performed/observed		

DISCHARGE CRITERIA:

1. Client/caregiver will demonstrate understanding of CHF and self-care management.
2. Client will integrate diet modifications, medications, and any prescribed exercise regimen into daily living plan.
3. Client's vital signs, weight and cardiovascular status at baseline for client.

SIGNATURE/TITLE

Review Questions and Activities

1. What are some of the possible barriers that older women with a chronic condition might have in obtaining health care? Think about ways that the nurse might facilitate access to needed services.

2. What are the major secondary conditions experienced by older individuals who have arthritis or cancer?

3. What are the major fracture sites associated with osteoporosis? Think about how these can affect the person's functioning and level of independence.

4. What are the most effective methods to assess chronic pain in older adults?

5. What are some ways in which the combined effects of chronic illness can affect the older individual's quality of life?

6. How does social support assist those who are chronically ill?

7. If the nurse observes signs that suggest that the client is depressed, what actions would be appropriate to take?

8. If you, as a nurse in a home health agency, were designing an assessment protocol to be implemented with all clients experiencing chronic illness, what factors would you consider essential

to measure? What other factors would be identified for assessment on an as-needed basis?

9. The nurse is frequently questioned by clients with functional limitations about resources that would support their participation in such community activities as attending church-related activities and senior centers. Where might the nurse find answers to these questions?

10. In planning any intervention for older individuals with chronic illness, why is it important to consider the individual as an important component of the team?

11. Discuss the social, political, and economic implications of living with (a) cancer and (b) osteoarthritis.

12. Explore the Internet web sites www.nof.org and www.cancer.org. What type of information did you find that would be helpful to (a) health care professionals and (b) clients and their families?

13. How can you serve as an advocate for those with chronic illnesses today? At school? In the community? In your work place? In public policy?

14. What is your vision of care for those with chronic illnesses in the twenty-first century?

References

Agency for Health Care Policy and Research. (1998, July). Studies examine health care needs and access to care for people age 80 and older. AHCPR Research Activities No. 217. Washington, DC: Author.

American Cancer Society. (1998). *Cancer: basic facts* [On-line]. Available: http://www.cancer.org/statistics/cff98/basicfacts.html#is.

Anthony, J., & Aboraya, A. (1992). The epidemiology of selected mental disorders in later life. In J. Birren, R. Sloane, & G. Cohen (Eds.), *Handbook of mental health and aging* (2nd ed., pp. 27–73). San Diego, CA: Academic Press.

Baird, S. B., McCorkle, R., & Grant, M. (Eds.). (1991). *Cancer nursing: A comprehensive textbook*. Philadelphia: Saunders.

Bandura, A. (1997). *Self-efficacy: The exercise of control*. New York: W. H. Freeman.

Beck, A., & Beck, R. (1972). Screening depressed patients in family practice: A rapid technique. *Postgraduate Medicine, 52,* 81–85.

Belza, B. L. (1996). Fatigue. In S. T. Wegener, B. L. Belza, & E. P. Gall (Eds.), *Clinical care in the rheumatic diseases* (pp. 117–119). Atlanta: American College of Rheumatology.

Belza, B., Henke, C., Yelin, E., Epstein, W., & Gilliss, C. (1993). Correlates of fatigue in older adults with rheumatoid arthritis. *Nursing Research, 42,* 93–99.

Bolla-Wilson, K., & Blecker, M. L. (1989). Absence of depression in elderly adults. *Journal of Gerontology, 44,* 53–55.

Bradley, L. A. (1996). Cognitive-behavioral therapy for chronic pain. In R. J. Gatchel & D. C. Turk (Eds.), *Psychological approaches to pain management: A practitioner's handbook* (pp. 131–147). New York: Guilford Press.

Brandt, K. D., & Slemenda, C. W. (1993). Osteoarthritis: Epidemiology, pathology, and pathogenesis. In H. R. Schumacher, Jr. (Ed.), *Primer on the rheumatic diseases* (10th ed., pp. 184–188). Atlanta: Arthritis Foundation.

Bressler, R. (1993). Adverse drug reactions. In R. Bressler & M. D. Katz (Eds.), *Geriatric pharmacology* (pp. 41–62). New York: McGraw-Hill.

Brody, E. M., & Kleban, M. G. (1983). Day-to-day mental and physical health symptoms of older people: A report of health logs. *Gerontologist, 23,* 75–85.

Buckelew, S. P., Parker, J. C., Keefe, F. J., Deuser, W. E., Crews, T. M., Conway, R., Kay, D. R., & Hewett, J. E. (1994). Self-efficacy and pain behavior among subjects with fibromyalgia. *Pain, 59,* 377–384.

Callahan, L. F. (1995). Awareness of the prevalence and impact of arthritis: The role of health professionals. *Arthritis Care and Research, 8,* 63–66.

Callahan, L. F. (1996). Impact of rheumatic disease on society. In S. T. Wegener, B.L. Belza, & E. P. Gall (Eds.), *Clinical care in the rheumatic diseases* (pp. 209–213). Atlanta: American College of Rheumatology.

Casey, D. (1994). Depression in the elderly. *Southern Medical Journal, 87,* 559–563.

Cook, A. J. (1998). Cognitive-behavioral pain management for elderly nursing home residents. *Journal of Gerontology, 53,* P51–P59.

Cronan, T. A., Groessl, E., & Kaplan, R. M. (1997). The effects of social support and educational interventions on health care costs. *Arthritis Care and Research, 10,* 99–110.

Crook, J., Rideout, E., & Browne, G. (1984). The prevalence of pain complaints in a general population. *Pain, 18*(1), 299–314.

Davis, G. C. (1991). *Refinement of the chronic pain experience instrument.* Unpublished report submitted to National Center for Nursing Research, National Institutes of Health.

Davis, G. C. (1998, January). *Aging and the chronic pain experience.* Paper presented at the Nursing Research Conference: Research for Clinical Practice, University of Arizona, Tucson, AZ.

Davis, G. C., Cortez, C., & Rubin, B. R. (1990). Pain management in the older adult with rheumatoid arthritis or osteoarthritis. *Arthritis Care and Research, 3,* 127–131.

Davis, G. C., & Raudonis, B. (1998). Chronic disease-related resources. In M. O. Hogstel (Ed.), *Community resources for older adults* (pp. 193–220). St. Louis: Mosby.

Davis, G. C., & White, T. L. (2000). Planning an osteoporosis education program for older adults in a residential setting. *Journal of Gerontological Nursing, 26*(1), 16–23.

Davis, M. A. (1988). Epidemiology of osteoarthritis. *Clinical Geriatric Medicine, 4,* 241–255.

Diamond, M., Catanzaro, M., & Lorensen, M. (1997). Chronic illness issues and the older adult. In E. A. Swanson & T. Tripp-Reimer (Eds.), *Chronic illness and the older adult* (pp. 1–30). New York: Springer.

Downe-Wamboldt, B. (1991). Stress, emotions, and coping: A study of elderly women with osteoarthritis. *Health Care for Women International, 12,* 85–98.

Ekblom, A., & Hansson, P. (1988). Pain intensity measurements in patients with acute pain receiving afferent stimulation. *Journal of Neurology, Neurosurgery and Psychiatry, 51,* 481–486.

Ferrell, B. A., Ferrell, B. R., & Osterweil, D. (1990). Pain in the nursing home. *Journal of the American Geriatrics Society, 38,* 409–414.

Fried, L. P., & Guralnik, J. M. (1997). Disability in older adults: Evidence regarding significance, etiology, and risk. *Journal of the American Geriatrics Society, 45,* 92–100.

Fries, J. F., Spitz, P. W., & Kraines, R. G. (1980). Measurement of patient outcome in arthritis. *Arthritis and Rheumatism, 25,* 1048–1053.

Fry, P. S., & Wong, P. T. P. (1991). Pain management training in the elderly: Matching interventions with subjects' coping styles. *Stress Medicine, 7,* 93–98.

Gallagher, D. (1986). The Beck depression inventory and older adults: Review of its development and utility. In T. Brink (Ed.), *Clinical gerontology: A guide to assessment and intervention* (pp. 149–163). New York: Haworth Press.

Getzen, T. E. (1992). Population aging and the growth of health expenditures. *Journal of Gerontology: Social Sciences, 47*(3), S98–S104.

Given, B. A., & Given C. W. (1998). Executive summary for grant no. 5R01 NR/CA01915-05 [On-line]. Available: http://www.fcs.chm.msu.educ/exec1.htm.

Grant, M., Anderson, P., Ashley, M., Dean, G., Ferrell, B., Kagawa-Singer, M., Padilla, G., Robinson, S., & Sarna, L. (1998). Developing a team for multicultural, multi-institutional research on fatigue and quality of life. *Oncology Nursing Forum, 25,* 1404–1412.

Guccione, A. A., Felson, D. T., Anderson, J. J., Anthony, J. M., Zhang, Y., Wilson, P. W. F., Kelly-Hayes, M., Wolf, P. A., Kreger, B. E., & Kannel, W. B. (1994). The effects of specific medical conditions on the functional limitations of elders in the Framingham Study. *American Journal of Public Health, 84*(3), 351–358.

Haber, D. (1994). *Health promotion and aging.* New York: Springer.

Habernam, M. R. (1998). Implementing the FIRE planning grant: Introduction. *Oncology Nursing Forum, 25,* 1389–1390.

Hamdy, R. C. (1992). Osteoporosis: The problem. *Southern Medical Journal, 85* (Suppl 2), 2S4–2S6.

Hamm, B. H., & King, V. (1984). A holistic approach to pain control with geriatric clients. *Journal of Holistic Nursing, 2*(1), 32–36.

Hawley, D. J. (1996). Health status assessment. In S. T. Wegener, B. L. Belza, & E. P. Gall (Eds.), *Clinical care in the rheumatic diseases* (pp. 25–31). Atlanta: American College of Rheumatology.

Herr, K. A, & Mobily, P. R. (1991). Complexities of pain assessment in the elderly: Clinical considerations. *Journal of Gerontological Nursing, 17*(4), 12–19.

Hogan, C. M. (1997). Cancer nursing: The art of symptom management. *Oncology Nursing Forum, 24,* 1335–1341.

Holzman, A. D., Turk, D. C., & Querns, R. D. (1986). The cognitive-behavioral approach to the management of chronic pain. In A. D. Holzman & D. C. Turk (Eds.), *Pain management: A handbook of psychological treatment approaches* (pp. 31–50). New York: Pergamon Press.

Husaini, B. A., & Moore, S. T. (1990). Arthritis disability, depression and life satisfaction among black elderly. *Health and Social Work, 15,* 253–256.

Jensen, M. P., Karoly, P., & Braver, S. (1986). The measurement of clinical pain intensity: A comparison of six methods. *Pain, 27,* 117–126.

Katz, P. P., & Yelin, E. H. (1993). Prevalence and correlates of depressive symptoms among persons with rheumatoid arthritis. *Journal of Rheumatology, 20,* 790–796.

Keefe, F. J., & Van Horn, Y. (1993). Cognitive-behavioral treatment of rheumatoid arthritis pain: Maintaining treatment gains. *Arthritis Care and Research, 6,* 213–222.

King, M. B., & Tinetti, M. E. (1995). Falls in community-dwelling older persons. *Journal of the American Geriatrics Society, 43,* 1146–1154.

Kleerekoper, M. (1999). Osteoporosis: Protecting bone mass with fundamentals and drug therapy. *Geriatrics, 54*(7), 38–44.

Kowarsky, A., & Glazier, S. (1997). Development of skills for coping with arthritis. An innovative group approach. *Arthritis Care and Research, 10,* 121–127.

Kremer, E., & Atkinson, J. H. (1983). Pain language as a measure of affect in chronic pain patients. In R. Melzack (Ed.), *Pain measurement and assessment* (pp. 119–127). New York: Raven Press.

Landis, S. H., Murray, T., Bolden, S., & Wingo, P. A. (1998). Cancer statistics, 1998. *CA: A Cancer Journal for Clinicians, 48*(1), 6–29.

Ling, S. M., & Bathon, J. M. (1998). Osteoarthritis in older adults. *Journal of the American Geriatrics Society, 46,* 216–225.

Lorig, K., & Fries, J. F. (1995). *The arthritis helpbook* (4th ed.). Reading, MA: Addison-Wesley.

Lorig, K., & Associates. (1996). *Patient education: A practical approach* (2nd ed.). Thousand Oaks, CA: Sage.

Management of Cancer Pain Guidelines Panel. (1994). *Management of cancer pain. Clinical practice guideline no. 9.* AHCPR publication no. 94–0592. Rockville, MD: Agency for Health Care Policy and Research, U.S. Department of Health and Human Services, Public Health Service.

McConnell, E. S. (1997). Conceptual bases for gerontological nursing practice: Models, trends, and issues. In M. A. Matteson, E. S. McConnell, & A. D. Linton (Eds.), *Gerontological nursing: Concepts and practice* (2nd ed., pp. 3–73). Philadelphia: Saunders.

McHorney, C. A., Ware, J. E., Lu, J. F. R., & Sherbourne, C. D. (1994). The MOS 36-Item Short Form Health Survey (SF-36): 3 tests of data quality, scaling assumptions, and reliability across diverse patient groups. *Medical Care, 30,* 40–66.

Meenan, R. F., Gertman, P. M., & Mason, J. H. (1980). Measuring health status in arthritis: The Arthritis Impact Measurement Scales. *Arthritis and Rheumatism, 23,* 146–152.

Meenan, R. F., Mason, J. H., Anderson, J. J., Guccione, A. A., & Kazis, L. E. (1992). AIMS2: The content and properties of a revised and expanded Arthritis Impact Measurement Scales health status questionnaire. *Arthritis and Rheumatism, 35,* 1–10.

Melzack, R. (1975). The McGill Pain Questionnaire: Major properties and scoring methods. *Pain, 1,* 277–299.

Melzack, R. (1987). The short-form McGill Pain Questionnaire. *Pain, 30,* 191–197.

Melzack, R., & Katz, J. (1992). The McGill Pain Questionnaire. In D. C. Turk & R. Melzack (Eds.), *Handbook of pain assessment* (pp. 152–168). New York: Guildford Press.

Melzack, R., Katz, J., & Jeans, M. E. (1985). The role of compensation in chronic pain: Analysis using a new method of scoring the McGill Pain Questionnaire. *Pain, 23,* 101–112.

Mock, V., Ropka, M. E., Rhodes, V. A., Pickett, M., Grimm, P. M., McDaniel, R., Lin, E., Allocca, P., Dienemann, J. A., Haisfield-Wolfe, M. E., Stewart, K. J., & McCorkle, R. (1998). Establishing mechanisms to conduct multi-institutional research—fatigue with patients with cancer: An exercise intervention. *Oncology Nursing Forum, 25,* 1391–1397.

Moldofsky, H., Jue, F. A., & Saskin, P. (1987). Sleep and morning pain in primary osteoarthritis. *Journal of Rheumatology, 14,* 124–128.

Mor, V. (1987). *Hospice care systems: Structure, process, costs, and outcomes.* New York: Springer.

Morris, J. N., Suissa, S., Sherwood, S., Wright, S. M., & Greer, D. (1986). Last days: A study of the quality of life of terminally ill cancer patients. *Journal of Chronic Diseases, 39,* 47–62.

Mosley, T., Grothues, C., & Meeks, W. M. (1995). Treatment of tension headache in the elderly: A controlled evaluation of relaxation training and relaxation training combined with cognitive behavioral therapy. *Journal of Clinical Geropsychology, 1,* 175–188.

Moss, M. S., Lawton M. P., and Glicksman, A. (1991). The role of pain in the last year of life of older persons. *Journal of Gerontology: Psychological Sciences, 46,* P51–P57.

Newman, S. P., Fitzpatrick, R., Lamb, R., & Shipley, M. (1989). The origins of depressed mood in rheumatoid arthritis. *Journal of Rheumatology, 16,* 740–744.

O'Leary, A., Shoor, S., Lorig, K., & Holman, H. R. (1988). A cognitive-behavioral treatment for rheumatoid arthritis. *Health Psychology, 7,* 527–544.

Parker, J. C., Frank, R. G., Beck, N. C., Smarr, K. L., Buescher, K. L., & Phillips, L. R. (1988). Pain management in rheumatoid arthritis patients: A cognitive-behavioral approach. *Arthritis and Rheumatism, 31,* 593–601.

Parmelee, P. A., Katz, I. R., & Lawton, M. P. (1991). The relation of pain to depression among institutionalized aged. *Journal of Gerontology, 46,* 15–21.

Pincus, T., Summey, J. A., Soraci, S. A., Jr., Wallston, K. A., & Hummon, N. P. (1983). Assessment of patient satisfaction in activities of daily living using a modified Stanford Health Assessment Questionnaire. *Arthritis and Rheumatism, 26,* 1346–1353.

Piper, B. F., Dibble, S., Dodd, M. J., Weiss, M. C., Slaughter, R., & Paul, S. (1998). The Piper Fatigue Scale: Psychometric evaluation in women with breast cancer. *Oncology Nursing Forum, 25,* 677–684.

Preston, S. H., & Martin, L. G. (1994). Introduction. In L. G. Martin & S. H. Preston (Eds.), *Demography of aging* (pp. 1–7). Washington, DC: National Academy Press.

Public Health Service (PHS). (1991). *Healthy people 2000: National health promotion and disease prevention objectives.* DHHS Publication No. PHS 91-50212. Washington, DC: U.S. Government Printing Office.

Puder, R. S. (1988). Age analysis of cognitive-behavioral group therapy for chronic pain outpatients. *Psychology and Aging, 3,* 204–207.

Radloff, L. (1977). The CES-D Scale: A self-report depression scale for research in the general population. *Applied Psychological Measurement, 1,* 385–401.

Rejeski, W. J., Ettinger, Jr., W. H., Martin, K., & Morgan, T. (1998). Treating disability in knee osteoarthritis with exercise therapy: A central role for self-efficacy and pain. *Arthritis Care and Research, 11,* 94–101.

Ries, D. (1987). *Health care coverage by age, sex, race, and family income: U.S. 1986.* Washington, DC: National Center for Health Statistics.

Riley, G. F., Potosky, A. L., Lubitz, J. D., & Kessler, L. G. (1995). Medicare payments from diagnosis to death for elderly cancer patients by stage of diagnosis. *Medical Care, 33*(8), 828–841.

Robert Wood Johnson Foundation. (1996). *Chronic care in America: A 21st century challenge.* Princeton, NJ: Author.

Roberto, K. A. (1994). The study of chronic pain in later life: Where are the women? In K. A. Roberto (Ed.), *Older women with chronic pain* (pp. 1–7). New York: Haworth Press.

Roberts, B. L., Matecjyck, M., & Anthony, M. (1996). The effects of social support on the relationship of functional limitations and pain to depression. *Arthritis Care and Research, 9,* 67–73.

Roy, R. (1986). A psychosocial perspective on chronic pain and depression in the elderly. *Social Work in Health Care, 12,* 27–36.

Shaw, R. (1992). Nursing research: Threats to reliability and validity in gerontology. *Journal of Gerontological Nursing, 18*(8), 31–37.

Sinclair, V. G., Wallston, K. A., Dwyer, K. A., Blackburn, D. S., & Fuchs, H. (1998). Effects of a cognitive-behavioral intervention for women with rheumatoid arthritis. *Research in Nursing and Health, 21,* 315–326.

Sofaer, S., & Abel, E. (1990). Older women's health and financial vulnerability: Implications of the Medicare benefit structure. *Women and Health, 16*(3/4), 47–66.

Speckens, A. E., & Van Hemert, A. M. (1995). Cognitive behavioral therapy for medically unexplained physical symptoms: A randomized controlled trial. *British Medical Journal, 311,* 1328–1332.

Stevenson, J. S. (1997). Health promotion for chronically ill elders. In E. A. Swanson & T. Tripp-Reimer (Eds.), *Chronic illness and the older adult* (pp. 31–61). New York: Springer.

Stewart, A., & Ware, J. (1992). *Measuring functioning and well being: The medical outcomes study approach.* Durham, NC: Duke University Press.

Taal, E., Rasker, J. J., & Wiegman, O. (1996). Patient education and self-management in the rheumatic diseases: A self-efficacy approach. *Arthritis Care and Research, 9,* 229–238.

Taxel, P. (1998). Osteoporosis: Detection, prevention, and treatment in primary care. *Geriatrics, 53*(8), 22–40.

Taylor, C. B., Bandura, A., Ewart, C. K., Miller, N. H., & Debusk, R. F. (1985). Raising spouse's and patient's perception of his cardiac capabilities following a myocardial infarction. *American Journal of Cardiology, 55,* 635–638.

Turk, D. C., Meichenbaum, D., & Genest, M. (1983). *Pain and behavioral medicine: A cognitive-behavioral perspective.* New York: Guilford Press.

Turk, D. C., Rudy, T. E., & Stieg, R. L. (1987). Chronic pain and depression: I. "Facts." *Pain Management, 6,* 17–25.

Verbrugge, L., & Patrick, D. (1994). Seven chronic conditions: Their impact on U.S. adults' activity levels and use of medical services. *American Journal of Public Health, 85,* 173–182.

Wegener, S. T. (1996). Sleep disturbance. In S. T. Wegener, B. L. Belza, & E. P. Gall (Eds.), *Clinical care in the rheumatic diseases* (pp. 121–124). Atlanta: American College of Rheumatology.

Williamson, G., & Schulz, R. (1992). Pain, activity restriction and symptoms of depression among community-residing elderly adults. *Journal of Gerontology, 47,* 367–372.

Wolfe, F. (1995). Health Status Questionnaires. *Rheumatic Disease Clinics of North America, 21,* 445–464.

Woo, B., Dibble, S. L., Piper, B. F., Keating, S. B., & Weiss, M. C. (1998). Differences in fatigue by treatment methods in women with breast cancer. *Oncology Nursing Forum, 25,* 915–920.

Yesavage, J. (1986). The use of self-rating depression scales in the elderly. In E. Poon (Ed.), *Clinical memory assessment of older adults.* Washington, DC: American Psychological Association.

Yesavage, J. A., Brink, T. L., Rose, T. L., Lum, O., Huang, V., Adey, M., & Leirer, V. O. (1983). Development and validation of a geriatric depression screening scale: A preliminary report. *Journal of Psychiatric Research, 17,* 37–49.

Resources

American Cancer Society: **www.cancer.org**

American College of Rheumatology: **www.Rheumatology**

American Fibromyalgia Association: **www.afsafund.org**

Arthritis Foundation: **www.arthritis.org**

Fibromyalgia Network: **www.fmnetnews.com**

National Cancer Institute: **www.nic.nih.gov**

National Osteoporosis Foundation: **www.nof.org**

Spondylitis Association of America: **www.spondylitis.org**

CHAPTER 17

Management of Medications

Janice A. Knebl, DO, CMD, FACP

COMPETENCIES

After completing this chapter, the reader should be able to:

- Describe the reasons for polypharmacy and how to prevent it.
- Define pharmacodynamic and pharmacokinetic changes in the older client.
- Describe common medication interactions.
- Explain the special differences and considerations when administering medications to older adults.
- Discuss the value and problems associated with generic medications.
- Analyze the effects of medications commonly prescribed to older adults.

MAKING THE CONNECTION

Refer to the following chapters to increase your understanding of medication management:

Polypharmacy

The ability to prevent, cure, and/or manage symptoms of certain diseases with medication is one of the major achievements of modern medicine. However, the challenge of appropriately utilizing our everexpanding medication array has become more and more complex, particularly in older adults. Studies have shown that older clients may respond differently than younger clients to medications because of the effects of normal aging (Montamat, Cusack, and Vestal 1989). In addition, there is a direct correlation between advancing age and the number of drugs prescribed (Chutka, Evans, Fleming, & Mikkelson, 1995)

Pharmacotherapy represents one of the most important ways in which the practice of geriatric medicine differs greatly from conventional medical care (Monane, Monane, & Semla, 1997). Multiple diseases, environmental factors, and genetic variation combine with normal physiological changes of advancing age to affect drug metabolism, efficacy, and toxicity (Montamat et al., 1989). In addition, older adults are the largest users of pharmaceuticals, receiving 30% of all written prescriptions—twice as many as the general population—and 40% of all over-the-counter drugs (Piraino, 1995). Older clients are two to three times more likely to experience an adverse drug reaction than are younger clients (Nolan & O'Malley, 1988a). Older clients underreport their symptoms, and the signs of disease or reaction may be subtle and not addressed promptly. This problem combined with atypical presentations and chronic illness results in an underestimation of adverse drug reactions (Klein, German, Levine, Feroli, & Ardery 1984).

Think About It

Why do you think there are increasing numbers of older adults taking so many prescription and over-the-counter medications?

Polypharmacy has been defined in multiple ways. *Healthy People 2000* (1990) defined polypharmacy as the concurrent use of multiple prescription drugs and over-the-counter medications and considered it the principal drug safety problem in the United States. Other definitions include the number of drugs taken; the measure of appropriateness, such as the prescription, administration, or use of more medications than indicated; or when the medication regimen includes at least one unnecessary drug (Monane et al., 1997). Determination of the frequency of polypharmacy in older adults is made difficult by the varied definitions of the problem. In one study, criteria were developed to measure the frequency with which respondents aged 65 and older answered the 1987 national medical Expenditure Survey as a means of measuring inappropriate prescribing for community-dwelling older adults. Based on this sample, the investigators concluded that 6 million older Americans (almost 25% of the population) were exposed to possibly inappropriate medication use (Wilcox, Himmelstein, & Woolhandler, 1994).

Polypharmacy has many consequences, including **adverse drug events,** drug-drug interactions, drug-disease interactions, drug-nutrient interactions, the duplication of therapy, decreased quality of life, and unnecessary financial and societal costs. An estimated 3%–10% of all hospital admissions for older clients were caused by adverse drug effects (Chrischilles, Segar, & Wallace, 1992). Advanced age, female gender, lower body weight, hepatic or renal insufficiency, polypharmacy, and a history of prior drug reactions are all associated with an increased risk of adverse drug reactions (Chutka et al., 1995). Drugs most frequently associated with adverse drug reactions are listed in Box 17-1.

In 1991, Beers and his colleagues at the University of California at Los Angeles published the first explicit criteria identifying inappropriate medication use and prescribing in nursing facility residents (Beers, Ouslander, Rollingher, Reuben, Brooks, & Beck, 1991). These criteria were designed for the sickest of the older population. Since the creation of the criteria, new medications have come to the marketplace and new scientific information has become available about the effects and side effects of many medications in older populations. Beers updated his explicit criteria for determining potentially inappropriate medication use by older adults in 1997 (Beers, 1997). These criteria defining inappropriate drug use are a helpful tool when prescribing and administering pharmaceuticals to the older population in an attempt to avoid adverse drug reactions.

BOX 17-1   Medications Associated with Adverse Reactions in Older Adults

- Digoxin
- Calcium channel blockers
- Sympathomimetics/antihistamines
- Nonsteroidal anti-inflammatory drugs
- Benzodiazepines
- Antidepressants
- Beta blockers
- Diuretics
- Corticosteroids
- Theophylline
- Neuroleptics

Pharmacodynamics

Pharmacodynamics is the study of drug effects at the receptor level. It has also been referred to as what a drug does to the body. Pharmacodynamic changes appear to be caused by the effects of normal aging, but the mechanisms are not well understood. As aging occurs, some drugs demonstrate enhanced efficacy, while others show diminished activity. Potential explanations for these differences include alterations in the blood-brain barrier or possible target organ dysfunction.

Research Focus

Citation:

Beers, M. H. (1997). Explicit criteria for determining potentially inappropriate medication use by the elderly. *Archives of Internal Medicine, 157,* 1531–1536.

Purpose:

This study updates and expands explicit criteria defining potentially inappropriate medication use by older adults. These criteria define medications that should be avoided in ambulatory older adults, doses or frequencies of administration that should generally not be exceeded, and medications that should be avoided in older adults known to have any of several common conditions.

Methods:

Literature search of articles written on guidelines for the use of medications in older adults as well as controlled clinical trials. Six nationally recognized experts participated in a survey initially and then a face-to-face full-day meeting to rate the use of medications in an older population.

Findings:

The panel identified 14 medications whose adverse outcomes in geriatric clients was considered severe and therefore not recommended in this population. Additionally, the panel also identified 35 drugs or categories of drugs that are inappropriate in persons with any of 15 known medical conditions. Outcomes of 17 of these were considered severe.

Implications:

Explicit criteria provide useful tools for assessing the quality of prescribing medications to older adults. These criteria may be used in drug utilization review, as the basis for educational materials, and to assess the quality of prescribing and potential risk from prescribing to vulnerable populations.

Whether this is a consequence of normal aging or caused by underlying disease is not known.

An example of altered pharmacodynamics in aging is the decreased adrenergic receptor response resulting in less pronounced bradycardia when beta-adrenergic blockers are used and less tachycardia when older clients receive isoproterenol (Vestal, Wood, & Shand, 1979). This differential effect in the older client may be caused by a decreased number of high-affinity receptors and a decreased sensitivity to those receptors (Montamat & Davies, 1989; Pan, Hoffman, Pershe, & Blaschke, 1986; Scarpace 1986; Vestal et al., 1979); Even though the effects of beta-adrenergic agonists and antagonists appear to diminish with aging, the clinical significance of these findings is not known.

In contrast, an increased receptor response is noted with use of benzodiazepines (Castleden, George, Marcer, & Hallett, 1977), opiates, or warfarin (Shepherd, Hewick, Moreland, & Stevenson, 1977). Thus, benzodiazepines produce increased sedation, opiates increase the analgesic effect and respiratory suppression, and warfarin enhances the anticoagulant effect in older clients (Chutka et al., 1995). Particular attention should be given to the prothrombin time/INR (international normalization ratio) when adjusting warfarin. Although normal aging is not a contraindication to oral anticoagulant therapy, factors such as gait instability, a history of falling or syncope, peptic ulcer disease, concomitant drug therapy, and poor **adherence** to drug regimen increase potential adverse effects.

Pharmacokinetics

Pharmacokinetics is the study of drug absorption, distribution, protein binding, hepatic metabolism (biotransformation), and renal excretion. Changes in pharmacokinetics with aging may cause higher drug concentrations at the site of action. Knowledge of the normal age-related changes in disposition should lead to more rational drug dosing. Table 17-1 lists the altered pharmacokinetics in aging.

Drug Absorption

There is currently no evidence that normal aging affects drug absorption to any significant degree. There is an increase in gastric pH, decrease in gastric emptying, diminished intestinal blood flow, and impaired intestinal motility (Cusack & Vestal, 1986). Medications such as ketoconazole, itraconazole, and iron supplements are absorbed better in an acid medium, so with decreased gastric acid secretion with advancing age, this may affect absorption, but this has not been proven. In addition, older adults have a 30% decrease in the mucosal surface area of the small intestine (because of flattening of

TABLE 17-1 Factors Affecting Pharmacokinetics in Older Clients

Factor	Normal Aging
Absorption	No change affecting drug
	Increased gastric pH
	Decreased gastrointestinal motility and gastrointestinal blood flow
Distribution	Decreased total body water, lean body mass, serum albumin, and body fat
Hepatic metabolism	Decreased liver size, liver blood flow, and enzyme activity
Renal clearance	Decreased renal blood flow, glomerular filtration, and tubular secretion

intestinal villi) and a 40% reduction of blood flow in the small intestine (Cusack & Vestal, 1986). However, despite these age-related changes, no clinically significant decreases in drug absorption attributable to normal aging have been detected. Conditions that can occur more commonly in the older population, such as various types of gastrointestinal disorders, malabsorptive states, partial resection of the small bowel, and the concomitant administration of multiple drugs, have been shown to decrease drug absorption. Antacids, for example, can decrease the absorption of cimetidine, digitalis, tetracycline, phenytoin, iron, quinolones, and ketoconazole (Chutka, Evans, Fleming, & Mikkelson, 1995).

Drug Distribution

Drug distribution depends on body composition, plasma protein binding, and blood flow. Age-related changes affecting drug distribution include reduced lean body mass, relative decrease in total body water, reduced serum albumin, and increase in the percentage of body fat (Vestal & Dawson, 1985). Lean body mass accounts for 82% of ideal body weight in a younger individual, compared to 64% in an older adult. The proportion of adipose tissue increases with age from 18% to 36% in men and from 36% to 48% in women (Bruce, Andersson, Arvidsson, & Isaksson 1980; Forbes & Reina, 1970; Novak 1972). Between the ages of 20 and 80 years, total body water (both intracellular and extracellular) decreases by as much as 15% (Chutka et al., 1995).

Implications for drug therapy based on the body composition changes outlined include the following. Digoxin is not very fat soluble and does not distribute in adipose tissue. Therefore, a reduction in lean body mass

and a decrease in total body water result in elevated serum digoxin levels as long as dose and creatinine clearance remain constant in normal older adults. Examples of fat-soluble drugs are barbiturates, phenothiazines, benzodiazepines, and phenytoin. As a result of the higher percentage of body fat in older clients, these drugs can be stored in this depot, resulting in a prolonged **half-life.** Drugs such as lithium, aminoglycosides, and cimetidine are water soluble and because of reduced total body water have higher serum concentrations in older clients. When diuretics are used, the extracellular fluid volume can be reduced even further.

Protein Binding

Plasma protein binding can affect drug distribution, especially for drugs that are highly protein bound. Albumin concentrations are minimally decreased in normal aging and therefore not clinically significant (Campion, DeLabry, & Glynn, 1988). However, older individuals with multiple chronic diseases often have significant reductions in serum albumin (Woodford-Williams, Alvarez, Webster, Landless, & Dixon, 1964). When serum albumin is reduced, the number of available binding sites is reduced, resulting in increased amounts of free drug that is biologically active. Most drug levels measure total drug (bound and unbound), and therefore serum levels may not be accurate in the face of hypoalbuminemia. However, it is only the free (unbound) drug that is capable of binding to its receptor site of activity or of undergoing biotransformation or elimination. Additional examples of drugs that are highly protein bound are listed in Box 17-2.

Diminished blood flow as a result of normal aging can affect the amount of drug delivered to the various organ sites. Cardiac output decreases by about 1% per year after the age of 30, with hepatic blood flow declining from 0.3% to 1.5% per year (Wynne et al., 1989). Therefore, the amount of blood flow delivered throughout the body can change according to the cardiac output and distribution of blood flow.

BOX 17-2 Examples of Medications with High Protein Binding

- Phenytoin
- Many nonsteroidal agents
- Furosemide
- Warfarin
- Diazepam
- Digoxin

Hepatic Metabolism

The transformation of drugs that enter the body depends on the activity of hepatic enzymes, the hepatic blood flow, and the number of functioning liver cells. Despite normal liver function testing in older clients, all of the determinants of hepatic metabolism can be significantly altered. As mentioned earlier, hepatic blood flow declines with aging and is further reduced in the face of congestive heart failure. There are two phases of hepatic metabolism that account for the biotransformation of drugs. Some phase I enzyme reactions involve oxidation, reduction, or hydrolytic reactions. Phase I reactions involving the cytochrome P-450 enzyme system are also known as the mixed-function oxidase system. A decline in phase I metabolism is often noted in older adults, inasmuch as several of the enzymatic reactions of the P-450 system slow considerably with advancing age (O'Malley, Crooks, Duke, & Stevenson, 1971; Vestal et al., 1975).

Phase II enzyme reactions involve the conjugation of a drug by glucuronidation, sulfation, or acetylation, usually resulting in a pharmacologically inactive metabolite. Phase II metabolism is generally unaffected by aging (Chutka et al., 1995). Procainamide is metabolized by acetylation. Clients may be fast or slow acetylators and probably have been so throughout life. The clinician must use trial and error along with good judgment to determine which client requires which dose of drug.

Table 17-2 shows examples of phase I and phase II biotransformation. Diazepam and alprazolam undergo oxidative (phase I) metabolism, which produces active metabolites, contributing to a prolonged duration of action in older clients. In contrast, lorazepam, oxazepam, and triazolam undergo conjugation (phase II metabolism), which is unaffected by normal aging, does not result in active metabolites, and is not associated with an appreciably increased duration of activity with aging

(Chutka et al., 1995). Both enzyme induction and enzyme inhibition of drug metabolism can occur in older adults. While in animal models enzyme induction usually declines with aging, some studies have shown that cigarette smoking induces hepatic microsomal enzyme activity (Campbell, & Hayes, 1974; Vestal et al., 1975).

Therefore, older smokers would metabolize theophylline to a greater extent, potentially producing inadequate levels of the drug. Serum levels should be used for dosing adjustments, particularly in older clients with a drug like theophylline, with its narrow toxic-therapeutic range.

Cimetidine, on the other hand, inhibits microsomal enzymes (cytochrome P-450) (Drug Interaction Facts, 1985). Simultaneous use of theophylline and cimetidine decreases theophylline clearance. However, this occurs to the same extent in young and older adults. Table 17-3 lists examples of drugs inducing or inhibiting cytochrome P-450.

Renal Elimination

The most predictable age-related pharmacokinetic change is the reduced rate of elimination of drugs by the kidneys. Glomerular filtration rate and renal tubular secretion diminish with aging (Cockcroft & Gault, 1976; Rowe, Andres, Tobin, Norris, & Shock, 1976). Normal renal function testing [for example, blood-urea-nitrogen (BUN) and creatinine] do not reflect actual renal function in older clients. The BUN is a reflection of protein intake, hepatic metabolism and detoxification of ammonia, and renal clearance. Decreased protein intake may cause a low BUN unrelated to renal function. Creatinine is dependent on the amount of muscle mass, which decreases with normal aging, especially in a thin, older adult with muscle wasting. As a result, serum creatinine may be falsely low in the face of actual declining renal function. To obtain an accurate measure of renal function, the Cockcroft-Gault formula is used to calculate creatinine clearance (Cockcroft & Gault, 1976). See Box 17-3.

TABLE 17-2 Medications Undergoing Biotransformation

Phase I	Phase II
diazepam (Valium)	temazepam (Restoril)
chlordiazepoxide (Librium)	oxazepam (Serax)
flurazepam (Dalmane)	lorazepam (Ativan)
alprazolam (Xanax)	triazolam (Halcion)
quinidine (Quinidex)	
theophylline (Theo-dur)	
nortriptyline (Pamelor)	
propranolol (Inderal)	
ethanol (alcohol)	

TABLE 17-3 Medication Interactions Affecting the Mixed-Function Oxidase (Cytochrome P-450 System)

P-450 Inducers	P-450 Inhibitors
Phenobarbital	Cimetidine
Rifampin	Influenza vaccine
Phenytoin	Erythromycin
Carbamazepine	Allopurinol
	Metronidazole

BOX 17-3 The Cockcroft-Gault Formula

- For a male:

    Creatinine clearance =

    $$\frac{(140 - \text{age}) \times \text{weight (kg)}}{72 \times \text{serum creatinine}}$$

- For a female:

    Creatinine clearance =

    $$\frac{(140 - \text{age}) \times \text{weight (kg)}}{72 \times \text{serum creatinine} \times 0.85}$$

The formula is accurate in ambulatory and hospitalized clients but may be less useful in nursing facility residents for unknown reasons (Drusano, Munice, Hoopes, Damron, & Warren, 1988). Creatinine clearance predictably declines linearly with aging in cross-sectional studies. This decline in renal function is less predictable in longitudinal studies (Rowe et al., 1976). Box 17-4 lists drugs that are predominantly eliminated renally. Drugs that undergo renal elimination with a narrow therapeutic range should be monitored with serum levels when available (for example, aminoglycosides, digoxin, lithium, and procainamide).

Drug Interactions

Drug interactions fall into three categories: drug-drug, drug-disease, and drug-nutrient. The following discussion addresses each interaction and its effect on the older adult.

Drug-Drug Interactions

As the number of drugs administered to an older adult increases, an increased incidence of reactions between

---

BOX 17-4 Medications with Decreased Renal Elimination in Old Age

- Digoxin
- Lithium
- Most antimicrobials
- Cimetidine
- Procainamide
- Aminoglycosides
- Chlorpropamide

---

drugs occurs. Drug-drug interactions may be defined as the combining of two or more drugs such that the potency or efficiency of one drug is significantly modified by the presence of another (Ellenhorn & Stemad, 1966). Some of the drug-drug interactions are predictable, based on the altered pharmacodynamics and pharmacokinetics (Lamy, 1986). For example, the amount of digoxin available for action is increased with the concurrent administration of quinidine because of a reduction in the renal excretion of the digoxin (lanoxin) (Sloan, 1986). Therefore, digitalis toxicity is more likely to occur when these two drugs are administered together because of the combined cardiac effects of both drugs.

A recent study by Goldberg and his colleagues on review of emergency department records looking at potential drug-drug interactions found that clients over 50 years of age receiving two or more medications were at substantial risk for an adverse drug-drug interaction and half of these would be attributable to medications administered or prescribed in the emergency department (Goldberg, Mabee, Chan, & Wong, 1996). They also noted that the potential for an adverse drug reaction in this population increased from 13% to 82% as the number of medications increased from two to seven or more (Goldberg et al., 1996).

Drug-Disease Interactions

Common sense dictates that drugs used to treat a disease may well worsen another disease or negate its treatment or possibly trigger another medical problem (Lamy, 1986). For example, the use of timolol (Timoptic) ophthalmic solution for glaucoma has been reported to cause symptomatic bradycardia, heart block, and decompensated congestive heart failure in older clients. These drug-disease interaction effects may necessitate the discontinuation of the medication.

Antihistamines and anticholinergics are widely available in cocktail multi-ingredient cold, allergy, and sleep aids. These could cause urinary retention in an older male client with benign prostatic hyperplasia or delirium in someone with an underlying dementing disorder (Koford, 1985). Clinical entities noted to have a higher relative risk of drug-disease interactions include hypertension, congestive heart failure, diabetes mellitus, and renal failure (Goldberg, Mabee, Chan, & Wong, 1996).

Drug-Nutrient Interactions

Drugs have been shown to interfere with the nutritional status of older adults in four basic ways: the suppression or stimulation of appetite, an alteration in nutrient digestion and absorption, an alteration in metabolism or utilization of a nutrient, and alteration in the excretion of that nutrient (Roe, 1986). Older adults are at particular risk because of the pathophysiological changes related to aging, multiple chronic diseases, endocrine dysfunction, alcoholism, and the common ingestion of restricted diets, either by prescription or choice (Thomas, 1995).

Antipsychotic agents (including lithium carbonate), antianxiety agents, and antihistamines can stimulate appetite or, as with some of the newer antidepressants, depress appetite.

The absorption of several antimicrobial agents, such as tetracyclines and certain fluoroquinolones, may be decreased by chelation with dietary cations (for example, Ca, Mg) found in milk and dairy products (Trovato, Nhulicek, & Midtling, 1991). The absorption of other often prescribed antibiotics may be reduced by food (for example, certain pencillins and tetracyclines), delayed by food (for example, sulfonamides), or remain unaffected by food (for example, ampicillin and amoxicillin) (Thomas, 1995). Still other antimicrobials have their absorption enhanced by the presence of food (for example, griseofulvin, nitrofurantoin) (Welling & Tse, 1982).

There is an enhanced excretion of certain ions (for example, K, Mg, and Zn) during the administration of thiazide and other type diuretics. Laxatives such as bisacodyl (Dulcolax), phenolphthalein, and mineral oil decrease glucose and thiamine uptake (Oppeneer & Vervoren, 1983), with mineral oil containing laxatives also impairing the absorption of fat-soluble vitamins.

Food can alter the bioavailability of some medications, reducing their efficacy. Older nursing facility residents, for example, may be receiving enteral formulas that could affect absorption of the medication. Another hazard includes occlusion of an enteral feeding tube when medication is instilled during the course of formula infusion. In a study conducted by Cutie, Altman, and Lendel (1983), several cough and cold medicines, formulated as elixirs, formed gelatinous masses capable of clogging a tube. Concurrent administration of phenytoin with continuous enteral tube feedings may lower the serum concentration and therefore its therapeutic effectiveness (Bauer, 1982).

Malnutrition can alter the pharmacokinetics of many drugs. Subclinical malnutrition may contribute to the increased incidence of drug toxicity seen in older adults (Rikans, 1986). In fact, nutritional hazards in older clients are greatest in those with preexisting subclinical nutritional deficiencies and in those being treated for chronic illness (Rikans, 1986).

Generic Medications

All medications have three names: chemical (e.g., acetylsalicylic acid), generic (e.g., aspirin), and trade name (e.g., Bayer, St. Joseph's). The name for **generic med-**ications is determined by a national council and the trade name (brand name) is invented by the pharmaceutical company.

Think About It

Do you think generic medications are safe for older adults? Why are they often given generic medications?

The introduction of generic drugs has increased competition in the pharmaceutical industry and reduced health care costs. Generic drugs by law must meet the standards for effectiveness, safety, purity, and strength that the original drug met. The total bioavailability of a generic drug may not vary from that of the brand drug by more or less than 20%. However, 20% can be a significant difference in a drug with a narrow therapeutic range. When the drug in question has a narrow therapeutic range, substituting one generic formulation for another whose bioavailability differs markedly is to cause therapeutic failure or toxicity, particularly in older clients (Piraino, 1995). For older clients, the most problematic generics include carbamazepine, phenytoin, digoxin, quinidine, and theophylline (Piraino, 1995).

With the advent of Medicare Health Maintenance Organizations (HMOs), these health plans are increasingly requiring that older clients receive medications from a formulary whose content is strongly influenced by cost. However, drugs within a given class may have differing side effects that make substitution medically inadvisable. Among H_2 blockers, for example, cimetidine is remarkable for its role in a large number of drug interactions and in causing confusion in older clients. Since cimetidine has become an available generic drug, it might be chosen as the H_2 blocker by the health plan formulary, and in some cases the physician may not know that the substitution had been made.

Lamy (1986) has suggested that there are critical clients, diseases, and drugs for which generic substitution should not be allowed. He further stated that clients age 75 and older should not have substitutions made. Therefore, nurses need to be aware if an older client's prescriptions have been filled with a generic drug, advocate for the client by consulting with the physician, and observe for any side effects or lack of efficacy of the drug.

Medication Administration

Oral medications can be either tablets or capsules containing the drug, active ingredients, and inactive ingredients such as fillers, lubricants, dyes, or gelatin. Tablets come in many forms, such as chewable, coated, effervescent, lozenges, and sublingual; whereas capsules only come in two forms, either hard or soft gelatin.

Some medications may also be controlled-release systems to deliver the ingredients in a constant amount over a long time period. Therefore, these should not be crushed and tablets or capsules should not be broken without consulting a physician, pharmacist, or drug reference manual. The long action of the medication could be destroyed because all the drug could be released at once and be dangerous to the client. In addition, the protective coating on the tablet could be destroyed and cause irritation to the stomach. Examples of some common medications that should not be crushed include Cardizem CD (diltiazem), Dulcolax (bisacodyl), Feosol (ferrous sulfate), Theo-dur (theophylline), and Symmetrel (amantadine). Medications may also come as an elixir or liquid delivery system that can be most helpful in clients who require tube feedings or have swallowing dysfunction.

> ### *Nursing Tip*
>
> When administering oral medications to older adults:
> - Assess ability to swallow first.
> - Identify the client by nameband in addition to asking the name.
> - Raise the head of the bed or have the client sit up.
> - Have the client take a few sips of the liquid before giving the medicine to moisten the mouth and esophagus and make swallowing easier.
> - Give the medications one at a time and schedule multiple medications at different times.
> - Ask the client to drink at least 6–8 ounces of fluid (if allowed), preferably water, with the medication.
> - Stay with the client until you are sure the medication has been swallowed (see Figure 17-1).

Problems of Self-Administration

Most older adults continue to live at home and are responsible for taking their own medications. There are many reasons why problems develop when medications are self-administered. One reason cited by Myers, Meier, and Walsh (1984) is the failure of health care personnel to give clear instructions on how and when to take each medication ordered. Myers et al. (1984) gave a number of reasons for failure to take medications correctly, including the failure of the physician or pharmacist to inform the client of the exact time to take a drug or the expected side effects of the drug. Other reasons found were forgetfulness by the client and the lack of funds to purchase the medication. Pepper and Robbins (1987) found that multiple prescriptions and complex regimens, for example, medications at many different times of the day contribute to lack of adherence. Over 25% of older clients incorrectly take prescription medicines as instructed on the medication bottle labels. In addition, an estimated 10% of older clients swap prescription medications with friends and relatives (Collet, 1988).

Older adults often take over-the-counter drugs along with prescription medications without consulting their physicians about the effects of adding the extra drug and without even realizing that over-the-counter purchases are drugs. Failing vision contributes to the inability of many older adults to read instructions on drug labels. Pharmacists often neglect to determine the client's ability to understand or remember how and when to take the drug.

Studies of ambulatory clients in a family practice clinic found some of the reasons for problems in self-administering medications by older clients included errors of omission, failure to take the entire prescription, obtaining drugs from more than one physician (thus taking drugs that interact adversely), and failure to understand how to take the drug (Myers et al., 1984). Other problems of self-medication arise when people take large doses of laxatives daily, various medications for colds frequently, and antacids regularly. These clients never consider that this information should be reported to the prescribing physician. In

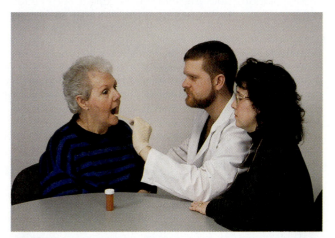

FIGURE 17-1 Checking the client's mouth if unsure the medication has been swallowed.

CLINICAL ALERT

All older adults should know the following about their prescribed medications:

- *Name of the drug*
- *Why the medication was ordered*
- *When to take the medication, for example, before meals, after meals, with meals, or at bedtime*
- *Whether to take the medication with or without food*
- *Major side effects of the medication*
- *What to do if any side effects occur*
- *Whether the medication is to be swallowed, chewed, or placed under the tongue*

fact, if not directly asked about the purchase or use of over-the counter medication, older clients will not readily provide this information.

If the older adult has poor vision, the pharmacist should be requested to use large bold print on the medication label. Clients should also ask the pharmacist to provide a large-print information sheet. Most pharmacists now provide such information sheets with all new prescriptions. These sheets include the following information:

- Name(s) of the medicine
- Ordered dose
- How to take
- Possible side effects
- Other drugs that should not be taken concurrently
- What to do if adverse effects occur

Also, containers that are easily opened are usually preferred by older adults. Older clients should be reminded to tell each of their physicians about all of the drugs they are taking. In fact, they should bring all of their medications in a "brown bag" for review during every physician's appointment. This process should include both prescription and over-the-counter medications. Before purchasing over-the-counter drugs, the physician and/or pharmacist should be consulted about possible drug interactions with prescribed medications. The trend toward **alternative therapies,** such as herbs and natural hormones, is increasing in all age groups, including older adults. Because of polypharmacy in the older population, therefore, clients should discuss all substances they are taking with their physicians (see Figure 17-2).

Nursing Interventions in Client Education

Wade and Finlayson (1983) have divided nursing interventions to reduce the occurrence of adverse drug reac-

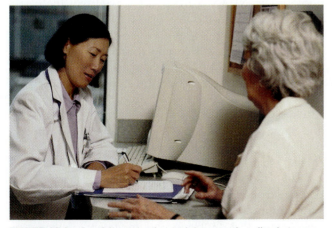

FIGURE 17-2 Carefully evaluating and documenting all substances a client may be taking.

tions into three domains: vigilance, accountability, and responsibility. Vigilance is the constant assessment by the nurse of the client's response to drugs or an adverse or toxic effect. This is done in the hospital, nursing facility, and community environments. The nurse should always maintain a high index of suspicion in older clients receiving multiple drug regimens. This requires knowledge of **pharmacogeriatrics,** careful observation, judgment, and appropriate documentation. The nurse is accountable for all aspects of medication administration. The consideration of accountability takes on **medicolegal** issues in today's health care environment.

Lastly, nurses are responsible for teaching clients about their medications, including self-administration techniques and behaviors to remove any barriers to adherence (Schwertz & Buschmann, 1989). Schwertz and Buschmann outlined several nursing actions to reduce adverse drug reactions:

- Establish a baseline health and drug history.
- Monitor physiological status prior to administering new drugs.
- Consider pharmacokinetics and pharmacodynamics.
- Monitor for polypharmacy.
- Consider nonpharmacological treatment modalities.
- Initiate medication education and teaching.
- Assess physical abilities.

Knowledge about the differences between young and older adult learners is imperative to the effectiveness of nursing interventions in reducing adverse drug events and improving adherence. Adult learners tend to be self-directed and learn more readily if the knowledge can be applied in solving an immediate problem (see Figure 17-3). Also, previous life experiences and cultural backgrounds can be very important in teaching older clients, allowing them to integrate new information on a familiar foundation and belief system (Collett, 1988).

Effects of Medications Commonly Used by Older Adults

Medication therapy in an aging population needs to take into account the interrelated changes in various organ systems and the variability of physiological changes found among people as they age. Some of the differences in the effects of drugs in older adults have been outlined in the pharmacokinetic and pharmacodynamic sections. Prescribing practices should include the

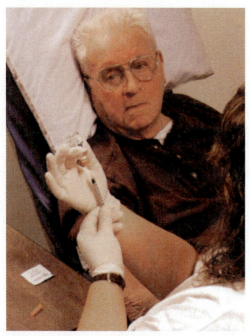

FIGURE 17-3 Learning insulin self-administration.

principles of pharmacokinetics, pharmacodynamics, disease states, aging factors, drug interactions, and client-related factors such as adherence (see Figure 17-4).

Cardiotonic Drugs

Digitalis-related toxicity occurs more frequently in older adults than in younger clients and is often difficult to recognize. Toxicity is frequent because of a marked reduction in the rate of its renal clearance. Also, the volume of distribution for digoxin is reduced in older adults because of diminished muscle mass; therefore, the loading dose should be reduced (Cusack, Kelly, O'Malley, Noel, Lavan, & Horgan, 1979). The maintenance dosage needs to be

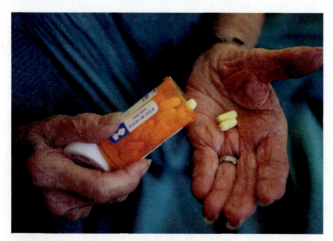

FIGURE 17-4 Careful prescribing practices, client education, and client cooperation are critical factors in managing medications with older adults.

adjusted in accordance with the glomerular filtration rate (creatinine clearance) (Montamat & Davies, 1989).

Classic symptoms of digitalis intoxication such as nausea, anorexia, and visual disturbances may occur; however, symptomatic cardiac arrhythmias, conduction disturbances, and confusion are more common initial manifestations (Passmore & Johnston, 1991; Smith, Janz, & Erker, 1992). Therefore, digoxin toxicity should be suspected in an older digitalized client with substantial weight loss and nonspecific symptoms or possibly dysrhythmia.

Any digitalis drug causes a higher incidence of toxicity in the presence of low serum potassium or magnesium levels that accompany treatment with thiazide or loop diuretics, such as hydrochlorothiazide (HydroDiuril) or furosemide (Lasix). The potential for digoxin toxicity may also be enhanced when drugs such as verapamil hydrochloride, amiodarone, propranolol hydrochloride, or quinidine are used concomitantly (Rodin & Johnson, 1988).

Plasma digoxin concentrations do not accurately reflect the level of drug activity. Some older clients are more sensitive to the effects of digitalis than others and may exhibit evidence of digitalis toxicity with serum therapeutic drug concentrations (Chutka et al., 1995). Performing electrocardiography is a much better way to monitor for possible digoxin toxicity.

Antiarrhythmic agents have a low therapeutic index. Alterations in their kinetics place older adults at a higher risk than younger clients. In the case of quinidine, clearance is reduced along with prolongation of the elimination half-life (Montamat & Davies, 1989). Therefore, monitoring of plasma levels for some of these drugs becomes essential in the older adult.

Antihypertensive Agents

Hypertension is the second most prevalent (40%) chronic disease process reported in older adults; arthritis (49%) is the most common (*A profile*, 1999, p. 13). Third National Health and Nutrition Examination Survey (NHANES III) data showed that there is a progressive rise in the average systolic blood pressure with advancing age, whereas diastolic blood pressure peaks during the sixth decade and falls thereafter (Burt et al., 1995). In the Framingham Heart Study isolated systolic hypertension, defined as systolic BP > 160 mm Hg with diastolic BP < 95 mm Hg, accounts for 57% of cases of hypertension in men between the ages of 65 and 89 years and two-thirds of cases among women in this age group (Wilking, Belanger, Kannel, D'Agostino, & Steel, 1988).

High blood pressure in an older client should be confirmed by several supine and standing blood pressure readings before treatment with medication is begun (see Figure 17-5). Overzealous treatment of hypertension in older clients may cause orthostatic hypotension,

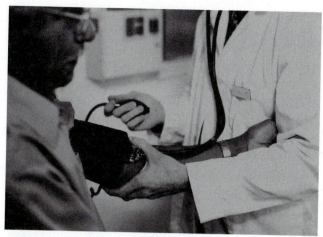

FIGURE 17-5 Supine and standing blood pressures should be taken before antihypertensive medication is given.

which could result in falls, altered mental states, or renal and cardiac physiological alterations.

An initial approach to treatment of hypertension in an older client should include a review of all medications being taken to rule out drug-induced hypertension. Reduction of salt intake, weight reduction, restriction of alcohol to less than 1.5 ounces/day, and exercise are other nonpharmacological recommendations to make.

Because of the heterogeneity of the older population when initiating pharmacological antihypertensive therapy, the coexistence of other disease states and conditions needs to be considered. Adherence, cost, and potential side effects need additional considerations.

Diuretics are effective in lowering blood pressure in older clients, but consideration should be given to use of the lowest effective dose. As a group, diuretics are the least costly and have a long duration of action, making once-a-day dosing possible. Thiazides are commonly prescribed as diuretics and antihypertensive agents. Thiazides cause potassium loss in older clients and may also produce **hyponatremia.** When thiazides are used in combination with angiotensin-converting enzyme (ACE) inhibitors, antihypertensive activity is enhanced; however, the risk of renal impairment increases (Chutka et al., 1995).

Centrally acting adrenergic inhibitors include methyldopa hydrochloride (Aldomet) and clonidine hydrochloride (Catapres). Caution should be exercised when utilizing these agents in an older client because of the troublesome side effects of orthostatic hypotension, dry mouth, impotence, and sedation. Peripherally acting alpha-adrenergic blocking agents include prazosin hydrochloride (Minipress), doxazosin (Cardura), and terazosin (Hytrin) (Pharmacy Corporation of America, 1997). These agents have been useful not only in the treatment of hypertension but also for the symptoms of benign prostatic hyperplasia.

Beta-adrenergic blocking agents may be suited to the older hypertensive client with angina or post–myocardial infarction, choosing cardioselective agents such as metoprolol (Lopressor) or atenolol (Tenormin). However, primary among the disadvantages are central nervous system disturbances such as depression and confusion, symptomatic bradycardia, and possible development of heart failure. Messerli, Grossman, and Goldbourt (1998) reviewed 30 years of the literature on beta blockers as a first-line therapy for hypertension in older adults and concluded that beta blockers should not be considered appropriate first-line treatment of uncomplicated hypertension in the older hypertensive client.

The ACE inhibitors include benazepril hydrochloride (Lotensin), captopril (Capoten), enalapril (Vasotec), lisinopril (Prinivil), moexipril hydrochloride (Univasc), quinapril hydrochloride (Accupril), ramipril (Altace), fosinopril (Monopril), and trandolapril (Mavik) (Pharmacy Corporation of America, 1997).

The ACE inhibitors have shown efficacy in controlling hypertension and reducing left ventricular hypertrophy in older clients (Tuck et al., 1988). Utility has also been shown in decreasing pre- and afterload in congestive heart failure and in the management of diabetic nephropathy.

Calcium channel blockers are available in three classes: diphenylalkylamines (verapamil hydrochloride), benzothiazepines (diltiazem), and dihydropyridines (nifedipine, felodipine, isradipine, amlodipine besylate, and nicardipine hydrochloride). All are effective in the treatment of hypertension and coronary artery disease, but each class has several unique features. The diphenylalkylamines have negative inotropic activity, prolong conduction through the atrioventricular (AV) node, and can therefore lead to heart block. Verapamil also can cause significant constipation in an older client (Chutka et al., 1995). The benzothiazepines also can exert an effect on conduction that can lead to bradydysrhythmias in the older client. The dihydropyridines have a more vascular-specific action and tend to produce vasodilation. Adverse effects include flushing, headache, tachycardia, and peripheral edema. As a group, the calcium channel blockers tend to be well tolerated by older clients; however, the cost of many of these agents may limit their use in some clients (Montamat & Abernethy, 1989).

Analgesics

Chronic pain is common in older adults (Helme & Gibson, 1997). A 1997 Louis Harris telephone survey found that one in five older Americans (18%) are taking analgesic medications regularly (several times a week or more), and 63% of those had taken prescription pain medications for more than 6 months (Cooner & Amorosi, 1997). Previous studies have suggested that 25%–50% of community-dwelling older adults experience important pain problems (Crook, Rideout, & Browne, 1984; Mobily, Herr, Clark, & Wallace, 1994). In addition, it has been estimated that 45%–80% of those residing in nursing facilities have substantial pain that is undertreated (Ferrell, Ferrell, & Osterweil, 1990; Ferrell, Ferrell, & Rivera, 1995).

The most common treatment of pain in older adults involves the use of analgesic drugs (Foley, 1994). Although older adults are more likely to experience adverse reactions, analgesic drugs are safe and effective for use by the older population (Popp & Portenoy, 1996).

Analgesics such as acetaminophen and salicylates (aspirin) are available over the counter and are used to relieve not only the discomfort of arthritis-related pains but also nonspecific pain such as headaches and oral pain. If taken in large amounts, salicylates can cause tinnitus and hearing loss (Mongan, Kelly, Wies, Porter, & Paulus, 1973). If renal function is impaired, an increased serum level of salicylate results and if liver function is impaired, an increased risk of acetaminophen toxicity occurs.

The chronic use of nonsteroidal anti-inflammatory drugs (NSAIDs) is associated with a high frequency of adverse effects in older clients (AGS Panel on Chronic Pain in Older Persons, 1998). For those aged 60 and older, the risk reaches 3%–4%, and for those aged 60 and older with a history of gastrointestinal bleeding, the risk is about 9% (Greenberger, 1997). The NSAIDs are frequently used in the management of osteoarthritis, rheumatoid arthritis, and other chronic inflammatory diseases. These drugs, such as ibuprofen (Motrin, Advil), inhibit prostaglandin synthesis that can affect other organ system functioning, such as renal blood flow and gastrointestinal mucosal protection. Unfortunately, the majority of older clients who develop NSAID-induced gastropathy remain asymptomatic prior to the complication (Jones & Schubert, 1991). For most clients with mild to moderate pain from degenerative joint disease, acetaminophen provides satisfactory pain relief with a much lower risk of side effects than with NSAIDs (Avorn & Gurwitz, 1995; Bradley, Brandt, Katz, Kalasinski, & Ryan, 1991).

The use of opioid drugs for chronic non-cancer-related pain remains controversial, but they are probably underutilized in the treatment of older clients (Popp & Portenoy, 1996). The doses of opioid analgesic medications needed for the treatment of non-cancer-related chronic pain are often smaller than those used for cancer-related pain. Monitoring the side effects of opioid treatment should focus on neurological and psychological functions such as sedation, concentration, and the ability to drive (AGS Panel on Chronic Pain in Older Persons, 1998). See Table 17-4 for a list of the opioid analgesic drugs.

TABLE 17-4   Opioid Analgesic Drugs

Short Acting	Long Acting
morphine sulfate (Roxanol, MSIR)	sustained-release morphine (MS Contin, others)
codeine (plain, Tylenol with codeine, others)	sustained-release oxycodone (Oxycontin)
hydrocodone (Vicodin, Lortab, others)	transdermal fentanyl (Duragesic)
oxycodone (Percodan, Tylox, others)	
hydromorphone (Dilaudid)	

Geriatric Psychopharmacology

Psychotropic medications are generally categorized as antipsychotics, antidepressants, and sedative/hypnotic agents. When prescribing psychotropic medications for older clients **(geriatric psychopharmacology),** factors of altered pharmacodynamics and pharmacokinetics are especially important because of the potential adverse effect on the central nervous system and risk of falls, confusion, altered functional abilities, and loss of independence. Common behavioral and/or mental disorders in the older outpatient population are dementia, depression, substance abuse, and psychosis. In the long-term care setting dementia exists in 50%–70% of the residents, followed by organic personality, organic psychosis, and affective disorders (Tariot & Sunderland, 1997).

Antipsychotics

Neuroleptic agents are the drugs most widely used for behavior problems and the most effective. However, in the older client they may be associated with significant toxicity, even when given at relatively low doses (University of Minnesota, 1997). In a study by Buck (1988), over half of the nursing facility residents studied were prescribed at least one psychotropic agent. This study predated the Omnibus Budget Reconciliation Act of 1987's (OBRA '87) implementation of prescribing parameters for psychotropic medication use in long-term care facilities. Each nursing facility must ensure that every resident's drug regimen is free from unnecessary drugs and dosages, undue adverse consequences, and any psychoactive drug administered for the purposes of discipline or as a chemical restraint (Elon & Pawlson, 1992). Studies performed after the implementation of OBRA '87 revealed that antipsychotics were decreased from 70% to 30% (Ray et al., 1993; Rovner et al., 1992).

When antipsychotic medication is considered in older clients, a comprehensive assessment will ensure that the antipsychotic drug therapy is necessary to treat a specific symptom or condition. Clients taking antipsychotic agents should receive gradual dose reductions, drug holidays, side effect monitoring, and behavioral programming in an effort to discontinue these medications if possible (Lamy & Michocki, 1988).

The antipsychotic agents or neuroleptics can be beneficial in the treatment of psychosis, paranoid illness, and agitation associated with dementia. The choice depends on the syndrome being treated and the client's other clinical problems. Prior to initiating therapy, a thorough evaluation should exclude any underlying acute or new medical illness. In general, antipsychotic medications should be prescribed at doses 30%–50% of those for younger clients (Thompson, Moran, & Nies, 1983a). The dosage is then titrated gradually until the therapeutic goal is reached or until adverse side effects develop (Raskind, 1993)

Haloperidol, with high antipsychotic effect per milligram of drug (for example, high potency) is more likely to produce tardive dyskinesia compared with thioridazine, an antipsychotic agent, with lower antipsychotic activity per milligram (for example, low potency). On the other hand, thioridazine is more likely to produce anticholinergic adverse effects such as dry mouth, urinary retention, constipation, and central anticholinergic delirium as well as orthostatic hypotension (Raskind, 1993). See Table 17-5 for a listing of other antipsychotic agents.

Antidepressants

The prevalence of depression in older adults varies depending on the criteria used for diagnosis and the population studied. A large study of community-dwelling older adults showed that mild to moderate depressive symptoms are more common (24%) than major depression (less than 1%) (Blazer, Hughes, & George, 1987). Major depression is present in 5%–13% of hospitalized clients and in 12%–20% of nursing facility residents (Abrams, Teresi, & Butin, 1992; Koenig, 1991). Diagnosis of clinically significant depression should follow the criteria established in the *Diagnostic and Statistical Manual of Mental Disorders,* 4th edition (American Psychiatric, 1994). The goals of treating depression in the older client includes alleviating depressive symptoms, reducing risk of recurrence and relapse, decreasing morbidity and mortality, and improving quality of life (DasGupta, 1998).

Box 17-5 lists the commonly recommended drugs for treatment of depression in older adults. Tricyclic antidepressants, which have been the primary therapy for depression in older adults in the past, are associated with frequent side effects. They can produce a variety of cardiac side effects; such as an increase in heart rate, prolonged p-R interval, QRS duration, QT time, and flattening of the T wave, and noncardiac side effects such as orthostatic hypotension and dry mouth. They remain effective and tolerated when monitored effectively and when choosing those with fewer side effects, such as nortriptyline and desipramine (Thompson, Moran, & Nies, 1983b).

TABLE 17-5 Antipsychotic Medications	
Traditional Antipsychotics	**Atypical Antipsychotics**
High potency	risperidone (Risperdal)
haloperidol (Haldol)	clozapine (Clozaril)
thiothixane (Navane)	olanzapine (Zyprexa)
thioridazine (Mellaril)	sertindole (Seraquil)
Moderate potency	
molindone (Moban)	
loxapine (Loxitane)	

BOX 17-5 Drugs in the Treatment of Depression

Tricyclic antidepressants
  Tertiary amines
    amitriptyline (Elavil, Endep)
    imipramine (Tofranil)
    doxepin (Adapin, Sinequan)
  Secondary amines
    nortriptyline (Pamelor, Aventyl)
    desipramine (Norpramin)
Selective serotonin reuptake inhibitors (SSRIs)
  fluoxetine (Prozac)
  sertraline (Zoloft)
  paroxetine (Paxil)
  citalopram hydrobromide (Celexa)
Serotonin norepinephrine reuptake inhibitors
  venlafaxine (Effexor)
Atypical antidepressants
  trazodone (Desyrel)
  bupropion (Buspar)
  nefazodone (Serzone)
Monoamine oxidase inhibitors (MAOIs)
  phenelzine (Nardil)
  tranylcypromine (Parnate)

Fluoxetine, paroxetine, and sertraline have become first-line agents for the treatment of depression in older clients because of their favorable adverse effect profiles, once-daily dosing schedule, and safety in cases of overdose (DasGupta, 1998). These SSRIs are highly selective for serotonin receptors and have little effect on other neurotransmitter systems, resulting in fewer adverse effects (Nemeroff, 1994). Most adverse effects associated with SSRIs are mild and include gastrointestinal symptoms (for example, nausea, anorexia, diarrhea, flatulence, and constipation), headache, agitation, insomnia, somnolence, and sexual dysfunction (DasGupta, 1998). When initiating therapy the recommendation to "start low and go slow" is best followed when treating older depressed clients.

Atypical antidepressants include trazodone, bupropion, and nefazodone. All of these agents have been used in older populations. Other agents such as the MAOIs are not first-line drugs for depression in older clients (DasGupta, 1998).

Antianxiety Agents, Sedatives, and Hypnotics

On review of the literature it is estimated that 10%–20% of older adults experience clinically significant symptoms of anxiety (Sheikh, 1992a). Anxiety disorders are classified into various diagnostic categories that include disorders (for example, panic, generalized anxiety, obsessive-compulsive, posttraumatic, and anxiety) and phobias (for example, agoraphobia, social, simple). General principles of management include knowledge of the disorder, sensitivity to the client, education of the client, and reassurance that relief is possible (Sheikh, 1992b).

Benzodiazepines have been the mainstay of anxiolytic therapy. Short-half-life benzodiazepines such as lorazepam, oxazepam, and temazepam are preferred because they are inactivated by direct conjugation in the liver, a mechanism that does not seem to be affected by aging (Moran, Thompson, & Nies, 1988). In addition, these drugs are relatively less lipophilic and, therefore, are less prone to accumulate in fatty tissues of older adults compared with more lipophilic drugs such as diazepam (Sheikh, 1992b). From literature review it appears that older clients are prescribed benzodiazepines at a rate disproportionately high to their percentage in the population. Given the probability that if taken for long periods of time, even short-acting benzodiazepines tend to accumulate in older adults. Any use of benzodiazepines in this population should be for specific indications and time limited, preferably less than 6 months (Sheikh, 1992b).

Buspirone is an anxiolytic with partial serotonin-agonist properties that has been well tolerated by older clients. It is less sedating than diazepam and does not cause withdrawal symptoms when discontinued. It is important to remember that buspirone may take 3–4 weeks before its therapeutic effects become manifest (Sheikh, 1992b).

Sleep disorders occur frequently in older adults. In fact, adults age 65 and older receive approximately 35% of all prescription sedatives (Dement, Miles, & Carskadon, 1982). Currently, there are several classes of medications used as sedative compounds. Of those, chloral hydrate and antihistamines (for example, benadryl), although relatively benign as far as addiction potential, are not very effective, and the sedative properties are quite temporary with nightly usage (Wooten, 1992). Antihistamines also have a number of side effects such as decreased cognitive function, decreased daytime alertness, and anticholinergic side effects (Reite, Nagel, & Ruddy, 1990). Antidepressants derive most of their sedative potential from antihistaminic properties and therefore have the same side effects as mentioned. However, trazodone is selective, has no anticholinergic or antihistaminic activity, and is quite useful as a hypnotic, especially when benzodiazepines cannot be used (Wooten, 1992).

The most favorable drug class available for sedative compounds are the benzodiazepines (Wooten, 1992). However, long-acting sedatives such as flurazepam should be avoided in older adults (Bliwise, Seidel, Greenblatt, & Dement, 1984). Choices should include agents such as temazepam, alprazolam, oxazepam, and estazolam because of shorter half-lives. Caution is also indicated with the use of these drugs in the older adult because of the risk of falls that can occur with the use of benzodiazepines. Pharmacological management of insomnia is only a part of the treatment approach that also needs to include behavioral and sleep hygiene approaches.

Summary

Over the past quarter century knowledge of the physiological changes that occur in the older adult has broadened. Better prescribing parameters have been developed, based upon the pharmacodynamic and pharmacokinetic alterations that occur. This improved knowledge base in geropharmacology will assist practitioners in caring for the aging population. However, further clinical research is needed regarding medication effects in the oldest and sickest nursing facility population.

Nurses assist older clients in many different settings: hospitals, nursing facilities, clinics, adult day programs, senior centers, and through home health care agencies. Nurses need to obtain an accurate medication history and should question the need for all of the drugs being

CARE PLAN

CASE STUDY

Mr. Pasquale Castanadez is an 84-year-old nursing facility resident. Prior to his admission 2 months ago, he was living in an SRO (single room occupancy) hotel in the city. He has an eighth-grade education and has worked at odd jobs throughout his entire life. At one point in his life, Mr. Castanadez was homeless. He considers himself "a survivor" and says, "I'm like a cat; I have nine lives."

Mr. Castanadez was found wandering outside his apartment. The ambulance brought him to the emergency department. He was diagnosed with dehydration, hypothermia, delirium, and atrial fibrillation. His medical history is very unreliable. There are no family members or friends to contact or confer with. Suspicions include alcohol abuse, abuse/neglect, and peripheral vascular disease.

Mr. Castanadez exhibited belligerent behaviors, including hitting, spitting, and kicking of staff. He also yelled and cursed in the emergency department.

After Mr. Castanadez was sedated, diagnostic tests were performed and medication management decisions were made in support of his medical diagnoses and behaviors. The local social services department was involved to determine whether Mr. Castanadez would be a harm to himself or others, a determining factor in placement after the emergency department admission.

Newly ordered medications included IV one-half normal saline with D_5W 60 cc/hr, digoxin, Haldol (haloperidol), Colace, and a multivitamin.

Three days later, Mr. Castanadez scored 15 points out of 30 on the Mini-Mental State Exam, indicating the possibility of dementia (<23/30 strongly suggests dementia). He was discharged to the nursing facility, the IV was discontinued, and after 2 weeks he was placed on more medications. Besides the digoxin, Haldol, Colace, and multivitamin, he now takes Ativan for anxiety, a sleeping pill, a potassium supplement, Lasix (furosemide), and Haldol as needed for agitated behavior or resistance to personal hygiene care. He now takes eight types of medications daily.

A 6-month follow-up examination showed that Mr. Castanadez is lethargic and despondent. He sleeps throughout the day and stays up at night. He is unable to swallow most of his medications or refuses to take them. He thinks he is "in jail" and confuses daytime with nighttime. He ambulates with moderate assistance. In addition, his Mini-Mental State Exam score has declined to 13/30 and he has become nearly immobile.

ASSESSMENT

Lifestyle, social support, and health status are highly integrated. Mr. Castanadez's environment, philosophy on life, and age predisposed him to health-related problems. His emergency department entry into the health care system led to events that required nursing facility placement. His overall decline in the nursing facility setting necessitates a close examination of its cause. Scrutinizing his medication regimen may optimize his ability to adapt to the new environment. Although three nursing diagnoses have been selected to include in his care plan, there are several more of equal priority. Can you list some of them?

NURSING DIAGNOSIS

Risk for injury related to cognitive and physical deterioration.

Outcomes:

Mr. Castanadez will:

- *Experience zero falls.*
- *Be safely assisted and ambulated by staff.*
- *Manifest normal laboratory results, vital signs, and no infection.*
- *Participate in meaningful activities.*

(continues)

CARE PLAN *continued*

Planning/Interventions:

The nurse will:

- *Assess for gait and balance and respiratory, urinary tract, or other infections.*
- *Teach staff [certified nursing assistants (CNAs)] how to effectively ambulate Mr. Castanadez.*
- *Ensure that food, fluid, and elimination needs are met every 2 hr.*
- *Examine most recent laboratory results and vital signs for abnormalities.*
- *Check for digoxin toxicity (labwork and review atypical presentation).*
- *Consult with physician/advanced nurse practitioner on reducing the number of medications to those that are absolutely necessary.*
- *Identify with Mr. Castanadez meaningful activities as appropriate diversions; i.e., card games, checkers, and dice games.*

EVALUATION:

Mr. Castanadez will not fall or injure himself. He will be assisted in walking and toileting. He will select activities that are compatible with his likes and dislikes. Abnormal laboratory results and infectious processes will be ruled out as contributing factors for risk of injury. Medications will be reduced to only those that are necessary to prevent delirium on top of his dementia.

NURSING DIAGNOSIS

Nonadherence related to resistance and failure to take medications.

Outcomes:

Mr. Castanadez will:

- *Verbalize reasons for nonadherence with medications.*
- *Ingest medications necessary for wellness.*
- *Repeat basic information about his medications.*

Planning/Interventions:

The nurse will:

- *Explore reasons for nonadherence, i.e., lethargy related to several potential factors, including malnutrition, overmedication, or digoxin toxicity.*
- *Collaborate with physician/advanced nurse practitioner, psychiatric clinician, and dietitian on evaluating and managing Mr. Castanadez's medication and behavior more effectively.*
- *Obtain nutrition profile screening for malnutrition.*
- *Obtain digoxin level.*
- *Check electrolytes, liver function tests, T_3, T_4, and thyroid-stimulating hormone (TSH).*
- *Assess behavioral patterns over the past month.*
- *Examine as-needed usage of Haldol.*
- *Propose increased fiber and fluid to reduce usage of Colace; suggest reducing Haldol in conjunction with a supportive behavioral plan; increase activity when lethargy decreases; decrease sleep medication and utilize nonpharmacological methods such as exercise and a bedtime snack.*

EVALUATION:

Mr. Castanadez's lethargy and deterioration are related to possible medication toxicity. The nurse will collaborate with the health care team to rigorously evaluate the medication regimen. A plan will be established and implemented for optimum medication, nutritional, and behavioral management. He will become involved in the process.

(continues)

CARE PLAN *continued*

NURSING DIAGNOSIS

Impaired adjustment related to emotional state, demonstration of nonacceptance of health status change, and failure to achieve optimal sense of control.

Outcomes:
Mr. Castanadez will:
- *Verbalize feelings about nursing facility placement.*
- *Verbalize adaptation to nursing facility routines.*
- *Participate in two therapeutic recreational group activities weekly.*
- *Control and perform morning care with minimal supervision.*

Planning/Interventions:
The nurse will:
- *Encourage Mr. Castanadez's verbalization of feelings about the nursing facility.*
- *Collaborate with the Activities Director on appropriate group activities for him.*
- *Teach self-care skills to Mr. Castanadez.*

EVALUATION:
Mr. Castanadez will attend therapeutic recreational activities twice weekly. He will perform self-care activities in the morning with minimal assistance to give him some sense of control over personal care. He will begin to make positive statements about his new home.

NURSING DIAGNOSIS

Sleep pattern disturbance related to use of sleeping medication, life change, medication regimen, and unfamiliar environment.

Outcomes:
Mr. Castanadez will:
- *Experience 6–10 hr nighttime sleep, uninterrupted.*
- *Verbalize a sense of perceived restfulness.*
- *Reduce use of sleeping medication to half the dose.*
- *Participate in an exercise and activity plan.*

Planning/Interventions:
The nurse will:
- *Assess Mr. Castanadez's level of daily activity.*
- *Assess laboratory results related to anemia and thyroid function.*
- *Collaborate with physical therapy and the Activities Director to establish an exercise regimen and activity plan.*
- *Establish a safe outdoor ambulation program.*
- *Discourage daytime napping.*

EVALUATION:
Mr. Castanadez will participate in an exercise and activity program. He will ambulate outdoors and refrain from daytime napping. Abnormal laboratory results will be diagnosed and treated and the need for sleeping medication will be reduced by half.

taken. This is particularly true when the nurse discovers changes in the older client's mental or physical status. Also, many times the nurse is the only health care provider evaluating the client in the home environment, where medication bottles can be reviewed with attention to prescribing physician, expiration dates, number of medications, and ability of the client to access the medication. Nurses can and should play a major role in the reduction of polypharmacy and adverse drug reactions in the older client.

Review Questions and Activities

1. State one reason why the older adult is more likely to experience an adverse drug reaction.

2. Define pharmacodynamics and pharmacokinetics.

3. Discuss three important pharmacodynamic properties of warfarin when prescribed for an older client.

4. Why is drug distribution altered with age?

5. Which phase of hepatic metabolism is affected with aging?

6. Identify three drugs that undergo phase I metabolism in the liver.

7. How can decline in renal function in an older client be assessed?

8. Name two reasons an older client might not follow the prescribed medication regimen.

9. State at least six facts older adults should know about their prescribed medications.

10. Discuss examples of clinical signs and symptoms of digoxin toxicity in an older client.

11. Identify two potential side effects of NSAID use in an older client.

12. Discuss medication management of depression in the older adult.

References

Abrams, R. C., Teresi, J. A., & Butin, D. N. (1992). Depression in nursing home residents. *Clinics in Geriatric Medicine: Psychiatric Disorders in Late Life, 8*(2), 309–322.

AGS Panel on Chronic Pain in Older Persons. (1998). The management of chronic pain: Clinical practice guidelines. *Journal of American Gerontological Society, 46,* 635–651.

American Psychiatric Association. (1994). *Diagnostic and statistical manual of mental disorders* (4th ed.). Washington DC: American Psychiatric Association.

A profile of older Americans 1999. (1999). Washington, DC: American Association of Retired Persons and the Administration on Aging, U.S. Department of Health and Human Services.

Avorn, J., & Gurwitz, J. H. (1995). Drug use in nursing homes. *Annals of Internal Medicine, 123,* 195–204.

Bauer, L, A. (1982). Interference of oral phenytoin absorption by continuous nasogastric feedings. *Neurology, 32,* 570.

Beers, M. H. (1997). Explicit criteria for determining potentially inappropriate medication use by the elderly. *Archives of Internal Medicine, 157,* 1531–1536.

Beers, M. H., Ouslander, J. G., Rollingher, I., Reuben, D. B., Brooks, J., & Beck, J. C. (1991). Explicit criteria for determining inappropriate medication use in nursing homes. *Archives of Internal Medicine, 151,*1825–1832.

Blazer, D., Hughes, D. C., & George, L. K. (1987). The epidemiology of depression in an older community population. *Gerontologist, 27,* 281–287.

Bliwise, D., Seidel, W., Greenblatt, D. J., & Dement, W. (1984). Nighttime and daytime efficacy of flurazepam and oxazepam in chronic insomnia. *American Journal of Psychiatry, 141,*191–195.

Bradley, J. D., Brandt, K. D., Katz, B. P., Kalasinski, L. A., & Ryan, S. I. (1991). Comparison of an antiinflammatory dose of ibuprofen, an analgesic dose of ibuprofen and acetaminophen in the treatment of patients with osteoarthritis of the knee. *New England Journal of Medicine, 325,* 87–91.

Bruce, A., Andersson, M., Arvidsson, B., & Isaksson, B. (1980). Body composition. Prediction of normal body potassium, body water and body fat in adults on the basis of body height, body weight and age. *Scandinavian Journal of Clinical and Laboratory Investigation, 40,* 461–473.

Buck, J. A. (1988). Psychotropic drug practice in nursing homes. *Journal of the American Geriatrics Society, 36,* 409.

Burt, V. L., Whelton, P., Roccella, E., Brown, C., Cutler, J. A., Higgins, M., Horan, M. J., & Labarthe, D. (1995). Prevalence of hypertension in the US adult population. Results from the third national Health and Nutrition Examination Survey. 1988–1991. *Hypertension, 25,* 305–313.

Campbell, T. C., & Hayes, J. R. (1974). Role of nutrition in the drug-metabolizing enzyme system. *Pharmacological Reviews, 26,* 171–197.

Campion, E. W., DeLabry, L. O, & Glynn, R. J. (1988). The effect of age on serum albumin in healthy males: Report from the Normative Aging Study. *Journal of Gerontology, 43,* M18–M20.

Castleden, C. M., George, C. F., Marcer, D., & Hallett, C. (1977). Increased sensitivity to nitrazepam in old age. *British Medical Journal, 1,* 10–12.

Chrischilles, E. A., Segar, E. T, & Wallace, R. B. (1992). Self-reported adverse drug reactions and related resource use: A study of community-dwelling persons 65 years of age and older. *Annals of Internal Medicine, 117,* 634–640.

Chutka, D. S., Evans, J. M., Fleming, K. C., & Mikkelson, K. G. (1995). Drug prescribing for elderly patients. *Mayo Clinic Proceedings, 70,* 685–693.

Cockcroft, D., & Gault, M. H. (1976). Prediction of creatinine clearance from serum creatinine. *Nephron, 16,* 31–41.

Collett, C. (1988, November). Assessing the patient education needs of the elderly. *Medical Times,* pp. 95–99.

Cooner, E., & Amorosi, S. (1997). *The study of pain and older Americans.* New York: Louis Harris and Associates.

Crook, J., Rideout, E., & Browne, G. (1984). The prevalence of pain complaints in general population. *Pain, 18,* 299–314.

Cusack, B., Kelly, J., O'Malley, K., Noel, J., Lavan, J., & Horgan, J. (1979). Digoxin in the elderly: Pharmacokinetic consequences of old age. *Clinical Pharmacology and Therapeutics, 25*(7), 772–776.

Cusack, B. J., & Vestal, R. E. (1986). Clinical pharmacology: Special considerations in the elderly. In E. Calkins, P. J. Davis, & A. B. Ford (Eds.), *The practice of geriatrics* (pp. 115–134). Philadelphia: Saunders.

Cutie, A. J., Altman, E., & Lenkel, L. (1983). Compatibility of enteral products with commonly employed drug additives. *Journal of Parenteral and Enteral Nutrition, 7*(2), 186–191.

DasGupta, K. (1998). Treatment of depression in elderly patients: Recent advances. *Archives of Family Medicine, 7*(May/June), 174–180.

Dement, W. C., Miles, L. E., & Carskadon, M. A. (1982). "White Paper" on sleep and aging. *Journal of American Geriatrics Society, 30,* 25.

Drug Interaction Facts. (1985). *Facts and comparisons.* St. Louis, MO: Author.

Drusano, G. L., Munice, H. L., Hoopes, J. M., Damron, D. J., & Warren, J. W. (1988). Commonly used methods of estimating creatinine clearance are inadequate for elderly debilitated nursing home patients. *Journal of American Gerontology Society, 36,* 437–441.

Ellenhorn, M. J., & Stemad, F. A. (1966). Problems of drug interactions. *Journal of the American Pharmaceutical Association, NS6,* 62–65, 68.

Elon, R., & Pawlson, L. G. (1992). The Impact of OBRA on Medical practice within Nursing Facilities. *Journal of the American Gerontology Society, 40,* 958–963.

Ferrell, B. A, Ferrell, B. R., & Osterweil, D. (1990). Pain in the nursing home. *Journal of the American Gerontology Society, 38,* 409–414.

Ferrell, B. A., Ferrell, B. R., & Rivera, L. (1995). Pain in cognitively impaired nursing home patients. *Journal of Pain Symptom Management, 10,* 591–598.

Foley, K. M. (1994). Pain management in the older. In W. R. Hazzard, E. L. Bierman, J. P. Blass, W. H. Ettinger, & J. B. Halter (Eds.), *Principles of geriatric medicine and gerontology* (3rd ed., pp. 317–331). New York: McGraw Hill.

Forbes, G. B., & Reina, J. C. (1970). Adult lean body mass declines with age: Some longitudinal observations. *Metabolism, 19,* 653–663.

Goldberg, R. M., Mabee, J., Chan, L., & Wong, S. (1996). Drug-drug and drug-disease interactions in the ED; analysis of a high-risk population. *American Journal of Emergency Medicine, 14,* 447–450.

Greenberger, N. J. (1997). Update in gastroenterology. *Annals of Internal Medicine, 12,* 827–834.

Healthy people 2000: National health promotion and disease prevention objectives. (1990). Publication No. 91-50212. Washington DC: Department of Health and Human Services.

Helme, R. D., & Gibson, S. J. (1997). Pain in the older. In T. S. Jensen, J. A. Turner, & Z. Wiesenfeld-Hallin (Eds.), *Proceedings of the 8th world congress on pain: Progress in pain research and management* (pp. 919–944). Seattle: IASP Press.

Jones, M. P., & Schubert, M. L. (1991). What do you recommend for prophylaxis in an elderly woman with arthritis requiring NSAIDs for control? *American Journal of Gastroenterology, 86*(3), 264–268.

Klein, L. E., German, P. S., Levine, D. M., Feroli, E. R., & Ardery, J. (1984). Medication problems among outpatients: A study with emphasis on the elderly. *Archives of Internal Medicine, 144,* 1185–1188.

Koenig, J. G. (1991). Depressive disorders in older medical inpatients. *American Family Physician, 44,* 1243–1250.

Koford, L. L. (1985). OTC drug overuse in the elderly: What to watch for. *Geriatrics, 40*(10), 55–60.

Lamy, P. P. (1986). Drug interactions in the elderly. *Journal of Gerontological Nursing, 12*(2), 36–37.

Lamy, P. P., & Michocki, F. J. (1988). Medication management. *Clinics in Geriatric Medicine, 4*(3), 623–639.

Messerli, F. J., Grossman, E., & Goldbourt, U. (1998). Are beta-blockers efficacious as first-line therapy for hypertension in the elderly. *Journal of the American Medical Association, 279*(23), 1903–1907.

Mobily, P. R, Herr, K. A., Clark, M. K., & Wallace, R. B. (1994). An epidemiologic analysis of pain in the older. The Iowa 65+ Rural Health Study. *Journal of Aging Health, 6,* 139–145.

Monane, M., Monane, S. & Semla, T. (1997). Optimal medication use in elder: Key to successful aging. *West Journal of Medicine, 167,* 233–237.

Mongan, E., Kelly, P., Wies, K., Porter, W. W., & Paulus, H. E. (1973). Tinnitus as an indication of therapeutic serum salicylate levels. *Journal of the American Medical Association, 226,* 142–145.

Montamat, S. C., & Abernethy, D. R. (1989). Calcium antagonists in geriatric patients: Diltiazem in elderly persons with hypertension. *Clinical Pharmacology and Therapeutics, 45,* 682–691.

Montamat, S. C., & Davies, A. O. (1989). Physiological response to isoproterenol and coupling of beta-adrenergic receptors in young and elderly human subjects. *Journal of Gerontology, 44,* M100–M105.

Montamat, S. C., Cusack, B. J., & Vestal, R. E. (1989). Management of drug therapy in the elderly. *New England Journal of Medicine, 321,* 303–309.

Moran, M. G., Thompson, T. L. II, & Nies, A. S. (1988). Sleep disorders in the older. *American Journal of Psychiatry, 145,* 1369–1378.

Myers, M., Meier, D., & Walsh, J. (1984). Pharmacology: General principles. In C. Cassel & J. Walsh (Eds.), *Geriatric medicine.* New York: Springer-Verlag.

Nemeroff, C. B. (1994). Evolutionary trends in the pharmacotherapeutic management of depression. *Journal of Clinical Psychiatry, 55*(suppl 12), 3–15.

Nolan, L., & O'Malley, D. (1988a). Prescribing for the elderly. Part I. Sensitivity of the elderly to adverse drug reactions. *Journal of Gerontology Society, 36,* 142–149.

Novak, L. P. (1972). Aging, total body potassium, fat free mass and cell mass in males and females between ages 18 and 35 years. *Journal of Gerontology, 27,* 438–443.

O'Malley, K., Crooks, J., Duke, E., & Stevenson, I. H. (1971). Effect of age and sex on human drug metabolism. *BMJ, 3,* 607–609.

Oppeneer, J. E., & Vervoren, T. M. (1983). *Gerontological pharmacology.* St. Louis: Mosby.

Pan, J. Y. M., Hoffman, B. B., Pershe, R. A., & Blaschke, T. F. (1986). Decline in beta-adrenergic receptor-mediated vascular relaxation with aging in man. *Journal of Pharmacology and Experimental Therapeutics, 239,* 802–807.

Passmore, A. P., & Johnston, G. D. (1991). Digoxin toxicity in the aged: Characterizing and avoiding the problem. *Drugs Aging, 1,* 364–379.

Pepper, G. A., & Robbins, L. J. (1987). Improving geriatric drug therapy. *Generations, 12*(1), 57–61.

Pharmacy Corporation of America. (1997). *Guide to preferred drugs in long term care: A comparative formulary for geriatric specialists.* Hudson, OH: Author.

Piraino, A. J. (1995). Managing medication in the elderly. *Hospital Practice, 15*(June), 59–64.

Popp, B., & Portenoy, R. K. (1996). Management of chronic pain in the elderly: Pharmacology of opioids and other analgesic drugs. In B. R. Ferrell &

B. A. Ferrell (Eds.), *Pain in the elderly* (pp. 21–34). Seattle: IASP Press.

Raskind, M. A. (1993). Geriatric psychopharmacology: Management of late-life depression and the noncognitive behavioral disturbances of Alzheimer's disease. *Psychiatric Clinics of North America, 16*(4), 815–827.

Ray, W. A., Taylor, J. A., Meador, K. G., Lichtenstein, M. J., Griffin, M. R., Fought, R., Adams, M. L., & Blazer, D. G. (1993). Reducing antipsychotic drug use in nursing homes. A controlled trial of provider education. *Archives of Internal Medicine, 153*(6), 713–721.

Reite, M. L., Nagel, K. E., & Ruddy, S. R. (1990). *The evaluation and management of sleep disorders.* Washington, DC: American Psychiatric Press.

Rikans, L. E. (1986). Minireview: Drugs and nutrition in old age. *Life Sciences, 39*(12), 1027–1036.

Rodin, S. M., & Johnson, B. F. (1988). Pharmacokinetic interactions with digoxin. *Clinical Pharmacokinetics, 15,* 227–244.

Roe, D. A. (1986). Drug-nutrient interactions in the elderly. *Geriatrics, 41*(3), 57–74.

Rovner, B. W., Edelman, B. A., Cox, M., & Shmuely, Y. (1992). The impact of antipsychotic drug regulations on psychotropic prescribing practices in nursing homes. *American Journal of Psychiatry, 149,* 1390–1392.

Rowe, J. W., Andres, R., Tobin, J. D, Norris, A. H., & Shock, N. W. (1976). The effect of age on creatinine clearance in men: A cross-sectional and longitudinal study. *Journal of Gerontology, 31,* 155–163.

Scarpace, P. J. (1986). Decreased beta-adrenergic responsiveness during senescence. *Federal Proceedings, 45,* 51–54.

Schwertz, D. W., & Buschmann, M. T. (1989). Pharmacogeriatrics. *Critical Care Nursing Quarterly, 12*(1), 26–37.

Sheikh, J. I. (1992a). Anxiety and its disorders in old age. In J. E. Birren, R. B. Sloane, & G. Cohen (Eds.), *Handbook of mental health and aging* (2nd ed., pp. 411–426). San Diego: Academic Press.

Sheikh, J. I. (1992b). Anxiety disorders and their treatment. *Clinics in Geriatric Medicine: Psychiatric Disorders in Late Life, 8*(2), 411–426.

Shepherd, A. M., Hewick, D. S., Moreland, T. A., & Stevenson, I. H. (1977). Age as a determinant of sensitivity to warfarin. *British Journal of Clinical Pharmacology, 4,* 315–320.

Sloan, R. (1986). *Practical geriatric therapeutics.* Oradell, NJ: Medical Economics Books.

Smith, H., Janz, T. G., & Erker, M. (1992). Digoxin toxicity presenting as altered mental status in a patient with severe chronic obstructive lung disease. *Heart Lung, 21*(1), 78–80.

Tariot, P. N., & Sunderland, T. (1997). *Aggression in patients with dementia.* Abcomm Inc., Champaign IL, pp. 1–17.

Thomas, J. A. (1995). Drug-nutrient interactions. *Nutrition Reviews, 53*(10), 271–281.

Thompson, T. L, Moran, M. G., & Nies, A. S. (1983a). Drug therapy: Psychotopic drug use in the elderly (first of the papers). *New England Journal of Medicine, 308*(3), 134–138.

Thompson, T. L., Moran, M. G., & Nies, A. S. (1983b). Drug therapy: Psychotropic drug use in the elderly (second of two parts: review article). *New England Journal of Medicine, 308*(4), 194–199.

Trovato, A., Nhulicek, D. N., & Midtling, J. E. (1991). Drug-nutrient interactions. *American Family Physician, 44,* 1651–1658.

Tuck, M. L., Griffiths, R. F., Beh, M. B., Johnson, L. E., Stern, N., & Morley, J. E. (1988). UCLA geriatric grand rounds. Hypertension in the elderly. *Journal of the American Geriatrics Society, 36*(7), 630–643.

University of Minnesota. (1997). *Alzheimer's disease: The primary care and total care perspective* (pp. 1–38). Minneapolis, MN: University of Minnesota Office of CME.

Vestal, R. E., & Dawson, G. W. (1985). Pharmacology and aging. In C. E. Finch & E. L. Schneider (Eds.), *Handbook of the biology of aging* (2nd ed.). New York: Van Nostrand Reinhold.

Vestal, R. E., Norris, A. H., Tobin, J. D., Cohen, B. H., Shack, N. W., & Andres, R. (1975). Antipyrine metabolism in man: Influence of age, alcohol, caffeine and smoking. *Clinical Pharmacology and Therapeutics, 18,* 425–432.

Vestal, R. E, Wood, A. J. J., & Shand, D. G. (1979). Reduced beta-adrenoceptor sensitivity in the elderly. *Clinical Pharmacology and Therapeutics, 26,* 181–86.

Wade, B., & Finlayson, J. (1983). Drugs in the elderly. *Nursing Mirror, 156,* 586–592.

Welling, P. G., & Tse, F. L. S. (1982). The influence of food on the absorption of antimicrobial agents. *Journal of Antimicrobial Chemotherapy, 9,* 7–27.

Wilcox, S. M., Himmelstein, D. U., & Woolhandler, S. (1994). Inappropriate drug prescribing for the community-dwelling elderly. *Journal of the American Medical Association, 272,* 292–296.

Wilking, S. V. B., Belanger, A., Kannel, R. B., D'Agostino, R. B., & Steel, K. (1988). Determinants of isolated systolic hypertension. *Journal of the American Medical Association, 260*(23), 3451–3455.

Woodford-Williams, E., Alvarez, A. S., Webster, D., Landless, B., & Dixon, M. P. (1964). Serum protein patterns in "normal" and pathological aging. *Gerontologia, 10,* 86–99.

Wooten, V. (1992). Sleep disorders in geriatric patients. *Clinics in Geriatric Medicine: Psychiatric Disorders in Late Life, 8*(2), 427–439.

Wynne, H. A., Cope, L. H., Mutch, E., Rawlins, M. D., Woodhouse, K. W., & James, O. F. W. (1989). The effect of age upon liver volume and apparent liver blood flow in healthy man. *Hepatology, 9,* 297–301.

Resources

Center for Drug Evaluation and Research: `www.fda.gov./cder/`

Commission for Certification in Geriatric Pharmacy: `www.ccgp.org`

CHAPTER **18**

KEY TERMS

Alcoholics Anonymous (AA)

catatonic

cognition

computerized axial tomography (CAT) scan

disorganized

electroconvulsive therapy (ECT)

lethality (high, moderate, low)

monoamine oxidase inhibitors (MAOIs)

Narcotics Anonymous (NA)

neuroleptic malignant syndrome (NMS)

over-the-counter (OTC) medications

paranoid

pseudodementia

psychopharmacology

reality orientation

reminiscence therapy

selective serotonin reuptake inhibitors (SSRIs)

substance abuse

substance dependence

tricyclic antidepressants (TCAs)

validation therapy

Mental Health Issues

Susan Ellen Margolis, PhD, RN

COMPETENCIES

After completing this chapter, the reader should be able to:

- *Analyze the role of psychopharmacology in the older client.*
- *Discuss risk factors related to depression.*
- *Analyze symptoms of depression in older adults that nurses must be aware of when assessing their physical and mental status.*
- *Describe specific assessment techniques for the depressed older client.*
- *Identify risk factors for suicide.*
- *Differentiate between active and passive suicidal ideation.*
- *Discuss lethality issues and interventions for the suicidal older client.*
- *Compare and contrast delirium and dementia.*
- *Give specific examples of dementia.*
- *Describe schizophrenia and specific assessment and intervention concerns in the older client.*
- *Discuss the use of legal and illegal substances that may lead to abuse in the older client.*

MAKING THE CONNECTION

Refer to the following chapters to increase your understanding of mental issues:

- **Chapter 3** *Changes in the Health Care Delivery System Affecting Older Adults*
- **Chapter 4** *Developmental Aspects of Aging*
- **Chapter 6** *Psychological Aspects of Aging*
- **Chapter 17** *Management of Medications*

Assessment and Diagnosis

The focus of this chapter is mental disorders that are commonly found in the older population. The major disorders are depression, organic mental disorders, schizophrenic disorders, and substance abuse disorders. Older individuals often have many complicating factors because they are dealing with more than one disease simultaneously. Other factors include multiple medications, drug interactions, situational concerns, and substance abuse. For these reasons it is sometimes difficult to diagnose mental disorders in this age group.

Unlike peering at an x-ray and seeing a broken bone, the assessment and diagnosis of mental health disorders are complicated by many intervening factors. These factors include the use of several practitioners, many different medical problems, and possibly numerous medications and treatments. Along with many different social concerns, such as transportation and economic considerations, there are also several losses associated with aging. Decreased independence and financial constraints may play a significant role in health care access and treatment.

The importance of a complete history and physical examination cannot be overstated. The first step when assessing any potential mental disorder is to rule out any underlying medical condition. This process includes a thorough physical examination and laboratory testing to include a complete blood count, urinalysis, thyroid levels, and electrolyte panel. The next step is the "brown bag" examination. The client (or family member) should be asked to bring in a sack all of the medications the client takes. This should include any herbs, vitamins or nutritional supplements, all prescription medications (to include all bottles of insulin), all **over-the-counter (OTC) medications,** and any lozenges, suppositories, and nasal and pulmonary sprays/inhalers. Many times the use of multiple medications alone has accounted for mental status changes, especially in older adults.

After the medication problems are recognized, what can be done about them? A list should be made of each medication, the practitioner who prescribed it, and for what it was given. After giving a complete list to all practitioners, it is important to determine if they would like to change any doses or medications. Finally, the revised list of medications, the prescribing practitioner's name and phone number, the reason the medication is being given, and the times to take the medication should be given to the client and family. The revised list should be sent to each of the prescribing practitioners. This will help them in coordinating future care and looking for possible drug interactions.

Once it has been established that there is no underlying medical condition to cause the observed mental status changes and polypharmacy considerations have been examined, a detailed history is needed. Because the client may be a poor historian or too depressed or confused to answer questions, a family member or close friend may be needed to give insight into the current situation. Issues of confidentiality will not be discussed here, but legal and ethical guidelines should be used when initiating and conducting the interviews.

The next step is making appropriate diagnoses. This chapter will examine diagnostic criteria. Because advanced practice nurses may have both diagnostic and prescriptive abilities, it is important to discuss these issues. In an attempt to have a universal language to discuss mental disorders and determine guidelines for diagnosis and treatment, the American Psychiatric Association (APA), along with suggestions from the World Health Organization (WHO), have consolidated mental disorders into specific categories. These are published by the APA in the *Diagnostic and Statistical Manual of Mental Disorders,* commonly referred to as the DSM-IV. Diagnoses are made on a multiaxial system as noted in Table 18-1.

Just by looking at the diagnoses in Table 18-2 for a hypothetical 89-year-old widowed male client, his problems and concerns can be identified. Major issues include medication management, safety concerns, nutritional issues, and suicidal ideation. If this multiaxial diagnosis list followed the client to each of his health care practitioners, the opportunity for comprehensive care and continuity would be possible.

Think About It

Depression is not a normal part of the aging process. What are some of the reasons for depression in older adults?

TABLE 18-1   Multiaxial System of Mental Disorders

Axis I	Clinical disorders; other conditions that may be a focus of clinical attention
Axis II	Personality disorders; mental retardation
Axis III	General medical conditions
Axis IV	Psychosocial and environmental problems
Axis V	Global assessment of functioning

Adapted from Diagnostic and Statistical Manual of Mental Disorders *(4th ed., pp. 25–35), 1994, Washington, DC: American Psychiatric Association.*

TABLE 18-2	Examples of the Diagnoses of an Older Client
Axis I	Major depressive disorder, recurrent, severe
Axis II	No diagnosis
Axis III	Congestive heart failure; eczema; glaucoma; hypertension; hypernatremia; S/P FX (no change after fracture) right humerus
Axis IV	Housing problems (two-story home)
Axis V	Current Global Assessment of Functioning (GAF) scale = 40 (major impairment in thinking, judgment, and mood) Past GAF = 60 (flat affect, isolative behaviors)

Depression

There was a time if a person were feeling "blue," that person would be labeled depressed. Part of the human condition is experiencing a wide range of events, some happy, some sad, and some that just *are*. It was once thought that all depressed feelings were the result of situations. This concept is more untrue in the older client than in any other age group. With increasing age, production of important neurotransmitters decrease. This is why medication that stimulates or replaces these chemicals can make a positive difference. Unfortunately, health care professionals fail to diagnose depression in almost 50% of depressed clients (Perez-Stable, Miranda, Munoz, & Ying, 1990). This fact is upsetting because it takes approximately 6 months to successfully treat an initial period of major depression. When untreated, depression reoccurs 75%–80% of the time (Hirschfeld & Goodwin, 1988). The DSM-IV criteria for a diagnosis of major depressive disorder may be found in Box 18-1.

BOX 18-1 Criteria for Major Depressive Episode

A. Five (or more) of the following symptoms have been present during the same 2-week period and represent a change from previous functioning; at least one of the symptoms is either (1) depressed mood or (2) loss of interest or pleasure. *Note:* Do not include symptoms that are clearly due to a general medical condition or mood-incongruent delusions or hallucinations.

1. Depressed mood most of the day, nearly every day, as indicated by either subjective report (e.g., feels sad or empty) or observation made by others (e.g., appears tearful).
2. Markedly diminished interest or pleasure in all, or almost all, activities most of the day, nearly every day (as indicated by either subjective account or observation made by others).
3. Significant weight loss when not dieting or weight gain (e.g., a change of more than 5% of body weight in a month) or decrease or increase in appetite nearly every day.
4. Insomnia or hypersomnia nearly every day
5. Psychomotor agitation or retardation nearly every day (observable by others, not merely subjective feelings of restlessness or being slowed down)
6. Fatigue or loss of energy nearly every day

7. Feelings of worthlessness or excessive or inappropriate guilt (which may be delusional) nearly every day (not merely self-reproach or guilt about being sick)
8. Diminished ability to think or concentrate, or indecisiveness, nearly every day (either by subjective account or as observed by others)
9. Recurrent thoughts of death (not just fear of dying), recurrent suicidal ideation without a specific plan, or a suicide attempt or a specific plan for committing suicide

B. The symptoms do not meet criteria for a mixed episode.
C. The symptoms cause clinically significant distress or impairment in social, occupational, or other important areas of functioning.
D. The symptoms are not due to the direct physiological effects of a substance (for example, a drug of abuse, a medication) or a general medical condition (for example, hypothyroidism).
E. The symptoms are not better accounted for by bereavement; i.e., after the loss of a loved one, the symptoms persist for longer than 2 months or are characterized by marked functional impairment, morbid preoccupation with worthlessness, suicidal ideation, psychotic symptoms, or psychomotor retardation.

From Diagnostic and Statistical Manual of Mental Disorders (4th ed., p. 327), 1994, Washington, DC: American Psychiatric Association. Used with permission.

It is evident that changes in mood and thinking are primary characteristics of depression. Just as there are differences in everyone, clients with depression differ in their emotional states. These differences may be based on cultural, ethnic, religious, or gender factors. When dealing with depressed individuals, one tends to find that *women are sad and men get mad*. This saying deals with gender differences and the different coping skills that are socially accepted for each group (Figures 18-1 and 18-2). The physical symptoms such as sleep impairment and appetite changes could easily be indicative of serious medical conditions. Therefore, it is necessary to first rule out any primary medical concerns.

Risk Factors

Current medical thought favors biological factors to explain the presence of depression. Specifically, chemical imbalances caused by the decrease of certain neurotransmitters are blamed. Genetic factors may be significant because depression is often seen in many members of the same family. It is important to assess the family history as well as the client's. Women have a higher incidence of depression than men (Hirschfeld & Goodwin, 1988). There is a strong correlation between alcohol/drug abuse and depression, not only in the client but in the family as well (Regier, Farmer, Rae, Keith, Judd, & Goodwin, 1990). This correlation is also applicable to past suicide attempts. If a family member has attempted suicide (whether or not the person was successful in carrying the attempt out), this may become a viable option for the client even if that client had no previous attempts. Situational life events also play a role in the development or severity of depression. Examples of these factors include lifestyle changes (retirement, relocation, and loss of spouse), stress such as financial constraints (fixed income, no savings), several chronic medical conditions, and legal problems (estate planning, competence concerns, local scams).

Assessment and Interventions

As discussed earlier, a complete history, including family history, is important. Asking about usual activities of daily living and any recent changes is important. Using the diagnostic criteria for depression is one way to ask about symptoms. There are also several depression scales (for example, Beck Depression Inventory, Geriatric Depression Scale, and the Center for Epidemologic Studies Depression Scale), which are easy to give and help to assess a client's condition. Depressed clients may appear to be confused and not perform well on a formal mental status exam because of stress and/or lack of interest. This condition is called **pseudodementia** and does not indicate a diagnosis of dementia such as Alzheimer's disease (Emmett, 1998). However, depression may also occur in early Alzheimer's disease so a specific diagnosis is essential.

There are many treatment options for depression. The main choices are psychotherapy, medication, and **electroconvulsive therapy (ECT).** These can be used singularly or in combination.

Psychotherapy consists of individual talk therapy, family therapy, group therapy (several clients), or a combination of any of these. These sessions are led by a mental health professional such as a psychiatric clinical nurse specialist, psychiatric nurse practitioner, licensed social worker, clinical psychologist, or psychiatrist. For group therapy there are often two therapists. The goals of the therapy are individualized to the client(s) involved. From behavior modification to adapting new coping skills or dealing with grief and loss issues, the sessions can be uniquely tailored to the current needs. Most family and group therapy sessions last from 1 to 6 months. Some are ongoing with new members joining and old members dropping out constantly. Group therapy uses the dynamics among group members

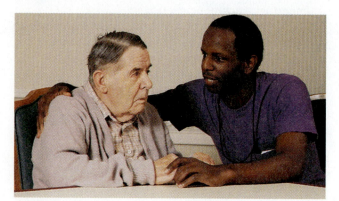

FIGURE 18-1   Signs of depression are signaled by changes in thinking and mood.

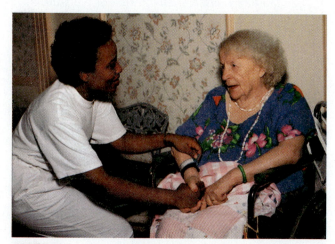

FIGURE 18-2   Differences in emotional states may be based on gender, ethnic, environmental, or religious factors.

as well as each individual's participation to promote growth (Yalom, 1995). **Reminiscence therapy** (talking about mostly pleasant past life events) and life review (being guided through perceived failures and regrets by a mental health professional) may be helpful to some older adults who are experiencing depression.

Medication intervention can be used alone or in conjunction with psychotherapy. There are several classes of antidepressants. These medications include **tricyclic antidepressants (TCAs), selective serotonin reuptake inhibitors (SSRIs), monoamine oxidase inhibitors (MAOIs),** and the newer atypical antidepressants. Besides the concern over side effects and drug interactions, one must keep in mind that the depressed client has an increased risk of suicidal ideation. This fact is important to consider when an overdose is a possibility. Many mental health practitioners limit the amount of antidepressants (and other potentially harmful medications) to 1 week's worth at a time. This restriction not only reduces the risk of overdose but also allows for an increased number of interactions with the health care professional.

This chapter will not discuss specific pharmacology issues but will discuss some aspects of **psychopharmacology.** An overview of the current classes of antidepressants and their nursing implications is needed, however. Antidepressants are not a quick fix and take 2–4 weeks to show any effects. Treatment periods are usually about 6 months for initial depressive episodes and from 1 to 2 years with persistent symptoms.

Tricyclic antidepressants are among the oldest forms of antidepressive medications. They work by blocking the reuptake of various neurotransmitters, including norepinephrine and serotonin. This action allows the chemicals to remain in the synaptic junction (the space between the neurons) for a longer period of time. The presence of these neurotransmitters aids in the feeling of well-being. Tricyclic antidepressants are associated with many side effects. Client education and frequent monitoring are essential. The most common side effects are the anticholinergic effects. These effects include dry mouth, constipation, tremors, blurred vision, postural hypotension, and sedation. As these effects increase the client's risk of falling, they are usually administered just before bedtime. Tricyclic antidepressants are frequently prescribed when there is a recent history of sleep impairment. Another serious side effect is urinary retention, which is especially important in men with benign prostatic hyperplasia. Questioning the client regarding any voiding problems is mandatory (Johnson & Wilson, 1989).

Monoamine oxidase inhibitors are a type of antidepressant that are seldom used now. They work by blocking various subtypes of monamine oxidase, which is the chemical responsible for breaking down norepinephrine, serotonin, and dopamine. Like the TCAs, these chemicals will now remain in the neuroleptic synapse longer. Common side effects include orthostatic hypotension, tachycardia, edema, dizziness, and agitation. It is imperative that clients taking MAOIs follow a strict diet low in tyramines (such as found in old cheeses) and avoid certain medications (such as those containing ergotamine). If they do not, the effects of a hypertensive crisis can be life threatening or even fatal (Bernstein, 1995).

Atypical antidepressants do not fall into a set drug category. Examples of these medications are trazadone and bupropion. Trazadone inhibits serotonin reuptake. Bupropion is a mild blocker of the reuptake of dopamine, norepinephrine, and serotonin. Side effects for both include dry mouth, dizziness, and drowsiness. Trazadone might also cause some gastrointestinal problems such as nausea and vomiting. Bupropion may cause an increase in the incidence of seizures, as much as ten times the incidence when used at doses over 450 mg. (*Physicians desk reference,* 1997)

The last class of antidepressant drugs are the selective serotonin reuptake inhibitors, better known as a SSRIs. This relatively new class of medications includes fluoxetine, paroxetine, and sertraline. They work by inhibiting the reuptake of serotonin, thus increasing its concentration in the neuroleptic synapse. The most common side effects of SSRIs are nausea, diarrhea, insomnia, dry mouth, tremors, and insomnia. These effects are why SSRIs are usually given in the morning right after breakfast, the time when clients are encouraged to be up and about, and the SSRIs help give them an early morning boost. A cautionary warning is indicated. Recent experiences have shown that clients with Parkinson's disease and possibly other tremulous disorders may have an exacerbation of their condition to the point of inducing Parkinsonian crisis. Dopamine receptor sites may be sensitive to these SSRIs and thus compete. Because tremors are one of the more common side effects of SSRIs, it might be wise to consider another class of antidepressant for these clients.

There are times when stimulants such as a pemoline, dextroamphetamine, and methylphenidate are useful. Usually other antidepressant therapies will be contraindicated. These medications are most likely to be used in clients who are very physically ill [cancer, human immunodeficiency virus (HIV), end-stage diseases]. These medications can have a quick, dramatic effect ranging from increased appetite to regaining an interest in usually pleasurable activities. As expected from a stimulant, they can cause insomnia and are usually administered in the morning and early afternoon. One side effect is tachycardia, so appropriate cardiac evaluation and monitoring are essential.

Dual antidepressive therapy is common. This type of therapy can include a mixture of psychotherapy and medications or the use of more than one antidepressant medication. If a client is having problems falling asleep at night and is also lethargic all day, a combination of a tricyclic, with its sedating qualities, might be given at bedtime and an SSRI, with its quality of insomnolence, might be given after breakfast. As the medications work in different ways, their synergistic effects can be quite valuable.

Electroconvulsive therapy (ECT) is not the usual first-line treatment for depression at any age. When it is used, it has an effective rate in clients age 65 and older and is sometimes safer than multiple medications taken over a long period of time. However, older adults may experience more memory loss for a period of time after the treatment. It is used in clients who have a treatment-resistant depression, not just those who experience recurrent bouts of depression that do respond to treatment. Electroconvulsive therapy is also used in life-threatening depressive situations such as acute suicidal ideation or a profound depression resulting in anorexia with dehydration. This therapy has changed dramatically over the years but unfortunately continues to carry a social stigma.

Only professionals skilled in this treatment modality should perform ECT. Usually a psychiatrist or neurologist accompanied by an anesthesiologist performs this treatment in a hospital or clinic setting. The client is given both an anesthetic and a muscle relaxant prior to this short treatment. Observing this procedure is usually anticlimactic. No longer are there the overt seizure activities once associated with ECT. The client is awakened shortly after the procedure is completed. There is usually some initial confusion and disorientation, but that eventually resolves. The ECT treatments are typically given every other day for 6–12 treatments. The results can be rapid and profound.

Suicide

Has anyone ever died of depression? The answer is a disturbing yes. This possibility makes it imperative to accurately diagnose and treat depression. Approximately 15% of severely depressed people commit suicide (Hirschfeld & Goodwin, 1988). Depressed people have 30 times the suicide risk compared to the general population. Suicide among older adults is particularly common. People age 65 and older account for 12% of the population, but they commit almost 20% of all suicides. Women make more suicide attempts, but men complete their attempts three times more often (Yesavage, 1992).

Risk Factors

As was mentioned earlier in the chapter, family history can have a great influence on the client's risk factors. If someone in the family attempted suicide, then the client would be at greater risk. If the client had a history of suicide attempts, the nurse would be even more concerned. Other risk factors include a client going from an inpatient to an outpatient status (referred to a psychiatric or state facility). Statistics show that the most vulnerable for risk of suicide are unemployed single males who live alone (Yesavage, 1992). Therefore, retired widowers are a high-risk concern.

Ideation

Suicidal ideation is the phrase used to describe the thought process of thinking about suicide. This is further broken down into active or passive ideation. Passive suicidal ideation is when the client might make a statement like "I'm ready to die. I wish the good Lord would just take me." This is heard often in long-term care settings. The client has feelings of helplessness and hopelessness and often worthlessness. These feelings are not uncommon in the depressed client. And who is the most likely person to commit suicide? The person who is depressed. What should the nurse do? The first thing is to spend some time with the client and acknowledge his or her feelings. Ask specifically if the client is thinking of hurting or killing himself or herself. There is a myth that asking the question will put the idea in their head. That is not true. If a person was not thinking about harming himself or herself, he or she will answer quite adamantly. If they are considering suicide, however, they will either refuse to talk about it or tell what they are contemplating. Research has shown that 80% of all people who have committed suicide told someone about it first. If a person talks about suicide, he or she has active suicidal ideation and action must be taken immediately. The person needs to know that the statement is taken seriously. An assessment is needed next. One should never leave a person with active suicidal ideation alone.

Lethality

In the United States the main means of suicide is by a gun. Other high-**lethality** methods include jumping and hanging. These methods are called **high lethality** because of the high completion of suicide by these methods. There is virtually no rescue time between the attempt and completion. Shooting is the attempt most likely to be fatal (Marzuk, Leon, Tardiff, Morgan, Stajic, & Mann, 1992). Most men who commit suicide use high-lethality methods.

Women use **moderate-lethality** methods more frequently. These include overdosing, use of carbon monoxide, and cutting one's wrists. The most common suicide attempt is by drug overdosing (Marzuk et al., 1992).

Methods of moderate lethality allow for some rescue time between the initial attempt and completion. People using moderate-lethality means are thought to be holding out some hope for rescue, not just from their suicide attempt but also from their current life situation.

Low-lethality methods are usually for getting attention and are used most frequently by young adults but occasionally by ill older adults as well. These methods include superficial skin slashing, banging one's head, holding one's breath, and trying to suffocate oneself in a pillow. Just because these methods are termed low lethality does not mean they should be confused with no lethality. There is still an attempt to do self-harm, and people have successfully killed themselves by these means, even though it is not as common.

Assessment and Interventions

There are certain questions that all potential suicidal persons should be asked:

1. How are you going to kill yourself?

2. Do you have the means (weapon, pills, . . .) to kill yourself?

3. When are you planning to kill yourself?

If the person obviously has a plan, the means, and the intent, then immediate steps must be taken. The more specific the plan is, the higher likelihood of an attempt (Marzuk et al., 1992). The person should not be left alone, not even to go to the bathroom. If the person is not an inpatient, he or she should be taken to the nearest psychiatric center or emergency department. Of course, the person may refuse to go. The legal system has several options to help protect the suicidal person. Many states have made suicide a crime. This situation allows the legal system to intervene and obtain needed help for the person. Other states prefer to give orders of protective custody or similar edicts to force a person to undergo a mandatory psychiatric evaluation. Using the 911 system can initiate the legal interventions.

If a person is an inpatient of a hospital or institution, it is still essential to assess the plan, means, and intent. Most institutions have set policies on dealing with all suicidal ideation. If a suicide attempt appears imminent, the client is put on constant one-to-one monitoring. The primary health care professional should be notified immediately so that drug therapy can be evaluated and initiated if indicated. Furthermore, all items that could be potentially used by the client to cause injury should be removed. These items include razors, jewelry with pins or sharp points, belts, shoe laces, metal eating utensils, mirrors, nails hanging pictures on the walls,

and nail files. In addition any OTC medications, aerosol sprays, and paint should be removed.

Organic Mental Disorders

The terms *delirium* and *dementia* are often confused and combined in the modern media (newspapers, magazines, lay journals). Both conditions involve alterations of **cognition.** Clients with both dementia and delirium may be disoriented and confused. It is the onset, level of consciousness, perceptions, and performance on mental status exams that differentiate between the two. Initially, two people may appear to have the same problem, but upon careful examination these two diagnoses can be differentiated.

> ### Think About It
>
> Why do many people (including family and health care providers) often assume that alterations in cognition (e.g., memory problems) in an 85-year-old person is Alzheimer's disease rather than delirium or some other kind of reversible dementia?

Differential Diagnoses

The DSM IV defines delirium as a "disturbance of consciousness that is accompanied by a change in cognition that cannot be better accounted for by a preexisting or evolving dementia" (American Psychiatric Association, 1994, p. 124). This condition has a rapid onset (hours to days) and is the result of a physical condition, substance use or withdrawal, effect of a toxin or medication, or any combination of these.

Dementia, on the other hand, is characterized by the "development of multiple cognitive defects (including memory impairment) that are due to direct physiological effects of a general medical condition, to the persisting effects of a substance, or to multiple etiologies (e.g. the combined effects of cerebrovascular disease and Alzheimer's disease)" (American Psychiatric Association, 1994, p. 133). The development of cognitive effects usually takes place over a period of several years. See Table 18-3.

Assessment

This is a situation that often requires family members and/or a significant other for a history. A mental status exam might not be possible initially. Obviously, a thorough medical examination is vital. There are several methods of examination to achieve a differential diagnosis for these dementias. A **computerized axial tomography (CAT) scan** can reveal brain abnormalities as a well as infarcts. Blood studies, such as a dopamine

TABLE 18-3 Differences between Delirium and Dementia

Factor	Delirium	Dementia
Onset	Rapid (hours to days)	Gradual (over years)
Level of consciousness	Fluctuates	Normal
Orientation	Confused, disoriented	Confused, disoriented
Affect	Fluctuates	Labile
Sleep	Disturbed	Usually normal
Memory	Impaired	Impaired
Cognition	Impaired	Impaired
Thought content	Incoherent, confused	Disorganized, delusional
Judgment	Poor	Poor
Insight	Present when lucid	None
Mental status exam	Poor, improves as a condition improves	Poor, worsens with time
Outcome	Reversible	Irreversible

levels, also are available. Up until very recently the only differential diagnosis for Alzheimer's disease was a post-mortem exam of the brain for the characteristic markers. Several years ago brain biopsies were conducted with great accuracy. This was an invasive examination usually done in early-onset dementia cases or in those cases where underlying medical conditions demanded differential diagnosis. Recently a new examination, which looks for specific markers in cerebrospinal fluid, was introduced and has produced a high rate of accuracy. This procedure is still invasive, but it offers new hope that, in time, markers in the blood will be found so that diagnosis will be secondary to a blood test rather than to a spinal tap or brain biopsy.

The commonly found types of dementia among older adults are Alzheimer's disease, vascular dementia, and Parkinson's disease.

Alzheimer's Disease

Alzheimer's disease is the most common type of dementia, affecting approximately four million Americans. Alzheimer's is a degenerative disease that affects the brain and the person's ability to think and reason. It is characterized by a gradual cognitive decline from forgetfulness to needing help with all the activities of daily living (Figure 18-3). This condition is irreversible and incurable although research on prevention and treatment continues.

Vascular Dementia

This condition was previously referred to as multi-infarct dementia (MID). Vascular dementia is characterized by a decrease in mental abilities associated with multiple strokes in the brain. This condition does not result in

continued deterioration unless there are further strokes. This condition is irreversible and incurable, although prevention of further strokes can maintain the status quo.

Parkinson's Disease

This disorder of the central nervous system is secondary to the lack of dopamine. Primary treatment is to use levadopa, which converts to dopamine in the brain. This disease is characterized by tremors, hesitancy and shuffling gait, stiffness, and speech impairment. During the late stages of Parkinson's disease, some clients develop dementia. The dementia and the disease are both treatable but irreversible and incurable.

Interventions

Interventions will be individualized for each client. For those clients with delirium, treatment for the underlying condition will be initiated. Continuous attempts at a mental status examination should be made, and results should improve with the resolution of the condition.

Treatment options for delirium are based on the underlying medical condition. Treatment could be in the form of antibiotics, antihistamines, and medications to block withdrawal symptoms, antitoxins, antidotes, or antivenoms. As the medical condition improves, so does the delirium. Delirium is reversible.

There is no cure for dementia. However, research continues to evaluate a number of medications that may delay disease progression. Some of the overt symptoms can be controlled through the use of psychotropic medications such as antipsychotic medications, antianxiolitic medications, and antidepressants. Medication needs to

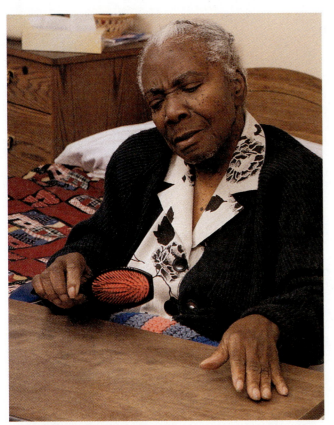

FIGURE 18-3 Alzheimer's disease is a common form of dementia characterized by a gradual cognitive decline that interferes with a client's ability to manage normal activities of daily living.

be well monitored and given at the lowest therapeutic dosage. Medication should be evaluated monthly (more often if indicated) and adjusted as needed. Side effects should be monitored carefully. The person with dementia may be unable to communicate problems so a proactive approach is essential to check for extrapyramidal symptoms, sedation, increased falling, increase of delusions, hallucinations, and fever. There is a rare effect of antipsychotic medications called **neuroleptic malignant syndrome (NMS).** This is characterized by a rapid onset of fever, confusion, and overt stiffness and rigidity of all muscles and joints. This problem is a potentially fatal situation, and a client with these symptoms should stop all psychotropic medication immediately and be sent to the nearest emergency department for treatment. This condition can occur after the first dose of an antipsychotic, the first week, or after several months, so constant evaluation is critical.

Besides administering and monitoring medications, nursing interventions include physical and emotional supportive care of the client and support of the family. Meeting the basic needs for nutrition, hygiene and grooming, and continued mobility are essential. The nurse should also assess, document, and report any changes in physical and mental status. **Reality orienta-**

tion (carefully reminding the client of reality) can be helpful in the early stages because people with dementia think about the past and they can be helped to think in the present if reminded. However, in the later stages it is important to accept people as they are as described by Feil (1982) in her work with **validation therapy** and to try not to bring them back to reality.

> ### *Nursing Tip*
>
> When caring for clients with Alzheimer's disease or other types of dementia:
> - Listen carefully to determine what the person is trying to say.
> - Be supportive, respectful, and concerned (the thinking process may be affected, but feelings usually remain).
> - Ask short questions one at a time and wait for a response.
> - Use reality orientation in the early stages and validation therapy in the later stages.
> - Do not argue with the client.
> - Use all needed interventions to provide a safe environment and to prevent falling or wandering out of the facility.
> - Listen to and be supportive of family members.

Schizophrenia

Schizophrenia is a mental disorder characterized by disturbed thought processes, altered perception, and labile affect (Hollandsworth, 1990). The DSM-IV (American Psychiatric Association, 1994) breaks down the behaviors and resulting dysfunctions listed in Box 18-2.

Schizophrenia is usually seen at an early age, when the person is in the early twenties. Differential psychiatric diagnoses were not as clear as they are today, and many persons were misdiagnosed 20–60 years ago. Now, a person is in the eighties, may have an inappropriate diagnosis (and possibly have been receiving inappropriate medications all along), or may never have been diagnosed with the problem in the first place. A thorough mental status exam with pointed questions is the first step toward an appropriate diagnosis. One thing that makes appropriate diagnosing more accurate at this time is our expanded use of technology. There are brain scans [positron emission tomography (PET) and CAT] that can actually examine differences in brain structures and functions that allow for a specific diagnosis of schizophrenia. These scans can also discern infarcts (strokes), which might add mitigating circumstances to current behaviors.

There is an important point to be made about older adults with schizophrenia. Just because they have schizophrenia does not mean that they do not have some

BOX 18-2   Diagnostic Criteria for Schizophrenia

A. *Characteristic symptoms:* Two (or more) of the following, each present for a significant portion of time during a 1-month period (or less if successfully treated):
1. Delusions
2. Hallucinations
3. Disorganized speech (e.g., frequent derailment or incoherence)
4. Grossly disorganized or catatonic behavior
5. Negative symptoms, i.e., affective flattening, alogia, or avolition

Note: Only one criterion A symptom is required if delusions are bizarre or hallucinations consist of a voice keeping up a running commentary on the person's behavior or thoughts or two or more voices conversing with each other.

B. *Social/occupational dysfunction:* For a significant portion of the time since the onset of the disturbance, one or more major areas of functioning such as work, interpersonal relations, or self-care are markedly below the level achieved prior to the onset (or when the onset is in childhood or adolescence, failure to achieve expected level or interpersonal, academic, or occupational achievement).

C. *Duration:* Continuous signs of the disturbance persist for at least 6 months. This 6-month period must include at least 1 month of symptoms (or less if successfully treated) that meet criterion A (i.e., active-phase symptoms) and may include periods of prodromal or active-phase symptoms). During these prodromal or residual periods, the signs of the disturbance may be manifested by only negative symptoms or two or more symptoms listed in criterion A present in an attenuated form (e.g., odd beliefs, unusual perceptual experiences).

D. *Schizoaffective and mood disorder exclusion:* Schizoaffective disorder and mood disorder with psychotic features have been ruled out because either (1) no major depressive, manic, or mixed episodes have occurred concurrently with the active-phase symptoms or (2) if mood episodes have occurred during active-phase symptoms, their total duration has been brief relative to the duration of the active and residual periods.

E. *Substance/general medical condition exclusion:* The disturbance is not due to the direct physiological effects of a substance (e.g., a drug of abuse, a medication) or a general medical condition.

F. *Relationship to a pervasive developmental disorder:* If there is a history of autistic disorder or another pervasive developmental disorder, the additional diagnosis of schizophrenia is made only if prominent delusions or hallucinations are also present for at least a month (or less if successfully treated).

From Diagnostic and Statistical Manual of Mental Disorders *(4th ed., pp. 285–286), 1994, Washington, DC: American Psychiatric Association. Used with permission.*

other problem that exacerbates their psychotic symptoms. Besides strokes, there are brain tumors, infections, postanesthesia delirium, traumatic events, and oxygen deprivation, to name just a few, that could cause exaggerated psychotic responses. Both a good medical examination as well as a mental status examination are essential. Also, even if diagnosed with schizophrenia, the signs and symptoms may not be as severe as in the twenties.

Schizophrenia can be seen in several different forms. Perhaps the most obvious is the **paranoid** type. The main characteristic is "preoccupation with one or more delusions or frequent auditory hallucinations" (American Psychiatric Association, 1994, p. 287). There are two main fears about a person in this state. First, the voices or delusions may convince people that they must destroy themselves. Unless quickly medicated, this person may take active steps toward suicide, often with fatal consequences. The second fear is that secondary to delusions and/or hallucinations, the person may act out violently. The weapon of choice is often a knife.

Another type of schizophrenia is the **disorganized** type. This type is characterized by disorganized speech, disorganized behavior, and flat or inappropriate affect. Persons with disorganized type of schizophrenia show a marked inability to perform usual activities of daily living such as preparing a meal, taking a shower and dressing, and taking medications as prescribed.

The **catatonic** type of schizophrenia is marked by a severe psychomotor disturbance. This client requires assistance with all activities of daily living. Because of the person's inability to initiate basic care (eating, drinking, toileting, bathing), the nurse needs to be especially concerned with fluid intake, output, and skin care needs. The diagnostic criteria for the catatonic type of schizophrenia are listed in Box 18-3.

Historical Perspective

In 1908, a Swiss psychiatrist, Eugen Bleuler, coined the term schizophrenia. This term comes from two Greek words: *schizo,* meaning "split," and *phren,* referring to

BOX 18-3 Diagnostic Criteria for 295.20 Catatonic Type

In this type of schizophrenia, the clinical picture is dominated by at least two of the following:

1. Motoric immobility as evidenced by catalepsy (including waxy flexibility) or stupor

2. Excessive motor activity (that is apparently purposeless and not influenced by external stimuli)

3. Extreme negativism (an apparently motiveless resistance to all instructions or maintenance of a rigid posture against attempts to be moved) or mutism

4. Peculiarities of voluntary movement as evidenced by posturing (voluntary assumption of inappropriate or bizarre postures), stereotyped movements, prominent mannerisms, or prominent grimacing

5. Echolalia or echoprazia

From Diagnostic and Statistical Manual of Mental Disorders *(4th ed., p. 289), 1994, Washington, DC: American Psychiatric Association. Used with permission.*

the mind. Thus, the *split mind* was the earliest understanding of this disorder. This definition has led to confusion among many students and young practitioners who have equated schizophrenia with a split personality, which is an entirely different situation. Schizophrenic clients have historically been the hardest group with which both families and the public must deal. This used to be the largest group of clients in institutionalized psychiatric settings. Now we find persons with schizophrenia to be among the largest group of the homeless mentally ill. Because of their social dysfunction and often paranoid ideation, trying to mainstream these individuals into conventional home or even group settings has been disappointing.

Assessment and Interventions

Nothing can take the place of a complete history, physical, and psychiatric examination. The schizophrenic person must be kept safe from self as well as others. This situation usually necessitates an initial period of hospitalization. Medications include lithium salts, available in many brand names and concentrations, and antipsychotics. All of these medications are usually started at low doses and titrated to therapeutic levels. This titration may take from several days to weeks depending on side effects, interactions with other medications, and other medical conditions. Persons with

schizophrenia have a poor compliance rate with taking their medications. This requires frequent follow-up by health care professionals to include medication counts and drug levels. Because these people have poor social skills, they are apt to live in other than traditional living arrangements, such as in group homes or shelters or on the street. Many county and state facilities have tried to answer this need by adding satellite clinics in areas of shelters and other alternative living sites. Understanding this population's poor adherence to medical regimens and subsequently frequent exacerbations helps health care workers cope with this very frustrating situation.

Substance Abuse

Substance dependence and substance abuse have different criteria according to the DSM IV. No matter how addicted a person is to caffeine and/or nicotine, this is listed under substance dependence, not abuse. Alcohol can fall under either category. This classification is also true for both legal and illegal substances. The diagnostic criteria of both dependence and abuse are listed in Boxes 18-4 and 18-5.

It is easy to see how prescription medications as well as caffeine and nicotine could fall into a pattern of dependence. Illegal drugs, specifically cocaine and marijuana, could also fall in this category. Older adults also have access to illegal drugs.

There are some notable differences between dependence and abuse. The effect of the substance on the person's every day life situation is the most dramatic. **Substance dependence** is characterized by behavioral, cognitive, and physiological symptoms of requiring a substance despite having no medical need to continue its use. **Substance abuse** changes a person's lifestyle to center around obtaining and using the substance to the point of not only neglecting major role obligations but also causing major problems in one's life. These problems can be directly caused by side effects of the substance (such as a impaired driving ability) or indirectly by making increasingly poor decisions secondary to impaired judgment.

Legal Substances

When an older adult initiates going to see a health care professional, it is usually because of current symptomology. The person expects some treatment to help immediately. Many health care professionals believe it is imperative to keep the client happy (with their care) and readily reach for the prescription pad. The older a person gets, the more medical problems one tends to have, and thus the number of health care specialists increase proportionally. Therefore, many health care

BOX 18-4 Criteria for Substance Dependence

Substance dependence is defined as a maladaptive pattern of substance use, leading to clinically significant impairment or distress, as manifested by three (or more) of the following, occurring at any time in the same 12-month period:

1. Tolerance, as defined by either of the following:
   (a) A need for markedly increased amounts of the substance to achieve intoxication or desired effect
   (b) Markedly diminished effect with continued use of the same amount of the substance

2. Withdrawal, as manifested by either of the following:
   (a) The characteristic withdrawal syndrome for the substance (refer to criteria A and B of the criteria sets for withdrawal from the specific substances)
   (b) The same (or a closely related) substance taken to relieve or avoid withdrawal symptoms

3. Substance often taken in larger amounts or over a longer period than was intended

4. A persistent desire or unsuccessful efforts to cut down or control substance use

5. A great deal of time spent in activities necessary to obtain the substance (e.g., visiting multiple doctors or driving long distances), use the substance (e.g., chain smoking), or recover from its effects

6. Important social, occupational, or recreational activities given up or reduced because of substance use

7. Substance use continued despite knowledge of having a persistent or recurrent physical or psychological problem that is likely to have been caused or exacerbated by the substance (e.g., current cocaine use despite recognition of cocaine-induced depression or continued drinking despite recognition that an ulcer was made worse by alcohol consumption)

Specify if:
- *With physiological dependence:* evidence of tolerance or withdrawal (i.e., either item 1 or 2 is present)

- *Without physiological dependence:* no evidence of tolerance or withdrawal (i.e., neither item 1 nor 2 is present)

From *Diagnostic and Statistical Manual of Mental Disorders (4th ed., p. 181), 1994, Washington, DC: American Psychiatric Association. Used with permission.*

professionals are treating the same person for a variety of symptoms, leading to polypharmacy and a lack of communication among all of the health care professionals involved in this one person's care. A full client history, including low pain tolerance and past drug dependence, might not be communicated among all professionals caring for this client.

The most likely legal substances that tend to be abused by older adults are analgesics, narcotics, sleep medications, and alcohol. Of greater concern is when there are two or more of these being taken at the same time. It is extremely important to ask detailed questions of the older adult regarding use of all substances. Clients should be requested to bring all of their medications in and ask them how they are taking them (which is not necessarily how they were prescribed). Often follow-up with the person's pharmacist can help establish patterns of use through calls for refills and multiple medications for pain or sleep disturbance.

Illegal Substances

Following major wars, such as World War II, Korea, and Vietnam, there has been an increase in illegal substance abuse by veterans. This abuse permeated the general population and came to a heated public debate (over the legalization of some drugs) in the 1960s. Many substances were originally smoked, and then shooting up became a popular way to "get high." As with legal substances, the interactions of two or more substances, including legal substances such as alcohol or prescription medications, could have fatal results.

Current illegal substance abuse includes amphetamines, opiates, cocaine, heroin, and other hallucinogenic substances. Marijuana abuse is often found in conjunction with these other substances. Another recent concern is inhalant abuse. Inhaling substances such as paint, epoxies, gasoline, and paint thinners has increased particularly among the older homeless person. These inhalants are easy to obtain and quite inexpensive. From the moment of inhalation, there is a quick reaction rate as the inhalant reaches the lungs and bloodstream. Many individuals' first experience with inhalants is their last. Some substances instantly coat the lungs and the person suffocates. Others experience an anaphylactic reaction. Still others have major irreversible brain damage.

BOX 18-5   Criteria for Substance Abuse

A. A maladaptive pattern of substance use leading to clinically significant impairment or distress, as manifested by one (or more) of the following, occurring within a 12-month period:

1. Recurrent substance use resulting in a failure to fulfill major role obligations at work, school, or home (e.g., repeated absences or poor work performance related to substance use; substance-related absences, suspensions, or expulsions from school; neglect of children or household)
2. Recurrent substance use in situations in which it is physically hazardous (e.g., driving an automobile or operating a machine when impaired by substance use)
3. Recurrent substance-related legal problems (e.g., arrests for substance-related disorderly conduct)
4. Continued substance use despite having persistent or recurrent social or interpersonal problems caused or exacerbated by the effects of the substance (e.g., arguments with spouse about consequences of intoxication, physical fights)

B. The symptoms have never met the criteria for substance dependence for this class of substance.

From Diagnostic and Statistical Manual of Mental Disorders (4th ed., pp. 182–183), 1994, Washington, DC: American Psychiatric Association. Used with permission.

Research Focus

Citation:

Byrne, G. J., Raphael, B., & Arnold, E. (1999). Alcohol consumption and psychological distress in recently widowed older men. *Australian New Zealand Journal of Psychiatry, 33*(5), 740–747.

Purpose:

To examine alcohol consumption in 57 older (average age 74.5) recently widowed men and their married counterparts.

Methods:

Self-reports from the sample on alcohol consumption, grief, and anxiety.

Findings:

Alcohol consumption was significantly greater in frequency in recently widowed men. Recently widowed men drank two and one-half time more alcoholic drinks per day than their married counterparts. But there was no relationship between levels of grief and alcohol consumption.

Implications:

Older widowers are a high-risk group for alcohol abuse and for recognition of issues regarding grief and death of spouse.

Assessment and Interventions

The importance of a thorough medication/substance history cannot be overemphasized. Direct questions must be asked about possible illegal substances. Nurses can begin with a statement such as, "There are some questions that I must ask everyone. Some may not be applicable to you. I want you to remember that what you tell me is confidential, but it is extremely important for you to tell me the truth for me to best help you."

Having said this, the nurse cannot rely completely on the older adult, or even a family member, to tell everything, especially related to substance abuse. Skills of observation (such as paint around the nostrils or patting a pocket constantly for reassurance that some substance is still there) are essential. It is appropriate to ask direct questions.

Treatment options must be individualized based on the person, medical condition, and situation. When people reach 80 years of age, their liver may decrease in size and

have less blood flow, which prolongs the half-life of some drugs (Lonergan, 1996). This change makes breaking down substances of any kind a longer and more difficult process. Substances tend to stay in the older adult's system for a greater amount of time. Because of the concern for hepatic shutdown or at very least impairment, all detoxification efforts must be under strict supervision with emergency medical back-up. This is why people age 80 years and older are usually hospitalized during detoxification procedures. Because of complicating medical factors, such as a cardiac or renal problem, the medical interventions and monitoring that can only be done in an inpatient setting are crucial. After detoxification procedures are completed, the older adult may find support in a variety of places. Usually drug rehabilitation units have aftercare that includes periodic drug testing and individual and group therapies. Many health care professionals insist on **Alcoholics Anonymous (AA)** or **Narcotics Anonymous (NA)** or similar types of support groups. These groups are listed in the yellow pages of the phone book and should be offered to all post–substance abuse persons. There are support groups specifically for the older adult where socialization skills, without drugs or alcohol, are introduced.

CARE PLAN

CASE STUDY

Gene McCardle is a 76-year-old man who lives in an apartment in the city. He has resided there since his wife died 8 years ago. Mr. McCardle was once employed at a local factory as a toolmaker. He thoroughly enjoyed his job and actually wished he had continued working after retiring at 65. Mr. McCardle took care of his wife for 2 years before she succumbed to breast cancer. Those 2 years, as he stated, "were the hardest thing I ever had to do."

Mr. McCardle's lifestyle changed slowly after his wife became ill and died. He stopped going to baseball games and socializing with many of his friends. When asked, he responds, "Every time I see Lou and Alice, it reminds me of my wife. It kills me to see them and I wish I was dead."

Mr. McCardle's medical history includes hypertension (since 1970), many years of angina, and CABG (coronary artery bypass graft, 1998), depression from abnormal bereavement (since 1995), folic acid deficiency (identified in 1996), and benign prostatic hyperplasia (BPH, since 1992). He religiously takes an over-the-counter (OTC) sleeping medication at night. Other medications related to Mr. McCardle's diagnoses include Elavil (amitriptyline), folate (folic acid), Isoptin (verapamil), and Benadryl (diphenhydramine) self-prescribed.

The most significant lifestyle changes in Mr. McCardle's life comprise alcohol abuse, social isolation and withdrawal from friends, and physical inactivity. His dietary habits also have changed, increasing processed and convenience foods and high-sodium choices. Neighbors and friends feel that Mr. McCardle has changed and become a recluse. Although they care, his friends have stopped trying. One neighbor called Mr. McCardle's daughter, who lives 500 miles away, to inform her of the changes: "Better get yourself out here before he does something bad to himself. I think he is slowly killing himself, suicidal too."

ASSESSMENT

Mr. McCardle has not adjusted to his wife's death or to his retirement. In an attempt to cope with the pain and loss, he is using alcohol and drugs. He is at high risk for suicide. Risk factors include age (older than 75), race (white), living alone, widowhood, and bereavement. Although we do not know Mr. McCardle's income and whether he has a history of attempted suicide, both low income and history of attempted suicide would increase his risk. Luckily, Mr. McCardle's neighbor called his daughter, which may have saved his life. Selective important aspects of his care plan are illustrated.

NURSING DIAGNOSIS

Dysfunctional grieving related to wife's death, as evidenced by prolonged changes in eating and sleeping patterns and activity level.

Outcomes:

Mr. McCardle will:

- *Acknowledge negative lifestyle changes.*
- *Express feelings about his wife's death.*
- *Resolve the issues causing prolonged and maladaptive grieving.*

Planning/Interventions:

The nurse will:

- *Assess Mr. McCardle's affective and cognitive functioning.*
- *Assess activity level and functional status.*
- *Assess nutrition and sleep patterns.*
- *Evaluate medication and dosages for effectiveness.*
- *Consult with physician/advanced psychiatric clinician on Mr. McCardle's behaviors and medication therapy.*
- *Arrange for more frequent psychiatric interventions, i.e., psychiatric counseling.*

(continues)

CARE PLAN *continued*

EVALUATION:

Mr. McCardle will express feelings associated with his losses of his wife and job. He will acknowledge negative coping mechanisms and commit to improving his quality of life. With increased psychiatric services, careful attention to medication regimen, and improved nutritional choices and increases in activity, he will change his life.

NURSING DIAGNOSIS

Risk for violence: self-directed, related to unemployment, widowhood, and evidence of alcoholism, substance abuse, and suicidal ideation.

Outcomes:
Mr. McCardle will:
- *Acknowledge the danger in sleeping pills and alcohol.*
- *Recognize that substance abuse does not solve his problems, only camouflages it.*
- *Stop the use of alcohol and sleeping pills.*

Planning/Interventions:
The nurse will:
- *Assess suicide risk level.*
- *Facilitate Mr. McCardle's expression of his substance abuse as a problem.*
- *Explain the drug–drug interactions of Benadryl, Elavil, and alcohol, especially on the central nervous system.*
- *Begin to explore unresolved feelings associated with the cause for substance abuse.*
- *Refer Mr. McCardle for psychiatric counseling and Alcoholic Anonymous.*
- *Contact Mr. McCardle's daughter for participation and presence in this critical situation.*

EVALUATION:

As a first important step, Mr. McCardle will recognize his problem with substance abuse. He will then explore the causes for the abuse. If he expresses a true detailed plan for suicide, it is the nurse's responsibility to facilitate more intensive care in the appropriate setting, such as a mental health treatment facility. The daughter's involvement will provide the social support necessary to positively influence his situation.

NURSING DIAGNOSIS

Altered role performance related to change in usual patterns of responsibility, undesired retirement, substance abuse, and depression.

Outcomes:
Mr. McCardle will:
- *Acknowledge that he is capable of employment opportunities.*
- *Explore new or modified roles and activities related to toolmaking or other interests.*

Planning/Interventions:
The nurse will:
- *Assist Mr. McCardle in identifying interests.*
- *Assist in listing employment sources given Mr. McCardle's interests.*

EVALUATION:

Mr. McCardle will identify his interests and seek employment. *Retirement* does not necessarily mean unemployment. Consequently, Mr. McCardle will overcome feelings of stereotypical myths about aging and retirement.

Summary

As nursing moves into realms of specialization and advanced practice, the need to function cooperatively with other health care professionals is essential. Understanding the criteria behind the psychiatric diagnosis also helps guide documentation. Medicare, Medicaid, and other health care billing entities look for criteria-based documentation when involved in utilization review for care and payment. With all health care workers looking at the same criteria for documentation and care, the client is more likely to have continuity of care as well as valid documentation of the disease/treatment progression.

Untreated depression, with its sad consequences of relapse and possible suicide, is prevalent among older adults. Depression is caused by many factors including losses, which can be in the form of a spouse, independence, housing, and/or health. A decrease in the amount of neurotransmitters also affects an older adult's likelihood of experiencing depression. Depression is treatable, and the sooner treatment is started, the more positive the outcome. Treatment options include psychotherapy, medications, and ECT.

Organic mental disorders, such as delirium and dementia, can have similar presentations. There are factors such as onset and level of consciousness that help to determine the difference. Quick, appropriate treatment can reverse delirium. Dementia is irreversible, although overt symptoms can usually be controlled by medications.

Schizophrenia is frustrating for both clients and health care providers. The thought disorders can be overt and scary. Medication can control the symptoms, but unfortunately, most clients with schizophrenia have a poor adherence rate. Careful and frequent monitoring of these clients is critical.

Substance abuse disorders occur at a high rate in the older adult population. Part of this problem is a direct result of the increased number of health care practitioners the clients see and the large amount of medications they receive. Polypharmacy alone accounts for many instances of mental health problems. The use of multiple pain medications or taking them longer than is needed has also contributed to the substance abuse problem. Alcohol and illegal substances together cause the older adult to become quite vulnerable to potential substance abuse. It is important to ask all clients very pointed questions about any possible substance use, dependence, and abuse. When substance abuse is discovered, the older client must be carefully monitored in a protected health environment to reduce the risks involved with detoxification procedures.

Mental health disorders such as depression, delirium, dementia, schizophrenia, and substance abuse do not always occur in isolation. Delirium can be secondary to substance abuse. Depression can occur with dementia. A schizophrenic client can become suicidal. The key to all of this is to be sure of the client's condition by a thorough history, physical, and mental status examination. Assessment of all medications and substances, including all prescriptions, OTC medications, and legal and illegal substances, is very important. By being knowledgeable about a client's current condition, nurses are better able to give the best care and provide, through appropriate documentation, the continuity of good care that results in a positive outcome for the client.

Review Questions and Activities

1. What complications might be expected from an older client receiving medications from several health care practitioners and why?

2. What are some of the risk factors of an adult person in relation to depression?

3. Name four symptoms of depression that an older adult client might exhibit.

4. How would the nurse assess a client for depression?

5. What are the risk factors for suicide?

6. Name three highly lethal methods of suicide and how the nurse would assess a client for high risk.

7. What interventions should be used with an older adult client who is suicidal? What if they resisted?

8. Compare and contrast delirium and dementia.

9. Name two types of dementia and their characteristics.

10. Describe schizophrenia and specific assessment and intervention concerns in the older adult.

11. How are legal and illegal substances related to substance abuse problems in the older adult?

References

American Psychiatric Association. (1994). *Diagnostic and statistical manual of mental disorders* (4th ed.). Washington, DC: Author.

Bernstein, J. G. (1995). *Drug therapy in psychiatry* (3rd ed.). St. Louis: Mosby.

Emmett, K. (1998). Nonspecific and atypical presentation of disease in the older patient. *Geriatrics, 53*(2), 50–60.

Feil, N. (1982). *Validation*. Cleveland, OH: Edward Feil Productions.

Hirschfeld, R. M. A., & Goodwin, F. K. (1988). Mood disorders. In J. A. Talbot, R. E. Hales, & S. C. Yudofsky (Eds.), *Textbook of psychiatry* (pp. 403–441). Washington, DC: American Psychiatric Press.

Hollandsworth, J. G. (1990). *The physiology of psychological disorders*. New York: Plenum Press.

Johnson, G. F. S., & Wilson, P. (1989). The management of depression: A review of pharmacological and non-pharmacological treatments. *Medical Journal of Australia, 151,* 397–406.

Lonergan, E. T. (1996). *Geriatrics*. Stamford, CT: Appleton & Lange.

Marzuk, P. M., Leon, A. C., Tardiff, K., Morgan, E. B., Stajic, M., & Mann, J. J. (1992). The effect of access to lethal methods of injury on suicide rates. *Archives of General Psychiatry, 49,* 451–458.

Perez-Stable, E. J., Miranda, J., Munoz, R. F., & Ying, Y. W. (1990). Depression in medical outpatients: Under-recognition and misdiagnosis. *Archives of Internal Medicine, 150*(5), 1083–1088.

Physicians desk reference (51st ed.). (1997). Montvale, NJ: Medical Economics Data Production Company.

Regier, D. A., Farmer, M. E., Rae, D. S., Keith, S. J., Judd, L. L., & Goodwin, F. K. (1990). Comorbidity of mental disorders with alcohol and other drug abuse. *Journal of the American Medical Association, 264*(19), 2511–2518.

Yalom, I. D. (1995). *The theory and practice of group psychotherapy* (4th ed.). New York: Basic Books.

Yesavage, J. A. (1992). Depression in the elderly. *Postgraduate Medicine, 91*(1), 255–262.

Resources

Alzheimer's Association: **www.alz.org**

Alzheimer's Disease Education and Referral Center: **www.alzheimers.org**

National Guideline Clearinghouse (for clinical practice guidelines): **www.guideline.gov**

UNIT 5

The Dilemma of Long-Term Care

PERSPECTIVES...

Long–term care, including hospice and home health, provides more opportunities than any other areas of nursing. The nurse has flexibility in scheduling visits, more autonomy in decision making, more opportunities for teaching patients and involving family members in the care of clients, and adequate time for discharge instructions when necessary. The client is cared for holistically and client's needs are adapted within their environment. There is also more time and opportunity to provide care based on the client's culture.

One of the greatest rewards of long-term care practice is the relationship between the client and family. The majority of clients relate wonderful stories of the past, often rich in history. Being a good listener sometimes helps the client as much as a specific skill. Older adults who are confined often have a limited number of visitors, and loneliness and depression may occur. The nursing care also provides help and support for the family members. For example, many family members are spouses, and getting out is just as difficult for them as for the home health client. The home health nurse is often the only social support the client and family have.

Nursing care includes educating clients and their families about the medications, conservation of energy, spread of infection, nutrition, skin care, and signs and symptoms to report among other aspects of total care. Most clients want to stay at home as long as they can and some want to remain there until they die. Hospice home health care assists the client to do that with the support and love of family members. Long-term home care allows clients a quality of life that they may not otherwise have as well as dignity during their last days.

CHAPTER 19

Nursing Facilities

Mildred O. Hogstel, PhD, RN, C

COMPETENCIES

After completing this chapter, the reader should be able to:

- *Name and describe the services of five different classifications of nursing facilities.*
- *Describe the role of the registered nurse in the nursing facility.*
- *Identify the functions of the certified nurse aide (CNA).*
- *Evaluate the role of the training coordinator in nursing facilities.*
- *Explain the differences in Medicare and Medicaid payments for nursing facility care.*
- *Discuss the methods of paying for long-term care.*
- *Analyze federal and state regulations for nursing facilities.*
- *Describe the purpose of the ombudsman program in nursing facilities.*
- *Explore to what extent wellness promotion and prevention of disease are provided in nursing facilities.*
- *Discuss the implications of medical malpractice in nursing facilities.*

MAKING THE CONNECTION

Refer to the following chapters to increase your understanding of long-term care:

Classification and Types of Services

Long-term care, which includes nursing facility care, will be one of the major health care issues and concerns in the twenty-first century as older adults increase in numbers and longevity. Only 4.2% of people age 65 and older lived in a nursing facility in 1996, but for people age 85 and older, the percentage increased to 19.8% (*A profile*, 1999). This chapter will focus on the delivery and regulation of care in those types of facilities.

Nursing facilities changed tremendously in the twentieth century, from something called an "old people's home" in the early to mid 1900s to a type of facility in the 1990s that provided care equivalent to that given in a hospital for certain residents needing skilled care. In 1996 there were 16,706 nursing facilities in the United States with more than 1.78 million beds. New York had the highest occupancy rate (98%) and Texas had the lowest (77%) (Bectel & Tucker, 1998). The lower percentage could reflect the fact that there are other types of facilities and services meeting the needs of dependent older adults, such as assisted-living facilities. Another factor is funding because much of nursing home care is paid for by **Medicaid**, a federal and state program, and most states have implemented a **Community Based Alternative (CBA)** program that allows people eligible for nursing facility care under Medicaid to be cared for in an assisted-living facility or at home with home health care assistance. The primary purpose of the CBA was to reduce state costs because nursing facility care is more expensive than assisted-living facilities or home care.

The major types of institutions that provide long-term care are listed in Table 19-1. All nursing facilities provide 24-hour care 7 days a week supervised by licensed nurses. The Director of Nurses is a registered nurse, who is ultimately responsible for the quality of care in the facility. All medical care is ordered and prescribed by a physician and/or advanced practice registered nurses, such as **gerontological nurse practitioners (GNPs)**, with prescriptive authority from the state.

Private ownership of nursing facilities is the most common form of proprietorship. Many health care corporations own chains of nursing facilities in various parts of the United States. Nursing facilities are also classified as *for-profit* or *nonprofit*. Many of these facilities are owned or affiliated with a religious or governmental agency (e.g., veterans).

Nursing Facility

Long-term health care facilities that receive Medicaid funds are classified as **nursing facilities (NF)**. Nursing facilities provide services to older adults who require institutionalization and nursing care directed by registered nurses or licensed vocational (practical) nurses. These older adults may need assistance with physical activities of daily living such as bathing and eating. They are given medications as prescribed by a physician and may need other continuous care such as catheter care. Custodial care such as assistance with bathing, eating, and dressing may be needed over a period of years because of multiple chronic illnesses and conditions of the residents. There is usually not strong emphasis on the rehabilitation potential of the resident, although maintenance of health status and prevention of further complications are important (see Figure 19-1).

Skilled Nursing Facility

Nursing facilities that receive **Medicare** funds are classified as **skilled nursing facilities (SNF)** and provide more skilled nursing care, such as tube feedings and

TABLE 19-1   Types and Services of Nursing Facilities

Facility	Services
Subacute care	Skilled care 24 hours a day by a team of health care professionals
Rehabilitation unit	All types of rehabilitative care, such as extensive physical and/or speech therapy following a cerebrovascular accident
Special care unit	A unit where specific kinds of residents are cared for (e.g., dementia care such as Alzheimer's disease)
Skilled nursing facility	Skilled care 24 hours a day provided under the direction and supervision of an RN or LVN. Residents need less extensive care than those in a subacute care unit.
Nursing facility	Supervised custodial care and support 24 hours a day
Skilled nursing unit, skilled nursing inpatient facility	A separate unit located in or on the same premises as a hospital

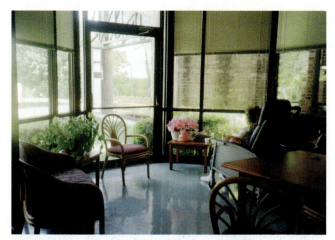

FIGURE 19-1 A resident looks outside from a large rural nursing facility.

sterile dressings. In addition to skilled nursing care (which is defined as care provided by a licensed nurse—RN or LVN), other skilled services such as physical therapy, respiratory therapy, speech-language pathology services, and occupational therapy are provided if needed, for the purpose of rehabilitation of the resident to the maximum extent possible. These types of services usually last less than 20 days, which is the length of time provided under Medicare Part A benefits without a copay.

Special Care Unit

Special care units (SCUs) are units in nursing facilities that provide specialized care and/or services to residents with specific needs. Some of the special needs are:

- Dementia, especially Alzheimer's disease, care in a dementia special care unit (DSCU)
- Mental illnesses and other acute episodic life crises
- Children and younger adults with long-term disabilities
- Residents with acquired immunodeficiency syndrome (AIDS)

These units usually have specialized equipment and activities to meet the needs of their residents. Staff on these units have inservice training that will help them to understand and care for their residents with specialized needs (Kovach, 1998).

Subacute Care Unit

Some free-standing nursing facilities have developed subacute care units (SUBs). This type of unit is designed for residents who require more intensive skilled care over a period of months, such as those who are ventilator dependent or need intravenous or other extensive kinds of therapy. These units are usually staffed by registered nurses 24 hours a day.

Hospital Skilled Nursing Unit/ Special Nursing Inpatient Facility

Some large hospitals have developed their own nursing facilities on the hospital premises. These provide the same or similar services as a separate free-standing skilled nursing facility. A hospital may have one or two units designated as **skilled nursing units (SNUs)** or **skilled nursing inpatient facilities (SNIFs)**. Length of stay is about the same as for an SNF because the primary payment mechanism for the older adult is Medicare. This type of unit is especially helpful for a hospital client who is ready to be discharged but needs a short period of rehabilitation before going home or perhaps back to an NF. The SNUs and SNIFs have the advantage of having all hospital services (such as laboratory and pharmacy) near when they are needed. It is also convenient for the resident's physician to visit more often.

Characteristics of Residents

The typical nursing facility resident is a female, widow, in her seventies or eighties, and has two or more chronic health conditions requiring nursing care and assistance (see Figure 19-2). However, there are more and more residents ages 90 to 100 or older. Many do not have close family members or regular visitors.

Think About It

Why are there more women than men in nursing facilities?

Major Health Problems

Cardiovascular problems and congestive heart disease are major reasons for admission. Coronary thrombosis and cerebrovascular accidents often change active older adults into people who can no longer care for themselves. Many older adults are admitted to a skilled nursing facility for a period of rehabilitation after surgery.

Orthopedic problems are prevalent. Arthritis and osteoporosis are conditions that cause pain and prevent independence in the physical activities of daily living. Fractures are common and require a long period of recovery. Elective surgery for knee or hip replacement requires periods of rehabilitation and daily physical therapy. Older adults with diabetes, blindness, glaucoma, and emphysema require supervised environments.

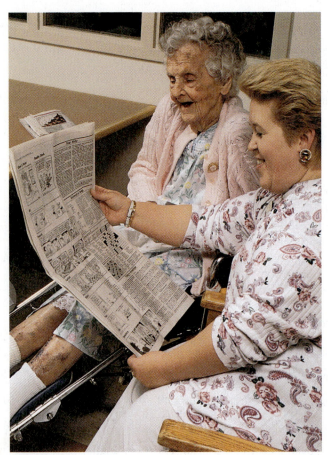

FIGURE 19-2   A 95-year-old resident who enjoys the company of staff.

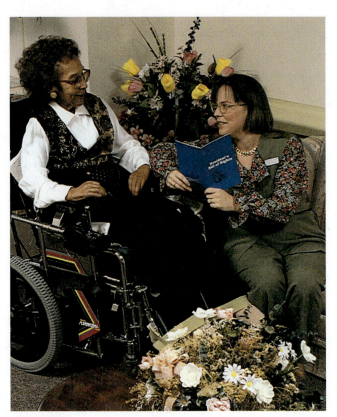

FIGURE 19-3   The resident receives a full explanation of resident's rights as part of the admissions process.

Hypertension often adds to the complications of other conditions. There are various mental health problems, such as organic mental disorders, confusion, and depression, that require nursing facility care. The number of residents diagnosed as having dementia of the Alzheimer's type also is increasing. Many older adults are admitted to nursing facilities because they no longer can live alone and still follow prescribed medications and diet.

Ask Yourself

- Have you ever spent some time in a nursing facility?
- What were your impressions?
- What changes, if any, would you like to have suggested to the administration and/or other staff?

Admission to a Nursing Facility

If the decision is made to admit the older adult to a nursing facility, the necessary forms must be completed. Physicians' orders must be received when the resident is admitted. A history and physical examination are required within 48 hours after admission. If the older adult is transferred from a hospital to the nursing facility, a summary of the hospital stay is needed. Every form that is signed by the responsible party should be completed in duplicate and copies retained by the family. Upon completion of the forms, the nursing facility has entered into an agreement with the family and the rights and responsibilities of the nursing facility and the family have been agreed upon. Nursing facilities must furnish information on the **Resident Bill of Rights**, a major component of the **Omnibus Budget Reconciliation Act (OBRA) of 1987** (Figure 19-3). Many nursing facilities have an enlarged copy of this Bill of Rights framed and displayed in a prominent place in the lobby of the nursing facility. The family has the freedom to select the pharmacy to be used. Medical care and supervision are furnished by the admitting physician or the resident may elect to transfer to the Medical Director of the nursing facility. Information is also collected regarding the name of the resident's dentist and which ambulance service and funeral home are preferred if needed. The resident and/or responsible party must be informed about their right to prepare a Directive to Physician (living will) and Medical Power of Attorney, which has been required since the Federal Patient Self Determination Act was passed in 1991. However, there should be no pressure by the staff to complete such a form.

It is essential that the admission process include a complete orientation and tour of the facility services,

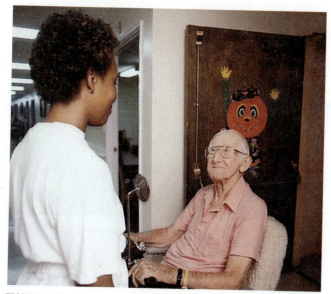

FIGURE 19-4 A comprehensive admissions process is one that includes sensitivity and awareness to the older adult's ability to adapt to a new environment successfully.

programs, and requirements for the resident and family if at all possible. The first 48 hours in the nursing facility can make an important impact on the resident's adaptation to a new environment (Figure 19-4). Older adults can experience anxiety, stress, confusion, and depression when changing from one environment to another one. This problem of **relocation** or **translocation syndrome** (which may include temporary confusion) is especially true if they moved from home to acute care hospital to rehabilitation hospital to nursing facility over a period of a few weeks.

Administration and Staffing

The ultimate quality of resident care, atmosphere of the facility, organization and coordination of all departments, and morale of personnel are major goals and responsibilities of the administrator and Director of Nursing. Each state differs in general educational requirements of the administrator. Most states require specific courses in nursing home administration, an intern period, and state **licensure**.

Some nursing care facilities experience high staff turnover, short staffing as a result of illness, a lack of transportation for personnel to get to the facility, and a demand for **certified nurse aides (CNAs)** that is greater than the supply. Staffing is a major problem. Supervisory personnel, especially registered nurses, are responsible for ensuring that all staff provide quality care to residents. Working conditions are often difficult because of low staffing and the multiple needs of chronically ill residents and their families. It is not easy to manage personnel and maintain quality care when there is frequent employee turnover.

Personnel

There are a variety of staff members employed in nursing facilities. The major categories are nursing, social work, dietary, activities, housekeeping, and environmental control. Other health care professionals may be employed full time or as part-time consultants as required by state laws according to the size of the facility.

Nursing

Federal and state standards usually define the minimum requirements for licensed nursing staff in nursing facilities. Minimal standards are suggested for the number of residents per nurse. However, the number of CNAs needed to give adequate nursing care is not clearly defined. A registered nurse must be on duty 8 hours a day 7 days a week during the day and be on call 24 hours a day. The facility must have a licensed vocational (practical) nurse on duty for each shift. In some states only registered nurses may start intravenous fluids, give intravenous medications, and insert nasal gastric tubes. The director of nursing must be a registered nurse and cannot also function as the inservice coordinator or be responsible for training the nurse aides. Bedside nursing or personal care is provided by CNAs who must be supervised by licensed nursing personnel. Medications are given only by licensed nurses. There are programs in some states that provide for **certified medication aides (CMAs)** after completing a course on medications beyond the CNA training. This type of assignment must be supervised closely. Professional nurses should be alert to state legislation that allows such practices and monitor this issue carefully because they are ultimately legally responsible for safe quality care.

The director of nursing is responsible for the overall quality of nursing care of the residents. The director works closely with administrative personnel to ensure that the standards of nursing care are maintained. The scope and standards of gerontological nursing practice as developed by the American Nurses' Association should be implemented and maintained by the professional nursing staff (*Scope and standards*, 1995). All medications, treatments, and transportation of residents to and from hospitals must be ordered by physicians or advanced practice nurse practitioners. A copy of all telephone orders must be forwarded to physicians, signed, and returned to the resident's chart. The director of nursing serves as an important liaison between the resident, family, and physician. Any changes in the condition or need for new treatment of the resident must be reported to the physician and the family. Some nursing facilities have 24-hour registered nurse coverage. However, if not, a registered nurse who is on call for the skilled nursing facility during the evening or night hours is notified of any changes in the condition of the residents or if any unusual incidents occur. Many times, the

Research Focus

Citation:

Atchison, J. H. (1998). Perceived job satisfaction factors of nursing assistants employed in midwest nursing homes. *Geriatric Nursing, 19*(3), 135–137.

Purpose:

To determine the characteristics and perceptions of nursing assistants in nursing homes in relation to job satisfaction.

Methods:

A two-part questionnaire composed of eight questions related to demographics and a job diagnostic survey. The subjects were 283 nursing assistants in 24 nursing facilities.

Findings:

Major concerns were job security, potential for growth and development in their jobs, socialization, and challenge in their work. The subjects were primarily single, female, ages 16–49, worked more than 35 hours a week, high school graduates, certified, and employed in the nursing facility less than 1 year.

Implications:

Inservice and support groups for assistants are suggested to reduce stress. Incomes were close to poverty level so salary is an important factor. With higher wages and more benefits, turnover was lower. Increased social or special activities for assistants and their families are important.

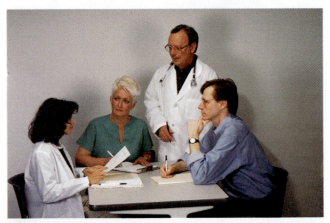

FIGURE 19-5 Members of the health care team work together for the benefit of the resident.

registered nurse will need to return to the nursing facility to observe and interpret changes in the condition of a resident. Expertise in assessment skills and nursing care are needed in nursing facility settings.

The assessment of each resident is the function of the professional and licensed nursing personnel in the nursing facility. As mentioned previously, several departments will assist in resident assessment. The professional nurse assesses the residents and identifies their individual problems, abilities, and needs. The assessment of mobility, independence in the physical activities of daily living, and degree of assistance required provides a baseline for planning nursing care and assigning staff to care for the residents.

Resident assessment involves a summary of the resident's ability to function physically, emotionally, mentally, and psychosocially. From this assessment, goal-directed therapy is planned for each resident. The prevention of further disabilities and rehabilitation are part of goal-directed therapy. With the use of a summary

of the resident assessment, an individualized interdisciplinary care plan is prepared for each resident. These summaries are also helpful in evaluating nursing care. Comprehensive care is continued for each resident, and the various departments within the nursing facility collaborate in this care (Figure 19-5). Physical therapy and speech/language pathology services are available within the facility, or the facility may request these services from other health care agencies.

More **gerontological clinical nurse specialists (GCNSs)** and GNPs are needed in nursing facilities to provide assistance in assessment, care planning, intervention, and teaching. Some are employed by nursing facility medical directors, as staff on a part-time basis, or as consultants. Several nursing organizations have worked for and obtained "direct reimbursement from Medicare Part B regardless of geographic location" (Facundus, 1998, p. 1). These individuals are usually required by state law to be registered with the Board of Nurse Examiners as an advanced practice nurse. These specialists could improve the quality of health care and life for nursing facility residents. Nursing facilities are often not able to find or pay for these types of specialists.

Other Personnel

The nursing facility is required to employ a pharmacist as a consultant. A monthly review of all medications is made. The validation of the effectiveness of the medications is a responsibility of the nurse. The pharmacist is available to furnish up-to-date data regarding medications and their effects. The pharmacist is responsible for monitoring or reviewing the system of drug administration for each resident.

A registered dietitian plans the regular menus for the residents as well as special diets. Eating and feeding problems, including likes and dislikes of foods, are considered when the diet is planned. Therapeutic diets such as low sodium, diabetic, high protein, bland, and

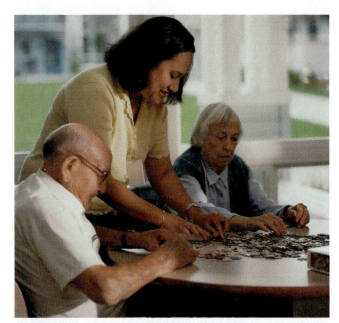

FIGURE 19-6 The activities director is responsible for planning and supervising a variety of activities for the residents.

blended are planned by the dietitian, who also assists in the evaluation of their effectiveness. The dietitian is responsible for the maintenance of standards in the kitchen.

Each facility is required to have a medical director to provide medical care to those residents who do not have a regular physician, to provide emergency care to residents when needed, and to participate in interdisciplinary meetings and activities. A dentist and **podiatrist** are also required to be available to residents.

A social worker is required in all facilities with more than 120 beds to counsel with the resident and family regarding concerns and problems related to the resident's total care. The activities director works closely with the nurses and social worker assessing residents' leisure time interests and needs. The activities director plans and directs social activities, religious services, exercise programs, and pet therapy and teaches and supervises crafts to residents (Figure 19-6).

A number of other persons are employed in the area of environmental services to maintain the equipment, cleanliness, and general operation of the facility. In some areas, 24-hour security personnel are employed to protect the residents and visiting family members from possible criminal dangers in the environment.

Some nursing facilities also contract with a variety of other consultants. For example, even though mental illness is not a primary diagnosis for most residents, a number of them have mental health problems such as depression in addition to physical problems. Rarely do nursing facility staff have specific educational preparation and/or experience in geropsychiatry. Therefore, nursing facilities contract with individuals such as geriatric psychiatrists,

geropsychiatric clinical nurse specialists, and gerontological psychologists and/or counselors to provide needed mental health diagnosis and treatment. Medications appropriate for older adults may be needed (e.g., antidepressants) together with individual and/or talk therapy. Other consultants may be sought to assist with inservice training for all staff or to facilitate family support groups.

Orientation, Training, and Supervision of Staff

Orientation to the physical facilities, the staff, and the departments within the facility assists new personnel in becoming a part of the organization. During their first day, new personnel should become acquainted with policies, other personnel, and the role that each member of the staff fills. New employees should not be expected to assume total responsibility for resident care immediately or to perform the same amount of work that will eventually be their assignment. New employees need to become acquainted with the functions of the facility and the responsibilities they will have. They should learn about the kinds of residents who are in their specific nursing facility.

Certified nurse aides who seek employment in a new institution have completed courses and received certificates in the care of older adults. This type of training is available through high schools and community colleges. Whatever the previous preparation, there must be a well-planned orientation period. The rights of residents and the confidentiality of resident records must be stressed to new nurse aides. These employees often have not considered the ethical and legal aspects of nursing care.

Information on aging should be part of the orientation process and should be presented frequently in inservice education programs. New aides should understand that their role is a supportive one and that the residents' wishes and needs should be met if at all possible. Supervisory staff members are responsible for assessing and managing residents' problems.

Even though aides may present certificates of training, it is essential that their skills be evaluated by a member of the nursing staff when they give nursing care. A safe practice in one facility might not be a safe practice in another home.

Aides with certification of training are usually assigned to another experienced aide to learn about the specific residents and their needs. Licensed personnel are responsible for evaluating the previous experience and training of the aides.

The job description for each employee dictates the amount of training required. Personal care skills should be taught in the classroom and not on the job. Training can consist of various types of instructional media, such as films and slides, and the demonstration and practice of procedures before the aides begin caring for residents. Supervisory nursing personnel should continue to evaluate all aides in their care of residents.

Federal and state laws require a certain amount of inservice training for all categories of personnel. This training is usually on site and in addition to any continuing education required for individual license renewal of professional staff members such as registered nurses. Such inservice training should be realistic and related to the specialized needs of older adults. Suggested essential topics of inservice training for all levels of nursing staff are shown in Box 19-1. A registered nurse, other than the director of nursing, or a licensed vocational (practical) nurse is usually responsible for the planning, implementation, and evaluation of these educational programs.

Inservice education is not a substitute for orientation. Many of the same topics should be covered in inservice education programs as in the orientation. These programs should be provided for all personnel, professional or paraprofessional, and should be scheduled at convenient times so that all employees can attend.

Planning inservice education programs is the responsibility of the inservice coordinator. The coordinator should work with supervisory personnel and involve them in the programs. Few programs are for aides only. Staff should especially be provided with the knowledge and skills to care for emergencies (see Table 19-2) when they arise (Duchemin, Clark, & Keeber, 1991).

An understanding of the aging process is important. Programs on the process of aging should be presented during the year. Simulated situations in which aides participate in role playing help them experience the limitations of their residents. The discarded glasses of older adults can be prepared with colorless nail polish, the lenses made dirty, or the sides clouded so the aides have difficulty seeing. By wearing thick gloves, the aides can experience limitations of the hands and fingers in eating, shaving, or even cleansing themselves after elimination. If the aides experience these limitations, they will have a better understanding of some of the physical restrictions in their older residents. Programs on death and dying are also important. A good question to ask is "What would you like done for you if you were dying?" At the end of the discussion there is generally a good summary of the kind of care the dying resident needs. The inservice coordinator should not present all the programs. Other staff members and/or outside speakers should share their philosophy and knowledge about caring for the residents.

Some inservice education programs should be concerned with the health and welfare of the personnel. Programs on cancer detection, blood pressure screening, and family planning are of value to the personnel. Special programs on fire prevention, disaster preparedness, and personal health maintenance are also helpful to the personnel and their families.

The professional staff should be alert to the fact that routine and repetitious care for older adults who are sick and dependent is not an easy assignment. Many complaints and frustrations are transmitted by residents to aides. The professional staff should be a source of physical and emotional support to the aides. The need to provide positive reinforcement to aides is important. The nurse supervisor should help aides express their feelings about particularly difficult residents and recognize that a resident's family may be making it difficult for them to care for the resident.

There are incidents of abuse of residents in nursing facilities. Programs should be planned to discuss the ethical and legal responsibilities of the nursing facility staff and the consequences of the discovery of abuse. The neglect of residents is also a major concern in nursing facilities. The open recognition of these two major concerns tends to lessen the incidence of abuse or neglect.

BOX 19-1 Sample of Essential Topics for Inservice Education for Nursing Facility Staff

- Common emergencies of geriatric residents and how to prevent them; for example, falls, choking on food or medicines, injuries from restraint use; recognizing sudden changes in physical condition, such as stroke, heart attack, acute abdomen, and acute glaucoma; and obtaining emergency treatment

- Universal precautions regarding the transmission of microorganisms from one person to another

- Assessment and nursing interventions related to the common physical and psychological changes of aging for each body system

- Communication techniques and skills useful when providing geriatric care, such as skills for communicating with the hearing impaired, visually impaired, and cognitively impaired; therapeutic touch; and recognizing communication that indicates psychological abuse

- Geriatric pharmacology, including treatment for pain management and sleep disorders

- Common mental disorders with related nursing implications

- Ethical and legal issues regarding advance directives, abuse and neglect, guardianship, and confidentiality

- How to cope with death and dying

There are many excellent videotapes and books for nurse aide training. A book should be provided to each aide to refer to for information on nursing care. A sense of owning the book, if this is possible, influences the feelings of worth the aides have. Registered nurses should realize that the quality of nursing care is ultimately their responsibility and must continually observe, supervise, and evaluate the care given by technical nursing staff.

Payment Mechanisms

The cost of long-term care in a nursing facility can be very expensive. Annual costs range from $30,000 to $80,000 or more, not including physician visits and care as well as medications and other special health care needs. The primary methods of paying for nursing facility care are listed in Box 19-2.

Medicare

Many older adults and their families do not realize that Medicare does not pay for nursing facility care except for a limited number of days and only if the resident needs specialized skilled care such as physical therapy after a fracture. One of the major problems facing older adults is the potentiality of having to pay for long-term care in a nursing facility for many years.

Medicaid

Medicaid is a federal (60%) and state (40%) type of assistance to eligible people who qualify based on assets and income. If older adults receive Social Security benefits or a small pension, this amount can be supplemented by Medicaid payments to the nursing facility. The administrative staff of the nursing facility has information available and will give family members instructions about how to apply for assistance. Application for Medicaid assistance is made at the local level by the resident or by the family member who is responsible for the financial

BOX 19-2   Methods of Paying for Nursing Facility

- Medicare
- Medicaid
- Long-term care private insurance
- Veterans' Affairs
- Private pay

arrangements. Medicaid approval is granted based on financial assets, including bank accounts, real estate, and personal income of the resident. Each state may have different requirements. If Medicaid assistance is approved, a certificate of need is granted and payments are made to the nursing facility to supplement the payments made by the resident.

If the older adult is accepted for Medicaid assistance, the monthly Social Security check will be paid to the resident or to the responsible family member. The resident or family retains a small amount (e.g., $45) of the check, which can be used for clothing and personal supplies for the resident. Medicaid payments supplement the money received from the family to pay for the services at the nursing facility. The daily rate of charge for nursing facility care is determined by state regulations when residents are on Medicaid. The average Medicaid per diem reimbursement for nursing facility care in 1995 was $84 (Bectel & Tucker, 1998). Medicaid also will pay for needed prescription drugs for each recipient. Pharmacists work closely with physicians and families to provide direct billing to the Medicaid office for payment of these prescription drugs. The nursing facility is responsible for furnishing commonly prescribed medications such as aspirin, antacids, and laxatives, as well as supplies such as nasal gastric tubes, urinary catheters, drainage bags, dressings, and tube feedings, to residents who qualify for Medicaid assistance.

Medicaid funds are paid only to nursing facilities that meet Medicaid standards. Physicians' services are paid for by Medicare, other insurance, or the family. Reimbursement for these fees is applied for through Medicare or Medicaid. Physicians must bill Medicare directly. Standard fees are authorized for physicians' services. In some situations the income of older adults changes during the years or their savings may be reduced to such a small amount that they will qualify for Medicaid assistance later.

Long-Term Care Insurance

Some private insurance companies provide insurance that will pay for long-term care, including care in a nursing facility. It is very important, however, that older adults and their families study the costs and benefits of these insurance plans before purchasing one of them.

Veterans' Affairs (VA)

Veterans who have chronic health problems can receive short-term care (e.g., several months) for rehabilitation purposes in a VA hospital that has an SNU or in a private nursing facility. However, long-term care for veterans with service-connected diseases or disabilities can be provided for as long as needed in a nursing facility.

Private Pay

Private pay is also an option, and some people are able to pay the total cost either until the long-term care insurance becomes effective or until personal financial resources are used up and they become eligible for Medicaid. Some nursing facilities accept private pay residents only.

Regulations and Oversight

Regulations are based on federal and state laws that mandate specific requirements related to staffing levels, quality of care, and building and environmental safety and cleanliness.

State Licensure

Licensure of the facility is required by a specific state regulatory agency. Licensure denotes that the nursing facility has maintained specific minimal standards and is frequently inspected for observance of fire and safety codes, sanitation standards, health codes, and the maintenance of approved methods of purchasing and preparing foods. Guidelines for licensure are legislated at both the federal and state levels. Certain state agencies are designated as licensing agencies for long-term health care facilities. The title of the agency varies from state to state, but its function is to oversee the care of older adults in nursing facilities. These standards cover building construction, number of qualified personnel, maintenance of health standards, operation of the home in compliance with medical and nursing standards, and the number of older adults who can be cared for within the facility. The state is the licensing agency; private pay homes are also licensed by the state agency. The in-

ability of the home to maintain minimal standards could mean that the facility will pay penalties and/or lose its license. Minor infractions must be corrected within a 30-day period. The level of care provided to the residents is also considered a part of the licensing process.

The administrator must have a current state license as a nursing facility administrator. State laws define the type and number of hours of education the administrator must have to qualify for licensure. The successful completion of state licensing examinations is required before licensure is approved. Yearly relicensure is granted upon the submission of proof of attendance at workshops or seminars related to nursing facility administration. Many nursing facilities have several employees who are licensed as administrators. Registered nurses and licensed vocational or practical nurses must have current licenses. All employees are required to have current health cards issued by the local health department and based on state standards. Personnel are especially screened for tuberculosis and sexually transmitted diseases and often are required to have a hepatitis B vaccination.

Federal Medicare Conditions of Participation

The OBRA of 1987, implemented on October 1, 1990, came about as a result of the efforts of a number of national organizations, such as the American Nurses' Association (ANA), the American Association of Retired Persons (AARP), and the National Citizens Coalition for Nursing Home Reform (NCCNHR) (Strumpf, Evans, and Schwartz, 1990). The major requirements of this federal legislation are listed in Box 19-3. While all of these regulations are important, the major ones will be discussed.

BOX 19-3   Federal Omnibus Budget Reconciliation Act (OBRA) of 1987

Sample of Requirements (effective October 1, 1990, with OBRA 1990 Additions)

A. Staffing
1. RN (at least one) 8 hours a day, 7 days a week (waiver available)
2. LVN/LPN 24 hours a day, 7 days a week (waiver available)
3. Social worker (at least one) if 121 or more beds
4. Nurse aides must have 75 hours of training within first 4 months of employment
5. Must check state registry before hiring nurse aides

B. Quality of care
1. Comprehensive admission assessment signed by RN within 14 days of admission
2. Written care plans after comprehensive assessment
3. Quality assessment and assurance committees required
4. Must justify medical need for physical and chemical restraints
5. Cannot admit mentally ill or retarded unless certified by state as needing such care

C. Other
1. Residents' rights all important
2. Patient Self Determination Act must be discussed with patient and/or family on admission

Staffing

Staffing regulations include at least one registered nurse during the day shift 7 days a week. Also, a licensed nurse is required on site 24 hours a day. A social worker is required if the home has 121 or more beds. A major change has been the increased amount of education for nurse aides. They must have a minimum of 75 hours of training within the first 4 months of employment and pass written and clinical tests. All nurse aides who have met these requirements must be listed on a state registry, and an employer must check this registry before employing them. The intent of this regulation is to be sure that the nurse aides have been certified regarding training and testing and that they have not been convicted of a felony or other wrong-doing. While training and testing for nurse aides have progressed well in most areas after a slow start, requirements for registered nurses should include more content on management and supervision of staff.

Admission Assessment

Another section of the OBRA regulations relates to quality of care (see Box 19-3). These include a comprehensive admission assessment of each resident by a registered nurse, written care plans based on a comprehensive assessment, and quality assessment and management committees. These regulations have been easier to implement because many of them were already in place.

Restraints

The need to justify the use of both physical and chemical restraints was addressed by the OBRA regulations. Too many restraints had been used in nursing homes, primarily for the convenience of the staff, though stating that they were for the safety of residents. Most research has demonstrated that the use of restraints does not prevent falls (Gross, Shimamoto, Rose, & Frank, 1990). Nurses have always known that physical restraints are used as a last resort, must be specifically ordered by the physician, and require more nurse time because of the need to assess the resident frequently to prevent complications.

The regulations stated that restraints should only be used if needed for the medical benefit of the resident (e.g., for a resident who might pull out a nasogastric feeding tube if not restrained) or in the case of bed rails to help the resident move in bed. Restraints should not be used to keep a resident who can walk from being ambulatory (e.g., a resident with a diagnosis of dementia of the Alzheimer's type (DAT) who wanders; he or she needs to walk). The number of restraint-reduced nursing homes is increasing (Coberg, Lynch, & Mavretish, 1991). Alternatives to restraints are discussed more completely in the Accidents section later in this chapter.

Chemical restraints, primarily psychotropic medications such as sedatives, hypnotics, antianxiety agents, and neuroleptics, also have been used in the past to control the behavior of hyperactive, wandering, agitated residents. The OBRA regulations state that these medications should only be given to residents who require them for a specific diagnosis. This regulation has increased the number of mental status assessments being performed in nursing facilities by psychiatrists and geropsychiatric nurses. When appropriate, there is a referral for further evaluation and treatment. The outcome has been beneficial because many older adults are receiving treatment they might not have otherwise received. Also, the reduced number of psychotropic medications is generally beneficial to the health of the older adult.

Mental Illness

Another regulation relates to the fact that persons whose primary medical diagnosis is mental illness or mental retardation should not be in nursing facilities. Organic mental disorders, such as Alzheimer's disease, are excluded because they are physical diseases. There are two reasons for this: (a) residents cannot receive adequate treatment for mental problems in nursing homes because that is not these institutions' purpose and (b) residents with these diagnoses often disturb the other residents. An evaluation program—Pre-Admission Screening and Annual Resident Review (PASARR)—has been used to determine if these residents should be in the nursing home or if they could be cared for more effectively in another setting. The PASARR program may also help to provide state mental health services for some residents.

Levels of Care

All nursing homes are now referred to as nursing facilities (NF) or skilled nursing facilities (SNF). Another focus was to determine the level of care and thus reimbursement by Medicaid, based on residents' "impairment and disability rather than on medical diagnosis" (Boondas, 1991, p. 311). In addition, a comprehensive instrument was developed through research to record health data about residents upon admission, yearly, and whenever there is a change in resident's status. This **minimum data set (MDS)** is used to assign residents to the appropriate level of care (Morris et al., 1990). This process determines resource requirements for each resident based on that person's individual characteristics and needs (Boondas, 1991). Therefore, this case mix classification based on MDS "is a method that will provide a more equitable system of payment, and an improved staffing pattern consistent with the case mix and an improved understanding of care time requirements" (Boondas, 1991, p. 311).

Implementations

Revised guidelines and waivers for many of these regulations have made the nursing facility reform law less effective than was originally planned. Although the federal government passed the OBRA law in 1987, the exact guidelines for implementing the law were very slow in being distributed and the method of implementation was vague. Some guidelines were only available late in the summer of 1990 before the law was to take full effect in October 1990. Also, the federal government did not provide for additional funding, primarily through Medicaid, to implement many of the requirements. Therefore, states with major budget problems did not have the Medicaid money available to help nursing facilities meet the federal guidelines. Nor do most states have other services or facilities for the treatment and care of chronically mentally ill older adults.

National Accreditation

Voluntary **accreditation** may be received from the Joint Commission on Accreditation of Healthcare Organizations (JCAHO). The nursing facility owner and/or administrator will determine whether this type of accreditation is sought because it is voluntary. Nursing facilities are usually members of state and local nursing facility associations. Membership in the American Health Care Association or the American Association of Homes and Services for the Aging is also available.

The Ombudsman Program

An **ombudsman** is a specially trained and certified volunteer or professional who advocates for quality of care in nursing facilities. Volunteers are supervised by professional staff ombudsmen who are part of the regional aging services network supported by the state Department on Aging. The Ombudsman program is mandated by the Older Americans Act of 1965 and funded by state and federal governments. The purposes of the Ombudsman program are to:

- Provide information to residents and families about rights and procedures and help identify additional resources in or out of the facility

- Investigate and resolve complaints by or on behalf of nursing facility residents

- Work with residents, families, friends, and facility staff to resolve complaints and difficulties

(Adapted from material provided by the Ombudsman Certification Training Regional Training Modules, Office of the State Long-Term Care Ombudsman, Texas Department on Aging.)

Residents and families should try to resolve problems and differences with the facility staff whenever possible. When this is not possible, or when the resident or family is unsure, a local ombudsman should be called. The ombudsman volunteer or regional staff ombudsman will assess the concerns and recommend possible courses of action. Often, the ombudsman can resolve the problem without involving other groups or agencies. Sometimes, the resident council or family support group is involved in the resolution. When the ombudsman cannot help resolve the problems, or when it involves serious abuse or neglect, the complaint is referred to the appropriate state agency. In all situations, the complaint is handled confidentially and information is not released without permission of the resident or legal guardian. The ombudsman is also a good source of information about selecting a long-term care facility, eligibility criteria, and other services for older adults needing this type of care.

Volunteer Organizations

There are national and state volunteer organizations that monitor the quality of care in nursing homes and provide information and support for family members of nursing home residents. The groups also are strong advocates for federal and state legislation to protect nursing home residents. Some of these organizations are:

- National Citizens' Coalition for Nursing Home Reform

- National Alliance for Senior Citizens

- National Conference of Gerontological Nurse Practitioners

There are state organizations with similar goals and activities.

Nursing Issues and Concerns

There are several special issues related to safety and quality of care in nursing facilities. Accidents, such as falls, skin care, and a sudden change in condition need to be reported and monitored carefully.

Acute Medical Emergencies

Acute medical emergencies occur among older adults in the nursing facility as well as in the community. These emergencies may involve acute illnesses, such as a myocardial infarction or a cerebrovascular accident, or accidents such as falls. See Table 19-2 for symptoms, possible causes, and emergency interventions for the most common medical emergencies. Immediate assessment and emergency treatment may be provided in the nursing facility, but the resident usually will require transfer to a nearby hospital for further evaluation and treatment.

TABLE 19-2 Common Medical Emergencies Among Older Adults in Nursing Facilities

Problems	Symptoms	Possible Causes	Interventions*
Myocardial infarction (MI) and/or cardiac arrest	Sudden behavior change, e.g., confusion, disorientation (probably before chest pain, nausea, vomiting, dyspnea, cyanosis, absence of pulse/respiration)	Long-term cardiovascular problems	Initiate cardiopulmonary resuscitation (CPR) if needed (if no "Do Not Resuscitate" order) and call 911 for ambulance
Choking, obstructed airway, and/or aspiration	Coughing, dyspnea, cyanosis, hand to throat	Past stroke, other neurological damage, edentulous, dysphagia, dilated esophagus	Assess type and degree; suction; Heimlich maneuver (if needed); call 911; continue to assess temperature and lung sounds; teach feeding techniques
Stroke (CVA)	Long-term cardiovascular problems, hypertension	Numbness in extremities, falling, slurred speech, ptosis of eyelids, blurred vision	Assess vital signs, neurological signs (especially pupils), hand grip; seek immediate medical treatment
Acute abdominal pain	Severe pain, nausea and vomiting, jaundice, elevated pulse and respiration	Possibly ruptured peptic ulcer or gall bladder, intestinal obstruction or rupture, internal hemorrhage	Assess vital signs and abdomen
Falls	Pain, bleeding, extremity out of alignment, unconscious	Dizziness, postural hypotension, medications (e.g., cardiovascular, psychotropic)	Assess vital signs and possible injuries before moving, especially head and extremities
Acute closed-angle glaucoma	Sudden severe pain in and around eyes, blurred vision, nausea and vomiting	Chronic open-angle glaucoma	Take to ophthalmologist as soon as possible
Fever >99°F†	Increased pulse, respiration, dehydration, dry lips, sunken eye sockets, decreased urination, decreased appetite, confusion	Infection, possibly infection of urinary tract or upper respiratory tract, including pneumonia	Call physician for further diagnostic tests and/or orders
Sudden behavioral change	Severe confusion, combative, withdrawal	Adverse medication effect, fever, myocardial infarction	Call physician for further diagnostic tests and/or orders

*In any emergency 911 should be called. The attending physician and at least one family member should be notified as soon as possible in all of these situations.
†Note that 99°F (rather than 101°F) should be referred for further evaluation because of the normal lower body temperature in older adults.

Accidents

The environment should be made safe so that the resident is not injured. A study of incident reports is a good method of determining the most common causes of accidents. Appliances used in assisting the person with walking, such as canes or walkers, should be kept in the same place when not in use so that they may be located quickly. The terrain where the person is likely to walk should be level; inclines or steps should be clearly marked with signs and yellow colors and should have handrails.

Falls

Safety measures should be closely monitored. A resident's poor vision and unsteady gait, as well as unsafe surroundings such as wet floors, dim lights, and furniture in the way, tend to increase the likelihood of accidents. Residents who are able to walk independently should not be restricted just because they might fall, but safety must be maintained in the environment. With adequate supervision, residents should remain mobile for as long as they can. Gross et al. (1990) found that most falls occurred "between 8:00 a.m. and 5:00 p.m. with peaks at 10:00 a.m. and noon" and that most "falls occurred in patients' rooms" (p. 22). Each institution should identify its residents at high risk for falling and plan specific measures for prevention in their nursing care plans. Morse (1997) has developed a Fall Scale that evaluates resident risk for falling. The major categories are:

- History of falling
- Secondary diagnosis
- Ambulatory aid
- Intravenous therapy/heparin lock
- Gait
- Mental status

Institutional Assessment of Older Residents Who are at High Risk for Falling

Name _____ Room # _____ Age _____

Factor	Assessment
1. Previous falls	No _____ Yes* _____ Number _____
	Reason _____ Outcome _____
2. Recent admission (one to two weeks)	Yes*_____ No _____
3. Mental status	
a. orientation	Person* if no _____ Place* if no _____ Time _____
b. memory	Immediate* if no _____ Recent* if no _____ Remote_____
c. diagnosis of cognitive impairment	Yes*_____ No _____
4. Ambulation/devices	Alone _____ With assistance*_____
	Instability of gait* _____
	Cane* _____ Walker* _____ Wheelchair*_____
5. Elimination	Urine: continent _____ incontinent*_____
	frequency*_____ urgency*_____
	Feces: continent _____ incontinent*_____
	diarrhea* _____
6. Vision	Acute _____ Limited* _____ Blind*_____
	Cataracts* (without surgery) _____ Glaucoma*_____
	Macular degeneration*_____
7. Hearing	Acute _____ Limited _____
	Severely limited*_____
8. Medication*	Drug Dose Time
Affecting ambulation, blood pressure, mental status (one point for each routine medication)	
9. Psychological	Attempts to ambulate independently*_____
	Uncooperative* _____ Agitated*_____
10. Physical factors	Age* (if >80) _____ Male _____ Female*_____
	Caucasian* _____ Black _____ Hispanic _____
	Height* (if <5'5") _____ Poor balance*_____
	Dizzy* _____ Cardiovascular problems*_____
	Neurological problems*_____
	_____
Total number of risk factors	
Total possible high-risk points = 34 + medications	*The greater the number, the greater the risk. Initiate the high risk for falling intervention program in Box 19-4 when one or more of the risk factors are present.

FIGURE 19-7   Institutional assessment of older residents who are at risk for falling.

A similar form that can be used to assess a resident's risk for falling is found in Figure 19-7 and a high risk for falling intervention program is provided in Box 19-4.

CLINICAL ALERT

Prevent Falls

They can be devastating and life-threatening to older adults who may have weak bones and other major health problems.

Choking

Nursing home residents sometimes choke on food during mealtimes. Donahue (1990) warns that "all patients should be carefully assessed during meals until they are judged as being low risk for choking" (p. 7). Refer to Donahue (1990), Hogstel and Robinson (1989), or Kolodny and Malek (1991) for specific techniques to aid in feeding the older adult who has difficulty swallowing. Supervision by the staff while residents are eating in the dining room is a necessity. The residents' mealtimes are not the best times for the staff to take their own meal breaks. The Heimlich maneuver for choking can be administered (if needed) to residents who are sitting in chairs or wheelchairs in the dining room. Residents may choke because their swallowing reflex is often depressed; they talk, cough, or laugh frequently while eating; they forget or are unable to chew food adequately; or they eat too quickly. Residents who eat in their own rooms should be checked frequently by the staff to ensure that they do not choke on food. Residents who eat in bed should be kept in a semi-Fowler's position for at least 1 hour after meals. This prevents regurgitation and possible aspiration of food or fluids, which is common in many older adults who have a dilated esophagus or hiatal hernia (Hogstel & Robinson, 1989). The head of the bed should also be elevated for residents receiving gastric tube feedings.

Burns

Inadequate orientation and supervision of new personnel could cause the unsafe use of whirlpool baths. They might allow the temperature of the water to be too hot or too cold. Because older adults have a lower metabolism and decreased perception of heat and cold, they are more subject to hypothermia or hyperthermia and skin injuries when the water is too cold or hot.

BOX 19-4   High Risk for Falling Intervention Program

1. Label the rooms of high-risk residents so they are obvious to staff but not visitors.

2. Keep the door open as much as possible and have all staff look in the room each time they walk by.

3. Check the resident at least every 15–20 minutes 24 hours a day.

4. Attach the signal cord to the resident's gown so light or buzzer will come on when it is pulled out of the wall when the resident tries to get out of bed. Label lights of high-risk residents' rooms at the nurses' station (red or orange).

5. Answer the signal light or buzzer as soon as possible.

6. Anticipate and meet elimination needs (especially in the early morning and between 10 PM and 6 AM).

7. Locate the resident in a room with a television monitor or as close to the nurses' station as possible.

8. Stagger breaks for personnel so that the unit is well covered at all times.

9. Use families and volunteers (if available) on the units during feeding and medication time because many falls occur when nursing staff are busy.

10. Keep the intercom system open to the resident's room during the night shift so moaning or movement by the resident can be heard.

11. Keep the bathroom light on at night if the resident is ambulatory.

12. Use restraints, if ordered, as a last resort and follow institutional policy regarding observing and releasing intervals.

13. Remind all staff of the severe problem of accidental falls through in-service education.

14. Display posters with fall prevention guidelines in the nurses' station and lounge.

15. Obtain movement monitors for beds and wheelchairs of residents prone to falling.

Compiled from "Point by Point: Predicting Elders' Falls," by E. Berryman, D. Gaskin, A. Jones, F. Tolley, and J. Macmullen, 1989, Geriatric Nursing, 10(4), pp. 199–201; "Monitoring Risk Factors," by Y. T. Gross, Y. Shimamoto, C. L. Rose, and B. Frank, 1990, Journal of Gerontological Nursing, 16(6), pp. 20–25; "How to Reduce Falls," by M. Hernandez and M. Miller, 1986, Geriatric Nursing, 7(2), pp. 97–102; and "Is Your Patient About to Fall?," by E. Lund and M. L. Sheafor, 1985, Journal of Gerontological Nursing, 11(4), pp. 37–41.

Special Nursing Needs

Residents in long-term care facilities are vulnerable to many changes in their ability to maintain a constant state of normal functioning. Many diseases that they have are chronic, and even vigorous preventive measures or treatment is unable to prevent deterioration. Common changes of aging will occur, but measures can be taken, such as an exercise group for those in wheelchairs or reminiscence groups to prevent depression and help the resident adapt to the aging process and to prevent complications. The nurse encounters a number of common problems in the process of implementing nursing care in the nursing home.

Skin Problems

The aging process produces many changes in the skin of older adults. Loss of subcutaneous tissue, decreased elasticity, and increased fragility cause many problems. The use of drying powders, too much soap, and immobility lead to skin breakdown. A daily bath does not increase dryness of the skin, as previously thought. Essential areas of the body, such as the face, axillary areas, and genital region must be bathed as often as needed. Nurse aides are often accustomed to using a large amount of soap when bathing residents; this procedure should be avoided with older adults. Also, older adults are not as agile as younger adults and therefore cannot dry their lower extremities, especially their feet, very well. The aides should cleanse and dry the areas between the toes very well, often a difficult process with residents who have contractures or severe arthritis. Older adults are extremely sensitive to temperature changes and require extra warmth when being bathed, a fact that CNAs may not realize.

The identification of areas that are prone to skin breakdown and special massage of these areas lessen the potential for breakdown. For residents who are confined to bed and unable to move independently, a specific schedule of turning at least every two hours or more often if high risk will relieve pressure to sensitive areas. Linens should be changed as soon as possible when they become soiled. The use of special pressure-relieving beds; alternating air, water, or sand mattresses; egg-crate-shaped foam-rubber mattresses; or sheepskin pads decreases pressure on sensitive areas such as the scapulae, coccyx, sacrum, ischial tuberosities, iliac crests, heels, and ankles. Care should also be taken to protect the sensitive skin and cartilage of the ears when the immobile resident is positioned on the side. Numerous bruises often can be observed on the skin of older residents, especially those in their nineties and hundreds. Gentle handling is essential. It is necessary to obtain assistance from other personnel in turning, moving, or transferring residents out of bed when the residents are unable to help themselves. Older residents also bruise themselves. They bump bedrails, wheelchairs, and doors, and even rub their own dry skin vigorously. Short fingernails and thin protective gloves prevent self-inflicted scratches. The extent of any skin breakdown should be described accurately as to appearance, size, and depth. Pressure ulcers should be assessed frequently and documented according to stage (Figure 19-8). Daily observations of the treatment and healing process are recorded in the nurses' notes. It is much easier to prevent skin breakdown than to treat the problem areas later.

Bowel and Bladder Control

Physical problems often hinder residents from having control over elimination, although many types of incontinence can be diagnosed and treated. Older adults may be unable to communicate this need or to go to the bathroom independently. A schedule of bowel and bladder training will assist residents in achieving control or at least remaining dry. New products similar to disposable pants (the term *diaper* should not be used) are available for incontinent adult residents. These products help the residents remain ambulatory, keep their skin dry, and control odors. Cleaning the residents well after elimination is essential. To prevent skin breakdown and assist in the control of odors in the nursing facility, residents confined to bed or wheelchair should be checked at least every 2 hours, genital areas should be washed and dried thoroughly (when needed), and linens should be changed often. Very lightly dusted powder or cornstarch can be used in areas that are slightly irritated where skin touches skin, such as in the groin or under the breasts. Powder or cornstarch should not be used directly on the genital area of the woman or man. Soiled linens should be placed in tightly covered containers and emptied frequently. This essential and frequent change of linens demands ample linen supplies.

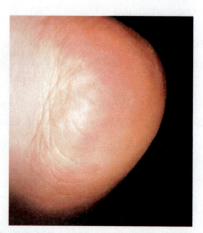

FIGURE 19-8   Detailed assessment and documentation of the signs of skin breakdown are important elements in providing good care to residents.

Immobility and Contractures

Exercises are important for residents who are partially immobile and/or unable to move independently. The professional nursing staff should teach the nurse aides and show them how to provide normal range of motion during the resident's bath. Proper positioning of residents in bed and in wheelchairs will help maintain range of motion in the joints. Daily activities should be planned to keep the residents as mobile as possible. The activities director can provide exercise classes for residents, including ball tossing and games that residents in wheelchairs can play. The nursing staff assists in preparing the residents for these activities. Ambulatory residents are encouraged to walk in groups about the halls or outdoors in safe protected areas with the supervision of a staff member or volunteer.

Residents who have had strokes or fractures require rehabilitative measures to help them become mobile again. Self-help devices need to be checked frequently to ensure that the devices are in good repair. Wheelchairs, crutches, and walkers have many parts that wear out and require repair. Realistic goals are set with the residents and the goals are updated frequently. The general goal is to maintain maximum activity. The concept of rehabilitation to reach maximum potential despite physical problems and handicaps is just as important for the nursing facility resident as for residents in other settings.

Food and Fluid Needs

Appetites change and older adults may forget that they need to drink fluids. Sometimes they lose the sense of thirst. Fluids should be offered to residents at least every 2 hours when they are checked, turned, or moved by the aides. Dietary restrictions sometimes discourage residents from eating their meals. Suggestions may be made to change some of the foods on their diets. Dietary changes may also be needed because of dentures and mouth problems. Good oral hygiene before and after meals is important and will help make eating more pleasant. Lemon and glycerine are no longer used for mouth care because they are drying to the mucous membranes. Other disposable mouth care products are now available that have a pleasant taste and can be used to cleanse the gums and teeth and keep the mucous membranes of the oral cavity moist. Referral to a dentist may be necessary to correct poorly fitting dentures. Residents who have changes in memory or who forget to eat when meals are served need prompting first and help in eating when needed. Stiffness in their fingers may prevent residents from opening containers, using silverware, or cutting food. Poor vision may make it impossible for the older resident to see the food that is on the tray. Taste buds may not be as sensitive as they used to be, and therefore appetites may be poor. Some residents are on caloric-restricted diets, which also creates the need to weigh residents weekly. A more common problem is decreasing weight because of depression (potentially suicidal), anorexia, or functional difficulties in eating.

General Hygiene

Fingernails should be kept clean and short. Aides are allowed to cut fingernails. Toenails require the attention of a podiatrist or the professional nurse because of the possibility of trauma, which may cause infection and slow healing because of decreased circulation to the lower extremities. Shaving and hair care are also part of daily care. Residents should be dressed and out of bed most of the day, if at all possible, because self-esteem is enhanced by appearance. Residents should be encouraged to make decisions about the clothing they wish to wear. Many times residents forget to change clothes because they have failing vision or a decreased sense of smell.

Changes in Behavior

Regression, hostile behavior, memory loss, disorientation, and confusion are disturbing to the family and the staff. Assessment of the cause of the behavior is essential before the type of nursing intervention is determined. In some communities, a geropsychiatric nursing consultant or multidisciplinary team has made their services available to nursing facilities on a regular or emergency basis. They help the nursing facility staff plan for and give care to residents who have psychotic episodes or who experience sudden major aggressive or disruptive behavior. This plan can prevent the need to send the resident to a hospital emergency department, which often makes the resident even more aggressive or hostile and where adequate geropsychiatric services usually are not available (Tierney, Cronin, & Scanlon, 1986). Methods other than drugs to control or modify behavior should be considered. The techniques of facilitative communication, sensory stimulation, and reality orientation can be used to improve some of these conditions.

Wandering Behavior

Wandering behavior is a common concern in many nursing facilities. Wandering is usually caused by organic factors (e.g., Alzheimer's disease, vascular dementia, or medications) or environmental factors (e.g., over- or understimulation) (Davidhizar & Cosgray, 1990). Some nursing facility residents have wandered away (**elopement**) from the nursing facility, become lost, and been returned to the home by strangers or the police. Others, not as fortunate, have been struck by an automobile or train or found dead alongside a road.

The mental status of all new residents should be assessed on admission to the nursing facility to determine those who might be at high risk for wandering.

Davidhizar and Cosgray (1990, p. 281) recommend using specific interventions (see Box 19-5) with those residents who tend to wander.

Coberg et al. (1991) recommend to "redirect energies of agitated or wandering patients" (p. 133). They also recommend a wooden lounge chair with an exaggerated downward tilt of the seat back that makes getting up more difficult. An enclosed, outside courtyard decorated with tables, chairs, plants, and flowers also allows the wanderer to walk and exercise in a safe and relaxing environment. Buzzers on all unsupervised doors that lead outside alert the staff that a resident has left the building. A number of electronic security systems also are available (Melillo & Futrell, 1998; Negley, Molla, & Obenchain, 1990).

Sexuality

Obvious sexual behavior in older adults is often disturbing to nurses, staff, other residents, and visitors in nursing facilities. However, the staff in one nursing facility showed exceptional understanding. They personally purchased a double bed for a couple who had recently married and moved to the facility. They had both been residents of another facility but were asked to leave when they decided to marry (M. O. Hogstel, personal communication, 1999). There should be inservice education for staff members on this topic. They should have the opportunity to explore their own beliefs about sexuality so that they can learn to accept the sexual behavior of older residents, who are so often thought of as being sexless. Cognitively alert consenting residents have the right to participate in sexual activities, although family members may disagree.

Death and Dying

Caring for a dying resident is stressful for the staff. Older adults who have lived many years in a nursing facility become, in effect, part of the family. Staff members may lessen the impact of death of a resident by inservice education and by exploring their feelings about death and dying. The policies in each nursing facility dictate whether residents are sent to a hospital to die or whether they will remain in the facility. Physician decisions, family wishes, and perhaps resident requests also determine whether to move the resident to a hospital. In any case, a skilled nursing facility is qualified to care for residents who are dying. In some instances, eligible residents receiving hospice services through Medicare are provided care and support by community hospice personnel in the nursing facility.

Planning Nursing Care

The licensed nurse who is assigned to the unit is responsible for overseeing the care of each resident. There are specific functions for which the professional nurse is responsible. Rehabilitative measures prescribed by the physical therapist will be supervised by the nurse. Each nurse aide is responsible for the care of a specific number of residents. The aide becomes familiar with the likes and dislikes of these residents and is able to manage their environment. One nursing facility uses a checklist for the physical activities of daily living for each resident. Each shift has a checklist for each resident, and the form is a part of the resident's record. This checklist is an excellent guide for the identification of the kind of care each resident requires and is a means of validating that care is given.

Monthly resident care plans should be implemented for each resident. The aide is an important member of the team conference. The dietitian, social worker, activities director, registered nurse, and other licensed personnel are included in the conferences. The director of nursing is available for consultation if needed. A regular schedule for team planning permits the aides to meet with the team and to discuss the care needs of their residents each month. Aides have valuable information about their residents and are able to identify problems the residents are experiencing daily. Open lines of com-

BOX 19-5   Interventions for Wandering Behaviors

- Divert their attention to another activity.
- Use kind firmness.
- Install waist-high fences at doors.
- Place a sitting chair by the window.
- Use reality orientation (if appropriate).
- Be sure glasses and hearing devices are in use.
- Decorate the resident's room.
- Assign consistent staff.
- Encourage family visits.
- Use touch if appropriate.
- Plan activities for a short attention span.
- Encourage exercise.
- Use a rocking chair (rocking wheelchairs are available).
- Have a large clock and calendar in the room.
- Place alarms on exit doors.
- Do not use restraints.

munication among the team participants promote improved resident care. Goals for each resident can be established, and the team members who are responsible for the care are able to coordinate the care. The nurses and aides who are responsible for the continued care of the residents on all shifts will receive a summary of the nursing care goals for each resident.

Among the problems that are reported by the aides most frequently are disturbed behavior or difficulties with the physical daily activities of living. If consistent care if provided by all personnel, the residents' behavior problems may be corrected, their memory span may be increased, and their self-help abilities may be maintained. Consistency is a key word in teamwork for all personnel.

The licensed nursing personnel are responsible for making entries in the nurses notes. Validation of all care is of the utmost importance. Changes in the physical or mental condition of the resident are recorded as well as the time the physician was notified, visits by the physician, new orders, and the time the director of nursing and the family were notified of any changes. Physical and behavioral changes in the residents and the nursing actions initiated are accurately documented in the resident's record. The nurses' notes for the entire week will give a complete picture of the status of the resident. Whenever there are changes in the condition of the resident, the chart will reflect these changes. For example, one day of nurses' notes will reflect the self-care activities and the amount of assistance the resident requires. Elimination and skin conditions will be documented on another day. Each day another aspect of the resident is observed: the emotional and psychological state of the resident, the food and fluid intake, the interaction of the resident with the environment and during social activities, and the mobility of the resident. A weekly summary documentation reflects the diagnoses of the resident, the medication and treatments the resident has received, and the effectiveness of the regimen. Changes in the condition of residents in the skilled section of the nursing facility are either so small that it is difficult to notice them or the changes may be so dramatic that problem-oriented documentation is needed.

Legal Issues

There has been an increasing number of **medical malpractice** suits filed against nursing facilities in recent years. Fox (1997) noted that "by 1996 nursing home **litigation** was the most rapidly expanding area of litigation in the United States" (p. 8). This issue may be related to an increase in general medical malpractice cases and/or to residents and family members who believe that inadequate care resulted in harm, injury, and/or death. Per-

haps both factors are important. See Box 19-6 for a list of some of the most common causes for medical malpractice cases in nursing facilities.

Think About It

Why is there an increasing number of medical malpractice lawsuits against nursing facilities?

For these reasons, a sufficient quantity and quality of staff in nursing facilities are essential to provide the basic standard of safe care that residents and families have a right to expect. Interdisciplinary quality management committees in nursing facilities have the responsibility to evaluate possible problems in the environment and/or care and recommend specific methods to prevent potential lawsuits.

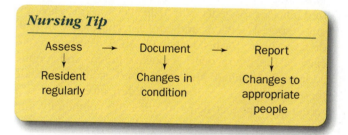

Nursing Tip

Assess → Document → Report

Resident regularly | Changes in condition | Changes to appropriate people

BOX 19-6   Samples of Causes for Medical Malpractice in Nursing Facilities

- Lack of prevention, treatment, and care of pressure ulcers (especially Stage IV ulcers resulting in septicemia and/or death)

- Inadequate safety factors in the environment and/or care that result in falls, fractures, head injuries, and possibly death

- Elopement (an individual wandering out of the home and becoming lost for a period of time, injured, and/or dying as a result of exposure or an accident)

- Choking while eating the wrong diet or being alone, resulting in death

- Inadequate assessing, documenting, and reporting of a resident's changing physical and/or mental status, resulting in severe progression of new or ongoing health problems

Emerging Needs and Trends

Adequate quality staffing in nursing facilities is a major concern and will continue to be a problem. There is a special need for more registered nurses. Professional nurses who are skilled in geriatric health assessment and management are needed in the nursing facility setting. Financial remuneration for professional nursing services in nursing facilities must be competitive with other health care facilities. However, the amount of money spent on health care is not reflected in the salaries of the caregivers in nursing facilities. In addition to better salaries, training and recognition programs for staff such as certificates, special awards, length of service awards, and birthday recognition will improve morale. A caring facility must be considerate of its employees if direct resident care is to be improved.

Many nursing facilities are expanding their services to include adult day services, respite care beds, specialized units for residents with Alzheimer's disease, hospice units, special services and care for chronically ill children, and care for residents with AIDS. The nursing facility of the future will be much different and require additional qualified and specialized staff to provide these specialized services. The **Eden alternative** is a recent concept that helps to bring the community into the nursing facility by adding live flowers, an aviary, and a fish tank and encouraging children to visit.

Changes in nursing facility payment mechanisms by Medicare and Medicaid as a result of the Balanced Budget Act of 1997 will influence the quantity and quality of resident care. Increases in federal and state regulations resulting from legislative efforts of various advocate groups (e.g., AARP) will also affect quality of care and costs.

Health Promotion and Wellness

Although the traditional role of the nursing facility has been to provide short-term skilled rehabilitation and long-term custodial care, there are concerns about other needs of residents for whom the facility is "home." There has traditionally been minimal focus on health promotion and wellness, although OBRA 1987 guidelines noted that the facility must provide sufficient staff to assist each resident to attain or maintain the highest practicable physical, mental, and psychological well-being. For example, vaccinations for pneumonia, influenza, and hepatitis B are available to residents. Exercise activities and good nutrition, which are very important in regaining and/or maintaining optimum health, are usually available. However, there is a need to provide more screening procedures, for example, mammograms, colon and osteoporosis screening, and prostate specific antigen (PSA) blood tests to detect disease early so that treatment can be initi-

ated just as these are available to individuals living in the community. Because these life-saving measures are now covered by Medicare, they should be available to nursing facility residents.

Mental Health Care

There continues to be a concern about the lack of mental health care services in nursing facilities. Although there are specific facilities and units in facilities that provide specialized staff, programs, and activities for residents with dementia (e.g., Alzheimer's disease), there is a need to identify, diagnose, and treat to the extent possible those residents with depression, anxiety disorders, paranoia, and schizophrenia.

Change in Payment Mechanisms

As a result of the Balanced Budget Act of 1997, nursing facilities receiving payment from Medicare for skilled services has changed to a prospective payment system (PPS) similar to how payments for hospital care changed in 1983. Also, the extent to which managed care organizations (MCOs) will be involved in Medicare and/or Medicaid payments is yet to be clarified and needs to be monitored closely.

Status of Federal and State Legislation

There has been an increasing number of both federal and state laws passed in recent years to protect health care consumers in managed care and in long-term care facilities, including nursing facilities. These trends are likely to continue as the baby boomers need this type of care because they may be more assertive in demanding quality health care.

Summary

Nursing facility care has been a traditional part of long-term care for almost a century. These facilities have changed tremendously, however, in recent years as they provide more types of services. The major classification of nursing facilities and units are nursing facility (NF), skilled nursing facility (SNF), special care unit (SCU), subacute care unit (SUB), and skilled nursing unit (SNU) or skilled nursing inpatient facility (SNIF). The most common description of residents are female, age 80, widowed, and having several chronic health care problems.

Administration patterns and type of staff are important in evaluating quality care and services. Most nursing facility care is paid for by Medicaid, a combined federal and state program, although some benefits are paid for by Medicare, Veterans' Affairs, and private pay. Private long-term care insurance policies are being encouraged to be purchased to decrease government costs as the population increases in number and longevity.

Nursing facilities are highly regulated, both by federal and state legislation and rules. National accreditation by the Joint Commission for the Accreditation of Healthcare Organizations is optional and expensive. A program funded by the federal government provides for professional and volunteer ombudsmen who are advocates and arbitrators for quality care for residents in nursing facilities. There are also state and national voluntary organizations that monitor and work to improve the quality of care in nursing facilities.

Licensed nurses play an essential role in nursing facilities as administrator, assessor, planner, teacher, and coordinator of essential nursing care. Care in nursing facilities is difficult but also challenging and rewarding because the nurse has more autonomy, control, and responsibility than in many other areas of nursing. Many of the residents have multiple disabilities and needs and are vulnerable to accidents and errors. New symptoms that develop suddenly must be promptly and adequately assessed and treated to prevent major complications and perhaps death.

The nursing facility will continue to change in the future as the health care needs of older adults change and new resources for care develop. Health promotion activities and mental health care are two areas that need to be expanded.

Review Questions and Activities

1. What percentage of the 65-and-older and 85-and-older age groups are in nursing facilities at any one time?

2. Describe five different types of nursing facilities.

3. Describe the demographics of the typical older adult in a nursing facility.

4. Give examples of major medical diagnoses of nursing facility residents.

5. Evaluate the sources of payment for nursing facility care.

6. Differentiate licensure and accreditation.

7. Describe the major requirements of OBRA 1987.

8. Evaluate the most common medical emergencies that occur in nursing facilities. How can they be managed?

9. What are some nursing interventions for the common long-term care problems encountered in a nursing facility setting?

10. Discuss the types and roles of staff in a nursing facility setting.

References

A profile of older Americans 1999. (1999). Washington, DC: American Association of Retired Persons.

Bectel, R. W., & Tucker, N. G. (Eds.). (1998). *Across the states. Profiles of long-term care systems* (3rd ed.). Washington, DC: American Association of Retired Persons Public Policy Institute.

Boondas, J. (1991). Nursing home resident assessment clarification and focused care. *Nursing and Health Care, 12*(6), 308–312.

Coberg, A., Lynch, D., & Mavretish, B. (1991). Harnessing ideas to release restraints. *Geriatric Nursing, 12*(3), 133–134.

Davidhizar, R., & Cosgray, R. (1990). Helping the wanderer. *Geriatric Nursing, 11*(6), 280–281.

Donahue, P. A. (1990). When it's hard to swallow. *Journal of Gerontological Nursing, 16*(4), 6–9.

Duchemin, K., Clark, J., & Keeber, M. (1991). Emergency procedures training program. *Journal of Gerontological Nursing, 17*(7), 6–9.

Facundus, R. (1998, Winter). The good news is—WE GOT IT! The bad new[s] is—now we have to document it! *NCGNP Newsletter, 58,* 1–2, 4.

Fox, S. C. (1997). *Primum Non Nocere* (First do no harm): Nursing home litigation, Part II. *Journal of Legal Nurse Consulting, 8*(4), 8–15.

Gross, Y. T., Shimamoto, Y., Rose, C. L., & Frank, B. (1990). Monitoring risk factors. *Journal of Gerontological Nursing, 16*(6), 20–25.

Hogstel, M. O., & Robinson, N. (1989). Feeding the frail elderly. *Journal of Gerontological Nursing, 15*(3), 16–20.

Kolodny, V., & Malek, A. M. (1991). Improving feeding skills. *Journal of Gerontological Nursing, 17*(6), 20–24.

Kovach, C. R. (1998). Nursing home dementia care units: Providing a continuum of care rather than aging in place. *Journal of Gerontological Nursing, 24*(4), 30–36.

Melillo, K. D., & Futrell, M. (1998). Wandering and technology devices. *Journal of Gerontological Nursing, 24*(8), 32–38.

Morris, J. N., Harnes, C., Fries, S. E., Phillips, C. D., Mor, V., Katz, S., Murphy, K., Drugouich, M. L., & Friedlob, A. S. (1990). Designing the national resident assessment instrument for nursing homes. *Gerontologist, 30*(3), 293–307.

Morse, J. M. (1997). *Preventing patient falls.* Thousand Oaks: Sage Publications.

Negley, E. N., Molla, P. M., & Obenchain, J. (1990). NO EXIT: The effects of an electronic security system. *Journal of Gerontological Nursing, 16*(8), 21–25.

Scope and standards of gerontological nursing practice. (1995). Washington, DC: American Nurses' Association.

Strumpf, N. E., Evans, L. K., & Schwartz, D. (1990). Restraint free care: From dream to reality. *Geriatric Nursing, 11*(3), 122–124.

Tierney, J. C., Cronin, A., & Scanlon, M. K. (1986). . . . And don't send her back! *American Journal of Nursing, 86*(9), 1011–1014.

Resources

Hospice Foundation of America: **www.hospicefoundation.org**

RN+ (fall prevention): **www.rnplus.com**

CHAPTER 20

Home Health Care

Deborah K. Fultner, MS, RN, CS

COMPETENCIES

After completing this chapter, the reader should be able to:

- *Define home health nursing.*
- *Define the purpose of home health nursing.*
- *Discuss the history of home health nursing.*
- *Explain the relationship of the demographics of older adults to home health nursing.*
- *Discuss the importance of the older adult's living arrangement.*
- *Describe the roles of the different disciplines in home health care.*
- *Discuss criteria for admission for home health care.*

MAKING THE CONNECTION

Refer to the following chapters to increase your understanding of home health care:

- **Chapter 2**   *Gerontological Nursing*
- **Chapter 3**   *Changes in the Health Care Delivery System Affecting Older Adults*
- **Chapter 12**   *Health Education*
- **Chapter 13**   *Assessment, Diagnosis, and Planning*
- **Chapter 17**   *Management of Medications*
- **Chapter 24**   *Community Organizations and Services*
- **Chapter 25**   *Ethical Theories and Principles*
- **Chapter 28**   *Trends and Future Needs*

History of Home Health Care

Home health care is an interdisciplinary service designed to meet the specific needs of people who require the assistance of medically skilled personnel to return to a baseline level of wellness. Nurses, physical therapists, occupational therapists, speech-language pathologists, home health aides, social workers, and, of course, the client comprise the interdisciplinary home health team. Home health nurses perform skilled care, monitor clients for exacerbation of disease processes, and provide education for self-care skills. Clients needing skilled care after hospitalization who meet specific criteria may receive home health services if there is no one in the home to provide care or if the care needed requires a skilled nurse. The nurse functions in the client's environment, and together, the nurse and client establish goals and formulate a plan of care based on a comprehensive assessment of the client, family, and environment. An improved quality of life for the client is possible when satisfaction and the client's well-being are the goals of home health care (O'Neill & Sorensen, 1991).

Since the implementation of diagnostic-related groups (DRGs) in the early 1980s and the advent of managed care, older adults have been discharged from hospitals *quicker and sicker*. To prevent readmission and premature long-term care institutionalization, physicians prescribed home health services.

The National Association of Home Care (NAHC) defines home health care as (Humphrey & Milone-Nuzzo, 1996, p. 3)

> services to the recovering, disabled or chronically ill person providing for treatment and/or effective functioning in the home environment. Home care can also assist in the provision of services to adults and children in danger of abuse or neglect. Generally, home care is appropriate whenever a person needs assistance that cannot be easily or effectively provided only by family members or friends on an ongoing basis for a short or long period of time.

One of the first formal nursing organizations in the home that made a contribution to public health nursing is credited to St. Vincent de Paul during the Renaissance. In the early seventeenth century de Paul organized nurses, known as the Sisterhood of the Dames de Charité, to visit the sick in their homes. As the number of nurses and clients increased, St. Vincent and Mademoiselle Le Gras formally organized the nurses. The nurses educated the caregivers on taking care of the poor and the sick, thus empowering them to provide the necessary care (Clemen-Stone, Eigsti, & McGuire, 1991).

In Europe, the period following the Renaissance saw nurses' status decline. This situation was in part because of a low social position of women and the lack of

scientific basis for medicine. Nursing lost its importance and social status because of the loss of the support of the church. Living conditions were poor, life expectancy was short, and mortality rates high. Hospitals were feared because only the very sick, poor, and homeless were admitted. Tuberculosis, yellow fever, cholera, and scarlet fever were epidemic and the hospitals were considered *pest houses*. Untrained men and women from the lower class provided care within the hospitals (Clemen-Stone et al., 1991).

The status of nurses changed in the nineteenth century with the Industrial Revolution. William Rathbone of Liverpool, England, set up a visiting nursing system with the help of Florence Nightingale in 1859. Rathbone's wife had been cared for in the home by skilled nurses and he was interested in helping the poor who were in need of health care. Florence Nightingale helped Rathbone establish a school for training nurses as visiting nurses. Nightingale trained nurses at the Liverpool Infirmary to care for the *sick poor*. These visiting nurses were the forerunners of what is known today as public health nursing (Clemen-Stone et al., 1991).

During the middle to late 1800s, home care became formally established in England and in the United States. The Industrial Revolution brought immigration to America from all of Europe to help meet the demands of industry. With the large influx of people, living conditions were crowded, money scarce, and sanitation a major problem. These conditions led to nurses visiting the sick in their homes. Groups of nurses in several large cities formed organizations to care for the poor. One of the nursing groups in Philadelphia began charging for their services. By the late 1800s, there were 21 visiting nurse organizations in the United States. As there were no standards— for practice or education—nurses formed what is now the American Nurses Association in 1896 (Clemen-Stone, et al., 1991).

Lillian Wald is known as the founder of public health nursing. Public health nursing was the earliest form of home care nursing in the United States. Wald emphasized family-focused nursing, health promotion, and prevention. After completing two years of nursing training at New York Hospital, Wald gave classes in home nursing and bedside nursing to women from the Lower East Side tenement district. Wald was dismayed at the poor sanitary conditions in the tenement district and believed that conditions would improve if people were taught about the care of the sick. In 1893 Wald established the Henry Street Settlement House. This development was inspired by Wald's experiences in the tenements. Needy persons had a place to receive care and it was funded by the wealthy. It was not associated with any religious organization or with just one physician. Wald believed that nurses could deliver better care if they worked independently and if they lived in the

TABLE 20-1	Growth of Home Health Care
1912	American Red Cross introduced visiting nurse program.
	County health departments developed programs that provided home health care nursing.
Early 1900s	Frontier nursing was established in rural Kentucky.
1941	The University of Syracuse offered home care program for clients discharged from the hospital.
1947	Montefiore Hospital Home Care Program was established in New York.
1958	The Chronic Disease Program of the U.S. Public Health Service established four elements for a home care program.
1961	The Community Health Services Facility Grant was established.
1965	Medicare and Medicaid were enacted.

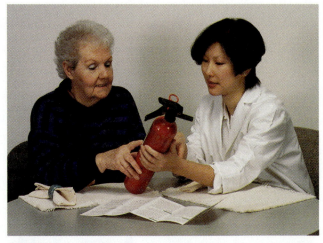

FIGURE 20-1 Educating the older client about safety, particularly in the home, is an essential nursing function that is facilitated with the use of visuals and clear step-by-step instructions.

neighborhood where they practiced. Wald also helped establish school nursing and rural health nursing. She was the founder and first president of the National Organization for Public Health (Clemen-Stone et al., 1991).

The idea of home visits began spreading across the United States. In 1898 the first governmental health department offered home visits through the Los Angeles Health Department. In 1909, home care benefits were offered to persons insured with the Metropolitan Life Insurance Company. Home care continued to grow throughout the country as a means to deliver health and illness care (see Table 20-1). Acute care was the focus of hospital care. Until 1965, the Visiting Nurse Association (VNA) was the major nursing organization delivering home care. With the passage of Medicare and Social Security, home health visits to older adults increased (McClain, 1995).

In the 1980s, the home care industry experienced a growth spurt because of the need to curb Medicare costs in acute care settings. The older population was increasing and, as a result, more were being hospitalized. At this same time, DRGs were implemented, which decreased the length of hospital stays and, as a result, older adults went home requiring continued care to recover fully (Figure 20-1). Diagnostic-related groups are one type of **prospective payment system (PPS)** that pays a specified amount of money based on the diagnosis. In 1986, the American Nurses Association (ANA) established the Standards of Home Health Nursing Prac-

tice (Box 20-1). Home health nurses are held to these standards in their practice (McClain, 1995).

The number of home care organizations continued to increase until the late 1990s. As of 1996, there were approximately 20,215 home care agencies in the United States. Of these, 10,027 were Medicare-certified home health agencies, 2,154 Medicare-certified hospices, and 8,034 home care organizations that did not participate in Medicare. More than 7 million individuals receive home care services because of acute illnesses, chronic illnesses, disability, or terminal illnesses (National Association, 1996).

The majority of home health agencies are hospital-based or freestanding proprietary agencies. In 1997 freestanding proprietary agencies comprised 47% of all agencies and hospital-based agencies were 26%. With the continuing changes in Medicare, the number of freestanding agencies has declined. Small rural agencies that have existed for only a few years are struggling financially because of Medicare's change in reimbursement guidelines in 1997. Home health continues to meet the needs of older clients and has as its goal to improve the quality of life of this group by (a) helping them to remain in their home, (b) increasing functional independence, and (c) teaching preventive health practices (National Association, 1996).

Demographics

The percentage of Americans age 65 and older has increased from 3.1% in 1900 to 12.7% in 1998. This represents 34.4 million persons 65 and older. By the year 2030, this number is projected to be 69.4 million. The older a person gets, the longer he or she is expected to live. For example, a person who was 65 in 1997 had an average life expectancy of an additional 17.6 years

BOX 20-1   ANA Standards of Home Health Nursing Practice

Standard I. Organization of Home Health Services
All home health services are planned, organized, and directed by a master's-prepared professional nurse with experience in community health and administration.

Standard II. Theory
The nurse applies theoretical concepts as a basis for decisions in practice.

Standard III. Data Collection
The nurse continuously collects and records data that are comprehensive, accurate, and systematic.

Standard IV. Diagnosis
The nurse uses health assessment data to determine nursing diagnoses.

Standard V. Planning
The nurse develops care plans that establish goals. The care plan is based on nursing diagnoses and incorporates therapeutic, preventive, and rehabilitative nursing actions.

Standard VI. Intervention
The nurse, guided by the care plan, intervenes to provide comfort, to restore, improve, and promote health, to prevent complications and sequelae of illness, and to effect rehabilitation.

Standard VII. Evaluation
The nurse continually evaluates the client's and family's responses to interventions in order to deter-

mine progress toward goal attainment and to revise the database, nursing diagnosis, and plan of care.

Standard VIII. Continuity of Care
The nurse is responsible for the client's appropriate and uninterrupted care along the health care continuum and, therefore, uses discharge planning, case management, and coordination of community resources.

Standard IX. Interdisciplinary Collaboration
The nurse initiates and maintains a liaison relationship with all appropriate health care providers to ensure that all efforts effectively complement one another.

Standard X. Professional Development
The nurse assumes responsibility for professional development and contributes to the professional growth of others.

Standard XI. Research
The nurse participates in research activities that contribute to the profession's continuing development of knowledge of home health care.

Standard XII. Ethics
The nurse uses the code for nurses established by the American Nurses Association as a guide for ethical decision making in practice.

Source: Reprinted with permission from American Nurses Association, Standards of Home Health Nursing Practice, *copyright © 1986 American Nurses Publishing, American Nurses Foundation/American Nurses Association, 600 Maryland Avenue, SW, Suite 100W, Washington, DC 20024-2571.*

(*A profile,* 1999). The fastest growing segment of this age group are persons 85 and older. This age cohort increased 33 times from 1900. From 2000 to 2030, the number of adults 65 and over is expected to increase from 13% of the population to 20% of the population. This is because of the baby boomers reaching age 65 in this time frame (*A profile,* 1999).

The minority population is also experiencing an increase in older adults. In 2030, 25% of the 70 million older adults will be minority persons. The gender ratio for older adults in 1998 was 143 women to 100 men. This ratio increases with age because women have a longer life expectancy than men. This disparity accounts for the marital status and living arrangements of older adults (*A profile,* 1999).

In 1998, approximately 3.4 million older adults were below the poverty level. Older women have a higher poverty rate than older men (12.8% and 7.2%, respectively). Older black women living alone experience the highest poverty rates at 49.3%. Older Hispanics have a poverty rate of 23.8% (*A profile,* 1999).

The impact of these demographics on home care means nurses will be caring for more people age 85 years and older, primarily women who live alone and who are poor. Home care nurses also will be caring for more minority persons, which means that knowing how to speak another language is important. Home care nurses will need to be familiar with diseases and chronic illnesses that affect women, especially the African-American older female. The challenge to keep older adults in their home is not an easy one. The older one gets, the more disabilities, chronic illnesses, and loss of functional status one experiences. There is also less chance that a family member will be able to provide the needed care because of age or possibly geographic location.

Teaching health promotion and prevention is one of the goals of home health nursing. The challenge is to teach older adults and their families considering their culture, age, and disabilities. The financial status of poor older adults presents a challenge because state funds, including Medicaid dollars, are needed to fund programs for this group. If these programs are not funded, the home health nurse will need to discover new and innovative ways to keep the older clients in their own homes and help them maintain a good quality of life.

Living Arrangements

Most older adults prefer living at home over any other living arrangements. Approximately 94% of older adults live in community households, either alone or with a relative. The remaining 6% live in nursing facilities or some type of group home for older adults. Of the 94% that live in the community, the majority live alone or with a spouse. The number of older persons under age 85 living with a relative other than a spouse is approximately 20%. That percentage increases with age (Atchley, 1997).

Aging in place is a concept that refers to remaining in one home throughout the majority of one's life. Assisted-living facilities, retirement homes, board and care homes, continuing care retirement communities, and congregate housing are alternatives to the older adult's own home. Even though these housing options are built specifically for the older adult, some of the freedom people have from living on their own is gone. Most of these facilities provide less space than an individual home, and older adults have to sacrifice some of their treasured mementos. They have to leave familiar surroundings and are faced with learning new addresses, phone numbers, and often, new persons with whom they do business, such as grocers, hairdressers, pharmacists, and bankers. Relocation can be very stressful and adaptation difficult. Moving is emotionally difficult and there can be negative psychological outcomes from relocation. If depression goes unrecognized, the older adult's state of mind can be mistaken for dementia, and the family or staff may believe the older adult should have even less freedom (McCann & Christiansen, 1996).

A move can cause more problems than remaining in the person's own home. Moving to a new location is difficult because of the physical aspect of going through years of collected treasures, packing and loading boxes, deciding what to do with many items, and adapting to a new place. Neighbors often have lived in the same place

for years, raised children together, experienced triumphs and failures, grown old together, and now watch out for each other. The older adults are sometimes surrogate parents or grandparents for younger couples who move into the neighborhoods.

There is also a downside of aging in place. Many homes need repairs and may be missing comforts, such as central air conditioning. Many neighborhoods experience changes in age and ethnic composition. A decline in functional status and vision and hearing often make adaptation and socialization difficult. The same is true when very young and childless couples move into the area. The older adult may not be valued in the community and isolation occurs because of the age differences. Some neighborhoods experience an increase in the crime rate and the older adult feels vulnerable and fearful. In spite of all these potential problems, most older adults still desire to remain in their own homes.

Home Health Personnel

Home health assumes an interdisciplinary approach to care. Nursing, physical therapy, occupational therapy, speech-language pathology, personal care, and social work are provided through home health. The interdisciplinary team works together to assist the client in regaining strength and returning to a prior level of wellness. The team collaborates with the client and family, especially the caregiver. The caregiver often provides the majority of the care until the care recipient can manage self-care activities.

Nurses

Preparation for home health nursing is at the bachelor's and master's levels. Advanced practice nurses (APN) are employed by home health agencies and generally function as case mangers or specialists in a specific area (for example, oncology nursing). Nurses with associate degrees (ADN) or diplomas also practice in home health nursing. Most agencies require registered nurses (RNs) to have at least one year of medical-surgical nursing. Licensed practical/vocational nurses (LPN/LVN) also work in home health in various positions. The LPNs/LVNs may perform most technical skills or tasks and reinforce education the RN has initiated. State nurse practice acts, licensing boards, and state laws governing home health agencies determine the type of care an LPN/LVN may deliver (Humphrey & Milone-Nuzzo, 1996).

Registered nurses function as case managers, team leaders, or primary care nurses depending on the model used by the home health agency. The RNs are the case mangers when occupational or speech-language pathologists are the only discipline needed for a client. Physical therapists stand alone, meaning they can admit the client to home health and serve as the case manager when an RN is not needed. Registered nurses are responsible for the admission assessment; initial education of the client and caregiver; writing the care plan that is submitted to the physician, Medicare, or insurance company; and ensuring the care plan is carried out. Registered nurses in home health are nurse generalists or specialists in areas such as diabetes management, intravenous therapy, cardiovascular home care, gerontology, wound care, and/or mental health nursing. Advanced practice nurses serve as consultants to other nurses, manage a specialty within the agency, are case managers for clients with complicated needs, or are experts in skilled areas and see clients with a particular skill or need. They may also be in an administrative position and manage a specialized program within the agency (Humphrey & Milone-Nuzzo, 1996).

The case manager or primary nurse is responsible for the treatment plan and all correspondence with the physician. They are responsible for following through with orders and reporting back to the physician the outcomes of treatment. In cases of private insurance, the case manager/primary nurse must also report to the case manager or utilization manager in the insurance company. All skills, services, and visits must be ordered by a physician for financial reimbursement by Medicare or an insurance company. In some agencies, communication with the physician or insurance provider is done by an LVN/LPN intake coordinator. The LVNs/LPNs take orders from the physician and then communicate them to the RN responsible for the case.

Enterostomal therapists (ETs) are nurses employed by an agency or contracted by an agency. They consult on cases or manage the part of the case that requires their skills. They stay in communication with the primary nurse or case manager and physician to move the client toward wellness. Education is a large part of their home health practice. They instruct clients and family members to manage and prevent skin breakdown and to perform ostomy care competently. Enterostomal therapists are also instrumental in helping the home health client and family members adjust psychologically to a changed body image.

Nurses specializing in cardiovascular care manage clients with complicated cardiac problems. With cardiac clients being discharged soon after an adverse cardiac event, the home care nurse plays a vital role in the rehabilitation process and assisting the client to maintain wellness. The cardiovascular home care nurse remains in close communication with the client's cardiac specialist and is competent in rapid assessment and detection of potential problems. The goal of the cardiovascular home care nurse is to reduce mortality and prevent future cardiac events (Asbour-Arnold & Jairath, 1998).

Intravenous therapy (IV) or home infusion therapy is another specialty in home health. Intravenous therapy in home health is used to provide IV antibiotics, hydration, transfusions, fluid and electrolyte replacement, pain management, parenteral nutrition, chemotherapy, and other types of IV therapies to home care clients. Many nurses are certified in placing and managing peripherally inserted central catheters (PICCs). This type of central venous access device can be used in the home when an IV line needs to remain in for longer than a peripheral catheter and an IV medication requires a central vein. Mobile x-ray companies are able to come to the client's home to take an x-ray of the line so correct placement can be confirmed. Other central access lines used in home health are the Port-A-Cath and the Hickman/Broviac. Small portable pumps are used in the home for IV therapy. Whenever possible, the home care nurse teaches the client or caregiver to manage the IV line and medications. The use of home infusion eliminates the need for the client to be in an ambulatory or acute care setting to receive the needed IV treatment (Humphrey & Milone-Nuzzo, 1996). Having nurses specialize in these areas allow clients to remain in their own homes to receive care that once was delivered only in an acute care setting. Close management of these clients also helps decrease hospital readmission and emergency department visits.

The ANA credentials nurses in home health nursing. The American Nurses Credentialing Center (ANCC) administers the certification program to nurses. Home health was established as a specialty area of practice by the ANCC in 1993. The certification exam for home health nurses is based on the home health care scope of practice and the home health standards of practice. The ANA developed the standards of home health practice for nurses to ensure that quality practice was delivered and maintained. Home health nurses are held to the standards of practice. Nurses wanting to be certified in home health care must meet certain educational and practice criteria. The examination covers broad categories of issues in home health practice. The ANCC sends the applicant a topical outline to study. The certification is valid for 5 years. At the end of the 5 years, the nurse may retake an exam for recertification or provide evidence of practice hours and continuing education hours in home health (Humphrey & Milone-Nuzzo, 1996).

Therapists

Therapists provide various types of therapy to the home health client when the client is unable to receive the therapy in an ambulatory setting. Therapy requires a physician's order and an appropriate diagnosis that indicates the need for therapy. Therapists are responsible for completing a care plan for the client that is submitted to

Medicare for approval for reimbursement. The aim of therapy is to assist the client to become as independent as possible within the limitations of the disease process. Therapists also suggest ways of modifying the client's environment to ensure safety.

Physical therapists (PTs) assist the client in ambulating and transferring in their own home. They provide education and instruction on exercises for muscle strengthening, improved balance, and transfer techniques. The PT assesses the home care client's environment for modifications needed that will facilitate ambulation and transfers within the home. This information is communicated to the physician and case manager. Assistive devices needed and the estimated length of the therapy regimen are also determined by the PT and communicated to the physician. Equipment and therapy plans require a physician's order for reimbursement by Medicare or private insurance. The PT works with the RN and **home health aide (HHA)** to ensure that the client remains safe and progresses toward the determined goal.

Physical therapy assistants (PTAs) are also used in home health. A PTA has a 2-year degree from a program approved by the American Physical Therapy Association or 2 years experience as a PTA and a satisfactory grade on a proficiency exam. This exam is sponsored by the U.S. Public Health Services. The PTA works under the supervision of the PT. The PT reviews the home care client's treatment plan and provides specific instructions for treatment. The PT must also be available by phone while the PTA is in the client's home (Campbell, 1995).

Occupational therapists (OTs) are prepared academically and clinically and must be board certified to work in home health. They work with home health clients to improve upper body strength and to use assistive devices that move the client toward independence. They help the client adapt to alternate ways of managing instrumental activities of daily living (IADL) and with coordination problems that interfere with independence or place the client at risk for injury (Ainsworth, 1995). See Figure 20-2.

Speech-language pathologists work with clients who have swallowing difficulties, cognitive speech problems, functional speech impairments, and voice and language disorders. A few medical diagnoses associated with the need for these services include strokes, head trauma, dysphagia, throat cancer, and Parkinson's disease. As with the other therapies, these services require a physician's order for home health and an appropriate diagnosis (Steele, 1995).

Home Health Aides

Home health aides are one of the most important members of the home care team because they see the client more than the other disciplines. As a result of this fre-

quency, the client feels comfortable with the aide and will often share concerns that the RN or therapist cannot elicit. The aide is responsible for providing personal care to the client and often finds skin problems or notices problems that are difficult for the RN to detect because of the limited time the RN is in the home for a visit (see Figure 20-3). Home health clients often feel the "nurse is too busy to bother" and, therefore, tells the HHA in hopes that the nurse will be informed by the aide.

Medicare requires that home health aides successfully complete a training and competency evaluation or pass a competency evaluation program. If an aide applies for employment in a Medicare home health agency and has not worked in an agency as a HHA for the past 24 months, he or she must repeat and successfully complete either the competency evaluation or the evaluation program. Home health agencies accredited by the Joint Commission on Accreditation of Healthcare Organizations (JCAHO) are also held to **Medicare Conditions of Participation.** The HHA must demonstrate competency in certain required skills and subjects taught in training (Apple & Truscott, 1995).

The RN must request an order for a HHA from the physician and justify the need for the aide. The home health aide visits are also to be intermittent. This means that the aide is to be in the home less than eight hours a

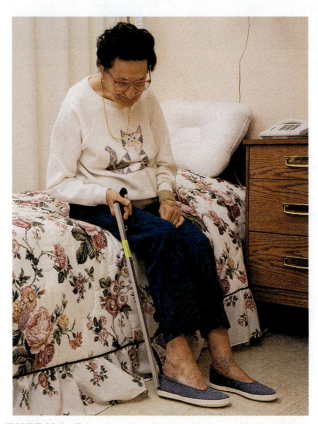

FIGURE 20-2 This woman is using an adaptive device that helps her better maintain her independence.

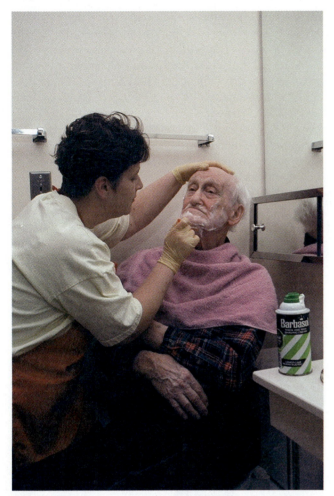

FIGURE 20-3   The home health aide can assist the nurse with client care through observation during time spent with the client.

day. The HHA responsibilities include providing personal care, assessing vital signs, and providing a clean and safe environment. Some health aides assist the client with exercises prescribed by a PT or OT. Teaching self-care to the client is a very important skill of the HHA. Home health clients need to be able to provide their own personal care at the time of discharge from the home health agency. The HHA may also remind the client to take daily medications but is not allowed to administer them. The HHA reports to the case manager and reports progress toward goals and any problems the client is experiencing. The RN supervises the HHA on a bimonthly basis (Apple & Truscott, 1995).

Personal care attendants (PCAs) may also be employed by home health agencies. Home health agencies hire PCAs for private duty cases where only a companion is required as opposed to someone who provides personal or skilled care. Letters of recommendation are generally the only requirements of PCAs. They are not required to have any formal or informal training, but individual agencies may provide an orientation and

some type of training. Duties performed by PCAs may include preparing light meals, assisting the client to the bathroom, assisting with dressing and ambulation, and in some cases, light housekeeping.

Social Workers

Social workers who work in home health must be prepared with a **Masters in Social Work (MSW).** Each agency requires different amounts of experience before working in home health. Social workers (MSW) assist the client in locating community resources that are needed at the time of admission to home health or when the client is discharged from the home health agency. Handicapped parking stickers, home-delivered meals, and chore services are a few of the services the social worker can help obtain. The social worker generally sees the client for one to two visits. If needed, the case manager can request additional visits by the social worker from the physician. In some agencies, the MSW provides short-term counseling therapy under a physician's order. Counseling for things such as long-term placement or caregiving issues also requires an order for reimbursement (Morgan, 1995).

Eligibility and Funding

Home health services are covered by Medicare, Medicaid, private insurance, managed care plans, and private pay. Persons of all ages are eligible for home health services. Criteria for services vary with the type of insurance individuals have. Medicare is the primary payer source for home health services because the majority of home health recipients are those persons age 65 and older. Medicare requires the home health client to (a) have a skilled need, (b) be confined to the home, (c) be unable to provide the skilled care alone, (d) require only intermittent care, (e) have a physician's order, and (f) receive care from a Medicare participating home health agency. If there is a caregiver present, he or she must be unwilling or unable to provide the skill required by the RN. Medicare establishes specific criteria for reimbursement for the physician, home health agency, disciplines providing care, and other entities (for example, medical supply companies) that provide goods or services to the client. The main purpose of eligibility criteria is to keep cost down and make providers accountable for services rendered. Other payer sources use Medicare criteria as a guideline for eligibility but have the flexibility to vary the criteria with individual circumstances (Rosenzweig, 1995).

Medicaid is delivered by each state and only mandated to pay for skilled services. Each state has its own criteria for reimbursement and can choose to pay however needs are best met. Generally, the RN is given a specified number of visits, based on the diagnosis and the needed skill. The RN stays in close touch with the Medicaid provider to report progress and request an increase or decrease in visits. Other funding sources of home health include Social Service block grants, Older Americans Act funds, and general state revenues. The dollar amount spent on home health by sources other than Medicare and Medicaid varies with each state. Veterans' Affairs, the Civilian Health and Medical Program for the Uniformed Services (CHAMPUS), and the Civilian Health and Medical Program of the Department of Veterans' Affairs (CHAMPVA) have their own coverage for home health and each covers different home health services (Rosenzweig, 1995).

Managed care companies have different methods of handling home health visits. Some companies approve only the admission assessment and, after reviewing it, approve a specified number of visits. Other companies approve a set number of visits based on the diagnosis, age of the client, family involvement, and nature of the needed skill. The home health agency stays in close communication with the case manager in managed care to report progress and request any changes in the original care plan.

Historically, home health services have been reimbursed by Medicare for services delivered to the client. Home health agencies submit their reports and charges to a **fiscal intermediary (FI)** that determines if criteria for reimbursement have been met. Once this is determined, the home health agency is reimbursed for the services. Services not covered include private duty nursing and personal care services if no RN or therapist is concomitantly delivering care. Occupational therapy and speech-language pathology services are not covered by Medicare unless there is an RN or PT also seeing the client. Home-delivered meals and the majority of medications are not reimbursable by Medicare (Rosenzweig, 1995).

The Health Care Financing Administration (HCFA) changed payments to home health care agencies to a prospective payment system in 1998. This system is similar to DRGs that are used for hospital reimbursement. This change in reimbursement has affected the care delivery system of home health. Care has to be delivered in a shorter amount of time, and caregivers are asked to play a more active role in the care. Medicare has developed a system to monitor outcomes to ensure that the home health client receives quality care that is delivered in an efficient and effective manner.

The Nursing Process

The nursing process is used to plan care for the home health client. All disciplines assess the client separately

and get together to coordinate the plan. The initial assessment is done by the RN who is the primary nurse or case manager. The RN can determine what other disciplines are needed if the physician has not requested them in the original order for home health services. All disciplines are responsible for knowing Medicare guidelines (or the guidelines of the payer source) for participation in home health. Once the entire plan is developed, it is phoned in to the physician for approval (Emlet & Crabtree, 1996).

Medicare requires a **plan of treatment (POT)** to be submitted for review and for reimbursement. The POT includes the skills to be performed by the RN and other disciplines. It also contains the frequency of visits per week, the expected goals, the potential that the client will reach the goals, and the conditions of discharge and a potential date. The original POT is mailed to the physician for a signature and then sent to an FI. The federal government has divided the country into 10 different regions, and each region has an insurance company that is responsible for delivering Medicare benefits. These regions are known as fiscal intermediaries. The FIs are responsible for ensuring that home health agencies adhere to Medicare guidelines and regulations (Humphrey & Milone-Nuzzo, 1996).

The Initial Visit

The first visit to see a client is made within 48 hours of the home health agency receiving an order from the client's physician. The home health agency first receives the order by phone followed by the written order via fax. Requests for home health care originate from hospitals, assisted-living facilities, or family members or the client can request care. The client's personal physician must determine if services are needed and then contact a home health agency. If the client is not covered by Medicare, the home health agency contacts the insurance company or health maintenance organization (HMO) to verify coverage of the ordered services.

The written order consists of the client's name, address, payer source, diagnosis, and treatment order. Typically, the home health nurse telephones the client to arrange a convenient time for the admission. This is also a good time to ask the client about family members who will be present for the admission. The caregiver and care recipient are viewed as part of the family process. Family members are needed to help add information to the history and present health status. Family members are also helpful if language, vision, or mobility are barriers to the admission process. With family members present, the nurse observes the interaction between family and client and assesses for strengths and weaknesses in the family process. Many times it is the family member who has been present during the hospital and discharge process and can provide valuable information to the home health nurse.

Required records must also be signed on the first visit. The client is required to sign a consent for treatment that includes the disciplines that will deliver care and the frequency of their visits. Advance directives can be signed if the client desires and if there is a witness other than a family member or the home health nurse present. The Patient's Bill of Rights is to be explained to the client and then signed by the nurse and client (Box 20-2). Agencies may have other forms specific to their agency. See Box 20-3 for federally required data.

Admission Assessment

The assessment on the initial visit sets the stage for all of the subsequent visits. The initial assessment includes the client assessment, an assessment of social support, environmental assessment, and an assessment of community resources used by the client (see Box 20-4). The purpose of this comprehensive assessment is to provide the home health nurse with a *picture* of the client. Each home health agency uses its own assessment form.

Older adults often have multiple diagnoses, chronic illnesses, and disabilities. Each part of the initial assessment is designed to aid the home health nurse to form a

---

BOX 20-2   Medicare Patient Rights

1. The patient has the right to exercise his or her rights as a patient of the Home Health Agency (HHA).

2. The patient's family or guardian may exercise the patient's rights when the patient has been judged incompetent.

3. The patient has the right to have his or her property treated with respect.

4. The patient has the right to voice grievances regarding treatment or care that is (or fails to be) furnished, or regarding the lack of respect for property by anyone who is furnishing services on behalf of the HHA, and must document both the existence of the complaint and the resolution of the complaint.

   - The HHA must investigate complaints made by a patient or the patient's family or guardian regarding treatment or care that is (or fails to be) furnished, or regarding the lack of respect for the patient's property by anyone furnishing services on behalf of the HHA, and must document both the existence of the complaint and the resolution of the complaint.

5. The patient has the right to participate in the planning of care.

   - The HHA must advise the patient in advance of the right to participate in planning the care or treatment and planning changes in the care or treatment.

6. The HHA must maintain written policies and procedures regarding advance directives.

7. The patient has the right to confidentiality of the client records maintained by the HHA.

8. The HHA must advise the patient of the agency's policies and procedures regarding disclosure of clinical records.

9. The patient has the right to be advised, before care is initiated, of the extent to which payment for the HHA services may be expected from Medicare or other sources, and the extent to which payment may be required from the patient. The HHA must inform the patient, orally and in writing, of:

   - The extent to which payment may be expected from Medicare, Medicaid, or any other Federally funded or aided program known to HHA;

   - The charges for services that will not be covered by Medicare; and

   - The charges that the individual may have to pay.

10. The patient has the right to be advised orally and in writing of any changes in the information provided under #9. The HHA must advise the patient of these changes orally and in writing as soon as possible, but no later than 30 calendar days from the date that the HHA becomes aware of a change.

11. The patient has the right to be advised of the availability of the toll-free HHA hotline in the state.

12. The HHA must advise the patient in writing of the telephone number of the home health hotline established by the State, the hours of its operation, and that the purpose of the hotline is to receive complaints or questions about local HHAs. The patient also has the right to use this hotline to lodge complaints concerning the implementation of the advance directives requirements.

Source: Reprinted with permission from Advanced Healthcare Services, Inc., Fort Worth, TX.

holistic view of the client and then develop an appropriate plan of care that meets the client's individual needs. Reimbursement from Medicare and insurance depend on the assessment of the client and the skilled needs identified by the nurse (Emlet & Crabtree, 1996).

Physical Assessment

The home health nurse performs a physical assessment to establish a baseline and confirm findings received in the discharge report from the facility and report any new findings. Knowledge of normal aging changes and atypical responses to disease processes are necessary for the home health nurse to assess and plan effectively for the home health client. Current complaints are elicited as well as the admitting diagnosis and a history of any major illnesses or surgeries. It is important to discover what the client knows about his or her own diagnosis so the nurse can determine teaching needs. The knowledge of the caregiver is also important to determine because the caregiver and client will be working together toward the same goal of reaching a maximum level of independence.

The home health nurse needs to spend time establishing rapport with the client and family on the first visit. It is important to understand the client's culture when eliciting information about physical health. Terms that are familiar to nurses are not always understood by the client. The client from another culture may not feel comfortable with someone in the home asking personal questions. Whenever possible, an RN who speaks the client's language and understands the client's culture is in the best position to obtain an oral history and explain the services to the client and family. Nurses need to be sensitive to the client's personal beliefs regarding health and illness.

Asking about medications is another area that may require extra time and good assessment skills. When older adults are asked to bring in medicines or bring a list of medications to a physician's office, they do not always think about over-the-counter (OTC) medications, the occasional pill taken from a previous prescription, or some of the spouse's medicine. The home is the ideal place to assess the client's medications. The home health nurse may ask about OTC medications or may ask the

---

BOX 20-3 What is OASIS?

Outcome Assessment Information Sets (OASIS) is required by the HCFA for all Medicare-certified HHAs and Medicaid home health providers in states where Medicare coverage requires agencies to meet the Medicare Conditions of Participation (COPs) (HCFA, 1999). Oasis is a group of data sets designed to measure client outcomes in home health care for outcome–based quality improvement (OBQI) (Shaughnessy, Crisler, Schlenker, & Hittle, 1998).

Over 12 years of research has been done on the collection of these data sets. In 1994 the first report measuring client outcomes from a 73-item data set was published, then expanded to a 79-item data set OASIS–A in 1995 (Shaughnessy et al., 1998). The information gathered was to be utilized for the Balanced Budget Act of 1997 (BBA). The plan was to develop a reliable case mix system by October 1, 1997, and have all Medicare-certified HHAs collecting the data and submitting it to the state by October 1998. There were items added and dropped, creating OASIS–B, still containing 79 items (Shaughnessy et al., 1998). The HCFA intends to use OASIS–B core data items to develop the PPS for home care agencies.

OASIS data sets include socio-demographics, environmental, support systems, health status, and functional status (Beacon Health, 1998). OASIS cannot "stand alone"; it does not form a comprehensive or complete assessment. OASIS must be integrated into the home health agency's comprehensive assessment (Beacon Health, 1998).

OASIS data are collected at the start of care (SOC), every 2 months following the SOC, but not earlier than 5 days before the end of the certification period, after an inpatient stay, significant change of client's condition, transfer to an inpatient facility, discharge from an agency, or death (*OASIS Education and Training*, 1999).

It is the admitting professional (RN, PT) who collects OASIS information at the SOC. Other OASIS data collection is done by the primary professional when follow-up, transfer to inpatient facility, or resumption of care is due. The last professional rendering care completes the discharge OASIS (HCFA, 1999).

OASIS will be done on a continual bases to generate objective and scientific reports on client care outcomes. It will be utilized to establish PPS and baselines for comparing HHAs with national references. Health care professionals in home care must fully understand the impact of OASIS on federal regulations. The importance of data collection and the time frame that it occurs are critical to a home care agency's survival.

Source: By Eileen M. Hermann RN, BSN, MSH, Director of Education, The Connecticut VNA, Wallingford, CT. Used with permission.

BOX 20-4   Components of a Home Health Assessment

Physical assessment
  Current complaints
  History of illnesses/surgeries
  Preventive health measures
Psychosocial assessment
  Family assessment
  Social support
  Assessment for depression/dementia
Financial assessment
  Type of health care coverage
  Medicaid, Food Stamps
  Adequate income for medications
Environmental assessment
  Assessment of home
  Assessment of risk factors for falls
  Neighborhood assessment-safety
  Home modifications
  Sanitation
Nutritional assessment
  Type and appropriateness of diet
  Vitamins
  Supplements

Current medications
  Prescriptions
  Over-the-counter medications
Functional assessment
  Physical activities of daily living
  Instrumental activities of daily living
Substance use
  Alcohol
  Tobacco
  Drugs
Assessment of community resources
  Home-delivered meals
  Transportation
  Adult day services
  Senior center services
  Support groups
Preventive health measures
  Screening
    Testicular
    Mammograms

client if he or she will "show me where you keep all of your medicines." Frequently, the nurse will find several bottles of outdated medications and possibly duplicates of medications because they have been prescribed by different physicians and possibly filled at different pharmacies. If one medication is the generic form and one is the brand name, there is a possibility that the client may not have realized this fact and is taking both medications. This problem can cause serious adverse effects for the older adult.

Asking the client about instructions for management of the disease process will assist the nurse in understanding the client's self-care methods. Often, a client is unable to comply with self-care management for various reasons but has not communicated this to the physician.

CLINICAL ALERT

Medication Assessment

Many older adults save their prescriptions if they do not take all of the medicine. The home health nurse needs to ask about all medications, including ones they are not presently taking but have in their home. This is an excellent opportunity for the nurse to teach the client about the danger of mixing medications and taking old medicines.

The relationship between the home health personnel and the client, the amount of time the home health personnel are able to spend with the client and family, and the milieu of the client's home facilitate communication about the client's issues surrounding self-care and management of the disease process.

Functional status is one of the best and most reliable determinants of well-being in the older adult. Physicians use functional status to determine a client's need for assistive devices, the client's ability to remain safe in the home, and the ability to perform self-care. If the older adult has a deficit in functional status, options for care include (a) a skilled nursing unit, (b) a rehabilitation unit, (c) a nursing facility, (d) home with a son or daughter, or (e) home with home health services. Functional status also determines if a physician will order nursing care, physical therapy, occupational therapy, or speech-language pathology services.

Functional status includes **physical activities of daily living (PADL)** and IADL. The older adult who experiences a deficit in functional status is more at risk than the older adult who has no interference in independence. One of the most important goals of home health is to enable older adults to live in their own home. The home health nurse enables the older adult to manage the functional deficit and help correct some of the deficiencies in the home through the use of community resources.

Research Focus

Citation:

Benesh, L., Szigeti, E., Ferraro, R., & Gullicks, J. (1997). Tools for assessing chronic pain in rural elderly women. *Home Healthcare Nurse, 15*(3), 207–211.

Purpose:

To identify a method of assessing pain in rural elderly women that was easy for them to describe and best characterize their pain.

Methods:

Four separate pain scales, the Visual Analog Scale (VAS), the Verbal Descriptor Scale (VDS), the 1 to 10 Pain Rating Scale, and the Pain Thermometer, were given to 40 women from a rural area in Minnesota. The women were 65 years and older and reported chronic pain from arthritis for at least 3 months. The women were asked to determine which scale best described their pain and was the easiest to complete.

Findings:

The Pain Thermometer was chosen by almost half (47.5%, $n = 19$) of the women in the study. The women indicated that this tool reflected their pain intensity accurately and was the easiest to complete.

Implications:

Home health clients often have chronic pain that is difficult to accurately describe. A standardized tool will aid the home health nurse to accurately assess the pain and implement interventions to decrease the pain.

CLINICAL ALERT

Signs and Symptoms of Abuse

Home health personnel must continually be alert for signs of abuse in the older adult. These signs and symptoms include (Morgan & McClain, 1995):

- *Unexplained neglect*
- *Unexplained/questionable fractures/injuries*
- *Fear/withdrawal/crying*
- *Weight loss (unexplained)*
- *Failure to thrive, depression*
- *Inadequate clothing/food*
- *Sudden inability to pay for medications*

Psychosocial Assessment

The psychosocial assessment consists of a mental status examination, assessment for depression, and assessment of available social and informal support. The mental status examination may consist of a few questions concerning orientation or may be one of many valid and reliable mental status assessment tools. Assessment for depression may also range from a question about how the care recipient is feeling emotionally to the use of a formalized instrument to measure depression.

A financial assessment is another part of the psychosocial assessment. Lack of funds for health care, medications, food, utilities, or transportation presents a barrier for self-care. The MSW or RN can contact various community agencies to assist older adults with financial management. Accessing agencies that provide resources is often difficult because of confusion about what agencies provide specific resources. Frequently, there are multiple phone numbers for services or one agency will refer a person to another agency for a particular resource only to discover that the agency's number has changed or it no longer provides the service. The system can be confusing and discouraging to the older adult who is already compromised physically or mentally.

Social support is a vital part of the older adult's well-being. Lack of social support can lead to depression that can then negatively affect the overall health status of the client. Many clients without adequate social support lack a reason for maintaining good health. Lack of social support can prevent access to needed health care such as physician visits, pharmacies, or grocery stores. Without the ability to access services, the older adult can have adverse physical and mental consequences. Social support consists of formal and informal persons who contribute to the client's well-being by providing some type of needed service. Informal support may refer to a family member who takes the client to the beauty shop or doctor's appointment or to a friend from the church who visits once every 1 or 2 weeks. Formal support often refers to community resources. Social support is determined by asking about family members or friends who help the client on occasion or phone or visit with some regularity. Clients involved in church, clubs, or senior citizen centers often have adequate support systems, but involvement in any of these activities does not necessarily equate with visits and assistance from others when the client is unable to leave home.

Environmental Assessment

The quality of life of the older adult is affected by his or her place of residence. The older adult's home is familiar and comfortable and holds valuable memories. Adults feel their needs are met in their own home. One aim of home health care is to avoid institutionalization of the older adult. Home health nursing assists clients to remain at home and return to a previous level of independence. An environmental assessment will assist in knowing what modifications need to be made to help keep the client safe in the home. The home health nurse enables the client to maintain wellness through self-care activities and prevention within physical and psychosocial limitations.

Ensuring safety for the home health client is a priority of the home health nurse. Falls are the major cause of accidents in persons age 65 and over and 20%–30% of falls lead to loss of mobility, independence, and increased risk of death. One-third of persons aged 75 and over who live in the community fall each year, and half of these experience more than one fall a year (Lange, 1996).

Reasons for falls in older people are multiple. Loss of agility, loss of strength, decreased visual acuity, disease processes, and medications are but a few reasons that older people are susceptible to falls. The home environment is also a major factor in falls. Unstable furniture, poor lighting, slippery floors, loose rugs, unsafe footwear, improper use of assistive devices, and lack of easy access to the bathroom or a phone are examples of environmental hazards. It is the interaction between the home health client and the environment that creates the risk for injuries related to falls (Fortin, Yeaw, Campbell, & Jameson, 1998). Assessment of strength and mobility of the client is critical in determining the ability of the older adult to perform PADL and lower the risk of falls. Deficits in muscle strength and neurological status also affect risk for injury. The home health nurse's assessment of the musculoskeletal and neurological systems aids in planning interventions and setting realistic goals of the client (Cho & Kamen, 1998; Neal, 1997).

The environmental checklist is a tool the home health nurse uses to assess for environmental hazards. Once unsafe areas are identified, the nurse and client plan interventions to modify the environment. The nurse also assesses for risk factors associated with falls that are not a part of the environment. Medications are an example of a potential risk factor associated with falls. Education on the side effects of medications can help prevent a fall. For the client who has decreased strength from a lengthy hospitalization or disease process, a physical and/or occupational therapist can provide exercises to increase the client's strength (Lange, 1996).

Planning

The planning phase of home health begins when the assessment is complete and the nursing diagnoses developed. The diagnoses are developed based on a combination of the medical diagnoses and the findings from the assessment. The diagnoses must be amenable to nursing interventions and the nursing interventions are to provide skilled care according to Medicare criteria.

There are two phases of the planning process—setting priorities and establishing goals. The priorities are based on the needs of the client and should start with physiological needs and advance to issues of self-actualization (Humphrey & Milone-Nuzzo, 1996). If the priorities do not complement the medical diagnoses, the RN must contact the physician for permission to alter the original order.

The goals are set collaboratively with the client and family. If the goals are set independently of the client, compliance with the plan may be jeopardized. The goals are to be specific and time limited. As home health is intermittent and short term, the goals need to be realistic, observable, measurable, and reflective of the problems identified in the assessment (Humphrey & Milone-Nuzzo, 1996).

Implementation

> ### Nursing Tip
>
> When teaching older adults, remember these points:
> - Adults retain new information when it is presented verbally and written.
> - After presenting the information verbally, leave written information in the home.
> - Use large block print on yellow or orange background.
> - Ask the client to tell you his or her explanation of the material presented.
> - For motor tasks, demonstration with return demonstration by the client is most effective.

Implementation involves intervention strategies and documentation. Intervention strategies must be skilled as defined by Medicare. Interventions include (a) teaching about a new disease process such as cause of the dis-

> ### Think About It
>
> Mrs. King, 86 years old, fell 3 weeks ago in her home and broke her left hip and wrist. She is being discharged from the skilled nursing unit in 2 days. She has received physical and occupational therapy for 10 days following surgical repair of both fractures. She will return to her home where she lives alone. Her physician is ordering home health services for insulin administration, personal care, and continued therapy. The home health nurse will admit her the afternoon she is discharged.
> - What functional deficits should the home health nurse assess Mrs. King for?
> - What should be included in the environmental assessment of Mrs. King's home?

ease, signs and symptoms, treatment, progression of the disease, and how to handle an exacerbation; (b) reinforcing teaching if needed to progress toward self-care; (c) instructions on all aspects of medication management such as brand and generic names, correct dosage to be taken, action of the medications, side effects to report, times of administration, and expected results of the medication; (d) wound care; and, (e) IV therapy/enteral therapy. Teaching is one of the main skills of the home health nurse because the assumption is that an informed client has the potential for being independent with self-care.

Documentation is the second phase of the implementation process. No matter what activities the nurse does, *if the documentation does not reflect those skills, Medicare will not reimburse the home health agency for the nurse, and the nurse is also jeopardizing her case with the client.* The phrase "if it's not documented, it's not done" is as true in home health care as it is in the acute care setting. Documentation carries even more importance because of reimbursement implications.

The nurse documents every visit (Figure 20-4). The visit note consists of an abbreviated assessment checklist, a place to note new problems identified in the visit, and an area to document the skill performed in the home, the client's response to the skill, and the client's progress toward the goals established in the original care plan.

Evaluation

The evaluation process consists of noting progress toward the client's goals. The documentation should reflect this progress and note when the goals are met. Documentation on the discharge form will also reflect if the goals were met. The RN and other disciplines should evaluate the progress on each visit and make adjustments to the care plan if needed to assist the client in reaching the goals. If goals are not met, the RN needs to evaluate the effectiveness of the care plan and the reasons for the client not achieving the goals, which should also be documented on the discharge form (Humphrey & Milone-Nuzzo, 1996).

Case Management

One goal of home health is to provide care that is effective and cost efficient. Case management is a model used by home health agencies to ensure care is delivered in this manner. Case management can improve client, physician, and payer satisfaction, demonstrate an increase in positive outcomes, and use resources effectively (Huggins & Phillips, 1998). One tool of the case management model is the **clinical pathway** or care map. Some home health agencies use clinical pathways to determine the number of visits a client will receive, the main activities of each discipline, and a time frame for delivery of care. Clinical pathways contain measurable outcomes, use of resources, and variances that occur in the treatment plan. A special nurse's note is developed that complements the clinical pathway (Figure 20-5) (Moulton, Wray-Langevine, & Boyer, 1997).

The pathways are developed collaboratively by nurses and physicians for each diagnosis. Clinical pathways are not to be used as recipes for treatment. As all clients are individual, revisions are necessary when the client is unable to meet the goals in the specified time. The case manager must decide the amount of time needed for each client. This time frame is determined by the case manager, physician, client, and payer source (Figure 20-6).

Variances from the care plan are evaluated and interventions modified to decrease the number of variances. Outcomes must be observable and measurable. The use of outcomes demonstrates an agency's ability to deliver care in a cost-effective and efficient manner. Outcomes are documented as they are met. They are also documented if not met. Outcomes can help the case manager determine problems in the care plan, the teaching process, the delivery of skills, or the assessment of the client and family (Figure 20-7) (Huggins & Phillips, 1998).

The use of clinical pathways is to serve as a framework for the nursing process. The care must still be individualized, and the disciplines seeing the client continually assess the client's response to the treatment plan and progress toward the goals (Moulton et al., 1997). The case manager is responsible for seeing that the clinical pathway is followed and for communicating with all disciplines caring for the client so that the care is coordinated and appropriate.

Community Resources

Community resources are an invaluable part of home health. Following the initial assessment, the home health nurse should recognize community resources that may be needed. Sometimes the need does not surface until a later visit or at discharge. For those resources needed at discharge, it is wise to make contact early so that when the nurses' visits have ended, there will not be a significant gap in time before the community resources are available.

The home health nurse needs to be familiar with community resources and how to access them. Knowledge of these resources is necessary to help meet the needs of the client. As the case manager, the RN is responsible for knowing what services the client requires to reach the goals of the care plan, maintain a specified

ADVANCED HEALTHCARE SERVICES, INC.
SKILLED NURSING VISIT NOTE

Date: _____ / _____ / ____

Time In: _____ Out: _____

Patient Name-Last, First:

Type of Visit: ☐SN ☐SN & Sup ☐PRN ☐Sup ☐Nonbillable

Medical Diagnosis:

Homebound Reason:

Skilled Service:

VITALS

T° _____ Resp. _____ ☐ Reg. ☐ Irreg.

Pulse: A _____ R _____ ☐Reg. ☐Irreg

Wt. _____ FSBS _____

NURSING ASSESSMENT/OBSERVATION SIGNS/SYMPTOMS
(Mark all abnormal with "X" and describe.)

B/P	LYING	SITTING	STANDING
Right			
Left			

Denote Location/Size of Wounds/Pres. Sores/Measure Ext. Edema Bil.

CARDIOVASCULAR
Fluid Retention	
Chest pain	
Neck vein distention	
Edema (specify)	
☐RUE ☐RLE ☐LUE ☐LLE	
Peripheral Pulses	
Other:	

RESPIRATORY
Rales	Rhonchi
Wheeze	Cough
Dyspnea	SOB
Orthopnea	
Other:	

DIGESTIVE
Bowel Sounds	
Anorexia	
Nausea	Vomiting
Epigastric distress	
Difficulty swallowing	
Abdominal distention	
Bowel Incontinence	
Colostomy	Diarrhea
Constipation	Impaction

INFECTION CONTROL
Universal Precautions	

GENITOURINARY
Burning	
Distention	Retention
Frequency	Urgency
Hesitancy	Hematuria
Incontin.	Catheter
Urine: Color _____	
Consistency _____	
Odor _____	
Pain	Discharge
Other:	

SKIN
Color:	
Jaundiced	
Temp	Chills
Decubitus	Wound
Rash	Itching
Turgor	
Other:	

PAIN
Origin:	
Location:	
Duration:	
Severity:	
Other:	

MUSCULOSKELETAL
Balance/Unsteady Gait	
Weakness	
Other:	

NEUROSENSORY
Syncope	Headache
Grasp: R _____	
L _____	

Movement:
☐ RUE ☐ LUE
☐ RLE ☐ LLE

Pupil	R _____
Reaction	L _____
Tremors	Vertigo
Speech Impairment	
Hearing Impairment	
Visual Impairment	
Decreased Sensitivity	
Other:	

EMOTIONAL STATUS
Disoriented	Lethargic
Agitated	Oriented
Comatose	Forgetful
Depressed	
Other:	

	#1	#2	#3	#4
Length				
Width				
Depth				
Drainage				
Tunneling				
Odor				
Sur.Tissue				
Edema				
Stoma				

INTERVENTIONS/INSTRUCTIONS (Mark all applicable with an "X". Circle appropriate item(s) separated by "/")

Skilled observation and Assessment	Chest physio./Postural drainage	IM injection	Evaluate diet/fluid intake
Foley care/Irrigation	Administration of B12	Psych. intervention	Diet teaching
Wound care/dressing	Preparation/Administration of Insulin	Observe S/S infection	Safety factors
Decubitus care	Teach/Adm.IVs/Clysis	Diabetic observation	Teach care - terminally ill
Venipuncture	Teach ostomy/ileo.conduit care	Teach diabetic care	Other:
Bowel/Bladder training	Teach/Adm.tube feedings	Observe/Teach meds - effects/side effects	
Digital exam with manual removal/Enema	Teach/Adm.care of trach.	Teach physiology/disease process	
Change NG/G tube	Teach/Adm.Inhalation Rx	Observe ADLs	

ANALYSIS OF FINDINGS/INTERVENTIONS _____

_____

_____

_____

_____

_____

_____

INSTRUCTION PROVIDED_____

_____

_____

EVALUATION AND PATIENT/CAREGIVER RESPONSE_____

_____

_____

_____

NEXT VISIT: _____ PLAN FOR NEXT VISIT : _____

CARE PLAN

Care Plan: ☐Reviewed/Revised with patient involvement ☐Outcome achieved ☐PRN order obtained **Medication status** ☐No change ☐Order obtained

Disc.Planning Discussed? ☐Yes ☐No ☐N/A Billable supplies recorded? ☐Yes ☐No Care Coor: ☐Phy ☐PT ☐ST ☐MSW _____

AIDE SUPERVISORY VISIT (Complete if applicable)

Aide: _____ ☐Present ☐Not present POC: Followed ☐Yes ☐No Updated: ☐Yes ☐No Aide is: ☐Punctual ☐Appro.Appear ☐Considerate ☐Thorough

POC Changes/Observation/Teaching: _____

PT/CG Comments: _____

Pt. ID#:	Patient Signature:	Nurse Signature/Title:	ID#

2015   White: Original   Yellow: Nurse   Rev 10/96

FIGURE 20-4 Skilled nurse's visit note. *Reprinted with permission from Advanced Healthcare Services Inc., Fort Worth, TX.*

Patient Name _____

ID # _____

Start of Care _____

CARDIAC/VASCULAR I CareMap
(CHF, Disorders in Cardiac Output)

ASSESS/OBSERVE EACH VISIT:

Complete cardiovascular assessment with vital signs, weight, lung sounds. Assess for fatigue, dyspnea, chest pain, cough, orthopnea, anorexia, mobility, emotional status, and orientation.

NURSING DIAGNOSES:

☐ 1. Fluid volume excess related to decreased cardiac output.
☐ 2. Activity intolerance related to decreased cardiac output.
☐ 3. Ineffective management of therapeutic regimen related to lack of knowledge of disease process, home management, activity/rest schedule, and pain.
☐ 4. High risk for impairment of skin integrity related to edema.
☐ 5. Ineffective individual/family coping related to responses to diagnosis and prognosis.

Collaborative Problems:

☐ 1. PC: Decreased Cardiac Output*
☐ 2. PC: Dysrhythmia
☐ 3. PC: Pulmonary Edema
☐ 4. PC: Deep Vein Thrombosis
　　*PC = Potential Complication

LONG-TERM GOALS:

☐ 1. Patient/caregiver will demonstrate understanding of disease process and self-care management.
☐ 2. Patient will have improved cardiac output.
☐ 3. Patient will minimize fluid retention.
☐ 4. Patient will have intact skin surface (or absence of S/S of infection from skin breakdown.)
☐ 5. Patient's vital signs, weight and cardiovascular status are normal for patient range for 3 weeks without major treatment plan changes.

GOAL	PROJECTED DATE	DATE MET	SIGNATURE
1			
2			
3			
4			
5			

RECOMMENDED FREQUENCY: $\dfrac{\text{3-4 wk x 2.2 wk x 3, 1 wk x 4}}{\text{(16 visits total)}}$

NOTE: It is anticipated that most patients may stabilize quickly and learn quickly, and meet all outcomes and long-term goals by the end of Visit 12. Some patients, however, will require additional visits. Visits 13-16 will be used to complete instruction not yet accomplished because of variances, to do additional teaching for concurrent diagnoses, to assess and evaluate cardiovascular status, and to monitor response to treatment.

Home Health CareMaps™ are designed to address the patient's acute episode of illness. Visit intensity and frequency may also be influenced by the patient's unique set of circumstances, including but not limited to the home environment, resources, presence of life-supporting therapies, and the presence of other chronic illnesses or limiting handicaps.

FIGURE 20-5 Example of a care map (or clinical pathway). *Reprinted with permission from the VNA of Essex Valley of New Jersey and VNA First of La Grange, IL.*

Visiting Nurse Association
of Essex Valley

CLINICAL PROGRESS NOTE

CARE MAP: CARDIAC/VASC I

T _____	RP _____	**EDEMA**
BP _____	R _____	R L
_____	LS (R) _____	I ___ I ___
_____	(L) _____	A ___ A ___
AP _____	WT _____	C ___ C ___

PATIENT NAME: _____   ID #: _____   VISIT DATE: _____   VISIT #: **1**

SUBJECTIVE FINDINGS: _____

CIRCLE OR FILL IN BELOW AS APPROPRIATE

CNS: L.O.C.:   alert   lethargic   other _____
Orientation: Person   Place   Time
Mood/Beh: Irritable   Restless   or Nervous?
Headache/Dizzy?   Location _____
Frequency _____

SKIN: Color: wnl   abnl   Turgor: wnl   taut   tenting
Cyanosis?   N   Y: lips   mucous membranes

CV: Pain?   N   Y: Chest?   N   Y
other location? _____
with exertion?   N   Y
freq. _____ duration _____
relieved by: rest?   N   Y
medications: N   Y _____
Palpitations?   N   Y _____
Other: _____

CP: S.O.B. at rest?   N   Y: After act.?   N   Y: Desc. _____
Orthopnea?   N   Y ___ # of pillows: ___   PND?   N   Y _____
Endurance: Good   Fair   Poor
Cough?   N   Y: Productive?   N   Y: Sputum?   N   Y: des. ___
Oxygen used?   N   Y: Rate _____ L/min., Freq/Dur ___
Equip: _____

GI: Food & Fluid intake: _____
BMs: freq. _____ wnl   ABN   Other:

GU: Nocturia?   N   Y: freq. _____
Output appropriate to intake and any medications?   N   Y
Other: _____

PV: Pedal pulses: L   wnl   faint   absent   R: wnl   faint   absent
T°:   L: Foot   warm   cool   Coloring: L: wnl   abn: _____
R: Foot   warm   cool   Coloring: R: wnl   abn: _____

MOBILITY: BB   WC   Amb. stdy/unstdy with assist of _____ persons &/or _____ device(s): _____

Medications: Changed?   N   Y   Pt. Knowledgeable?   N   Y   Compliant?   N   Y   Exhibiting side effects?   N   Y

CARE ELEMENTS		DONE	NOT DONE	COMMENTS
DISEASE PROCESS	Provide brief definition and causes of cardiac disease.			
MEDICATION	Establish basic medication schedule in writing and leave in home (name of medication, times.)			
NUTRITION/ HYDRATION	Assess prior knowledge regarding dietary and fluid restrictions.			
ACTIVITY	Avoid exertion; instruct frequent rest periods.			
SAFETY	Assess for environmental hazards, including O$_2$; provide emergency phone numbers.			
TREATMENTS	Weigh patient (on patient's own scale, if available.)			
TESTS	Ask MD for orders for electrolytes, digoxin level, others as indicated by medications/diagnosis.			
PSYCHOSOCIAL				
INTERDISCIPLINARY SERVICES/COMMUNITY REFERRALS	HHA, if unable to do ADLs; MSW for social factors interfering with care.			

PATIENT OUTCOMES		MET	NOT MET	EXPLAIN VARIANCE
	States definition of CHF.			
	Verbalizes understanding of simple medication schedule.			
	States/how when to call for help.			
	Identifies need to avoid exertion and to rest frequently.			
	Adequate cardiac output as evidenced by *pulse pressure >30 mm Hg; lungs clear; warm dry skin. (If not met, nurse will notify MD.)			

CHECK HERE FOR COMAP ☐

SIGNATURE _____

*Pulse pressure is the difference between the systolic and diastolic blood pressure.

FIGURE 20-6   Clinical progress note. *Reprinted with permission from the VNA of Essex Valley of New Jersey and VNA First of La Grange, IL.*

VNA Community Care Services
Patient Outcome Tool: Heart Failure

Patient Name: _____ Age: _____ Medical Record # _____

Sex: M F   Physician: _____ Payor: _____

Admit Date: _____ Day of Week: S- M - T - W - T - F- S Admit Time: _____ Admit RN: _____

Primary Dx(s): _____

Secondary Dx(s): _____

Primary Caregiver: Self _____ Spouse _____ Sibling _____ Friend _____ Other _____

Discharge Date: _____ Caregiver utilized to meet outcome(s)? Yes No

Discharge Reason: Independent at home _____ Refused services _____ Other _____

Rehospitalized R/T primary Dx _____ Rehospitalized R/T other Dx _____

Expected # Visits: 12 Visits   Recommended Frequency: _____ Expected LOS: _____

Outcome	Met at Admission Yes/No	Met at Visit 12 Yes/No	Met at Discharge Yes/No	Comments if no
1. Correctly verbalizes/demonstrates med adm. (dose, route, frequency)				
2. Meets or exceeds adm physiologic status (vital signs, lung and edema status)				
3. Correctly verbalizes: • control of their risks factors				
• management of their disease process				
4. Correctly verbalizes/demonstrates knowledge of: • when and how to seek medical intervention				
• community services available				
5. Meets or exceeds previous level of functioning: • bathing				
• mobility				
• dressing				
• toileting				
• eating				
6. Correctly verbalizes healthy coping mechanisms				
7. Correctly verbalizes or demonstrates: • obtain weight				
• prescribed diet				
• fluid restriction				
• evaluate edema				
• energy conservation				

RN Signature: _____ Date: _____

FIGURE 20-7 Patient outcome tool. *Reprinted with permission from the VNA of Lancaster County, PA.*

level of wellness, and avoid institutionalization. The community resources needed can be accessed by the nurse, the social worker, the client, or the client's caregiver. Enabling the client or caregiver to access community resources promotes independence and moves the client toward self-care.

Discharging the Client

The home health client is discharged when skilled services are no longer needed, the client is hospitalized, the client moves out of the service area, the client no longer meets Medicare criteria for home health, the physician discharges the client, or the client expires. The discharge requires an order from the physician. Each discipline (except the HHA) is required to get a discharge order from the physician.

Discharge planning begins on admission to home health. The nurse assesses resources currently in place and assesses resources that will be needed when the client no longer has home health. With each home visit, the nurse reviews the discharge plan and makes appropriate

Think About It

Mrs. Bobek recently had a stroke and her speech, coordination, and decision-making ability were affected. Mrs. Bobek lives with her husband who has Type II diabetes with peripheral neuropathy. Mrs. Bobek has been her husband's caregiver for the past 10 years. She checks his blood sugar three times a week, administers his insulin injections, and takes care of his feet to prevent skin breakdown. Because of Mrs. Bobek's stroke, she is no longer able to care for her husband. They have no relatives in the area. Mrs. Bobek's physician suggested that the couple move into an assisted-living facility until she recovers from the stroke. The physician ordered home health for the couple. An RN will check Mr. Bobek's blood sugar, give his injections, and assess his feet and legs for skin breakdown. A home health aide will provide both with personal care three times a week. Mrs. Bobek will receive home health services from an RN and physical and speech-language pathology services to assist in rehabilitation following her stroke.

When Mrs. Bobek regains her strength and ability to function without an RN or HHA, she and her husband want to move back to their home.
- What topics are to be a part of the RN's teaching plan for Mrs. Bobek?
- How will the RN evaluate Mrs. Bobek's readiness to resume providing care for her husband?
- What community resources might the RN recommend for the Bobeks?
- What services will Medicare continue to cover until Mrs. Bobek is fully recovered?

updates. Part of home health education is instructing the client to manage self-care activities and to take advantage of available resources. It is important for the client to know when home health services will be terminated.

All disciplines are responsible for carrying out the discharge plans. The HHA instructs the client or caregiver on self-care including bathing, dressing, and transfer techniques. Providing good skin care and observing for skin breakdown are also part of the educational process. Therapists working with the home health RN must document whether or not goals were met and the progress of the client. If all of the goals have not been met, some disciplines may continue to see the client if the physician extends the order beyond the original end date. A PT may stay in the home without the RN. If the OT or speech-language pathologist needs to continue therapy, the RN remains the case manager. The HHA can continue with a physician's order as long as another discipline is in the home and there is a documented need for the aide.

Think About It

Your home health client is a 76-year-old female with a 10-year history of congestive heart failure (CHF). You have seen her once a week for 7 weeks. She has been hospitalized at least once a year for an exacerbation of her CHF and went to the emergency department (ED) numerous times.
- Do you discharge her and readmit her after an exacerbation?
- Or do you continue to see her in hopes of decreasing her ED and hospital visits?

Ethical and Legal Issues

The home health nurse has an ethical duty to the home health client to maintain privacy and confidentiality of the client and the clinical records. The home health client has the right to privacy in that he or she can request to be left alone, can refuse intrusions into private affairs, and can expect that his or her case will not be discussed in public and that his or her name or picture will not be used for economic advantages of the home health agency. If a nurse wants to use the client's case, name, or picture, written permission must be obtained from the client prior to the information being used (Brent, 1997).

The home health nurse must be careful to protect the client's privacy when discussing the client at a case conference or with a colleague. For a nurse starting in home health, this point cannot be overemphasized. As nurses go from one client's home to another, it is easy to let slip the client's name. Sometimes a nurse must communicate with the agency or physician while with another client and it is important not to reveal another

CARE PLAN

CASE STUDY

Seventy-six-year-old Mary Franco was found on the floor of her home by her daughter, Marie. She was unable to respond. She was taken to the emergency department and diagnosed with Type 1 diabetes, having a blood sugar of 600. After stabilizing her condition over 2 days, Mrs. Franco spent 2 weeks in the hospital, where the nurses and doctors tried the effective use of insulin and diet management, taught self-administration of insulin along with foot care, what to do when feeling ill, and exercises related to diabetes and metabolic needs. Marie was able to take her mother home after 2 weeks. Mrs. Franco and her daughter were not interested in nursing facility placement.

Mrs. Franco's insulin therapy includes a premixed 70%/30% combination dose of regular ("short acting" appears clear) insulin and NPH ("intermediate acting" looks cloudy) given in a single shot twice daily. Her daughter has been instructed on how to prepare and give the insulin, with demonstration and repeated return demonstrations. Mrs. Franco is very capable and willing to learn how to give her own insulin because her daughter normally works during times of administration. She and her daughter have a very positive relationship.

Blood sugar levels are tested at 6 AM, 12 noon, and 6 PM, which Mrs. Franco is learning how to perform. Both daughter and mother are committed to the dietary regimen but are still learning the dietary exchange system.

Although Mrs. Franco is a willing learner, she confuses hypoglycemia with hyperglycemia and the associated symptoms. She also states that she can not understand why she should not clip her own toenails and she hopes to continue to do so.

ASSESSMENT

Mrs. Franco is a perfect candidate for home care support. After physician referral to a home care agency, the home care nurse will arrange for a 1½–2-hour evaluative visit. Family and client needs will be determined and a POC (plan of care) will be established collaboratively with Mrs. Franco, her daughter, her nurse and physician, and other members of the interdisciplinary team (dietitian, social worker). The overall goal is to optimize control over the diabetes, maintaining normal blood glucose levels (100–180), and prevent devastating complications such as cardiac and renal disease. The heart of home health care is teaching, teaching, and more teaching to client and family. In addition, promotion of independence and linking the client with appropriate community resources are vital to independence. The care plan reflects a community health focus. The insulin-dependent diabetes mellitus (IDDM) care pathway shows interventions, outcomes, and a summary of the visit with emphasis on the client/family goals and goal accomplishment.

The pathway is not filled in for this situation; check off what you think would be included. Use the traditional care plan as a guide.

NURSING DIAGNOSIS

Knowledge deficit related to hypoglycemia and hyperglycemia, blood glucose monitoring, and insulin administration.

Outcomes

Mrs. Franco will:
- *List signs and symptoms of hyperglycemia and hypoglycemia.*
- *Demonstrate all steps involved in insulin administration.*
- *Demonstrate all steps in blood glucose self-monitoring.*
- *Describe foot care and rationale.*
- *Make an appointment with the podiatrist.*

(continued)

CARE PLAN *continued*

Planning/Interventions

The nurse will:

- *Explain and give Mrs. Franco a list of signs and symptoms of hyperglycemia and hypoglycemia.*
- *Teach insulin preparation and administration, all steps broken down into small steps.*
- *Reinforce and teach blood glucose monitoring, all steps broken down into small steps.*
- *Explain effective foot care and rationale for foot care.*
- *Ensure the arrangement of podiatry appointment.*
- *Explore with Mrs. Franco aspects of a conservative exercise program.*

EVALUATION

Mrs. Franco has the will and ability to participate in her own diabetic care. Although she is newly diagnosed, she will learn about all aspects of her chronic disease. She will not cut her own toenails, understanding the critical importance involved if she cuts the skin and infects a toe. Blood glucose monitoring, an essential skill shown to be associated with positive diabetes management outcomes, will be carried out by Mrs. Franco twice daily. All goals will be accomplished within a 3-month period of time.

NURSING DIAGNOSIS

Risk for impaired skin integrity related to altered metabolic state.

Outcomes

Mrs. Franco will:

- *Assess her own skin with assistance from her daughter.*
- *Be able to identify a skin problem.*
- *Provide her own skin care.*
- *Maintain proper hydration and nutrition.*

Planning/Interventions

The nurse will:

- *Assess Mrs. Franco's skin using the Braden Scale.*
- *Refer to a dermatologist if assessment findings are abnormal.*
- *Teach Mrs. Franco and her daughter how to assess the skin and identify a problem.*
- *Explain the importance and connection between optimum skin integrity, drinking 8–10 glasses of water daily, dietary adherence, and normalization of blood glucose levels.*

EVALUATION

Mrs. Franco and her daughter will regularly screen for skin problems. They will be able to prevent or identify early any open areas or infections. They will adhere to nutrition and hydration guidelines consistent with healthy skin.

NURSING DIAGNOSIS

Risk of infection related to diabetes, a chronic disease.

Outcomes

Mrs. Franco will:

- *List signs and symptoms of infection for older adults, systemic (atypical presentation) and localized.*
- *Explain the effects of infection on blood glucose levels.*

(continued)

CARE PLAN *continued*

- *Describe when to call her physician/advanced practitioner.*
- *Describe what to do with diet and insulin on "sick days."*

Planning/Interventions

The nurse will:
- *Explain signs and symptoms of infection and the importance of observation.*
- *Describe an emergency situation such as diabetic ketoacidosis and calling 911.*

EVALUATION

Mrs. Franco will list the signs and symptoms of infection and the importance of prevention. She will verbalize what to look for and how to observe for these symptoms. Mrs. Franco and her daughter will explain how to respond and adjust to new problems and when to call 911.

client's name. There are circumstances where the home health nurse finds it necessary to discuss the client's case, but it is important not to compromise the privacy of the home health client.

Confidentiality refers to not sharing information about the home health client or allowing anyone to see the client's record unless permission is obtained from the client. One of the forms the home health client signs on admission addresses confidentiality. The home health client is assured that the case will only be discussed with the physician or another nurse for consultation purposes. Another issue of confidentiality is the disclosing of a diagnosis. There are some diagnoses that could potentially injure the home health client if certain persons were to be aware of the diagnosis. Some examples include AIDs and mental illnesses (Brent, 1997).

The home health nurse must also be careful with the client's records. It is not unusual for the nurse to take the records home overnight. The nurse is responsible for not allowing the records to sit out so that anyone could see the name of the client or the nature of the illness. This is also true within the home health agency. Different personnel handle the charts for various reasons and they, too, are held responsible for maintaining confidentiality. Breach of privacy or confidentiality could have legal ramifications. Nurses need to be knowledgeable of the state's nurse practice act and rules and regulations governing client privacy and confidentiality.

Paternalism is an ethical principle that needs discussing in home health care. The nurse, physician, and caregiver or family member often believe that they know what is best for the home health client. The client's wishes might be in opposition to others, but the client has the right to self-determination. Self-determination

corresponds to autonomy. If the client is mentally capable of making decisions, then he or she should be allowed to make autonomous decisions regarding health treatment. When the decisions made by the client will result in unsafe consequences, an ethical dilemma exists.

Beneficence applies to the home health nurse as goals are established and services obtained. It is the responsibility of the nurse to weigh the benefits, risks, and harm of the goals and services. An example is that of discharging a client from home health services. The nurse must weigh the benefits of discharging the client against any risks and harm that might occur because of the discharge (Cary, 1995). Unfortunately, there are no easy answers.

Home health care poses ethical and legal issues not found in the acute care setting or in a long-term care setting. Home health nurses need to be familiar with ethical decision-making models to guide them when dilemmas arise in home health. The nurse not only needs to be aware of the nurse practice act and standards of care but also needs to be knowledgeable of state laws governing assisted suicides and other matters of this nature (Robbins, 1996).

Think About It

- What ethical dilemma exists when the home health nurse believes the client should move to an assisted-living facility and leave his or her home of 50 years for safety reasons and the client adamantly opposes moving?
- How does the home health nurse justify allowing the client's self-determination and autonomy?
- What are the benefits and risks of each decision?

INSULIN DEPENDENT DIABETES MELLITUS

SKILLED NURSING PATHWAY

PATIENT NAME	PATIENT ID#
DATE OPENED	DATE CLOSED

STANDARD

The physical assessment standard and standard for nursing interventions are based on the Agency for Health Care Policy and Research (AHCPR) guidelines for nursing care of the patient with Insulin Dependent Diabetes Mellitus.

DISCHARGE CRITERIA

1. Client will demonstrate understanding of IDDM and self-care requirements
2. Client will demonstrate competent insulin management
3. Client will demonstrate integration of dietary requirements into daily life
4. Blood glucose levels will stabilize within an acceptable range of values.

NURSING DIAGNOSES (Choose appropriate diagnoses from the list below)

1. Knowledge deficit regarding disease process and self-care
2. Alteration in metabolism of glucose and production of insulin.
3. Knowledge deficit related to medications use.
4. Alteration of lifestyle secondary to disease.
5. Knowledge deficit related to dietary restrictions
6. Other (specify):

TEACHING TOOLS

Medication Teaching Sheets
IDDM Patient Teaching Packet

SN VISIT FREQUENCY
Recommended: 12-15 visits
Other Disciplines Active in Care Plan: ☐ PT   ☐ OT   ☐ ST   ☐ MSW ☐ HHA ☐ Other:

VARIANCE CODES:

A: Patient too physically impaired/ill   E: Equipment problems
B: Co-morbid interference   F: Pt/CG learning difficulties
C: Psychosocial issues interfering   G: Pt/CG decision
D: Caregiver limitations/difficulties   H: Does not apply (explain)

Nursing Pathway. This pathway includes first and second visits. *Courtesy of Connecticut VNA, Inc.*

INSULIN DEPENDENT DIABETES MELLITUS
PATIENT OUTCOME LOG: SKILLED NURSING

For each visit made, enter date of visit and place a check-mark (√) next to any outcomes achieved during the visit. If an outcome can not be achieved during this plan of care due to some interfering factor, enter a variance code from the list at the bottom of the page. Explain the use of a variance code in the "Explanation of Variances" area.

DATE OF VISIT:															
VISIT #	1	2	3	4	5	6	7	8	9	10	11	12	13	14	15
Patient will demonstrate insulin preparation															
Patient will demonstrate insulin administration and site rotation															
Patient will demonstrate skin care/skin inspection techniques															
Patient will demonstrate ability to order supplies and equipment independently															
Patient will verbalize methods for managing sick days															
Patient will verbalize preventive measures/ corrective actions to take for hypo/ hyperglycemia															
Patient will demonstrate ability to obtain and prepare foods within the prescribed diet															
Patient will state onset, peak, and duration of prescribed insulin															
Patient will state s/s of infection and implications of infection for the diabetic															
Patient will verbalize basic understanding of disease process and chronic complications of diabetes															
Patient will demonstrate ability to log, interpret, and respond to symptoms related to diabetes															
Patient will exhibit blood glucose values within an acceptable range															
Patient will demonstrate integration of a routine exercise and weight control program into daily living.															
Patient will verbalize understanding of need for ongoing dental, medical, and eye care services.															
Patient will identify family/community resources for support in management of diabetes.															
Other:															
Other:															
TOTAL GOALS MET THIS VISIT															
INITIALS OF RN															

EXPLANATION OF VARIANCES:

SIGNATURE BLOCK: NAME/TITLE _____ INITIALS _____
                     NAME/TITLE _____ INITIALS _____
                     NAME/TITLE _____ INITIALS _____
                     NAME/TITLE _____ INITIALS _____

TOTAL OUTCOMES MET: _____
TOTAL POSSIBLE: _____
%ACHIEVED (ACHIEVED/POSSIBLE):   _____

VARIANCE CODES:
A: Patient too physically impaired/ill   E: Equipment problems
B: Co-morbid interference   F: Pt/CG learning difficulties
C: Psychosocial issues interfering   G: Pt/CG decision
D: Caregiver limitations/difficulties   H: Does not apply (explain)

INSULIN DEPENDENT DIABETES MELLITUS
SKILLED NURSING PATHWAY

PATIENT NAME:		DATE	
PATIENT SIGNATURE:	INSURANCE TYPE/ PAYOR:	ID#	**VISIT 1**

CONFINED TO HOME DUE TO:	NOT CONFINED TO HOME DUE TO:
Unable to leave home w/o use of device/another person due to:	Attends **SOCIAL** adult day care program
Trips out of home are medically contraindicated due to:	Leaves home frequently without assistance
Experiencing extreme weakness/pain related to illness/surgery:	Leaves home for long periods of time without asst.
Cardio/respiratory tolerance to ambulate only ___ ft. due to:	Other:
Unsafe to leave home due to psychiatric illness:	
Other (specify):	

SUBJECTIVE DATA/PRIMARY COMPLAINT PER PATIENT:

VITAL SIGNS/ASSESSMENT STATISTICS/LAB VALUES

Temp	BP: lying/sitting/standing	PEDAL EDEMA:		LAB VALUES:
Resp	Right	Left instep	Right instep	O2 sat resting: activity:
Radial Pulse	Left	Left ankle	Right ankle	Protime INR
Apical Pulse	Abd Girth (cm)	Left calf	Right calf	FBS/RBS
Weight actual/reported:	Other:	pitting/non-pitting	pitting/non-pitting	Other:

NURSING ASSESSMENT/OBSERVATION: MARK ALL APPLICABLE WITH AN "X"; CIRCLE APPROPRIATE ITEM(S) SEPARATED BY "/".

CARDIOVASCULAR	GI/DIGESTIVE	GENITOURINARY	NEUROSENSORY
WNL	WNL	WNL	WNL
fluid retention	nausea/vomiting	distention/retention	headache
chest pain	epigastric distress	frequency/urgency	grasp:
neck vein distention	difficulty swallowing	hesitancy	left
(+) peripheral pulses L/R	abdominal distention	hematuria	right
abnormal heart sounds	diarrhea	bladder incontinence	pupil reaction
cyanosis	constipation/impact.	catheter:	left:
RESPIRATORY	bowel incontinence	burning/pain	right:
WNL	bowel sounds:	Discharge	seizures
lungs clear to auscultation	**MENTAL STATUS**	**NUTRITION**	tremors
lung sounds diminished:	alert/oriented	Appetite:	speech impairment
lung sounds absent:	lethargic	hydration:	hearing impairment
dyspnea/SOB	agitated	anorexia	visual impairment
orthopnea	forgetful	obesity	decreased sensitivity
crackles/rhonchi/wheeze	disoriented		syncope
cough: productive/non-prod.	comatose		
sputum:			

MS/MOBILITY		
Ambulates unassisted	Ambulating with assistance	weakness:
Ambulates with assistive device	Non-ambulatory	unsteady gait/fall risk

PAIN MANAGEMENT

No pain per client	Per patient, pain affects: sleep physical activity appetite emotions concentration other:
intermittent/continuous	Location of pain
sharp/dull/ache	Per patient, rate level of pain: LEAST 0 1 2 3 4 5 6 7 8 9 10 WORST

Pain treatment/effectiveness:

SKIN/WOUND CARE For all wound treatments, reference the Wound Assessment/Treatment Plan for assessment key and current Rx orders.

WNL	rashes	bruising	turgor: good /fair/poor
jaundice	diaphoretic	rash/itching	pressure ulcer/wounds

SEE WOUND ASSESSMENT/RX AREA BELOW

WOUND #	WIDTH cms	LENGTH cms	DEPTH cms	DRAINAGE	TUNNELING	UNDER- MINING	TISSUE DESCRIP.	TISSUE EDGES	SURR. SKIN
					___ cm ___ o'clock	___ cm ___ o'clock			
					___ cm ___ o'clock	___ cm ___ o'clock			

PRESSURE RELIEVING DEVICE: ☐ Not applicable OR specify type:

ADDITIONAL CLINICAL FINDINGS/NARRATIVE COMMENTS:

INTERPRETATION OF CLINICAL FINDINGS BY NURSE:

Pathway continued.

IDDM NURSING PATHWAY—VISIT 1
PAGE 2/2

MEDICATION MANAGEMENT:.
☐ Written medication information given to patient ☐ Adheres to medication regimen ☐ Verbalized dose/schedule
☐ Medications re-ordered: ☐ Med box prefill from (date) to (date)
☐ Medications assessed for side effects/contraindications/effectiveness. Medications instructed (specify):

TREATMENTS/PROCEDURES
☐ Medication administered by nurse(specify med, dose, route, site, response):

☐ Other treatment/procedure performed by nurse:

ALLIED HEALTH FINDINGS

☐ Impaired ADLs	☐ Psychosocial interference with care plan	☐ Speech/swallowing difficulties/impairment	Other:
☐ Impaired IADLs	☐ Financial issues impacting care plan	☐ Impaired cognition	
☐ Fall Risk	☐ Nutritional status impacting recovery		

☐ Consult with/make referral to/other action taken:

TEACHING/TRAINING

Instructions given to: ☐ Pt. ☐ PCG. ☐ Other:	Teaching/training regarding:	☐ Instructed ☐ Reinstructed	Retention verified via: ☐ demonstration ☐ verbal response	Level of understanding: ☐ Complete ☐ Partial ☐ None
Instructions given to: ☐ Pt. ☐ PCG ☐ Other:	Teaching/training regarding:	☐ Instructed ☐ Reinstructed	Retention verified via: ☐ demonstration ☐ verbal response	Level of understanding: ☐ Complete ☐ Partial ☐ None

CLIENT RESPONSE TO CARE Document response to treatments and interventions, progress toward discharge goals, and understanding of and compliance with treatments/interventions.

PLAN FOR NEXT VISIT: (include follow-up to treatments, interventions, and demonstrations) **Approx. Next Visit Date:**

COORDINATION OF CARE: Document case conference content on Conference Form ☐ CC WITH (NAME):
☐ TELEPHONE CALL TO:
Next MD appt:
Care Plan Management/Discharge Planning: Care Plan [ ] Reviewed and/or [ ] revised with patient/cg involvement;
Discharge plan [ ] formulated with patient/PCG [ ] Reviewed with patient/PCG

HOME HEALTH AIDE (CIRCLE ONE) ORIENTATION/SUPERVISION-- Name of HHAide:

Yes	No	Orientation/Supervision Activity	Yes	No	Orientation/Supervision/ Activity
		Patient care plan revised/updated/reviewed by nurse			Care given as per the aide care plan
		Patient care needs reviewed by aide prior to starting care			Standard precautions practiced by aide
		Pt/PCG participated in POC changes prior to implementation			Continued need for home health aide services
		Rapport between aide and Pt/cg satisfactory			Follow up required (specify)
Activities requiring specific instruction and return demonstration:			Other activities performed/observed		

DISCHARGE CRITERIA
1. Client will demonstrate understanding of IDDM and self-care requirements
2. Client will demonstrate competent insulin management
3. Client will demonstrate integration of dietary requirements into daily life
4. Blood glucose levels will stabilize within an acceptable range of values.

SIGNATURE/TITLE

Pathway continued.

INSULIN DEPENDENT DIABETES MELLITUS: SKILLED NURSING PATHWAY

PATIENT NAME:		DATE	
PATIENT SIGNATURE:	INSURANCE TYPE/ PAYOR:	ID#	**VISIT 2**

CONFINED TO HOME DUE TO:	NOT CONFINED TO HOME DUE TO:
Unable to leave home w/o use of device/another person due to:	Attends **SOCIAL** adult day care program
Trips out of home are medically contraindicated due to:	Leaves home frequently without assistance
Experiencing extreme weakness/pain related to illness/surgery:	Leaves home for long periods of time without asst.
Cardio/respiratory tolerance to ambulate only _____ ft. due to:	Other:
Unsafe to leave home due to psychiatric illness:	
Other (specify):	

SUBJECTIVE DATA/PRIMARY COMPLAINT PER PATIENT:

VITAL SIGNS/ASSESSMENT STATISTICS/LAB VALUES

Temp	BP: lying/sitting/standing	PEDAL EDEMA:		LAB VALUES:
Resp	Right	Left instep	Right instep	O2 sat resting: activity:
Radial Pulse	Left	Left ankle	Right ankle	Protime INR
Apical Pulse	Abd Girth (cm)	Left calf	Right calf	FBS/RBS
Weight actual/reported:	Other:	pitting/non-pitting	pitting/non-pitting	Other:

NURSING ASSESSMENT/OBSERVATION: MARK ALL APPLICABLE WITH AN "X": CIRCLE APPROPRIATE ITEM(S) SEPARATED BY "/".

CARDIOVASCULAR	GI/DIGESTIVE	GENITOURINARY	NEUROSENSORY
WNL	WNL	WNL	WNL
fluid retention	nausea/vomiting	distention/retention	headache
chest pain	epigastric distress	frequency/urgency	grasp:
neck vein distention	difficulty swallowing	hesitancy	left
(+) peripheral pulses L/R	abdominal distention	hematuria	right
abnormal heart sounds	diarrhea	bladder incontinence	pupil reaction
cyanosis	constipation/impact.	catheter:	left:
RESPIRATORY	bowel incontinence	burning/pain	right:
WNL	bowel sounds:	Discharge	seizures
lungs clear to auscultation	**MENTAL STATUS**	**NUTRITION**	tremors
lung sounds diminished:	alert/oriented	Appetite:	speech impairment
lung sounds absent:	lethargic	hydration:	hearing impairment
dyspnea/SOB	agitated	anorexia	visual impairment
orthopnea	forgetful	obesity	decreased sensitivity
crackles/rhonchi/wheeze	disoriented		syncope
cough: productive/non-prod.	comatose		
sputum:			

MS/MOBILITY

Ambulates unassisted	Ambulating with assistance	weakness:
Ambulates with assistive device	Non-ambulatory	unsteady gait/fall risk

PAIN MANAGEMENT

No pain per client	Per patient, pain affects: sleep physical activity appetite emotions concentration other:
intermittent/continuous	Location of pain
sharp/dull/ache	Per patient, rate level of pain: LEAST 0 1 2 3 4 5 6 7 8 9 10 WORST

Pain treatment/effectiveness:

SKIN/WOUND CARE   For all wound treatments, reference the Wound Assessment/Treatment Plan for assessment key and current Rx orders.

WNL	rashes	bruising	turgor: good /fair/poor
jaundice	diaphoretic	rash/itching	pressure ulcer/wounds
			SEE WOUND ASSESSMENT/RX AREA BELOW

WOUND #	WIDTH cms	LENGTH cms	DEPTH cms	DRAINAGE	TUNNELING	UNDER-MINING	TISSUE DESCRIP.	TISSUE EDGES	SURR. SKIN
					_____ cm _____ o'clock	_____ cm _____ o'clock			
					_____ cm _____ o'clock	_____ cm _____ o'clock			

PRESSURE RELIEVING DEVICE: ☐ Not applicable OR specify type:

ADDITIONAL CLINICAL FINDINGS/NARRATIVE COMMENTS:

INTERPRETATION OF CLINICAL FINDINGS BY NURSE:

IDDM NURSING PATHWAY—PAGE 2/2

MEDICATION MANAGEMENT:.

☐ Written medication information given to patient   ☐ Adheres to medication regimen   ☐ Verbalized dose/schedule
☐ Medications re-ordered: ☐ Med box prefill from (date) _____ to (date) _____
☐ Medications assessed for side effects/contraindications/effectiveness. Medications instructed (specify):

TREATMENTS/PROCEDURES

☐ Medication administered by nurse(specify med, dose, route, site, response):

☐ Other treatment/procedure performed by nurse:

ALLIED HEALTH FINDINGS

☐ Impaired ADLs	☐ Psychosocial interference with care plan	☐ Speech/swallowing difficulties/impairment	Other:
☐ Impaired IADLs	☐ Financial issues impacting care plan	☐ Impaired cognition	
☐ Fall Risk	☐ Nutritional status impacting recovery		

☐ Consult with/make referral to/other action taken:

INTERVENTIONS	√	INTERVENTIONS	√
Teach disease process; assess understanding		Teach/demonstrate insulin preparation and admin.	
Instruct on skin care/daily examination of skin for open areas; teach foot care; assess compliance		Instruct in all medication effects, side-effects, and contraindications; leave medication schedule in home	
Teach s/s of hypo/hyperglycemia and corrective action to take if noted		Teach role of ongoing dental care, eye care, and general medical care in disease management	
Teach finger stick blood glucose testing; teach interpretation of results		Teach site rotation and site rotation logs	
Instruct on s/s of infection and effect upon diabetes		Instruct on Medic-Alert bracelets and need to identify self as a diabetic	
Teach chronic complications of diabetes; assess for neuropathy, retinopathy, ASHD, UTI, et al		Instruct on insulin onset, peak, and duration and on the types of insulin available and their differences	
Instruct on management of sick days		Assess diet knowledge; have pt keep 3 day diet log	
Teach emergency procedures and identify family/social resources; identify environmental hazards		Teach _____ cal. ADA diet based on calorie needs, ability to purchase foods, and customary diet pattern	
Teach relationship of activity to bl glu levels and the role of regular exercise in disease management		Assess understanding and compliance to diet plan; teach relationship of food to blood glucose levels	
Teach proper handling/disposal of sharps		Other interventions:	

CLIENT RESPONSE TO CARE Document response to treatments and interventions, progress toward discharge goals, and understanding of and compliance with treatments/interventions.

PLAN FOR NEXT VISIT: (include follow-up to treatments, interventions, and demonstrations) **Approx. Next Visit Date:**

COORDINATION OF CARE: Document case conference content on Conference Form   ☐ CC WITH (NAME):
☐ TELEPHONE CALL TO:
Next MD appt:
Care Plan Management/Discharge Planning: Care Plan [ ] Reviewed and/or **[ ]** revised with patient/cg involvement;
Discharge plan [ ] formulated with patient/PCG **[ ]** Reviewed with patient/PCG

HOME HEALTH AIDE (CIRCLE ONE) ORIENTATION/SUPERVISION-- Name of HHAide:

Yes	No	Orientation/Supervision Activity	Yes	No	Orientation/Supervision/ Activity
		Patient care plan revised/updated/reviewed by nurse			Care given as per the aide care plan
		Patient care needs reviewed by aide prior to starting care			Standard precautions practiced by aide
		Pt/PCG participated in POC changes prior to implementation			Continued need for home health aide services
		Rapport between aide and Pt/cg satisfactory			Follow up required (specify)
Activities requiring specific instruction and return demonstration:			Other activities performed/observed		

SIGNATURE/TITLE

Pathway continued.

Future of Home Health Care

The home health industry is currently undergoing major changes. The majority of these changes are the result of the passage of the Balanced Budget Act of 1997 (BBA). Home care agencies, recipients, providers, insurers, and suppliers are affected. Some services are no longer covered by Medicare, reimbursement by Medicare to home health agencies has changed, and more changes are scheduled to occur. The changes to home health care are the result of the tremendous growth of the home health industry, the amount of Medicare dollars spent on home health care, and the discovery of fraud and abuse within the industry. Home health agencies are investigating new and innovative ways to deliver home health care that will continue to benefit the client while being cost-effective and efficient (Harris, 1998).

The result of some of the changes that occurred are more older adults being admitted to nursing facilities, more family members having to provide care, and an increase in the use of state-funded programs (Rosenzweig, 1995). Home health nurses are in an ideal position to be advocates for their clients and demonstrate the need for home health care. Registered nurses need to develop ways to deliver care that is less costly and yet results in the same quality of care.

Another issue surrounding home health care is the educational preparation of home health nurses. Associate degree and diploma programs do not always include home health or community health nursing in their programs. As home health nurses have some of the most autonomy of all specialties, it is imperative that they have the knowledge base on which to develop plans of care and make independent decisions that will provide the home health client with quality care that is cost-effective and efficient. Some universities have graduate programs that focus on home health care. It is important that home health nurses receive the needed education to practice home health care, whether that education is at the basic nursing education level or within the home health agency in a mentoring program.

Summary

As the older population increases, the health care field faces new challenges. People are living longer and wanting to remain independent. At this same time, funds for home health care for people age 65 years and older are decreasing. Nurses are challenged to develop new ways to deliver quality care to the older adult in the home. Nurses are also faced with demonstrating cost savings that are attributed to home health care. Continuing changes in the health care delivery system can be seen as a challenge and opportunity for nurses to become involved in public policy debates regarding health care issues.

The future of home health can be exciting and a time of recognition and growth for the home health nurse. The goal of home health care has not changed. It remains to help the older adult enjoy a good quality of life. As nursing enters the twenty-first century, the home health nurse will be an important part of assisting the older adult to remain as independent as possible for as long as possible in the home environment.

Review Questions and Activities

1. What is the purpose of home health care?

2. How do home health services assist older adults to remain in their own homes?

3. What are the criteria for admission to home health care?

4. What disciplines are involved in delivering home health care?

5. What is the relationship between functional status and home health for an older adult?

6. What are the positive aspects of case management?

7. What is the importance of documentation by all disciplines in home health care?

8. How does discharge planning in home health care differ from acute care?

9. How does Medicare determine coverage for home health care services?

10. How does a home health care agency protect a client's autonomy when nurses' notes and orders are faxed to the agency and accessible to everyone in the office?

References

Ainsworth, E. (1995). Role of occupational therapy in home care. In K. Morgan & S. McClain (Eds.), *Core curriculum for home health care nursing* (pp. 39–44). Gaithersburg, MD: Aspen.

American Nurses Association. (1986). *Standards of home health nursing practice*. Washington, DC: Author.

Apple, R., & Truscott, S. (1995). Role of homemaker/home health aide in home care. In K. Morgan & S. McClain (Eds.), *Core curriculum for home health care nursing* (pp. 57–65). Gaithersburg, MD: Aspen.

A profile of older Americans 1999. (1999). Washington, DC: American Association of Retired Persons and the Administration on Aging, U.S. Department of Health and Human Services.

Asbour-Arnold, S., & Jairath, N. (1998). Acute myocardial infarction: Early recognition and management from the home healthcare nurse's perspective. *Home Healthcare Nurse, 16*(6), 379–386.

Atchley, R. (1997). *Social forces and aging* (8th ed.). Belmont, CA: Wadsworth.

Beacon Health Corporation. (1998, May). An outline for staff education on the OASIS instrument. *Homecare Direction, 6*(5), 6–8.

Brent, N. (1997). Legalities in home care. *Home Healthcare Nurse, 15*(4), 256–258.

Campbell, S. (1995). Role of the physical therapy in home care. In K. Morgan & S. McClain (Eds.), *Core curriculum for home health care nursing* (pp. 5–38). Gaithersburg, MD: Aspen.

Cary, A. (1995). Ethical considerations for the home health nurse. In K. Morgan & S. McClain (Eds.), *Core curriculum for home health care nursing* (pp. 391–398). Gaithersburg, MD: Aspen.

Cho, C. Y., & Kamen, G. (1998). Detecting balance deficits in frequent fallers using clinical and quantitative evaluation tools. *Journal of the American Geriatrics Society, 46*(4), 426–430.

Clemen-Stone, S., Eigsti, D., & McGuire, S. (1991). *Comprehensive family and community health nursing* (3rd ed.). St. Louis: Mosby.

Emlet, C., & Crabtree, J. (1996). Introduction to in-home assessment of older adults. In C. Emlet, J. Crabtree, V. Condon, & L. Treml (Eds.), *In-home assessment of older adults* (pp. 1–16). Gaithersburg, MD: Aspen.

Fortin, J., Yeaw, E., Campbell, S., & Jameson, S. (1998). An analysis of risk assessment tolls for falls in the elderly. *Home Healthcare Nurse, 16*(9), 624–629.

Harris, M. (1998). Medicare and the nurse. *Home Healthcare Nurse, 16*(7), 435–437.

Health Care Financing Administration. (1999, January 25). Rules and Regulations. *Federal Register, 64*(15), 3747–3763.

Huggins, C., & Phillips, C. (1998). Using case management with clinical plans to improve patient outcomes. *Home Healthcare Nurse, 16*(1), 15–20.

Humphrey, C., & Milone-Nuzzo, P. (1996). *Orientation to home care nursing*. Gaithersburg, MD: Aspen.

Lange, M. (1996). The challenge of fall prevention in home care: A review of the literature. *Home Healthcare Nurse, 14*(3), 198–206.

McCann, J., & Christiansen, K. (1996). Home care. In A. Lueckenotte (Ed.), *Gerontologic nursing* (pp. 913–943). St. Louis: Mosby.

McClain, S. (1995). History of home health care nursing. In K. Morgan & S. McClain (Eds.), *Core curriculum for home health care nursing* (pp. 3–6). Gaithersburg, MD: Aspen.

Morgan, K. (1995). Role of social work in home care. In K. Morgan & S. McClain (Eds.), *Core curriculum for home health care nursing* (pp. 54–56). Gaithersburg, MD: Aspen.

Morgan, K., & McClain, S. (1995). Role of the registered nurse in home care. In K. Morgan & S. McClain (Eds.), *Core curriculum for home health care nursing* (pp. 7–12). Gaithersburg, MD: Aspen.

Moulton, P., Wray-Langevine, J., & Boyer, C. (1997). Implementing clinical pathways: One agency's experience. *Home Healthcare Nurse, 15*(5), 343–354.

National Association for Home Care. (1996). Inventory of home care agencies for total agencies, and HCFA, Health Standards and Quality Bureau and Bureau of Policy Development for Medicare-certified agencies. [On-line]. Available: www.nach.org/consumer/hcstats.html.

Neal, L. (1997). Basic musculoskeletal assessment: Tips for the home health nurse. *Home Healthcare Nurse, 15*(4), 227–233.

OASIS Education and Training. (1999, June). OASIS assessment reference sheet. [On-line]. Available:

http://www.hfca.gov.medicare/hsqb/oasis/ hhedtrng.htm.

O'Neill, C., & Sorensen, E. (1991). Home care of the elderly: A family perspective. *Advances in Nursing Science, 13*(4), 28–37.

Robbins, D. (1996). *Ethical and legal issues in home health and long-term care.* Gaithersburg, MD: Aspen

Rosenzweig, E. (1995). Trends in home care entitlements and benefits. *Journal of Gerontological Social Work, 24*(3/4), 9–29.

Shaughnessy, P., Crisler, K., Schlenker, R., & Hittle, D. (1998, June). Medicare OASIS: Standardized outcome and assessment information set for home health care. *Center for Health Services and Policy Research, Denver, CO,* OASIS-B1, 1–3.

Steele, H. (1995). Role of speech-language pathology services in home care. In K. Morgan & S. McClain (Eds.), *Core curriculum for home health care nursing* (pp. 45–53). Gaithersburg, MD: Aspen.

Resources

Home Care Association of America: **www.hcaa-homecare.com**

National Association of Home Care: **www.nahc.org**

Administration on Aging: **www.aoa.dhhs.gov**

National Institutes of Health: **www.nih.gov**

OASIS: **www.hcfa.gov/medicare/hsqb/oasis/hhregs.htm**

KEY TERMS

bereavement

certified hospice palliative nurse (CHPN)

continuum of care settings

curative care

dying well

end-of-life care

good death

holistic approach

hospice

interdisciplinary team

palliative care

physician-assisted suicide

symptom management

terminally ill

trajectory

wellness in dying

Hospice and Palliative Care

Barbara M. Raudonis, PhD, RN, CS

COMPETENCIES

After completing this chapter, the reader should be able to:

- *Describe the major issues driving the renewed interest in end-of-life care in the United States.*
- *Discuss the historical development of hospice care.*
- *Differentiate between the different models of hospice care.*
- *Discuss the philosophy and outcomes of end-of-life care.*
- *Explain the services provided by the hospice interdisciplinary team.*
- *Describe the hospice insurance benefit according to private insurers, health maintenance organizations, and Medicare.*
- *Apply nursing interventions related to dying, death, and bereavement.*
- *Define the difference between hospice and palliative care.*
- *Discuss trends in palliative care.*
- *Design new approaches to meet the end-of-life needs of older adults using a continuum of palliative care services.*

MAKING THE CONNECTION

Refer to the following chapters to increase your understanding of hospice and palliative care:

- **Chapter 3** *Changes in the Health Care Delivery System Affecting Older Adults*
- **Chapter 6** *Psychological Aspects of Aging*
- **Chapter 7** *Social Aspects of Aging*
- **Chapter 13** *Assessment, Diagnosis, and Planning*
- **Chapter 25** *Ethical Theories and Principles*
- **Chapter 26** *End-of-Life Decisions and Choices*

History of Hospice

Despite modern technology, Americans fear the pain of chronic illnesses such as cancer and becoming a burden on family and friends during the **trajectory** of the illness. However, only 450,000 clients had **hospice** services in the United States in 1996. Although hospices have provided compassionate **palliative care** for **terminally ill** persons and their families in the United States for over 20 years, many people are still not aware of these services. Hospices cared for only one of every two persons dying from cancer in America in 1995. Seventy-four percent of hospice clients were 65 years of age or older (Hospice Fact Sheet, 1998).

The rapidly aging population has refocused attention on the universal need for humane end-of-life care (*Peaceful death,* 1997). Aging adults have complex needs that require care across the **continuum of care settings:** hospitals, day services, home care, long-term care, and hospices. The National Hospice Organization's (NHO) census figures show that 77% of hospice clients died in their own personal residence, 19% died in an institutional facility, and 4% in other settings (Hospice Fact Sheet, 1998).

The public's perception of the process of dying in American hospitals frequently involves intense use of medical life support and inadequately relieved pain and suffering (Oddi & Cassidy, 1998). These perceptions were confirmed in a recent research study. The major findings of the multimillion dollar intervention Study to Understand Prognosis and Preferences for Outcomes and Risks of Treatment (SUPPORT) were that (a) increased efforts to improve communication about clients' preferences for end-of-life care to physicians did not have a significant impact on the care that is provided in hospitals and (b) improved communications alone is not enough in providing quality, compassionate care for the dying (SUPPORT, 1995). These dismal results have provided a focal point for innovative national initiatives to improve end-of-life care, federal funding for end-of-life research, private foundation financial support, and other action plans to improve the quality of end-of-life care in the United States.

However, the American public has already responded to their own fears about dying by approving initiatives such as in Oregon that permit **physician-assisted suicide.** This course of action was enabled by the U.S. Supreme Court ruling that the states maintain jurisdiction over the end-of-life issue of physician-assisted suicide. Other individuals continue to seek the services of Dr. Kervorkian to maintain control of their end-of-life experiences. The American Medical Association and the American Nurses Association oppose the concept of physician-assisted suicide.

Ask Yourself

What is your opinion of physician-assisted suicide?

Finally, the financial impact of the intense use of medical technology at the end of life has given insurance programs an incentive to explore alternative forms of care as a form of cost cutting. Together, all the above issues provide the background for the increasing interest in **end-of-life care.**

The Latin origin of the word *hospice* traces back to the word *hospis* and practices related to hospitality and hospitable. Pilgrims making the grueling journey to the Holy Lands during the Middle Ages found respite, food, and water at way stations alongside the roads. In addition, hospices were centers of refuge for poor, sick, and dying people. The universal metaphor that death is part of the journey of life that continues into eternity was an important Christian perspective during the Middle Ages (Stoddard, 1978). This metaphor continues to be used today.

The Sisters of Charity were influential pioneers in the historical development of hospice care. Sister Mary Aikenhead of the Irish Sisters of Charity opened Our Lady's Hospice in Dublin in 1879. This hospice provided care exclusively to the terminally ill. Later in 1905, the English Sisters of Charity opened St. Joseph Hospice in London. Decades later, St. Joseph Hospice provided the inspiration and clinical expertise for Dame Cicely Saunders' vision of care for the terminally ill (Amenta, 1986).

Dame Cicely Saunders is universally considered the founder of the modern hospice movement. Her education and clinical practice include those of nurse, social worker, and physician. She founded St. Christopher's Hospice in Sydenham, England, in 1967. Dame Saunders credits her early work at St. Joseph Hospice as the foundation for pain and **symptom management,** the hallmarks of hospice care (DuBoulay, 1984). Other important innovations were the use of oral medications to prevent pain rather than the traditional use of injections to relieve pain once it occurred. Finally, the **holistic approach** of including the dying individual and family's spiritual and psychological needs was identified and encouraged by Saunders and her colleagues (Lattanzi-Licht, Mahoney, & Miller, 1998).

St. Christopher's Hospice continues as the prototype for all hospices. The types of palliative care services offered at St. Christopher's Hospice continue to evolve. The inpatient care program began in 1967 and then the home care program followed in 1969. In December 1990 the St. Christopher's Hospice Day Center opened. The purpose of the day center is to improve the quality of life of terminally ill persons through a variety of programs in a nonmedical environment. English hospice and palliative care services do not require a time limit (for example, prognosis) for eligibility. Therefore, typical day center activities may include arts and crafts projects, outings, and beauty care. In addition, the traditional services offered include a review of symptom control and medications, respite for relatives and friends, companionship of people with similar problems, opportunities to talk to others without hurting family or friends, counseling and support, and help with personal hygiene (Hayward House, 1996; St. Christopher's Hospice, 1996). However, Dame Saunders cautions that St. Christopher's Hospice should not be cloned throughout the world. The principles of hospice and palliative care must be refined within the cultural context of the needs of the individuals the hospice serves.

Historically, the next landmark in the development of hospice care was the publication of Kubler-Ross's book *On Death and Dying*. Her seminal work identified the stages of dying and brought the needs of the dying and discussion of end of life to the public. Only now, 30 years later, are these issues "gaining critical mass attention" (Lattanzi-Licht et al., 1998, p. 46).

The first hospice in the United States was a home care program established in Connecticut in 1974. The Connecticut hospice home care program became the U.S. model of hospice care and originally did not have inpatient beds, in contrast to the St. Christopher prototype. Eventually, inpatient beds were added to the Connecticut Hospice, and it became the first independent hospice inpatient facility in the United States (Lattanzi-Licht et al., 1998). In the 1990s, it is now common to find freestanding inpatient hospices, inpatient hospice units within hospitals, and hospice-designated beds scattered throughout a hospital.

Approximately 3,200 operational or planned hospice programs exist in all 50 states, the District of Columbia, and Puerto Rico. During the last 10 years the annual growth of new hospices has averaged approximately 8% (*Hospice fact sheet*, 1998). However, many questions regarding the future of hospice care in the next few years and into the twenty-first century remain unanswered. Will hospice continue to exist as a separate entity in our health care system or will the diffusion of hospice principles become integrated into the traditional health care system as Dame Cicely Saunders envisioned (DuBoulay, 1984)? These questions are yet to be answered.

Philosophy and Goals of Care

Hospice is a philosophy of care for dying persons and their families that affirms life and empowers dying persons to live with dignity, alert and pain free, while in-

volving families and loved ones in giving care that emphasizes quality of life. In addition, the hospice team facilitates the establishment of an environment where dying persons and their families have satisfactory psychological and spiritual preparation for death. Figure 21-1 illustrates some of the end-of-life issues experienced by dying persons and their families. Suffering occurs when these issues are unresolved. Hospice care is designed to eliminate suffering at end of life regardless of its cause.

Inherent in the hospice philosophy is the belief that dying is a part of living. Dying and human suffering are the unique experiences of all individuals within the cultural and spiritual context of their lives. Therefore, it is necessary to understand the personhood of our dying hospice clients to meet their needs (Byock, 1996) and the goals of hospice care.

The traditional goals of hospice care are (a) to relieve the pain and suffering of the terminally ill, (b) to make possible a **good death,** (c) to help the family, and (d) to assist in the search for meaning (Storey, 1990). However, Byock (1996, 1997) suggested that **dying well** and **wellness in dying** better describe the positive end-of-life experience desired than the term good death. He conceptualizes dying as a stage in the human life cycle that involves developmental landmarks and specific tasks for the end of life (Byock, 1996). These landmarks are listed in Box 21-1. For further elaboration on the specific tasks related to the developmental landmarks, refer to the work referenced in Box 21-1. Byock (1996) stated that for there to be a sense of growth within the midst of dying, the experience must be

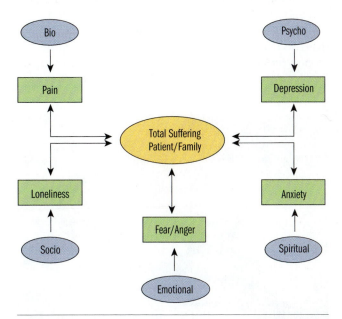

FIGURE 21-1 Bio/psycho/socio/emotional/spiritual human dynamics. *Courtesy of Gerald H. Holman, MD, FAAP, FRCPC, Crown of Texas Hospice, Amarillo, TX.*

BOX 21-1 Developmental Landmarks and Tasks for the End-of-life

- Sense of completion of worldly affairs: transfer of fiscal, legal, and formal social responsibilities

- Sense of completion in relationships with community: closure of multiple social relationships (employment, commerce, organizational, congregational); components include expressions of regret, expressions of forgiveness, acceptance of gratitude, and appreciation; leave taking: the saying of goodbye

- Sense of meaning about one's individual life: life review, the telling of "one's stories," transmission of knowledge and wisdom

- Experienced love of self: self-acknowledgment, self-forgiveness

- Experienced love of others: acceptance of worthiness

- Sense of completion in relationships with family and friends: reconciliation, fullness of communication and closure in each of one's important relationships; component tasks include expressions of regret, expressions of forgiveness

and acceptance, expressions of gratitude and appreciation, expressions of affection; leave-taking: the saying of goodbye

- Acceptance of the finality of life—of one's existence as an individual: acknowledgment of the totality of personal loss represented by one's dying and experience of personal pain of existential loss; expression of the depth of personal tragedy that dying represents; decathexis (emotional withdrawal) from worldly affairs and cathexis (emotional connection) with an enduring construct; acceptance of dependency

- Sense of a new self (personhood) beyond personal loss

- Sense of meaning about life in general: achieving a sense of awe; recognition of a transcendent realm; developing/achieving a sense of comfort with chaos

- Surrender to the transcendent, to the unknown— "letting go"

Source: *From "The Nature of Suffering and the Nature of Opportunity at the End-of-Life," by I. R. Byock, 1996,* Clinics in Geriatric Medicine, *12(2), pp. 237–252. Copyright 1996 by W. B. Saunders Company. Reprinted with permission.*

"important, valuable, and meaningful for the dying person and the family" (p. 251). See Figure 21-2.

The decade of the 1990s ushered in an era of increased accountability for the effectiveness and quality of care provided as well as for the resources used by all health care providers. The goals of hospice care were

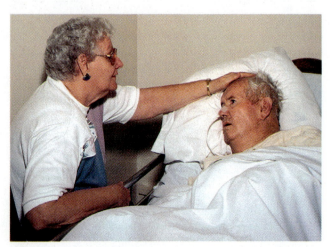

FIGURE 21-2 End-of-life tasks include the family as well as the client.

redefined in terms of outcomes of care. The NHO defined an outcome as "any result attributable to health services intervention and/or natural progression of disease or disability, including changes in physical, psychological, social and spiritual well-being and levels of function" (*A Pathway,* 1997, p. 1). The three end-result outcomes of hospice care are self-determined life closure, safe and comfortable dying, and effective grieving. Specific interventions and adequate lengths of stay as a hospice client are required for dying clients and families to achieve these outcomes (*A Pathway,* 1997). Figure 21-3 illustrates the outcomes of hospice care. Dying well is the overall goal and the end result of the interdisciplinary team's support of the dying person's self-determined life closure, safe and comfortable dying, and the family's effective grieving.

Services Provided

Major variations in the type and number of services available to hospice clients occurred during the early development of hospice care in the United States. However, when hospice services were included as part of the

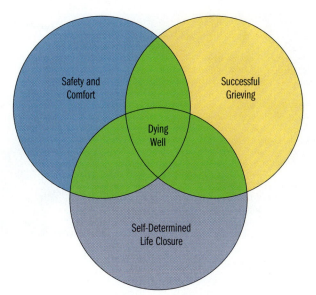

FIGURE 21-3 Outcomes of care supported by the interdisciplinary team. *Courtesy of Gerald H. Holman, MD, FAAP, FRCPC, Crown of Texas Hospice, Amarillo, TX.*

Medicare benefit, a basic level of service became the standard expectation throughout the country. To be Medicare certified, hospices have to meet the federally imposed standard level of services. These services are listed in Box 21-2.

The underlying assumption of all hospice services is the goal of comfort versus cure. Hospice care is palliative, or comfort, care. The NHO's definition of palliative care provides specific guidelines for hospice professionals to use in determining what type of interventions can be offered as part of their services. The critical com-

ponent in the NHO definition of palliative care is the agreement between hospice professionals, the client, and family caregiver that the goals of enhancing comfort and improving quality of life are met by the specific interventions. Both the NHO and World Health Organization's (WHO) definitions of palliative care are included in Box 21-3. Although similar, the two definitions contain different nuances so that when the definitions are taken together, hospice professionals have specific guidelines to follow when choosing appropriate interventions.

Interdisciplinary Team

The **interdisciplinary team (IDT)** is the foundation and hallmark of hospice care. The team meets regularly, usually once a week, to discuss and make plans to meet the complex physical, spiritual, emotional, and social needs of the dying person and family during the dying process and throughout the period of bereavement. The complexity of the needs of dying persons requires the strength of an interdisciplinary team approach (Eng, 1993). In addition, the interdisciplinary team is mandated by the Medicare regulations.

The core members of the interdisciplinary team include the dying person's personal physician, the hospice registered nurse, the hospice physician, social worker, clergy, certified nurse aides, and volunteers. Other team members, such as nutritionists, physical and occupational therapists, and speech-language pathologists, are included in the plan of care depending on the needs of the dying person and family. In addition, there is an increasing demand for complementary therapies. Some examples include art, music, massage, and aroma therapies.

BOX 21-2   Basic Level of Services Required to Become a Medicare Certified Hospice

General Provisions and Administration
Governing body
Medical director
Continuation of data
In-service training
Interdisciplinary group
Licensure
Professional management
Plan of care
Informed consent
Quality assurance
Volunteers
Central clinical records

Core Services
Nursing services
Medical social services
Physician services
Counseling services

Other Services
Physical therapy
Speech-language pathology
Home health aides
Short-term inpatient care
Occupational therapy
Medical supplies
Homemakers services

Source: *Adapted from* The hospice choice: In pursuit of a peaceful death, *by M. Lattanzi-Licht, J. J. Mahoney, and G. W. Miller, 1998, New York: Fireside.*

BOX 21-3　Definitions of Palliative Care

World Health Organization

The active total care of clients whose disease is not responsive to curative treatment. Control of pain, of other symptoms, and of psychological, social, and spiritual problems is paramount. The goal of palliative care is achievement of the best quality of life for clients and families. It affirms life and regards dying as a normal process. Palliative care neither hastens nor postpones death. It emphasizes relief from spiritual aspects of client care and offers a support system to help the family cope during the client's illness and in their own bereavement.

National Hospice Organization

The treatment that enhances comfort and improves the quality of the client's life. No specific therapy is excluded from consideration. The test of palliative treatment lies in the agreement by the client, the physician, the primary caregiver, and the hospice team that the expected outcome is relief from distressing symptoms, easing of pain, and enhancement of quality of life. The decision to intervene with an active palliative treatment is based on the treatment's ability to meet the stated goals rather than its effect on the underlying disease. Each client's needs must continue to be assessed, and all treatment options evaluated in the context of the client's values and symptoms.

Sources: *Adapted from* Cancer pain relief and palliative care *(Technical Report Series 804), 1990, Geneva: World Health Organization;* Introduction. Oxford textbook of palliative medicine *(2nd ed.), D. Doyle, G. Hanks, and N. MacDonald, Eds., 1998, Oxford: Oxford University Press; and* Standards of a hospice program of care, *1993, Alexandria, VA: National Hospice Organization.*

Counseling services are available for hospice clients and their families. After the death of the hospice client, survivors are followed up to a year after the death. **Bereavement** services are available to assist as needed in achieving effective grieving and healing (Figure 21-4).

Ask Yourself

How do you feel about the death of a newborn versus the death of an 85-year-old?

The roles and responsibilities of the core team members are common to all hospices. The primary responsibility of the team is to discuss, review, and revise the plans of care for clients and families (Eng, 1993). All team members serve as competent caregivers and educators

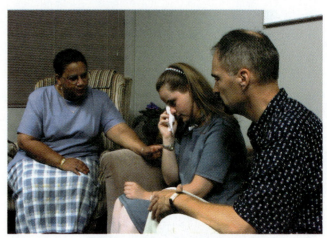

FIGURE 21-4　Bereavement counseling is available through hospice services for family members grieving the loss of a loved one.

within the context of their own discipline and role on the team. According to Eng (1993), the team's commitment to the educator and competent caregiver roles empowers the team to "realize goals, seek assistance to improve, and develop necessary skills in new members, enabling them to become vital members of the team" (p. 55).

Physician

The dying person's personal physician provides continuity of care and a trusting relationship developed over time. In addition, the physician knows the client's medical history and response to the previous treatments. The personal physician and the hospice team manage the pain and symptom control.

The hospice team physician frequently is the Medical Director of the hospice. Large hospices may have more than one physician on staff. The physician is an expert in palliative medicine and is able to educate the team members and serve as a consultant to the client's personal physician on pain and symptom management.

Registered Nurse

The hospice registered nurse provides direct client and family care. The nurse monitors each client's pain and symptom regimen and is able to make adjustments as needed. In addition, as a case manager, the nurse coordinates the care of the interdisciplinary team. This intense involvement with clients and their families provides the opportunity for the development of empathic nurse-client relationships. Raudonis (1995) found that the development of these empathic relationships was based on a reciprocal sharing of each other's personhood. Empathic relationships between some hospice nurses and clients positively impacted the client's physical and emotional well-being (Raudonis, 1993).

Hospice and palliative care are recognized as a specialized area of nursing practice. National certification in this specialty by the National Board for Certification of Hospice Nurses provides recognition of competence in basic hospice and palliative nursing knowledge (*Certification,* 1997). A nurse who meets the certification requirements becomes a certified hospice palliative nurse (CHPN).

Ask Yourself

What are your feelings about giving morphine to a former drug addict who has lung cancer with extensive metastasis to the bones and is experiencing severe pain?

Social Worker

The social worker assesses and identifies client and family needs and then finds resources to meet those needs. This professional is the link between the hospice team and community resources through both the dying and bereavement processes (Eng, 1993).

Think About It

What would you do if your hospice client's personal physician refused to increase the pain medication for an individual despite consistent pain levels of 8 on a scale of 0–10 for the past 3 days?

Clergy

Clergy identify and manage the issues of spiritual distress and provide spiritual guidance regardless of their religious affiliation. They may be asked to perform religious services including the funeral service. As members of the interdisciplinary team, their insight about dying persons and their families contributes to the discussion and plan of care (Eng, 1993).

Volunteers

Volunteers are an integral part of hospice services. Medicare regulations mandate the use of volunteers to augment hospice services. Volunteers complete required training programs offered by the hospice program. Volunteers regularly visit the hospice client and family providing a link to the outside community. Their visits allow family caregivers to attend to personal needs, shopping, respite, and relaxation even if for only a few hours. A strong bond frequently develops between hospice volunteers and the dying persons they serve. Eng (1993) attributed the bond to the person-to-person sharing rather than the more formal person-to-professional relationship. In addition, many volunteers have had hospice

Research Focus

Citation:
McCorkle, R., Robinson, L., Nuamah, I., Lev, E., & Benoliel, J. Q. (1998). The effects of home nursing care for patients during terminal illness on the bereaved's psychological distress. *Nursing Research, 47*(1), 2–10.

Purpose:
This landmark intervention study attempted to determine if specialized oncology home care nursing services provided to terminally ill clients with lung cancer positively impacted the bereavement outcome of psychological distress among surviving spousal caregivers, compared with other models of care.

Methods:
The study was a secondary analysis of data from a longitudinal study that used a prospective, controlled design that compared spousal dyads (final spousal sample equaled 91) who were assigned to an oncology home care group, a standard home care group, or an office control group.

Findings:
The results of the study indicate that initially psychological distress was significantly lower among the spouses of clients who had received the oncology home care intervention. This significant difference was sustained for 13 months after the oncology home care intervention. However, by the 25th month there were no significant differences among the groups.

Implications:
Implications of this study include the need to expand the focus of home care for terminally ill persons to also include the family caregiver to relieve their burden of care and enhance their own health, well-being, and healing through the grief process.

care for members of their own families, and this "connectedness through mutual tragedy" also contributes to developing meaningful relationships with hospice volunteers (Eng, 1993, p. 53).

Insurance Coverage

Historically, during the early years of the hospice movement few insurers paid for hospice services. In 1982 Congress mandated that hospice services become a

Medicare benefit. However, this initially was a temporary 3-year benefit. In 1986 Congress passed legislation that made hospice services a permanent part of Medicare coverage (Lattanzi-Licht et al., 1998).

To receive hospice services as a Medicare benefit, certain eligibility criteria must be met. An individual must have a life expectancy of 6 months or less. Although the NHO has developed guidelines to assist physicians in making these determinations, it is very difficult to project the future. Admission to hospice services requires a physician's order and certification by two physicians that the person has a terminal diagnosis with a 6 months or less life expectancy if the disease runs its normal course.

The evaluation for admission to hospice care includes documentation of the following conditions: progression of the disease, functional decline, and impaired nutritional status related to the terminal diagnosis. In addition, the client and the family must agree to the goal of palliative/comfort care rather than **curative care.** The hospice client must have a safe, supportive environment, including the availability of a family caregiver within the geographical boundaries served by the particular hospice. Depending on an individual's clinical status and environmental circumstances, the setting for hospice services may change from home care to inpatient unit to nursing facility. The hospice team will provide the continuity of care regardless of the setting.

Hospice services are available under Medicare Hospital Insurance (Part A). The services covered by the Medicare Hospice Benefit are summarized in Box 21-4. This coverage is only for those services related to the hospice diagnosis. Most coverage under Medicare is 100% insured without any deductible. A local hospice agency and/or Medicare can provide more specific and current guidelines.

The Medicare rules and regulations pay covered costs for two 90-day periods, followed by an additional 30-day period and an unlimited extension, if the client is recertified as terminally ill. Hospice nurses reassess the client at the end of each benefit period. Hospice clients have the right to stop hospice care at any time and revert back to their previous Medicare coverage. When a client stops hospice care any remaining days in that benefit period are forfeited. However, clients can re-elect the next benefit period at any time provided that they meet the eligibility criteria.

Some hospice clients have received services for longer than the 6-month prognosis. As discussed earlier, it is difficult to predict the future. Some individuals experience temporary levels of improvement with aggressive pain and symptom management. The hospice team carefully re-assesses all clients to determine if they meet the eligibility criteria. If a client's status no longer meets these criteria, the team will advise the client and family regarding appropriate services.

Nursing Interventions

Nursing interventions in hospice and palliative care are guided by the Standards of Hospice Practice and Professional Performance developed by the Hospice Nurses Association Task Force on Hospice Nursing Standards in 1995. These standards are summarized in Box 21-5. In 1998, the Hospice Nurses Association changed its name to the Hospice and Palliative Nurses Association to include all nurses working in the area of palliative care regardless of the setting.

It is beyond the scope of this chapter to discuss in detail the numerous nursing interventions implemented

---

BOX 21-4 Services Covered by the Medicare Hospice Benefit

- Interdisciplinary team of skilled professionals that focus on quality of life and client comfort, skilled pain management, symptom control, and education/counseling to reduce family stress

- One hundred percent coverage with no deductible on all home care visits, client's personal physician, hospice nurses on an intermittent basis, home health aides and homemaker services, medical social workers, chaplains, and volunteers

- Full coverage of medications for pain and symptom management related to terminal illness

- Physical, occupational, and speech-language pathology services

- Short-term inpatient care (usually 5–7 days), including respite care

- Continuous care during periods of medical crisis

- Full coverage of usual and customary supplies and equipment such as beds, commodes, and walkers

- Emotional, spiritual, and other counseling services to client and family members

- Nurse available for emergencies 24 hours a day, 7 days a week (on-call services)

- Bereavement counseling up to 1 year after client's death

to achieve the hospice client's and family goals and outcomes. The reader is advised to explore other texts and journal articles on pain and symptom management, end-stage disease processes, interdisciplinary collaborative practice, and grief and bereavement.

Nursing Tip

- Older adults are at risk for undertreatment of pain because of some changes of aging, age-related diseases, stereotypes, and myths.
- Assess older adults frequently for possible side effects and toxicity to pain medications. May need to adjust doses to prevent or decrease toxicity.
- Based on common physiological changes of aging, older adults are generally more sensitive to the effects of opioids. Peak effect is higher and the duration is longer; therefore, doses must be prescribed and monitored accordingly.

Using the *Standards of Hospice Nursing Practice* and the NHO document *A Pathway for Patients and Families Facing Terminal Illness,* intervention strategies will be described that can be used with all hospice clients and families.

Nursing Tip

- Assessment tools may have to be simplified or used more frequently with cognitively impaired older adults.
- Visual, hearing, and motor impairments may also require changes in the pain and other symptom assessment tools used.

Assessment is the critical component of effective palliative care. The first step upon admission to hospice care is that of a systematic and comprehensive assessment of the present and potential care needs of the client and family (Anderson, 1998). In hospice care the dying person and the family are considered the unit of care. Therefore, both must be the focus of any assessments. The NHO defined seven key assessment areas as follows:

- *Client disease state:* A person's disease state identifies pathologic conditions of the body that generate organic and/or behavioral disorders or abnormalities with specific etiologies, signs, and symptoms.

- *Client symptom state:* A person's symptom state includes subjective manifestations and objective signs of, or reactions to, a pathologic condition.

- *Client adaptation state and family adaptation state:* A person's adaptation state reflects the capacity to adjust emotionally and/or spiritually to changing environmental conditions or life circumstances.

- *Client functional state and family functional state:* A person's functional state reflects physical and/or social capacity to communicate, learn, and manage activities of daily living. Used here to also refer to the ability to understand and implement care requirements, such as treatment compliance.

- *Client/family resource state:* A client/family unit's resource state includes the scope of their environmental, legal, and financial capacity, including exposure to potential risk.

Summarizing the above definitions, nurses and other members of the interdisciplinary team assess four client-specific states: disease, symptom, adaptation, and functional states. In addition, two family-specific states are also assessed: adaptation and function. Finally, one state specific to the client/family unit of care is the resource state.

In addition to using the above definitions as a guiding framework, other guidelines include systematic and consistent use of the same scales to assess pain and

---

BOX 21-5 Standards of Hospice Nursing Practice and Professional Performance

Standard I. Assessment: The hospice nurse collects client and family data.

Standard II. Diagnosis: The hospice nurse analyzes the assessment data in determining diagnosis.

Standard III. Outcome Identification: The hospice nurse identifies expected outcomes individualized to the client and family.

Standard IV. Planning: The hospice nurse develops a nursing plan of care that prescribes interventions to attain expected outcomes.

Standard V. Implementation: The hospice nurse implements the interventions identified in the plan of care.

Standard VI. Evaluation: The hospice nurse evaluates the client's and family's progress toward attainment of outcomes.

other symptoms to communicate clearly and document the client's condition and needs. Use of such scales enables the nurse to evaluate the response to medications and other interventions. Revisions to the plan of care can be made based on the nurse's evaluations and role of client/family advocate for the needed changes. In addition, consistent use of the same assessment forms regarding emotional, spiritual, social, psychological, and cultural needs will provide consistent and comprehensive data for the plan of care. If all members of the team use the same assessment scales, communication and delivery of care are enhanced.

Continuing to use the NHO pathway as a guideline, three intervention strategies are identified and defined:

- *Treat:* To address, eliminate, or lessen an active problem using a skilled assessment and therapeutic intervention.

- *Prevent:* To avoid a possible problem through a skilled assessment and therapeutic intervention.

- *Promote:* To encourage growth or a higher level of wellness through a skilled assessment and therapeutic intervention.

These strategies will assist the hospice nurse in developing specific palliative care interventions for the hospice client and family from the time of diagnosis to death (Anderson, 1998).

All three strategies focus on quality of life. The third strategy of promoting growth can be used to promote the healing of relationships. Figure 21-5 illustrates the dimensions of end-of-life spirituality. The dying person's relationships with God (or other supreme force), nature, family, friends, community, and inner self may need healing. The hospice nurse and other members of the interdisciplinary team provide a compassionate, caring, and healing environment by listening, sharing, laughing, and praying (if requested) with each family (Holman, 1998). Byock (1996) encourages the hospice team to help hospice clients and their families convey and acknowledge the following five things: "Forgive me. I forgive you. Thank you. I love you. Good-bye" (p. 249).

Nursing practice focuses on the human responses to health, illness, and the full range of human experiences through the application of scientific knowledge within a context of caring relationships that facilitate health and healing (*Nursing's social,* 1995). Nursing interventions to the human response to dying (approaching death) can be categorized according to the biological response, the psychological response, and the spiritual response (*Guidelines,* 1997).

Assessment of client and family needs or desires in each of the above categories is essential for implementing effective interventions. Interventions applicable

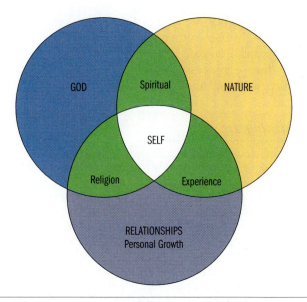

FIGURE 21-5   End-of-life spirituality. *Courtesy of Gerald H. Holman, MD, FAAP, FRCPC, Crown of Texas Hospice, Amarillo, TX.*

to the biological response to dying include use of pharmacological and nonpharmacological methods for pain and symptom management to provide comfort and alleviate suffering, emphasis on comfort measures, and use of complementary therapies. Massage, music therapy, and aroma therapy are a few examples, but interventions are not limited to these.

Interventions applicable to the psychosocial response to dying include all forms of therapeutic communication used with client/family and the hospice team; crisis intervention; teaching client/family, staff, and community; use of conflict resolution strategies with client/family, staff, and the hospice team; and use of reflection, story telling, and empathetic listening. Interventions during the provision of hospice services and after the death are provided to prevent complicated or pathological bereavement. Interventions applicable to the spiritual response of dying include touch with intent, therapeutic touch, massage, acupressure, visualization, guided imagery, prayer, and relaxation techniques (Figure 21-6).

CLINICAL ALERT

- *When clients are taking opioids, constipation is an anticipated problem. Rigorous assessment and maintenance of a bowel care program will minimize this side effect.*

- *Acute situations, for example a bowel obstruction, might require an emergency intervention such as surgery to relieve pain but not cure the terminal condition.*

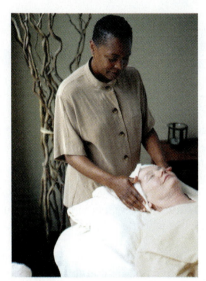

FIGURE 21-6 Therapeutic massage is an example of interventions used in the spiritual response of the dying.

End-of-Life Care in the Twenty-First Century

The arrival of a new century is an exciting opportunity to take time for reflection on the past, evaluate the present, and dream about visions for the future. How can hospice and palliative care evolve to meet the growing needs of an aging population that experiences multiple chronic illnesses that cannot be cured? The purpose of the following discussion is to stimulate new ideas and action. Knowing that it takes 2–5 years for the diffusion and utilization of new ideas, the reader is urged to act now so that end-of-life care will improve in the twenty-first century.

A vision of a continuum of palliative care already exists. Beltran and Coluzzi (1997) stated that comprehensive palliative care can be delivered in any setting. Empowering clients to self-determine their treatment options is a potentially cost-effective outcome of comprehensive palliative care. The above statements are congruent with the NHO-defined outcomes of palliative care. However, the paradigm shift occurs in dividing the continuum of medical treatments into three equal parts:

• Curative

• Chronic/restorative (active palliative care)

• Palliative (terminal/hospice) care.

According to Beltran and Coluzzi (1997, p. 50):

Curative therapies represent only about 30% of all medical interventions and include care of trauma,

obstetrical conditions, surgeries for acute conditions, some infectious disease programs, and approximately 50% of oncological care. Fully 70% of currently available medical treatments should be considered palliative, focusing on the management of chronic illnesses.

However, palliative care is not limited to physical needs. The WHO definition of palliative care (refer to Box 21-3) provides support for a comprehensive model by including the total care of chronically and/or terminally ill persons in their definition. The above statements also are congruent with the NHO definition of palliative care (refer to Box 21-3).

The uniqueness of the Beltran and Coluzzi (1997) comprehensive model of palliative care is the second or middle portion of the continuum: active palliative care. The two ends of the continuum: curative treatment (where a diagnosis occurs) and comfort palliative care (where death occurs) have been well established. Using the continuum approach provides a flexible transition between the stages. The interventions and treatment options flow directly from the primary goals of each stage on the continuum. The primary goal of the curative phase is reversal of the disease process and the prolongation of life. In the active palliative care phase the primary goals are fourfold: (a) clear delineation of the outcomes of therapy, (b) symptom control, (c) restoration of the level of function, and (d) treatment of comorbidities. Finally, in the third stage—comfort palliative care—the primary goals are symptom control and biopsychosocial and spiritual support. Hospice and palliative care nurses have the knowledge and expertise to practice in any phase of the continuum. Therefore, nurses must advocate throughout the health care system for this paradigm shift to develop a system that is responsive to the needs of those persons nearing the end of their life.

Using such a comprehensive model in the delivery of palliative care will enable persons whose chronic illness trajectory is more than 6 months in length to benefit from the comprehensive, interdisciplinary services palliative care can offer. In addition, the client as the focal point of the palliative care system will receive services in a meaningful context of relationships with family, friends, and a health care system that provides quality end-of-life care.

Summary

As previously discussed in the beginning of this chapter, end-of-life care has finally captured the attention of health care providers, insurers, government, policy

CARE PLAN

CASE STUDY

Florence Pearson is a 78-year-old woman who resides in a nursing facility. She has been diagnosed recently with colon cancer, metastasizing to the bladder and spine. After surgery, she has a colostomy and a urinary catheter in place. Mrs. Pearson refuses to look at her colostomy. She has been medicated for pain with Percocet (oxycodone and acetaminophen) with minimal relief. Other medications include prednisone, Beclovent inhalant, and a multivitamin. She has a long history of smoking and emphysema.

When the physician told Mrs. Pearson that she had cancer, she experienced disbelief and anger. Her daughter, who is a nurse, encouraged her hopefulness and suggested surgery. Mrs. Pearson agreed reluctantly: "I don't want to live my last days with tubes and bedridden. That's not who I am." She does not have a living will or any form of advance directives.

Mrs. Pearson is married. Her husband, Ralph, is on the Alzheimer's unit of the nursing facility for midstage disease. She was visiting him almost every day, yet he was beginning to be unable to identify her, especially if she visited him toward the end of the day.

The Pearsons loved playing pinochle and other card games with another couple at the nursing facility, Dorothy and Harry Bolton. Mrs. Pearson and Mrs. Bolton are best friends, although Mrs. Bolton has vascular dementia. The nursing facility has a swimming program that Mrs. Pearson and Mrs. Bolton have attended.

Mrs. Pearson's daughter will be taking her home to spend her last days. Both are comfortable with this decision.

ASSESSMENT

Mrs. Pearson is experiencing major life crises and changes: loss of health, loss of the husband she once knew, loss of friendship, and change in body image. Her decision-making ability seems to be influenced by her daughter. It is not uncommon that children of an aging or dying parent take control and influence major health decisions of the parent. In the absence of knowing what Mrs. Pearson's feelings are about end-of-life issues, her well-meaning daughter is robbing her freedom of choice in this very important matter. The following care plan illustrates four major aspects of Mrs. Pearson's care.

NURSING DIAGNOSIS

Chronic pain related to extensive tissue damage.

Outcomes:

Mrs. Pearson will:

- *Rate pain low on a pain scale (1 = low intensity; 10 = highest intensity).*
- *Exhibit relaxed facial expression, no irritability.*
- *Manifest a sleep pattern as close to her baseline pattern as possible, preferably 6–10 hours sleep, with perceived (verbalized) sleep as "good" or "restful."*
- *Show an appetite for food by eating at least half of each meal.*
- *Begin to explore how to return/modify previous activity level.*

Planning/Interventions:

The nurse will:

- *Assess pain and teach the daughter to assess pain at least four times daily.*
- *Consult with the physician/advanced nurse practitioner on the need for long-acting pain medication, such as Duragesic (fentanyl transdermal system).*
- *With Duragesic, monitor respiration and pulse rate for decreases in both; monitor for increased and excessive lethargy and changed mental status.*

(continued)

CARE PLAN *continued*

- *Notice facial and body movements for discomfort.*
- *Observe sleep pattern for quantity and quality of sleep.*
- *Teach relaxation exercises, deep breathing, meditation or prayer, visualization, and music strategies to reduce discomfort and promote sense of well-being.*
- *Probe with reference to interest in acupuncture and alternative therapies for pain management.*

EVALUATION:

Mrs. Pearson will rate pain as 0–2. Her facial and body movements will indicate relaxation and alertness. Pulse rate and respiration will fall within normal limits. Adequate sleep will be noted. Change in pain regimen will enhance pain management and return Mrs. Pearson to some of her previous activities. She will explore acupuncture as an adjunct therapy to promote control over remaining discomfort. She will spend the remaining days at home in comfort while maintaining the maximum quality of life possible.

NURSING DIAGNOSIS

Decisional conflict related to ambiguity and alternative actions being considered about course of illness and end-of-life quality.

Outcomes:

Mrs. Pearson will:
- *Decide on which end-of-life interventions are right for her.*
- *Discuss the interventions with the health care team.*
- *Formulate a living will and assign a medical power of attorney.*
- *Involve her daughter, as needed, in the decision, with focus on Mrs. Pearson's wishes.*

Planning/Interventions:

The nurse will:
- *Allow Mrs. Pearson to express her feelings about death and dying, along with her wishes about her care when she is unable to make such decisions.*
- *Explain the living will to Mrs. Pearson and answer any questions.*
- *Consult with and involve the social worker in this process.*
- *Offer to coordinate clergy involvement, if Mrs. Pearson agrees.*
- *Facilitate and coordinate an interdisciplinary meeting with Mrs. Pearson, her daughter, physician/ advanced nurse practitioner, and social worker.*
- *Advocate for Mrs. Pearson's end-of-life plans.*
- *Ensure that community resources complement Mrs. Pearson's wishes.*

EVALUATION:

Mrs. Pearson will be able to clarify her plans and wishes for end-of-life care. Her wishes will reflect her feelings (as opposed to her daughter's) about what is a "right" and "good" way to exit this world. Social worker, nurse, clergy, physician/advanced nurse practitioner, and community hospice resources will enact and advocate for Mrs. Pearson during this process.

NURSING DIAGNOSIS

Body image disturbance related to altered body part, as evidenced by not wanting to look at the colostomy.

(continued)

CARE PLAN continued

Outcomes:

Mrs. Pearson will:

- *Acknowledge that she has a colostomy.*
- *Look at and touch the colostomy.*
- *Express her feelings about having a colostomy.*
- *Participate in her own colostomy care.*

Planning/Interventions:

The nurse will:

- *Encourage Mrs. Pearson to express her feelings about the surgical alteration.*
- *Incorporate Mrs. Pearson into some aspects of assisting with her colostomy care, progressing to an increased level of involvement.*
- *Consult with the social worker and/or advanced practice psychiatric clinician.*
- *Involve Mrs. Pearson's daughter, if Mrs. Pearson is agreeable and if it is anticipated that the daughter will be a helpful and therapeutic force.*

EVALUATION:

Mrs. Pearson will express feelings of anger, loss, grief, and sadness over the loss of normal bowel elimination. As a result, she will have taken the beginning steps in the healing process and accept the change by examining, touching, and participating in her colostomy care. Social worker, advanced nurse practitioner, and Mrs. Pearson's daughter will play a supportive role in Mrs. Pearson's recovery and acceptance and positive image of an altered body part.

NURSING DIAGNOSIS

Risk for loneliness related to affectional deprivation and physical isolation in a new environment while recovering from surgery.

Outcomes:

Mrs. Pearson will:

- *Visit with her husband three times weekly, earlier in the daytime, as soon as she is able.*
- *Visit with her friend Mrs. Bolton for brief periods of time.*
- *Phone friends and relatives with whom she has had meaningful positive relationships.*
- *Explore activities that will be meaningful and fun but not exhausting.*

Planning/Interventions:

The nurse will:

- *Help Mrs. Pearson delineate two or three meaningful and realistic activities.*
- *Assist Mrs. Pearson's daughter in arranging for transportation.*
- *Assist Mrs. Pearson with visiting her husband and Mrs. Bolton and phoning others.*

EVALUATION:

Mrs. Pearson will not become socially isolated despite surgical tubes, colostomy, and moving back home. She will have visitors, phone contacts and, as soon as able, will visit her husband during the times when he is most alert and oriented.

HOSPICE AND PALLIATIVE CARE OF CONNECTICUT
COMPREHENSIVE INITIAL ASSESSMENT

PATIENT NAME:	DATE:	TIME IN: AM/PM
		TIME OUT: AM/PM
PRIMARY DX:	ID#	INS/PAYOR:

PRESENT ILLNESS	MEDICAL HISTORY
	When diagnosed w/present illness: □ Had Chemotherapy □ Had Radiation □ Had surgical intervention (specify)

ALLERGIES: □ None   □ PCN □ Sulfa □ ASA □ Other (list): _____

EMERGENCY CONTACT (Outside Of Home)
Name:_____
Relationship _____
Phone # _____Street Address _____Town _____ State ____ Zip _____
Primary Caregiver (name/relationship): _____ □ Assists with ADLs □ Provides Physical Care

INTERPRETER/ESCORT SERVICES
Interpreter Present If Needed? □ Yes □ NoIf no, explain: _____
Primary Language _____   Interpreter needed? □ Yes □ No
Escort Needed □ Yes □ No   **If yes**, what hours?

INFECTION CONTROL:
□ No evidence of infection upon admission   □ Infection present upon admission   Type:
□ Infection Control Report Completed

ADVANCED DIRECTIVES/HEALTH CARE CHOICES: patient/caregiver have executed:
□ Living Will   □ Health Care Agent (specify) _____
□ Power of Attorney (specify) _____   □ Conservator _____
□ Hospice benefit explained   □ Certification forms sent to MD/DO
DNR   □ Yes   □ No
Funeral Arrangements: □ Yes   □ No
    If yes, Funeral Home Name/Contact: _____
    Funeral Home Phone _____

REVIEW OF SYSTEMS: For all ROS items, make a (√) mark in the next to the assessment items indicated; circle items separated by a "/".

Temp	BP: lying sitting standing
Resp	Right
Radial Pulse	Left
Apical Pulse	Abd Girth (cm)
Weight actual/reported:	Other:

HEAD AND NECK	□ WNL	□ cataracts	□ glaucoma	□ blurred vision	□ glasses
	□ prosthesis R /L	□ contact lenses	□ jaundice	□ legally blind	□ dentures U/L/partial
	□ lesions	□ gum disease	□ deaf	□ hearing aid	□ hard of hearing
	□ discharge eyes/ears	□ ringing in ears	□ nasal congestion	□ nose bleeds	□ sore throat
	□ loss of smell	□ sinus problems	□ dysphagia	□ other:	
	Comments:				

CARDIOVASCULAR	□ WNL	□ anemia	□ cyanosis	□ DOE	□ orthostatic hypotn	□ leg cramps
	□ palpitations	□ radial pulses	□ varicosities	□ SOB	□ cap refill: <3sec/>3sec	□ pedal pulses
	□ pacemaker	□ other:				
	□ Edema:					
	□ Chest Pain: DESCRIBE:	□ anginal □ sharp	□ postural □ dull	□ localized □ ache	□ substernal □ radiating	□ vice-like
	Comments:					

Nursing pathways showing the various stages of hospice care and documentation. Included are the initial assessment, stages 2 and 3 of care, patient family outcomes, discharge summary and nurse pronouncement of death notice. *Courtesy of Connecticut VNA, Inc.*

HOSPICE COMPREHENSIVE INITIAL ASSESSMENT
Page 2

RESPIRATORY	☐ WNL	☐ orthopnea	☐ asthma	☐ wheezing	☐ cough	☐ smokes _____ ppd
	☐dyspnea	☐ congestion	☐ hemoptysis	☐ sputum (describe)		☐ other:
	Lung sounds:	☐ clear	☐ Other (describe):			
	Comments:					
INTEGUMENT	☐ WNL		☐ cold/clammy	☐ rashes		☐ bruises
			☐ jaundice	☐ turgor: good/ fair/ poor		☐ tattoos
	Denote location of specific skin conditions/wounds by completing the Wound Assessment and Treatment form.					
URINARY/ GASTROINTESTINAL	☐ WNL	☐ ostomy	☐ burning/pain	☐ urinary retention	☐ incontinence	☐ distention
	☐ prostate prob.	☐ urinary	☐ urinary	☐ exog. Obesity	☐ rectal bleeding	☐ heartburn
	☐ hemorrhoids	urgency	frequency	☐ anorexia	☐ abd rigidity/pain	☐ diarrhea
	☐ bowel sounds	☐ N/V	☐ constipation	☐ tarry stools	☐ other:	
	☐ catheter:	type:	size:			
	Comments:					
GYNECOLOGICAL/ GENITALIA	☐ WNL	☐ vaginal bleeding	☐ vaginal discharge	☐ breast pain		☐ breast discharge
	☐ breast lumps	☐ performs SBE	☐ STD/herpes	☐ birth control		☐ penile discharge
	☐ menses	Comments:				
HEMATOPOETIC/ ENDOCRINE	☐ anticoagulant therapy	☐ bleeding/bruising		☐ history of/active DVT		☐ anemia: Fe defic/pernic
	☐ thrombocytopenia	☐ Hemophilia		☐ other coagulation disorders		☐ hyper/hypo glycemia
	☐ enlarged thyroid	☐ other:				☐
	LAB VALUES:	☐ BLOOD GLUCOSE:		☐ HGB/ HCT		☐ PROTIME:
MS/MOBILITY	☐ WNL	☐ limited ROM	☐ gait disturbance	☐ amputation (specify)		☐ swollen joints
	☐ uses cane	☐ uses walker	☐ uses wheelchair	☐ uses crutches		☐ braces/prosthesis
	☐ crepitus	☐ symmetrical movement	☐ coordination impaired	☐ limited strength		☐ scoliosis/kyphosis
	☐ other:	Comments:				
NEURO/ EMOTIONAL/ BEHAVIORAL	☐ A&O x3	☐ flat affect	☐ slowed responses	☐ delusional/hallucinatory		☐ agitated/hyperactive
	☐ anxious	☐ depressed	☐ lethargic	☐ stuperous/comatose		☐ PERLA
	☐ paresis	☐ headaches	☐ speech/swallowing difficulty	☐ hearing deficit		☐ vertigo
	☐ paralysis	☐ tremors/spasms	☐ blackouts	☐ numbness		☐ neuralgia
	☐ neuropathy	☐ memory loss	☐ hand grasps unequal	☐ substance/ETOH use		☐ other
	Comments:					

Bereavement Issues:

☐ No spiritual/emotional concerns expressed   ☐ Family hx of mental/emotional problems   ☐ Loss of home (feared/actual)
☐ Health problems   ☐ Family hx of chemical dependence   ☐ Difficulty dealing with previous losses
☐ Dependent family members   ☐ Communication difficulties within family   ☐ Loss of constant companion/emotional support
☐ Children/adolescents in immediate family   ☐ Decision making difficulties   ☐ Loss of financial provision
☐ Concurrent life crisis/life losses   ☐ Reluctance to face facts of terminal illness   ☐ Other:

Bereavement Follow-up: Primary Bereaved _____

Relationship _____
Phone # _____ Street Address _____ Town _____ State ___ Zip _____

List Other Family Members: _____

_____

Comments: _____

_____
_____

Spiritual/Emotional:

☐ Questions of Meaning   ☐ Searching for alt. beliefs   ☐ Seeking spiritual aid   ☐ Struggling to find meaning in life or death
☐ Ethical dilemma   ☐ Loss of hope   ☐ Anxiety   ☐ Anticipatory Grieving
☐ Disturbed sleep   ☐ Situational depression   ☐ Guilt   ☐ Anger
☐ Social withdrawal

Comments: _____

_____
_____

Initial assessment pathway continued.

HOSPICE COMPREHENSIVE INITIAL ASSESSMENT
Page 3

Symptom Management
☐ Symptom control is satisfactory
☐ Respiratory distress_____
☐ Nausea/vomiting _____
☐ Weakness/fatigue _____
☐ Nutritional deficit _____
☐ Anxiety/emotional distress _____
☐ Sleep _____
☐ Mobility _____
Other: _____
_____
_____

Describe **pain** using the scale below, where 0 is no pain and 10 is worst possible pain

Location of Pain: Mark areas of pain on the diagrams below:

Current Pain:
Worst pain in the last 24 hours:
Best pain has been in the last 24 hours:
Per patient, is this an acceptable level of pain?

☐0 ☐1 ☐2 ☐3 ☐4 ☐5 ☐6 ☐7 ☐8 ☐9 ☐10
☐0 ☐1 ☐2 ☐3 ☐4 ☐5 ☐6 ☐7 ☐8 ☐9 ☐10
☐0 ☐1 ☐2 ☐3 ☐4 ☐5 ☐6 ☐7 ☐8 ☐9 ☐10
☐ Yes   ☐ No

DESCRIBE PAIN: ☐ Pain is continuous   ☐ Pain is intermittent
Other: _____
_____
_____
_____

PRECIPITATING/RELIEVING FACTORS (per pt/caregiver) _____
_____
_____

EFFECTIVENESS OF INTERVENTIONS FOR PAIN/COMMENTS _____
_____
_____

NUTRITIONAL ASSESSMENT— Complete for all Clients; *Evaluate need for dietitian referral for scores > 12*.

WEIGHT: HEIGHT:

NUTRITIONAL PARAMETERS	SCORE
Diet at Home: 0= Regular 1= Soft 2= Thickened Liquids 3= Cardiac Diet 4= Diabetic /Renal ☐ Fluid Restriction (specify): ☐ Increased Fluids (specify)	
Appetite: 0= ☐ Good 2= ☐ Fair 4= ☐ Poor	
Self Care/Feeding 0= Able to feed self 2= Set meal, supervise 3= Partial feed 4= Total feed	
Nutritional Supplements: 0= No 4= Yes	
Tube Feeding/TPN 0= No 12= Yes Tube Feeding: Formula: _____ Rate: _____ per _____ Home TPN :Formula _____ Rate _____ per _____	
Difficulty Chewing 0= No 4= Yes	
Difficulty Swallowing 0= No 4= Yes* (if yes, evaluate need for SLP referral)	
Recent Weight Changes ☐ Obese ☐ Anorexic 0= No 4= Greater than 5% weight loss or gain in past month (involuntary) OR 10% weight loss* or gain in past 6 months (involuntary)	
☐ Evaluate for dietician referral based on score ☐ No need for dietitian referral ☐ Patient declines nutrition referral **NUTRITION ASSESSMENT SCORE:**	

Initial assessment pathway continued.

HOSPICE COMPREHENSIVE INITIAL ASSESSMENT
Page 4
Complete the Braden Scale© for predicting pressure sore risk; use the scale below to determine risk for pressure sore development.
HIGH RISK: Total Score </= 12   MODERATE RISK: Total Score 13-14   LOW RISK: 15-16 if under 75 years old OR 15-18 if over 75 years old.

RISK FACTOR	SCORES/ DESCRIPTIONS				SCORE
SENSORY PERCEPTION Ability to respond meaningfully to pressure related discomfort	1. COMPLETELY LIMITED— Unresponsive (does not moan, flinch, or grasp) to painful stimuli, due to diminished level of consciousness or sedation OR limited ability to feel pain over most of body surface	2. VERY LIMITED— Responds only to painful stimuli. Cannot communicate discomfort except by moaning or restlessness OR has a sensory impairment which limits the ability to feel pain or discomfort over ½ of body	3. SLIGHTLY LIMITED— Responds to verbal commands but cannot always communicate discomforrt or need to be turned OR has some sensory impairment which limits ability to feel pain or discomfort in 1 or 2 extremities	4. NO IMPAIRMENT— Responds to verbal commands. Has no sensory deficit which would limit ability to feel or voice pain or discomfort	
MOISTURE Degree to which skin is exposed to moisture	1. CONSTANTLY MOIST— Skin is kept moist almost constantly by perspiration, urine, etc. Dampness is detected every time patient is moved or turned	2. OFTEN MOIST— Skin is often but not always moist. Linen must be changed at least once a shift.	3. OCCASIONALLY MOIST— Skin is occasionally moist, requiring an extra linen change approximately once a day	4. RARELY MOIST— Skin is usually dry; linen only requires changing at routine intervals	
ACTIVITY Degree of physical activity	1. BEDFAST— Confined to bed	2. CHAIRFAST— Ability to walk severely limited or nonexistent. Cannot bear own weight and/or must be assisted into chair or wheelchair	3. WALKS OCCASIONALLY— Walks occasionally during day but for very short distances, with or without assistance. Spends majority of each shift in bed or chair.	4.WALKS FREQUENTLY— Walks outside the room at least twice a day and inside room at least once every 2 hours during waking hours	
MOBILITY Ability to change and control body position	1. COMPLETELY IMMOBILE— Does not make even slight changes in body or extremity position without assistance	2. VERY LIMITED— Makes occasional slight changes in body or extremity position but unable to make frequent or significant changes independently	3. SLIGHTLY LIMITED— Makes frequent though slight changes in body or extremity position independently	4. NO LIMITATIONS— Makes major and frequent changes in position without assistance.	
NUTRITION Usual food intake pattern 1. NPO-nothing by mouth 2. IV: Intravenously 3. TPN: Total parenteral nutrition	1. VERY POOR— Never eats a complete meal. Rarely eats more than 1/3 of any food offered. Eats 2 servings or less of protein (meat or daily products) per day. Takes fluids poorly. Does not take a liquid dietary supplement OR is NPO and/or IV for more than 5 days.	2. PROBABLY INADEQUATE— Rarely eats a complete meal and generally eats only about ½ of any food offered. Protein intake includes only 3 servings of meat or dairy products per day. Occasionally will take a dietary supplement OR receives less than optimum amount of liquid diet or tube feeding	3. ADEQUATE— Eats over half of most meals. Eats a total of 4 servings of 4 or more servings of protein (meat, dairy products) each day. Occasionally will refuse a meal, but will usually take a supplement if offered OR is on a tube feeding or TPN regimen, which probably meets most of nutritional needs	4. EXCELLENT— Eats most of every meal. Never refuses a meal. Usually eats a total of 4 or more servings of meat and dairy products. Occasionally eats between meals. Does not require supplementation.	
FRICTION AND SHEAR	1. PROBLEM— Requires moderate to maximum assistance in moving. Complete lifting without sliding against sheets is impossible. Frequently slides down in bed or chair, requiring frequent repositioning with maximum assistance. Spasticism, contractures, or agitation leads to almost constant friction.	2. POTENTIAL PROBLEM— Moves feebly or requires minimum assistance. During a move, skin probably slides to some extent against sheets, chair, restraints, or other devices. Maintains relatively good position in chair or bed most of the time but occasionally slides down.	3. NO APPARENT PROBLEM— Moves in bed and chair independently and has sufficient muscle strength to lift up completely during move. Maintains good position in bed or chair at all times.		
TOTAL SCORE					

Source: Barbara Braden and Nancy Bergstrom, copyright 1988

Initial assessment pathway continued.

HOSPICE COMPREHENSIVE INITIAL ASSESSMENT
Page 5

ADMISSION ADL ASSESSMENT	DEPEN	MOD depen	MIN depen	INDEP	ADMISSION IADL ASSESSMENT	DEPEN	MOD depen	MIN depen	INDEP
BATHING					MEAL PREP				
DRESSING					MEDICATION				
TOILETING					SHOPPING				
TRANSFERING					PERSONAL FINANCES				
FEEDING					TRANSPORTATION				
AMBULATION					LAUNDRY/CLEANING				
					TELEPHONE USE				

<u>Home Safety:</u> Complete checklist below; document follow-up to findings in at the end of the section.
Y= Safe (observed or in place)   **NA= does not apply**
N= Attention needed/action taken (describe in comments)

☐ Y ☐ N ☐ NA Handwashing, PPD use, blood/body fluid precautions
☐ Y ☐ N ☐ NA Sharps disposal and storage
☐ Y ☐ N ☐ NA Disposables/non-disposables cleaned/discarded/stored properly
☐ Y ☐ N ☐ NA Proper storage/disposal of medications
☐ Y ☐ N ☐ NA Medication labels present/readable
☐ Y ☐ N ☐ NA Able to manage own medication schedule
☐ Y ☐ N ☐ NA Scatter rugs secured or removed
☐ Y ☐ N ☐ NA Adequate lighting (indoors/outdoors)
☐ Y ☐ N ☐ NA Knowledge of planning for emergencies/natural disasters
☐ Y ☐ N ☐ NA Non-skid surfaces in bathroom/floors
☐ Y ☐ N ☐ NA Bars for toilet/tub/shower if appropriate
☐ Y ☐ N ☐ NA Functional smoke alarms
☐ Y ☐ N ☐ NA Emergency exit reviewed
☐ Y ☐ N ☐ NA Fire extinguisher available
☐ Y ☐ N ☐ NA Electrical cords in good condition/out of ambulation pathway

Child Safety:
☐ Y ☐ N ☐ NA Chemicals/medications out of reach of children
☐ Y ☐ N ☐ NA Telephone number for poison control posted/available
☐ Y ☐ N ☐ NA Hot objects/appliances out of reach/outlets have safety guards
☐ Y ☐ N ☐ NA Glass doors marked with decals
☐ Y ☐ N ☐ NA Toxic plants out of reach
☐ Y ☐ N ☐ NA Gates positioned at tops/bottoms of stairs/other locations
☐ Y ☐ N ☐ NA Syrup of Ipecac in home

Comments related to home safety assessment Document action taken for all positive (unsafe) findings: _____
_____
_____

☐   **Patient/Caregiver have received the Home Safety Handout**

Note: if assessment shows significant social/safety issues, evaluate for MSW referral.

HABITS:check and describe use:
☐ Alcohol:_____
☐ Nonprescription Drugs_____
☐ Smoking:_____
☐ Caffeine:_____
☐ Other:_____

MEDICATION MANAGEMENT
Is patient taking mediations from a pre-filled medication box?   ☐ Yes   ☐ No
If **yes**, who pre-fills the medication box?
          ☐ patient☐ other person (specify person/relationship) _____
Does the patient have the resources to purchase and obtain medications independently? ☐ Yes   ☐ No
If no, who assists the patient in buying/obtaining medications?_____

Equipment and Medical Supplies Management—write in any equipment/supplies in home or needed in the home:

Equipment Type:	Has	Needs	Medical Supplies:	Has	Needs

DME COMPANY/CONTACT NAME/PHONE NUMBER:_____
_____

Initial assessment pathway continued.

HOSPICE COMPREHENSIVE INITIAL ASSESSMENT
Page 6

INTERVENTIONS RELATED TO INITIAL VISIT:

INTERVENTIONS	√	CLINICAL INFORMATION/COMMENTS
PLAN OF CARE/DISCHARGE PLANNING		
Establish emergency procedures, instruct on when to call 911 vs. Hospice personnel; teach 24/7 availability of staff		
Begin long term planning		
Instruct on death at home procedures		
DISEASE MANAGEMENT:		
Instruct on expected disease process		
Discuss DNR status and process physician orders for DNR and nurse pronouncement as appropriate		
SYMPTOM MANAGEMENT		
Instruct on symptom management; assess effectiveness of interventions		
PSYCHOSOCIAL/EMOTIONAL		
Encourage pt/family to verbalize feelings.		
Assess bereavement risk factors and ability to cope with grieving process		
Make referrals as needed to address emotional, financial, bereavement, and/or spiritual needs.		
Assess coping with death/dying issues; begin to instruct on the availability of services to meet spiritual and emotional needs.		
Begin development of a bereavement plan		

MEDICATION MANAGEMENT
☐ Instruct on pain medications; increase dose/change route of medications to ensure pain control and symptom management; assess effectiveness of interventions
☐ Teach purpose/effects of medications; assess understanding and compliance(specify medications instructed)

OTHER INTERVENTIONS

COORDINATION OF CARE
☐ Conference with IDT members to establish the initial plan of care and facilitate hospice admission.
☐ Coordinate visits with other professionals and volunteers
Next MD appt:
☐ Case conference as needed (CIRCLE)   Bereavement Coordinator PT/ OT / MSW / ST / HHA/HM / Pastoral / Volunteer
Other:
☐ TELEPHONE CALL TO:

Discharge Goals—check all goals that apply:
☐ Disease extension/co-morbidity factors will be treated and/or prevented.
☐ Patient will achieve the optimal level of consciousness throughout the death/dying process.
☐ Patient will have an acceptable level of pain management and/or symptom control.
☐ Patient/family will demonstrate adaptive behaviors that are effective for them in dealing with death/dying
☐ Other (specify): _____

NURSE SIGNATURE/TITLE:

hospro\initdata   8/99

Initial assessment pathway continued.

HOSPICE AND PALLIATIVE CARE OF CONNECTICUT   **HOSPICE NURSING CARE PATHWAY**

PATIENT NAME:		-	DATE

PATIENT SIGNATURE:	INSURANCE TYPE/ PAYOR:	ID#	VISIT #

VITAL SIGNS/ASSESSMENT STATISTICS/LAB VALUES

Temp	BP: lying/sitting/standing	PEDAL EDEMA:		LAB VALUES:	
Resp	Right	Left instep	Right instep	O2 sat resting: activity:	
Radial Pulse	Left	Left ankle	Right ankle	Protime INR	
Apical Pulse	Abd Girth (cm)	Left calf	Right calf	FBS/RBS	
Weight actual/reported:	Other:	pitting/non-pitting	pitting/non-pitting	Other:	

LEVEL OF CONSCIOUSNESS

☐ ALERT/ORIENTED	☐ COMATOSE	☐ AGITATED	☐ OTHER:
☐ LETHARGIC	☐ ANXIOUS	☐ CONFUSED	

CURRENT CONCERNS (per patient/caregiver):

DOCUMENT OBJECTIVE FINDINGS/SYMPTOM MANAGEMENT:

☐ NUTRITION/HYDRATION:

☐ PAIN:

☐ SKIN CONDITION:

☐ RESPIRATORY COMFORT:

☐ ELIMINATION:

☐ OTHER SYMPTOMS/ASSESSMENT DATA:

Describe **PAIN** using the scale below, where 0 is no pain and 10 is worst possible pain
Current Pain: 0 1 2 3 4 5 6 7 8 9 10 | Worst pain in the last 24 hours: 0 1 2 3 4 5 6 7 8 9 10
Best pain has been in the last 24 hours 0 1 2 3 4 5 6 7 8 9 10 | Per patient, is this an acceptable level of pain? ☐ YES ☐ NO
PRECIPITATING/RELIEVING FACTORS (per pt/caregiver)/**EFFECTIVENESS OF INTERVENTIONS/COMMENTS**

SPIRITUAL ASSESSMENT:
☐ Pastoral Care active in POC ☐ No spiritual concerns expressed today by patient/caregiver
Comments:

EMOTIONAL ASSESSMENT:
☐ MSW active in POC ☐ No emotional concerns expressed today by patient/caregiver
Comments:

BEREAVEMENT ASSESSMENT:
☐ MSW active in POC   ☐ No bereavement risk factors identified today
Comments:

PATIENT/CAREGIVER RESPONSE TO PLAN OF CARE: ☐ Continue with current POC
☐ Changes (frequency/duration of services) required to POC (specify):
☐ Additional services/resources/specialty referrals required for care (specify):
PLAN FOR NEXT VISIT:

HOME HEALTH AIDE (CIRCLE ONE) ORIENTATION/SUPERVISION-- Name of HHAide:

Yes	No	Orientation/Supervision Activity	Yes	No	Orientation/Supervision/ Activity
		Patient care plan revised/updated/reviewed by nurse			Care given as per the aide care plan
		Patient care needs reviewed by aide prior to starting care			Standard precautions practiced by aide
		Rapport between aide and Pt/cg satisfactory			Continued need for home health aide services
					Follow up required (specify)
Activities requiring specific instruction and return demonstration:			Other activities performed/observed		

(OVER)   PAGE 1 OF 2

Stage 2 pathway.

HOSPICE CARE PATHWAY
Stage 2 Nursing Visit Sheet—for all visits during intermediate care up to Stage 3 (final)

INTERVENTIONS	√	CLINICAL INFORMATION/COMMENTS
PLAN OF CARE/DISCHARGE PLANNING		
Discuss and evaluate the POC with pt/caregiver		
Instruct on death at home procedures		
DISEASE MANAGEMENT:		
Instruct on disease symptoms/disease progression		
Instruct on pacing activity to patient tolerance		
Instruct on hazards of immobility, including respiratory complications and skin breakdown.		
Instruct on nutritional requirements for a dying person and instruct patient/family on diet as tolerated. Instruct on decreasing desire/need for food as disease progresses		
Review with pt/caregiver to call Hospice whenever necessary for assistance/questions		
SYMPTOM MANAGEMENT		
Instruct on symptom management; assess effectiveness of interventions		
Instruct on management of constipation; assess effectiveness of bowel regime.		
PSYCHOSOCIAL/EMOTIONAL		
Encourage pt/family to verbalize feelings.		
Assess bereavement risk factors and ability to cope with grieving process		
Make referrals as needed to address emotional, financial, and/or spiritual needs.		
Assess coping with death/dying issues; continue to instruct on the availability of services to meet spiritual and emotional needs.		

MEDICATION/SUPPLIES/EQUIPMENT MANAGEMENT   ☐ Written medication information given to patient

☐ Instruct on pain medications; increase dose/change route of medications to ensure pain control and symptom management; assess effectiveness of interventions
☐ Teach purpose/effects of medications; assess understanding and compliance(specify medications instructed)
☐ Assess effectiveness of current equipment in meeting patient/family needs.
☐ Order any required supplies/ equipment as patient condition changes
☐ Instruct on use of all supplies and equipment; assess safety in supply and equipment use.
☐ Other:

OTHER INTERVENTIONS

COORDINATION OF CARE

☐ Instruct on availability of respite care if needed   ☐ Coordinate visits with other professionals and volunteers
☐ Review visit information with IDT members   **Next MD appt:**
☐ Case conference as needed (CIRCLE) Bereavement Coordinator PT/ OT / MSW / ST / HHA/HM / Pastoral / Volunteer
Other:
☐ TELEPHONE CALL TO:

SIGNATURE/TITLE

Stage 2 pathway continued.

HOSPICE CARE PATHWAY
Stage 3 Nursing Visit Sheet—for all visits during final stage

INTERVENTIONS	√	CLINICAL INFORMATION/COMMENTS
PLAN OF CARE/DISCHARGE PLANNING		
Discuss and evaluate the POC with pt/caregiver		
Increase support services as needed		
DISEASE MANAGEMENT:		
Instruct on s/s of active dying, including increased secretions and apnea.		
Discuss arrangements for after patient death.		
Instruct on hazards of immobility, including respiratory complications and skin breakdown.		
Instruct on care of a bed-bound patient; instruct on personal care and positioning for comfort.		
Assess for nausea, vomiting, diarrhea, and constipation. Instruct on decreased desire for food/drink.		
Teach mouth care to increase patient comfort		
Review with pt/caregiver to call Hospice whenever necessary for assistance/questions		
SYMPTOM MANAGEMENT		
Instruct on symptom management; assess effectiveness of interventions		
PSYCHOSOCIAL/EMOTIONAL		
Encourage pt/family to verbalize feelings.		
Complete final arrangements		
Encourage pt/caregiver to resolve conflicts, if any, and to say goodbye.		
Assess coping with death/dying issues; continue to instruct on the availability of services to meet spiritual and emotional needs.		

MEDICATION/SUPPLIES/EQUIPMENT MANAGEMENT   ☐ Written medication information given to patient
☐ Instruct on pain medications; increase dose/change route of medications to ensure pain control and symptom management; assess effectiveness of interventions
☐ Teach purpose/effects of medications; assess understanding and compliance(specify medications instructed)
☐ Assess effectiveness of current equipment in meeting patient/family needs.
☐ Order any required supplies/ equipment as patient condition changes
☐ Instruct on use of all supplies and equipment; assess safety in supply and equipment use.
☐ Other:

OTHER INTERVENTIONS

COORDINATION OF CARE
☐ Instruct on availability of respite care if needed   ☐ Coordinate visits with other professionals and volunteers
☐ Review visit information with IDT members   **Next MD appt:**
☐ Case conference as needed (CIRCLE)   Bereavement Coordinator PT/ OT / MSW / ST / HHA/HM / Pastoral / Volunteer
Other:
☐ TELEPHONE CALL TO:

SIGNATURE/TITLE

Stage 3 pathway.

HOSPICE CARE PATHWAY—PATIENT/FAMILY OUTCOMES

Patient Name _____ ID# _____ .

Enter date met or variance code if not met:

VARIANCE CODES—

A: PATIENT TOO PHYSICALLY ILL/IMPAIRED
B: CO-MORBID INTERFERENCE
C: PSYCHOSOCIAL ISSUES INTERFERING
D: CAREGIVER LIMITATIONS/DIFFICULTIES
E: EQUIPMENT PROBLEMS
F: PT OR CG LEARNING DIFFICULTIES
G: PT/CG DECISION
H: DOES NOT APPLY

Nurse Signature Block:

Initial: _____	Signature/Title:_____
Initial: _____	Signature/Title:_____
Initial: _____	Signature/Title:_____
Initial: _____	Signature/Title:_____

Admission Visit	RN Initials	Met	Not Met	Explanation of Variances
Verbalizes hospice protocols				
Verbalizes correct medication schedule				
Verbalizes plan of care and services				
Verbalizes understanding of emergency procedures; states emergency plan				
Demonstrates safe use of equipment and supplies				

Stage 2 Hospice Care	RN Initials	Met	Not Met	Explanation of Variances
Verbalizes purpose and side effects of medications				
Demonstrates effective medication management				
Verbalizes measures to promote normal bowel elimination				
Verbalizes s/s of approaching death and plan for time of death				
Verbalizes s/s requiring medical intervention and those related to normal dying process.				
Identified family/social supports needed to manage advancing disease at home				
Verbalizes that spiritual support is adequate				
Freedom from complications related to decreased mobility				
Verbalizes that emotional needs are being met				
Verbalizes nutrition/hydration needs of a dying person				
Demonstrates effective symptom control				
Maintains maximum level of function				

Stage 3 Hospice Care	RN Initials	Met	Not Met	Explanation of Variances
Verbalizes s/s of active dying process				
Verbalizes understanding of plan for time of death; has resources in place for time of death				
Demonstrates/verbalizes effective symptom control				
Demonstrates effective medication management				
Verbalizes that emotional needs are being met				
Verbalizes that spiritual needs are being met				
Demonstrates/verbalizes activities to promote patient comfort				
Demonstrates safe use of supplies/equipment				

Patient/family outcomes pathway.

HOSPICE CARE PATHWAY
DISCHARGE SUMMARY

CLIENT NAME _____   Discharge Date: _____
CLIENT ADDRESS_____
PHYSICIAN NAME _____
PHYSICIAN ADDRESS_____

Reason for discharge:

☐ Condition Improved
☐ Moved out of area
☐ Self/family choice
☐ Placed in ECF
☐ Referred to Hospital Inpatient Care
☐ Referred to another agency in service area
☐ Client Died, Care of Sick
☐ Not taken up to services
☐ Died at home—Hospice Benefit
☐ Died in medical facility—Hospice Benefit
☐ Died, place unknown—Hospice Benefit

☐ Patient not under the care of a physician/not compliant to POC
☐ Prohibited by scope of service/agency medical policies
☐ Change in treatment plan requires new start of care
☐ **Emergency Discharge**: safety issues place client and/or agency staff in immediate jeopardy
☐ **Financial Discharge**: Refused to accept financial responsibility for costs in excess of insurance/government programs

Hospice Care Pathway Outcomes			
Self determined life closure	*Met*	*Not Met*	*Explanation of Variances*
Pt/family demonstrate freedom from coping, grieving, or existential problems related to approaching death			
Pt achieves optimal level of consciousness throughout death/dying process			
Pt/family exhibit adaptive behaviors that are effective in : • coping with and integrating the knowledge of approaching death • identify opportunities for working with grief reconciliation as separation is anticipated • preserving patient autonomy			
Safe and comfortable dying	*Met*	*Not Met*	*Explanation of Variances*
Disease extension/co-morbidity factors will be appropriately treated and/or prevented			
Treatment side effects will be treated/prevented			
Treatments will be tailored to patient/family functional capacity			
Crisis arising from resource deficits will be prevented			
Financial, legal, and environmental problems will be managed via appropriate resources/referrals and will not compromise care			
Effective grieving	*Met*	*Not Met*	*Explanation of Variances*
Problems with coping problems related to death/dying will be prevented/treated			
Patient/family will demonstrate adaptive behaviors that are effective for them in dealing with death/dying			
Family will successfully integrate the memory of their loved one into their lives.			

Signature/Title of Nurse _____

Discharge summary pathway.

NURSE PRONOUNCEMENT OF DEATH NOTE

CLIENT NAME	CLIENT ID #
DATE OF VISIT	TIME OF DEATH

FAMILY/OTHER CAREGIVERS PRESENT IN HOME (list names/relationships)

Nurse Pronouncement:
Absence of vital signs (pulse and heartbeat)
Cessation of respirations
Pupils fixed and dilated
Other findings:

	ASSESSMENT AND INTERVENTION	CLINICAL INFORMATION/COMMENTS
PLAN OF CARE/ DISCHARGE PLANNING	___ Reinforce that bereavement services are available, and that the hospice will be in contact with family/caregiver	
DISEASE PROCESS	___ Pronounce death, sign death certificate. ___ Call funeral home (specify name/contact) ___ Instruct family/caregivers on expected changes in condition/appearance of the body after death. Assess understanding. ___ Assist in preparing body for removal, if needed.	
MEDICATION, EQUIPMENT, AND SUPPLIES MANAGEMENT	___ Instruct on/assist with disposal of medications. ___ Complete the medication inventory/ disposal form ___ Call for removal of equipment as appropriate. ___ Instruct on storage/management of unused supplies.	
SPIRITUAL/ EMOTIONAL	___ Allow family/caregivers contact with patient. ___ Assess family/caregiver coping; allow/encourage expression of grief.	
COORDINATION OF CARE	___ Report death to primary physician ___ Report death to team/staff members: MSW HHA PT Chaplain Volunteer Others: ___ Coordinate with bereavement staff responsible for follow-up.	

Pronouncement Visit Outcomes	Met	Not Met	Explanation of Variances/Comments
Patient dies at home			
Family/caregivers express grief and verbalize that spiritual/emotional help is available			

A: Patient too physically impaired/ill
B: Co-morbid interference
C: Psychosocial issues interfering

D: Caregiver limitations/difficulties
E: Equipment problems
F: Pt/CG learning difficulties

G: Pt/CG decision
H: Does not apply (explain)

Signature of Nurse _____

OVER for MEDICATION DISPOSAL RECORD

Nurse pronouncement of death pathway.

NURSE PRONOUNCEMENT OF DEATH NOTE
MEDICATION DISPOSAL RECORD
PAGE 2/2

CLIENT NAME:	ID#

I. **MEDICATION INVENTORY**— List medications found in patient's home:

MEDICATIONS	QUANTITY IN HOME

II. **DISPOSAL OF MEDICATIONS**

The above medications have been disposed of by:

Nurse: _____   Date: _____

Family Member/Caregiver Name: _____   Date: _____

I have been requested to dispose of all the above medications, but decline to do so.

Family Member/Caregiver Name: _____   Date: _____

Witness: _____   Date: _____

Nurse pronouncement of death pathway continued.

makers, the media, and society as a whole. Questions regarding the quality, effectiveness, and cost of end-of-life care continue to arise. Models of care within the managed care environment continue to evolve. All the solutions to critical questions are not known. Therefore, research must continue in the area of end-of-life care, models of care that provide quality and cost-effective outcomes must be developed, and laws and policies that advocate for all to die well need to be formulated.

Review Questions and Activities

1. What are the options for end-of-life care for an 82-year-old man diagnosed with end-stage kidney failure?

2. How would you plan nursing interventions that can be implemented to help hospice clients experience safe and comfortable dying (one of the three major outcomes of hospice care)?

3. According to Dr. Ira Byock, dying can be a time of growth. Discuss the developmental landmarks of this last transition in life.

4. What are the roles and responsibilities of each member of the hospice interdisciplinary team?

5. What is the meaning of the statement: hospice care is palliative care but not all palliative care is hospice care?

6. Explore the following web sites on the Internet: National Hospice Organization at www.nho.org; the Last Acts Campaign to improve care and caring at the end-of-life at http://lastacts.rwjf.org, and the Agency for Health Care Policy and Research for a review of the clinical practice guidelines on the management of cancer pain in adults at www.ahcpr.gov.

7. Reflect on your own attitudes and beliefs regarding dying and death. What are your wishes regarding end-of-life care? Have you completed an advance directive? If not, why not?

8. What are the hospice benefits under the Medicare program?

9. What is your vision of palliative care for the twenty-first century?

10. Contact a hospice program in your community and interview a hospice nurse about his or her experiences caring for terminally ill persons and their families.

References

Amenta, M. O. (1986). The hospice movement. In M. O. Amenta & N. L. Bohnet (Eds.), *Nursing care of the terminally ill* (pp. 49–64). Boston: Little, Brown and Company.

Anderson, C. (1998). *Practice framework*. Unpublished manuscript. The University of Texas at Arlington, School of Nursing, Arlington, TX.

A pathway for patients and families facing terminal illness. (1997). Arlington, VA: National Hospice Organization.

Beltran, J. E., & Coluzzi, P. H. (1997, Spring/Summer). A model for comprehensive palliative care. *Talbert Journal of Health Care*, 47–57.

Byock, I. R. (1996). The nature of suffering and the nature of opportunity at the end-of-life. *Clinics of Geriatric Medicine, 12*(2), 237–252.

Byock, I. (1997). *Dying well: The prospect for growth at the end-of-life*. New York: Riverhead Books.

Cancer pain relief and palliative care (Technical Report Series 804). (1990). Geneva: World Health Organization.

Certification examination for hospice nurses: Handbook for candidates. (1997). New York: National Board for Certification of Hospice Nurses.

DuBoulay, S. (1984). *Cicely Saunders: Founder of the modern hospice movement*. New York: Amaryllis.

Eng, M. A. (1993). The hospice interdisciplinary team: A synergistic approach to the care of dying patients and their families. *Holistic Nursing Practice, 7*(4), 49–56.

Guidelines for curriculum development on end-of-life and palliative care in nursing education. (1997).

Arlington, VA: National Council of Hospice Professionals.

Hayward House. (1996). *Day care at Hayward House, City Hospital* (pamphlet). Nottingham, England: Author.

Holman, G. H. (1998). Dying well: Spiritual care at the end-of-life. *NOEP Informer, 15*(3), 4–6.

Hospice fact sheet. (1998). National Hospice Organization. [Online]. Available: http://www.nho. org/facts.htm.

Hospice Nurses Association Task Force on Hospice Nursing Standards. (1995). *Standards of hospice nursing practice and professional performance*. Pittsburgh, PA: Hospice Nurses Association.

Improving approaching death: Care at the end-of-life. (1997). Institute of Medicine. Washington, DC: National Academy Press.

Lattanzi-Licht, M., Mahoney, J. J., & Miller, G. W. (1998). *The hospice choice: In pursuit of a peaceful death*. New York: Fireside.

Nursing's social policy statement. (1995). Washington, DC: American Nurses' Association.

Oddi, L. F., & Cassidy, V. R. (1998). The message of SUPPORT: Change is long overdue. *Journal of Professional Nursing, 14*(3), 165–174.

Peaceful death. (1997). Washington, DC: American Association of Colleges of Nurses.

Raudonis, B. M. (1993). The meaning and impact of empathic relationships in hospice nursing. *Cancer Nursing, 16,* 304–309.

Raudonis, B. M. (1995). Empathic nurse-patient relationships in hospice nursing. *Hospice Journal, 10*(1), 59–74.

St. Christopher's Hospice. (1996). St. Christopher's Hospice Day Center. Handout. Sydenham, England.

Standards of a hospice program of care. (1993). Alexandria, VA: National Hospice Organization.

Stoddard, S. (1978). *The hospice movement: A better way of caring for the dying*. New York: Vintage Books.

Storey, P. (1990, February). Cancer update: Goals of hospice care. *Texas Medicine, 86,* 50–54.

SUPPORT Principal Investigators. (1995). A controlled trial to improve care for seriously ill hospitalized patients: The Study to Understand Prognoses and Preferences for Outcomes and Risks of Treatments (SUPPORT). *Journal of the American Medical Association, 274,* 1591–1598.

Resources ☐ ☒

Hospice Foundation of America: **www.hospicefoundation.org**

Hospice and Palliative Nurses Association: **www.hpna.org**

National Hospice and Palliative Care Organization: **www.nho.org**

UNIT 6

Community Health Care Resources

PERSPECTIVE . . .

Dorothy Gonzales, age 83, has been feeling extremely sad for the past 4–5 weeks. Her husband's death 2 years ago was almost more than she could bear. She had always loved to bake and cook and prided herself on winning several local baking contests over the years. She used to bake for seven children and her husband. Now cooking and baking for one seem like a waste of time. Also, arthritis has made cooking, baking, and other household tasks difficult to complete.

Mrs. Gonzales' children all live out of town, but they visit as often as possible. Every couple of weeks one or two stop by to visit and help with household chores. It has become apparent that Mrs. Gonzales is losing weight and having difficulty with grooming. She also complains of feeling tired. Mrs. Gonzales' children are concerned about her general condition, possible health care problems, lack of social contacts, and safety. They are busy with their families and work and do not know how or where to obtain the help she needs. Changes are necessary to improve the safety and quality of her life. What are her major needs? What referrals to community agencies might the nurse make? How would a primary care center meet her health care needs?

CHAPTER 22

Primary Care Centers

Marsha Cox, PhD, RN, CS, GNP, ANP
Libby High, NP, PhD(C), MS, BSN, RN

COMPETENCIES

After completing this chapter, the reader should be able to:

- *Identify three reasons why a health clinic that specializes in the older population is important.*
- *Differentiate among types of primary care clinics that cater to the older population's health needs.*
- *Complete a community assessment to determine medical necessity and financial feasibility for a new primary health care clinic for older adults.*
- *Define the differences among HPSA, MUA, and MUP.*
- *Identify the services to be offered in a primary health care clinic that focuses on older adult needs.*
- *Define the roles of key personnel necessary for the efficient operation of a primary health care clinic.*
- *Develop an organizational chart and necessary policies and procedures for a new primary health care clinic.*
- *Advertise a primary health care clinic appropriately and cost effectively.*
- *Identify and utilize effective negotiation skills for obtaining a professional position in a primary health care clinic for older adults.*
- *Identify and measure quality within the clinic, including client satisfaction and appropriate outcomes.*

MAKING THE CONNECTION

Refer to the following chapters to increase your understanding of primary care centers:

Types of Primary Health Care Centers

Geriatric **primary health care clinics** are designed to deliver care to predominantly Medicare enrollees. Most use an interdisciplinary approach incorporating services of physicians, midlevel providers such as **nurse practitioners** and physician assistants, social workers, dietitians, and pharmacists. Segregating and specializing care of older adults are important. Geriatrics is an evolving discipline and with the number of older adults increasing, developing an effective and efficient care delivery system is crucial. In addition to maintaining health status and preventing disease, an older adult may have chronic problems that must be evaluated and treated on an ongoing basis. There are several classifications of primary care centers for older adults. A **primary health care center** is a center that is set up as an outpatient facility of a hospital where older adults can obtain preventive health care services as well as diagnosis, treatment, and care of common medical problems. Private clinics or private practices with linkages to hospitals (for example, through **managed service organizations (MSOs)** also deliver primary care to Medicare enrollees. **Community nursing organizations (CNOs)** belong to a third class of primary care centers and provide nurse-managed care. The nurse working in these centers must be familiar with reimbursement issues, organizational structures, job descriptions, and marketing as well as the delivery of client care.

Primary Health Care Centers

Because a primary health care center is usually a hospital-based department, there is a two-tiered billing structure, a professional component and the technical component provided by the hospital. Reimbursement is on a cost basis for the technical component. Usually the centers do not make a profit, but they can provide advantages for the hospitals. Primary health care centers can (a) expand services into unserved or underserved areas, (b) provide comprehensive services for older adults, (c) provide expertise to other programs in the hospital that are designed for older adults, and (d) provide a competitive advantage by strengthening a continuum of care strategy (Reinberg, 1996).

Because most primary health care centers do not make a profit, establishing them must make sense financially. The Medicare population in the area must be unserved or underserved. There may be a high Medicare population where the hospital has low market share, overutilization of the hospital's emergency department or **urgent care center**, or difficulty finding Medicare physicians. The hospital may also desire to

establish excellence in the delivery of care to older adults. They may want to expand or perfect geriatric services. Senior health centers can benefit the hospital, community, clients, and physicians.

One large hospital system in a metropolitan area currently operates 13 primary health care centers specifically for older adults. There is also a geriatrics center that offers education, home visits, specialized clinics, and research. The system provides coordination of primary care, acute care, and long-term care for older adults in the area (Baylor Health Care System, 1998).

Think About It

- What are the advantages of providing primary health care centers specifically for older adults? Any disadvantages?
- Have health care outcomes been positively affected by specialized health care?
- Have nurse practitioners made a positive impact on the care of older adults? How much of the care is complementary to physician care and how much of the care is instead of the physician?
- What process is involved in opening a primary health care center?

Private Clinics and Centers

Hospitals, private physicians, and clinics set up alliances to deliver care to older adults. Separate identity is maintained, but common goals are reached in a cost-effective and efficient manner. Managed service organizations oversee the linkage and provide advantages to both parties in the form of group discounts on liability and malpractice insurance, health insurance for employees, office and medical supplies, billing and collections, payroll and human resources functions, marketing, managed care contracting, and quality assurance and utilization management. Each entity is reimbursed for the respective services rendered.

Community Nursing Organizations

The Health Care Financing Administration (HCFA) has provided funding for four CNOs: (a) Visiting Nurse Service of New York; (b) Healthy Seniors Program of Carondelet Health Network in Tucson, Arizona; (c) The Healthy Seniors Project at the Living at Home Block Nurse Program in St. Paul, Minnesota; and (d) Carle Clinic Association Community Nursing Organization in Urbana, Illinois. These programs provide nurse-managed care in a variety of settings. These sites provide specific Medicare benefits such as physical therapy, speech-language pathology services, occupational therapy, skilled nursing care, home health aides, social work, durable medical equipment, and outpatient therapies. They are reimbursed on a capitated payment plan that pays a set fee for each enrollee. All of the CNOs stress health promotion and disease prevention. Although nurse managed, members of the team include physicians (Burtt, 1998).

Medicare Reimbursement for Nurse Practitioners

Medicare reimbursement for nurse practitioners in primary health care centers was recently broadened to all settings (not just skilled nursing facilities and rural settings) in the Balanced Budget Act of 1997 (Public Law No. 105-33—Medicare). The new payment regulations allow nurse practitioners to be reimbursed for services in areas and settings authorized by state licensure laws. These laws vary state by state. When the professional fee is **unbundled** from other fees, the nurse practitioner may receive 80% of the actual charge or 85% of the physician fee schedule amount, whichever is less. Nurse practitioners will be unable to separate Medicare payments in **rural health centers (RHCs)** and **federally qualified health centers (FQHCs),** however, because those fees are designed to be all-inclusive and to include nonphysician professionals (American College, 1998).

Developing a Primary Health Care Clinic/Center for Older Adults

CLINICAL ALERT

- *Care for Medicare enrollees is regulated and those regulations must be known. The HCFA monitors care provided to Medicare recipients.*
- *The practice of nurse practitioners varies from state to state, and those regulations must be followed.*

Community Assessment

There may be several reasons why a person or an organization is considering opening a primary health care clinic for older adults. They may perceive a large older population in the geographic area or an unusually high number of hospitalized older adults. A community assessment is necessary to obtain tangible proof of the original perceived assumptions. The purpose of the community assessment is to determine medical feasibility and the potential for success of a new clinic.

Process

The sponsoring organization must first identify and define the motive and philosophy that surrounds the desire to undertake the project. Objectives need to be clear and feasible. The staff's current scope of practice along with involvement and history in the community needs to be clarified (Finnigan, 1996). Problems that may occur need to be evaluated carefully.

Community resources should be identified (e.g., the County Medical Society, the area Council of Governments, the Chamber of Commerce, and the closest HCFA office) to determine primary health care clinics already established that will be competitors. These clinics should be assessed for reception/billing staff as well as the health care providers concerning client populations, number of clients seen daily, ethnicity of the clients, types of client payment, services offered, and problems. Is the clinic perceived to be a success? Clinics that are already operational will provide much positive and negative information. There are many variables that can be manipulated in such a setting to turn negative perceptions into positive ones. Staff attitudes, medical provider competency, waiting room comfort, length of client wait, and even billing practices are all variables that can be improved.

Demographic information about the area where the new clinic will be located can be found on the Internet or by visiting an area Chamber of Commerce (usually for a fee), the local area Council of Governments, or the maps room of the city hall or county seat. A large geographical area around the new clinic site, about a 50-mile radius, needs to be assessed. What is the population, the employment rate, the availability of health care and hospitals, the ethnicity and age of the population, the mean income, the potential for growth, and the number of nonspecialist physicians in the area (available through the Internet to the state medical board)?

The assessment should be limited to the area where the proposed clinic will be located. A map will show census tracts of about a 5-mile radius in an urban area and a 25-mile radius (or more depending on the population) in a rural area. Most of the census information on the Internet is a projected approximation for current years (it will all be current again when the 2000 census data are available). Information about population numbers, age, ethnicity, employment, major employers, makeup of the households, and mean income should be obtained. Any percent of the 65-year-old and over population of 10% or more is encouraging. The types and numbers of physicians serving the area can be obtained from the state medical board. Because clinics need to be in various locations in the community where older adults live, location, accessibility, and safety are very important. Criteria for an effective site for a primary health care clinic for older adults are listed in Box 22-1.

BOX 22-1   Criteria for Selecting a Site for a Primary Health Care Clinic for Older Adults

- Located near an area where many older adults live (e.g., large retirement center)

- Adequate close parking, including parking for disabled people

- Easily accessible area from major freeways

- Accessible from public transportation routes (e.g., buses)

- Clinic transportation provided

- Adequate inside and outside lighting

- No or few stairs or step edges clearly marked with yellow or red

- Free from potential criminal activity for both clients and staff

- Security system, alarm system, secured front door

Federal Designation Programs

The **health professional shortage area (HPSA)** and **medically underserved area/population (MUA/MUP)** are geographical areas designated under federal programs administered by the Division of Shortage Designation (DSD), Bureau of Primary Health Care (BPHC), and U.S. Department of Health and Human Services (DHHS). Each has its own unique eligibility criteria and designation process. Information about areas or population groups designated in a certain state can be found at the Department of Health in each state.

There are incentive programs and federal grants that can be sought when an area has an HPSA or MUA/MUP designation (see Tables 22-1 and 22-2). Clinics that are established within one of these areas have a more relaxed regulatory mechanism and can be designated a *freestanding* clinic in some states. This type status allows a nurse practitioner or physician assistant to be the primary medical management person on site while the supervising physician is located miles away. Each state's specific rules and regulations can be checked through the state medical board. Information on freestanding clinics may include (but not be limited to) the type of medical provider who may work in one, the number of times the supervising physician must visit, the number of charts the supervising physician must review and sign, and the distance the supervising physician needs to be from the clinic.

Health Professional Shortage Areas

An HPSA is an area, facility, or population group with a shortage of primary care physicians (providers), as defined by a population-to-primary-care-physician ratio of at least 3,500:1 and other requirements specified in the federal designation criteria. Indicators of need for primary medical care such as the poverty rate, infant mortality rate, and fertility rate (live births per 1,000 female population) are also considered, as well as indicators of insufficient capacity to meet existing needs. The HPSAs can qualify designated areas and population groups for benefits.

Medically Underserved Areas/Populations

The MUAs/MUPs are areas or population groups with a quantifiable shortage of personal health services as defined by the U.S. Department of Health and Human Services designation area criteria. For MUAs, an index of medical underservice (IMU) score is calculated based on a statistical process that takes the individual area's poverty rate, percentage of older population, and primary care physicians per 1,000 population and compares it with national averages. Individual population groups in areas not qualifying as MUAs can qualify as MUPs using the IMU method or a process whereby the population group's usual local conditions are documented to result in a barrier to access to health care. The latter process requires the governor of the state to submit a recommendation to the federal government for MUP designation of the specific population group. The MUAs/MUPs can qualify designated areas and population groups for benefits under certain programs.

Business Plan for Opening a Primary Health Care Clinic for Older Adults

There are many factors to consider and evaluate when planning a new health care service in the community. Some of these factors are financing, site, and ancillary services such as equipment and supplies. However, one of the most important is to obtain an adequate number of qualified health care professionals to meet the needs of the population to be served.

Financing

If the financing of a new clinic is to be completed by a group of investors through a financial lending institution, there are several necessary steps to prepare for the loan acquisition. The group of investors meet with a business attorney to develop the type of organization, such as a corporation, partnership, or association. Once this process is determined, each individual will complete

TABLE 22-1 Health Professional Shortage Areas (HPSAs)

Name of Program Benefit	Nature of Benefit	Contact
Medicare Provider Incentive Payments (geographic HPSA sites)	10% Medicare bonus payment, Public Law (PL) 100-203, Section 4043	Division of Medicare, Health Care Financing Administration (HCFA) (in your state)
National Health Service Corps (NHSC) Placement Program (HPSA sites only)	NHSC Scholarship Program and NHSC Loan Repayment Program, Public Health Service (PHS) Act, Secs. 333 and 338B, provides scholarships and then scholarship forgiveness to those health professionals who work in HPSAs	Primary Care Provider (PCP) Placement Program, Bureau of Community Oriented Primary Care (within State Department of Health)
Rural Health Clinic (RHC) Act (nonurbanized areas only, HPSA and MUA sites)	PL 95-210 provides cost-based reimbursement for provider services under the Medicaid and Medicare programs	*Reimbursement information:* Medicare Division of HCFA, U.S. DHHS (in your state) *RHC and Medicare certification information:* State Department of Health
Physician Education Loan Repayment Program (HPSA only)	State-approved specialties may qualify certain physicians loan forgiveness of $18,000/year for up to 5 years for service in HPSA or state agency	Physician Education Loan Repay Program, State Higher Education Coordinating Board
Prescriptive Authority (HPSA, MUA/MUP, RHC/MUP sites)	Prescriptive authority for nurse practitioners and physician assistants in listed areas; varies by state	State Board of Nursing, State PA Licensure, State Department of Health
Community Scholarship Program (HPSA sites only)	Federal, state, and community partnership supports students in their third or fourth year of medical school, or PA or NP programs, who return to HPSA communities	Center for Rural Health Initiatives (CRHI)

Other federal programs using HPSA designations:

- Higher "Customary Charges" for New Physicians in HPSAs (PL 100-103, Sec. 4047)
- Nurse practitioner/midwifery training [PHS Act, Sec. 822(a)]
- Physician assistant training (Sec. 783)
- Residency training and fellowships in internal medicine, pediatrics, family medicine, dentistry [Secs. 784, 786(a), 786(b)]
- Area Health Education Center Program [Sec. 781(a)(1)] and mental health clinic traineeships [Sec. 303(d)]

Source: Adapted from information provided by the Texas Department of Health, July 1998.

Nursing Tip

Nurses should be aware of the business and financial aspects of health care delivery. Resources should be matched with needs. The best nursing care may never be delivered if the clinic or center cannot survive financially.

---

a financial statement and prepare for a credit check. The loan officer of the lending facility (bank or credit union) can assist with the types of information necessary to present in the business plan (Crow, 1996).

Lease/Purchase/Build the New Facility

The location and specifications of the new clinic and how the facility will be acquired should be determined

TABLE 22-2   Medically Underserved Area/Population Federal and State Benefits

Name of Program	Nature of Benefit	Contact
Community Health Centers (CHCs) MUA/MUP sites	Limited grant funds for operating costs of CHCs (PHS Act, Sec. 330)	Health Resources and Services Administration, Public Health Service, U.S. DHHS
Federally Qualified Health Centers (FQHCs) (MUAs/MUPs)	Cost-based reimbursement under Medicare and Medicaid programs (PHS Act, Secs. 329, 330)	Health Resources and Services Administration, Public Health Service, U.S. DHHS
Rural Health Clinic (RHC) Act (nonurban HPSA or MUA site, excludes MUP sites)	Cost-based reimbursement for medical care under the Medicaid and Medicare programs (includes NP, PA, midwife, psychologist, and social worker) (PL 95-210)	*Reimbursement information:* Medicare HCFA, U.S. DHHS *Medicare certification information:* Health Facility Compliance Division, Bureau of Licensure and Certification, State Department of Health
Limited Prescriptive Authority (HPSA, MUA/MUP, RHC/MUP sites)	Limited prescriptive authority for nurse practitioners and physician assistants in listed areas; varies by state	State Board of Nursing, State PA Licensure, State Department of Health
Physician Assistant Loan Repayment Program (rural HPSA or MUA site)	Repayment of educational loans for PAs agreeing to practice in rural HPSAs/MUAs at rate of $5,000/year	State Center for Rural Health Initiatives

Source: Adapted from information provided by the Texas Department of Insurance, July 1998.

(Blatchford, 1996). If the building is to be leased, a fair agreement should be discussed with the agent of the building. The process for needed repairs, handicap accessibility, rent, repair of the ventilation system, and use of any available equipment or office furniture should be discussed. The building should meet standards for security, fire safety, and sanitation. If the clinic is to be built, a reputable architect who has designed other medical facilities for older adults should be consulted.

Services Needed

Arrangements have to be made for (a) janitorial services; (b) insurance for contents, the building, and liability; (c) a telephone system that includes lines for fax, modem, and security; (d) medical waste disposal for biohazardous waste; (e) computer system; (f) start-up medical supplies and equipment; (g) office furniture; (h) office supplies; (i) security system; (j) professional services for consulting, attorney, and accounting; and (k) image development and advertising. Bids should include an initial cost, such as for a computer system, and a monthly maintenance cost, such as for computer supplies (Meyer, 1997).

Primary care providers (PCPs) will be needed to treat clients (e.g., physicians, nurse practitioners, and/or physician assistants). Salaries will be deter-

Think About It

A hospital is trying to determine whether it would be feasible to establish a primary health care center in an area of the city. They have evaluated census data and have determined that there are 3,000 people age 65 years and older in the defined area. The residents in the area currently obtain their health care needs by private physicians in the area. The planning committee seeks answers to the following questions before they proceed with plans to open the center. Are older adults moving into the area? Are the residents satisfied with the care they are currently receiving? If older adults did change to the health center, would there be concerns expressed by the primary and specialty physicians in the area? What is the anticipated use of health care center services? What is the cost of opening such a center?

mined based on many factors such as education, license, and individual factors.

Laboratory services are offered by area accredited medical laboratories that will pick up specimens and distribute results. Laboratories will usually provide a centrifuge and all specimen containers, vacutainers, and necessary supplies. Certain specimens will need to be refrigerated.

Primary Health Care Clinic Services

The clinic plan will include details about the types of services to be offered. For example, physician services, diagnostic testing of all types, emergency care if needed by clinic clients while there, and educational programs on wellness and health promotion for individuals and groups are usually provided.

Outpatient Services

By offering outpatient services, the clinic must determine the hours of operation and the type of staff that will be necessary to run the clinic. As with any diverse group, some older clients prefer early morning appointments (these are the persons that awake at 4:00 AM), and others do not want to get out of the house until afternoon. Clinic hours can be determined by client need and availability of staff. Some of the staffing hours need to be set aside for nondirect client activities such as data entry, billing, calling clients regarding procedures and laboratory reports, calls to pharmacies, and time for paperwork.

When older clients are seen medically in the outpatient clinic setting, about 50%–60% will be for acute conditions and 40%–50% for chronic recurring illnesses (see Table 22-3). The clinic must have the capability to draw blood tests and have most results reported in 1–4 days. Simple laboratory tests that can be completed in the office might be urine dipstick, blood glucose finger stick, stool for occult blood, hemoglobin and hematocrit, and microscopic wetpreps. Each state has regulations concerning competency and quality of these office laboratory tests. Usually a logbook that registers periodic test controls is helpful to maintain the integrity of the ongoing testing. Electrocardiograms must be immediately available as well as accessibility to x-ray equipment. Some clinics with trained **advanced cardiac life support (ACLS)** professionals may choose to have an emergency defibrillator and crash cart (Figure 22-1), while other clinics may prefer to call 911 and only administer cardiopulmonary resuscitation (CPR) and basic emergency drugs.

Sample medications that are donated to the primary care provider from pharmaceutical companies must be kept locked. Most are dangerous drugs that are dispensed through prescription only. Samples are dispensed in a fair and equitable manner. Sample drugs are especially helpful for older clients whose income may be minimal. A few days supply can be taken initially to monitor for adverse drug reactions, side effects, and effectiveness before the client fills an expensive complete prescription. The federal **Drug Enforcement Agency (DEA)** and the State Department of Public Safety regulate sample drugs. Basically the regulations are quite simple. The provider must (a) sign a receipt of acceptance from the pharmaceutical representative when samples are obtained and (b) make an entry into the client record of the date, type, and number of samples the client was given. A conscientious practitioner will follow the Board of Pharmacy rules and regulations and be sure that the samples are properly labeled with the client name and complete dosing instructions. There are no federal regulations on out-of-date drugs; however, some states and hospital facilities might have such regulations. Some clinic providers have special relationships with medical professionals who use out-of-date sample drugs for out-of-country mercy medical care. This is an ethical issue that needs investigation. Besides sample drugs, an outpatient clinic will need certain stock medications and vaccinations on hand. These are usually a one-time dose or a dose of medication that needs to be given immediately to prevent further illness or complication.

TABLE 22-3 Common Health Care Problems in Older Adults	
Acute Conditions	**Chronic Conditions**
Heart disease	Arthritis
Cancer	Osteoporosis
Stroke	Parkinson's disease
Chronic obstructive pulmonary disease	Visual and hearing problems
Pneumonia and influenza	Dementia

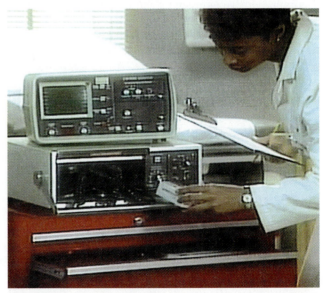

FIGURE 22-1 Medical crash carts, like this one, are used in some clinics that staff trained personnel.

Research Focus

Citation:

Boult, C., Boult, L., Morishita, L., Smith, S. L., & Kane, R. L. (1988). Outpatient geriatric evaluation and management. *Journal of the American Geriatrics Society, 46*(3), 296–302.

Purpose:

To describe the development and operation of a practical model of outpatient geriatric evaluation and management (GEM) for high-risk, community-dwelling older adults.

Methods:

Participants were community-dwelling Medicare beneficiaries age 70 years and older who were medically stable but had a high probability of repeated admissions to the hospital [P(ra) > .40] in the future (n = 248). The intervention was outpatient GEM. The measurements were demographic, clinical, and use-of-hospital characteristics of clients; nature and quality of GEM services; and satisfaction of clients and their established primary care physicians.

Findings:

At enrollment, the average client was 78.7 years old, took 5.0 long-term prescription medications, and was unable to perform 0.5 (of six) activities of daily living (ADL) and 1.4 (of seven) instrumental ADL. Many clients (71.3%) reported hospital stays during the previous year. Each of three interdisciplinary teams (physician, gerontological nurse practitioner, nurse, and social worker) performed comprehensive assessments and then provided primary care and case management to a case load of 45–52 clients. On average, GEM required 6 months, during which clients visited the GEM clinic 7.4 times, had 10.4 active problems addressed, spoke to GEM staff members weekly by telephone, and were referred to two other providers. Most clients (94.4%) completed the GEM program; 66.7% completed advance directives. Satisfaction with GEM was high among the clients and their established primary physicians. The cost of the GEM personnel averaged about $1,540 per client treated.

Implications:

This model of outpatient GEM provided 6 months of targeted intensive care at a reasonable cost. The satisfaction ratings of clients and their primary care physicians were high.

Examination tables within an outpatient clinic should be safe, low, padded, and convenient for older adults. It is often difficult for someone with painful joints or an unsure equilibrium to climb up on an elevated surface. Fall prevention that is emphasized in the clinic can be transferred to the client's own environment through role modeling. Stable footstools are essential. Tables and chairs with material that can be cleaned in case of incontinence decreases odor, bacteria, and embarrassment.

Finally, the outpatient clinic needs close parking. Entryways into the clinic should have rails, a minimum number of stairs, and handicap accessibility. Easy access to the receptionist is recommended. The older client should not be kept waiting but should see the PCP as quickly as possible. The waiting room chairs should be comfortable with arms to assist in standing.

Educational Services

Medicare will partially reimburse for educational materials developed for the older population. This material should exclude advertisements and be written with the older adult in mind. The **American Association of Retired Persons (AARP)** suggests using sharply contrasted type and background with at least a size 14 font print. Newsletters that target the needs and special problems of the older adult must provide a forum to teach and suggest solutions to a culturally and socioeconomically diverse group of people. A monthly newsletter with short concise articles written by the clinic primary care provider indicates to the client and the public that their needs are being met.

Newspapers often offer an Ask-A-Pro type section for the public to present questions and an expert to provide the answers. The expert as a form of interactive advertising usually pays for this forum. If the clinic decides to use this type of advertising, data on the continued educational needs of the population can be collected. Fees for this method can be $80–$200 per month depending upon the newspaper's circulation. Participation by a PCP is an excellent way to provide name recognition to the community.

Radio and television shows are often searching for articulate individuals to talk about specific services offered in the community. Volunteers appear to discuss the health care needs of older adults. This is an opportunity not only to educate the community but also to advertise.

Once a month educational programs at the clinic can provide many different benefits to the older client. A regular monthly schedule and refreshments may increase attendance. The first hour could be a presentation by a specialist on hypertension, diabetes, home safety, or advance directives. The following 15–20 minutes could provide a social time period where participants can interact and have refreshments. Games, such as Bingo, can be provided as an additional incentive to attend the program. A monthly meeting is not only educational but also provides a reason for a lonely individual to leave the house and interact with other people.

Health Fair and Mini-Screening Exams

Shopping malls in large and small communities have health fairs that attract medically oriented businesses that set up booths and present their products or services. During annual or biannual health fair events, primary health care clinics attract an audience by offering (a) to take blood pressure, (b) check blood glucose and cholesterol levels, (c) measure body mass index with height and weight, (d) test vision and hearing, and/or (e) offer influenza and pneumonia vaccinations (Figure 22-2). This type of interaction with the community helps to build trust and name recognition. When irregularities are discovered, the person being screened is encouraged to make an appointment for follow-up.

Other Services

The services offered by an interdisciplinary team are designed to meet the needs of older adults (Figure 22-3). However, each person must be treated as an individual and goals designed with that person in mind. The prices of services often are fixed within the guidelines of Medicare or an HMO. Convenience to the clients is important. Older adults sometimes rely on family, friends, or public transportation to get to the clinic and to other diagnostic testing centers and specialists' offices. Some centers are served by mobile mammography vans. Some centers

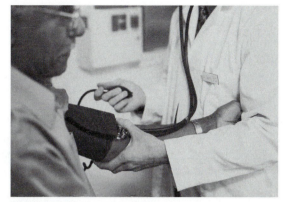

FIGURE 22-2   Free blood pressure screenings provide a community service and can attract new clients.

also have mobile retinopathy clinics and specialists (e.g., cardiologists, psychiatrists) on site on designated days. Some primary health care centers have early and late clinic times for clients who work or who depend on family members who work for transportation. Client satisfaction surveys are good sources of information about ways that the services can be modified to meet the needs of clients more effectively.

Organizational Development

Organization and management of the clinic should include competent staff who understand the policies and procedures, some of which are federally or state mandated. Informing those who could use the services of the clinic is an important part of the marketing strategy.

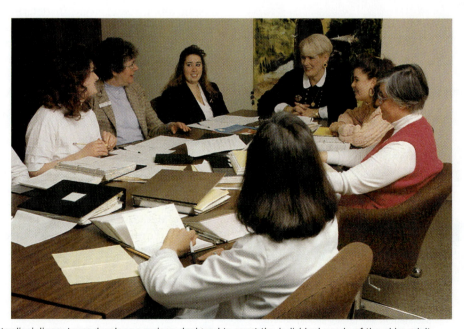

FIGURE 22-3   The interdisciplinary team develops services designed to meet the individual needs of the older adult.

Staffing

Staffing the outpatient clinic begins after a vision and philosophy are developed. Will the PCP be an on-site physician, nurse practitioner (NP), or physician assistant (PA) (O'Neill, 1996)? Whoever it is, the person must have a current job description for that facility, a file that proves licensure to practice in the state, a record of continuing education, a copy of prescriptive authority and DEA number, and Medicare, Medicaid, and HMO certification and/or contract. Some states require a NP or PA to have protocols for practice that have been signed by the supervising physician.

There is always the need for a personable receptionist with a good sense of humor and a clear voice. This person is usually the initial contact person with the clinic and must explain and repeat the same information many times, usually to different people. The receptionist needs a ready client smile, good telephone manners, and willingness to lead older adults through the process of medical management. Data entry and billing personnel must understand many intricate regulations. There is nothing more frustrating than having a claim denied because paper work is filled out incorrectly or precertification was not done. As rules and regulations become more complex, a knowledgeable, assertive billing person is good for business.

The primary care provider will need a nurse or **medical assistant (MA)** to gather brief subjective data from each client on admission along with vital signs, height, and weight. This person needs to have excellent communication skills, along with a sincere enjoyment of working with older people (Figure 22-4). The nurse or

MA will need to know how to do a venipuncture and an electrocardiogram (ECG), set up for procedures and wound care, handle pharmacy renewals, and keep accurate records. This person is responsible for the organization of the office and flow of the clients.

Ancillary personnel who are a vital part of a primary health care clinic team include a social worker, clinical pharmacist, dietitian educator, and a variety of therapists. A social worker (SW) may be asked to obtain long-term medications from a pharmaceutical company, at a discount if possible, or assist in finding different living accommodations for someone. The SW can bill through Medicare for completing a Mini-Mental Status Exam (MMSE), a Depression Survey, or for individual counseling. With the problem of multiple medications in many older clients, a clinical pharmacist might review medications and make suggestions that prevent adverse drug reaction or decreased effectiveness. There are several pharmacist-managed programs that can be reimbursed without direct physician oversight. These include programs for anticoagulation and antihypertensive therapies based on established treatment protocols. A dietitian educator is essential for developing food plans and lifestyle changes for the diabetic client or the person with specific nutrition problems. Occupational and physical therapists help older adults stay independent and help control pain through exercise and modification of behavior.

Policies and Procedures

The clinic scope and plan of care are documented in writing as guidelines to encourage continuity among providers of services. With written policies and procedures, a clinic employee can quickly determine the clinic's position and technique for handling multiple circumstances. Clinic policies and procedures should take into account the rules of various federal and state regulatory boards. Clinic policies and procedures must never contradict existing regulations but may add additional policy that fits the environment.

Organizational policies and procedures will include a statement about the scope of practice including the types of clients and remuneration that will be accepted in the clinic. A clear policy outlining the admission of a client to the clinic is suggested along with a policy on initial assessment and repeated reassessment or follow-up. Any Medicare or HMO standards such as the use of a **drug formulary** should be defined. The necessity of collaboration with a physician or specialist needs to be clarified along with a policy for referral. Any specific diagnostic procedures that are to be included on every or specific clients need to be considered. An example is that an **ankle-brachial index** is to be measured on all clients with leg pain, diabetes, or risk factors for athero-

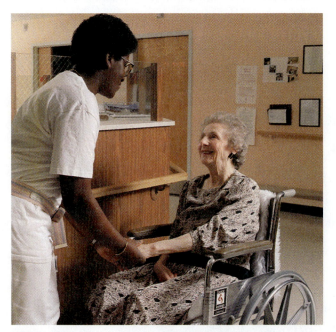

FIGURE 22-4 The medical assistant in any facility should have a sincere enjoyment of working with older adults.

sclerosis. If education and community involvement are important to the clinic, a policy that defines services is helpful.

An organizational chart should be identified so that all clinic employees are clear on supervision and hierarchy. With most primary health care clinics, a board of directors is the top regulatory entity. There may next be a **chief executive officer (CEO)** or office manager who oversees the financial aspect of the clinic. The PCP in the clinic supervises the clinic staff with the assistance of an office manager. A PCP, whether a physician or NP, should never be supervised by someone who is not involved with medical management decisions. Employment issues can be supervised by an office manager, but never medical issues. Peer review of medical modalities and the adherence to regulatory standards should be done only by a PCP's medical equal. Most state civil statutes clearly define the relationship of the physician and the NP or PA. Because of the fairly new role of the NP in the clinic and hospital-based setting, there have been major concerns about NPs being supervised by nurse administrators. This issue should be avoided at all costs so the NP feels confident in the medical management role. It is suggested that the NP join a group of area NPs to develop and regulate their practices according to joint acceptable standards (Sadaniantz, 1998). This is the way that physicians regulate and evaluate their own practices.

Marketing

In 1964 McCarthy designated the four P's as the way to plan marketing strategies. The "product" (and services) were designed to meet the unfilled needs and wants of the consumer. The "price" was determined by analyzing the consumer's ability to pay in relationship to supply. The "place of exchange" in the marketplace was then determined. The product was then "promoted" in some format. Additional P's were often added to the mix. "Packaging" the product became important and was an aspect of "promotion." An additional P representing people was sometimes added to the mix (Bennett, 1997).

In 1991 Robins gave marketing the four C's: customers, competitors, capabilities, and company. The satisfaction of the customer's needs remained the driving force. As marketing became more developed, the complexity of who customers were and what they expected in relationships became more defined. Customers were defined as internal (representing exchanges within the corporation) and external (representing exchanges of the products and services with the consumer of those products and services). Customers were often viewed as a collective, but now they are also looked at as individuals (Bennett, 1997).

Bennett (1997) proposed that the customer disposition has five dimensions: (a) value, (b) viability, (c) volume, (d) variety, and (e) virtue. Value not only is the price/product quotient but also encompasses the convenience, attributes of uniqueness, and brand status. Viability considers distance, availability, and acceptability of the product/service in terms of the expectations of the buyer. In a health care setting this may include not only the primary care clinic but also access to specialists and diagnostic testing. Volume is associated with both the amount of the product/service and the accompanying parts required with the purchase. For instance, some products come in packages of three when a customer may only need one. In a primary care clinic a new client may only want medication renewed but may be required to get a physical examination or diagnostic testing. Codes of practice are considered also. Variety is what gives customers choices with similar products/services. In addition to what the product/service looks like, choices can include insurance and collection. Brand switching is always a potential when there are several primary care centers in the area. Customers who share stories about their dissatisfaction with care can cause preconceived opinions in others. Virtue can be visualized by customers in the services and products they purchase. Customers may believe that their selection of products/services is the ultimate or optimum choice. The integrity of the buyer-producer relationship is important for a long-lasting and satisfying association (Bennett, 1997).

A relationship with a small advertising agency or creative group is essential for the positive image projection of the new clinic. A marketing package may include logo, image, initial introduction, continuing advertisement for the proposed clinic, and measurement of client satisfaction. Brochures distributed to community centers and churches will attract clients. A story about the clinic, those involved in the development, and the services offered to the older population will provide invaluable exposure in the media (e.g., newspaper). Coupons offering free mini-health screens may bring clients who decide to stay with the clinic. Community involvement in the needs of the older population adds validity to the purpose of the primary health care clinic.

Professional Development

Nurses, especially nurse practitioners, should clearly evaluate their options for a role in the clinic. The focus on measuring outcomes of medical and nursing care is increasing as customers seek quality care and health care costs continue to escalate.

Negotiation of a Professional Position

A nurse practitioner who is interested in working at a primary health care clinic or center must choose between several business options. A full partnership in a clinic would ensure equal opinion in decisions and an equal share in profits. On the reverse, a partnership acquires equal liabilities and financial and ethical responsibilities. A limited partnership may reduce liabilities and reward initiative and additional work practices (Crow, 1998). The nurse practitioner may decide that straight employment by the facility is most desirable. Hours of work will be set, along with salary, benefits, and possible incentives.

After determining the type of employment, the professional must come to the interview with specific ideas about what is acceptable employment (Anderson, 1998). One must be willing to sacrifice the employment if the condition is not met. It is ideal if one can develop one's own unique job description and terms for employment. Sadly, it is often found that nurses underestimate their desirability and worth to the rest of the medical community. This problem is found in the reluctance to ask for appropriate financial compensation and agreeing to take on too much responsibility.

It is important to have a clear understanding of how one's work will be evaluated. The person who will be completing the evaluation should provide a set of objectives that are clear and specific (Dove, 1998). Periodic off-the-record reviews will provide a sense of trust and predictability and allow the nurse practitioner a period to improve on deficits before the official evaluation. As stated previously, a nurse practitioner's medical management must be evaluated only by other nurse practitioners or physicians.

Outcome Evaluation

Management of the health and illness of an individual, family, or community by the NP includes not only medical management, such as a history and physical, diagnostic screening services, interpretation of data, prescriptive use of pharmaceuticals, and the use of referral services, but also nursing management, such as counseling, client education, health promotion, disease prevention, and evaluation of outcomes. Good health is everyone's goal, but views on what it is and how to get it differ enormously (Windsor, Baranowski, Clark, & Cutter, 1994). A provider of health and illness management services must include the health care recipients' perspective as well as positive health outcomes; otherwise the relevance of the service is lost along with participation and compliance.

The consumer public has been enlightened through the mass media to the facts that health care in the United States is the most expensive in the world but places little emphasis on proactive health promotion. The recipients of health care increasingly are using terms such as quality of life, quality of health care, and client satisfaction.

The NPs not only must justify and be accountable to the public that their medical management is effective (Brooten & Naylor, 1995) but also must justify the role of the NP and how it differs from that of the physician (Safriet, 1992). Additional rationale for evaluating client outcomes includes the justification of costs (Brown & Grimes, 1992) and the identification of variables that can have a positive or negative effect on outcomes (e.g., communication) (Knaus, Draper, Wagner, & Zimmerman, 1986). Edmunds (1991) insisted that for Congress to reimburse NPs independently, NPs must describe clearly the contributions they make to the health care delivery system. Legislators must be persuaded that the care provided by NPs is desirable, acceptable, and affordable.

The measurement of outcomes is as varied as the professional's imagination. The professional NP can, with the help of colleagues and the recipients of their service, determine expected and projected outcomes that need to be measured. The most obvious outcome is mortality and morbidity rates, while more creative ones include client knowledge, adherence to treatment, pain, mobility, physical status, mental attitude, general welfare, skin condition, objective and subjective evaluation of progress, return to work, or return office visits (Brooten & Naylor, 1995). Lang & Marek (1992) contributed examples of outcomes that reflect the unique contribution of nursing practice such as quality of life, home functions, family strain, goal attainment, utilization of services, safety, client satisfaction, and caring.

Finally, the NP must have a concern not just with clinical or physiological outcomes but also with measures of health-related quality of life, including physical and emotional functioning, general perceptions of health and well-being, and satisfaction with the process or care.

Summary

Many of the health care needs of older adults are being met in primary health care centers in the community. There are several types of primary health care centers: (a) health clinics, (b) private clinics, and (c) community nursing organizations. An interdisciplinary approach is working well. Older adults, physicians, nurse practitioners, physician assistants, social workers, pharmacists, health educators, and dietitians collaborate to obtain quality health outcomes. Medicare is the primary health insurance. Location of the primary health care center determines the type of reimbursement and the regulations for nurse practitioners. For example, in some states the degree of physician supervision for the nurse practitioner varies depending on geographical location, with the rural areas requiring less direct, on-site physician coverage.

A community assessment is necessary before developing a primary health care center for older adults. The marketplace for the exchange of services is defined and advertising strategies are chosen. When the primary care center is new, the nurse practitioner can often negotiate with administration regarding the functions of the position and the compensation (salary and benefits). To demonstrate the cost/benefit ratio of using the nurse practitioner in the primary care role, health outcomes must be identified. By demonstrating the achievement of those outcomes in an efficient and cost-effective manner, the nurse practitioner's contributions can be defined. Research related to the nurse practitioner's role in meeting health outcomes is imperative.

Older adults often require more time in the primary health care center because of their physical limitations and number of chronic health problems. Matching the client's needs with the best resource (e.g., member of the interdisciplinary team) to manage the concern can improve the quality of care as well as minimize the costs.

Review Questions and Activities

1. Why is a primary health care clinic that specializes in the older population important to health care delivery in the United States?

2. What are the different types of primary health care clinics that strive to meet the older population's health needs?

3. What are the components of a community assessment needed to determine medical necessity and financial feasibility for a new primary health care clinic for older adults?

4. What are the differences among HPSAs, MUAs, and MUPs?

5. What services are offered in a primary health care clinic and what personnel are needed to provide those services?

6. What policies and procedures must be incorporated into the operations of a primary health care clinic?

7. What are some of the marketing considerations in operating a primary health care clinic for older persons?

References

American College of Nurse Practitioners. (1998). *Summary of HCFA program memorandum*. [On-line]. Available: acnp@nurse.org.

Anderson, K. (1998). 16 tips for reaching agreement. *Nursing, 28*(7), 64.

Baylor Health Care System. (1998). *Primary care centers*. [On-line]. Available: http://www.bhcs.com.

Bennett, A. R. (1997). The five Vs—a buyer's perspective of the marketing mix. *Marketing Intelligence and Planning, 15*(2/3), 151–156.

Blatchford, W. (1996). Lease or purchase? *Denistry Today, 15*(1), 80.

Brooten, D., & Naylor, M. (1995). Nurses' effect on changing patient outcomes. *Image: Journal of Nursing Scholarship, 27*(2), 95–99.

Brown, S., & Grimes, D. (1992). *A meta-analysis of process of care, clinical outcomes, and cost effectiveness of nurses in primary care roles: Nurse practitioners and nurse midwives*. Washington, DC: American Nurses' Association Division of Health Policy.

Burtt, K. (1998). Nurses step to forefront of elder care. *American Journal of Nursing, 98*(7), 52–57.

Crow, G. L. (1996). The business of planning your practice: Success is no accident. *Advanced Practice Nursing Quarterly, 2*(1), 55–61.

Crow, G. L. (1998). The entrepreneurial personality: Building a sustainable future for self and profession. *Nursing Administration Quarterly, 22*(2), 30–35.

Dove, M. A. (1998). Conflict, process and resolution. *Nursing Management, 29*(4), 30–32.

Edmunds, M. (1991). Lack of evidence could exclude NPs from reimbursement-reform legislation. *Nurse Practitioner, 16*(5), 8.

Finnigan, S. (1996). Getting started in business: From fantasy to reality. *Advanced Practice Nursing Quarterly, 2*(1), 1–8.

Knaus, W., Draper, E., Wagner, D., & Zimmerman, J. (1986). An evaluation of outcomes from intensive care in major medical centers. *Annals of Internal Medicine, 104,* 410–418.

Lang, N., & Marek, K. (1992). *Outcomes that reflect clinical practice. National Institutes of Health, Patient Outcomes Research: Examining the effectiveness of nursing practice* (pp. 27–38) (DHHS publication No. 93-3411). Washington, DC: U.S. Government Printing Office.

Meyer, H. R. (1997). Capital spending, loan program on borrowed time? *Hospitals and Health Network, 71*(15), 61–62.

O'Neill, A. E. (1996). Geriatric care management: Nurse entrepreneur niche. *Nursing Spectrum, 6*(6), 11.

Sadaniantz, B. T. (1998). Nurses in collaborative practice: A local perspective. *Nursing Spectrum (New England Edition), 2*(3), 14.

Safriet, B. (1992). Health care dollars and regulatory sense: The role of advanced practice nursing. *Yale Journal on Regulation, 9*(2), 417–488.

Windsor, R., Baranowski, T., Clark, N., & Cutter, G. (1994). *Evaluation of health promotion, health education, and disease prevention programs* (2nd ed.). Mountain View, CA: Mayfield.

Resources

U.S. Census Bureau: **www.census.gov**

Elder Web: **www.elderweb.com**

CHAPTER 23

Hospital Outpatient Care and Services

M. Nelia Davis, RN, MSN

Debbie Schutkowski, LMSW, CCM, MS

COMPETENCIES

After completing this chapter, the reader should be able to:

- *Identify the reasons for the trend to outpatient care.*
- *Differentiate vertical from horizontal integration of health care systems.*
- *Identify the common uses of hyperbaric oxygen therapy.*
- *Discuss several types of preventive hospital outpatient services.*
- *Describe the primary purpose of rehabilitation programs.*
- *Identify types of outpatient services that concentrate on pain, incontinence, and sleep disorders.*
- *List sites for mobile health screening programs that would be convenient for older adults.*
- *Describe the role of the nurse in hospital outpatient programs for older adults.*
- *Describe the importance of an interdisciplinary approach and the role that each health discipline plays in gerontological health care.*
- *Recognize that older adults themselves, together with their family caregivers, play a major role toward successful and productive aging.*

MAKING THE CONNECTION

Refer to the following chapters to increase your understanding of hospital outpatient care and services:

- **Chapter 10** *Informal Support Systems*
- **Chapter 18** *Mental Health Issues*
- **Chapter 24** *Community Organizations and Services*

The Need for Outpatient Services

For the past 50 years, the primary setting for adult health care services has been in inpatient care settings. In 1997, "older people accounted for 36% of all hospital stays and 49% of all days of care in hospitals" with 6.8 days as the average length of a hospital stay (*A profile,* 1999, p. 14). Today, for a variety of reasons, medical and nursing care are being delivered through more **outpatient hospital services.** Sultz and Young (1999) discussed health systems based on vertical or horizontal integration. Vertical integration involves a variety of programs and services owned and operated by the system, on and off site of the major facility, that meet the needs of their clients through a continuum of care. Horizontal integration, on the other hand, concentrates on providing "the same goods or services" in volume through mergers and acquisitions of many facilities (Sultz and Young, 1999, pp. 102–103). Because of decreased lengths of hospital stays and the need for a broader range of services, vertical integration increased in the late 1990s. See Box 23-1. However, with decreasing payments to health systems from Medicare, hospitals have decreased and/or eliminated some of these services. Also, other factors such as **iatrogenesis,** or an "untoward event while hospitalized" (such as falls, im-

mobility, and/or incontinence), are more likely to occur in older adults the longer they are in the hospital (Ash, MacLeod, & Clark, 1998; Jacelon, 1999), so outpatient services may be the most appropriate if possible.

Older adults are especially vulnerable in a health care system that fails to focus on preservation and restoration of **functions.** They need a **comprehensive** approach to care and bridge between acute care and home-based or institutional long-term care. Many outpatient programs are designed to provide innovative and **interdisciplinary care** that is reimbursable under current structures. These programs seek to maximize independent function, promote health, and enhance quality of life for chronically ill older adults living in the community.

The aging of America has compelled both payers and providers to seek alternatives to inpatient care. The ability to treat clients in outpatient hospital settings has been hastened by the development of sophisticated diagnostic and therapeutic interventions that can be safely and effectively used in an outpatient setting.

Older adults usually prefer the lower cost and freedom associated with outpatient care settings. Current inpatient **reimbursement** limits health care providers the opportunity to observe the evolution of chronic medical conditions and its effects on the life of older adults. Outpatient services allow health care providers to see both the client's problems and progress from the medical as well as social and emotional aspects. Many illnesses treated in outpatient services are chronic in nature and cannot be eradicated or reversed. The primary purpose of therapies is to lessen the symptoms and improve functions as well as prevent further deterioration. To achieve this purpose, it is important to understand the client's activities, resources, and support systems. The goal is best accomplished through development of bonds between client and family and health care provider in a long-term relationship in an outpatient setting (Fihn & McGee, 1992).

BOX 23-1   Vertical Integration of Health Care Systems

Emergency department/trauma center

↓

Surgery

↓

Surgical intensive care unit

↓

Acute inpatient care

↓

Rehabilitation unit

↓

Skilled nursing unit

↓

Home health care

↓

Outpatient care (rehabilitation)

↓

Wellness and health education programs

↓

Social programs and activities

Think About It

How have these changes in hospital programs and services affected the employment status of nurses and other health care providers?

Categories of Services

There are numerous outpatient services that exist in current health care systems. This chapter will discuss outpatient care services frequently used by older adults. They include wound healing and hyperbaric centers, preventive services, cardiac rehabilitation, sports medicine, incontinence programs, pain clinics, and sleep laboratories.

Wound Healing and Hyperbaric Centers

Hyperbaric oxygen therapy (HBOT) involves 100% oxygen at two to three times the atmospheric pressure at sea level, which can result in arterial oxygen tension in excess of 2,000 mm Hg and oxygen tension in tissue of almost 400 mm Hg. Such doses of oxygen have a number of beneficial biochemical, cellular, and physiological effects (Tibbles & Edelsberg, 1996). "Hyperbaric oxygen therapy was first developed to treat divers and pilots experiencing the **'bends'** [boldface added]. By increasing the amount of oxygen in cells this therapy removes carbon dioxide and nitrogen from the circulatory system and helps destroy certain bacteria sensitive to high oxygen concentrations. The infusion of oxygen into the body promotes red blood cell growth and speeds healing. It can be specially effective in treating chronic wounds like those found in diabetic patients" (*Apple Extra,* 1998, p. 4). Bends is a painful condition in the limbs and abdomen related to decreased air pressure.

According to Tibbles and Edelsberg (1996), hyperbaric oxygen is used for problem wounds, especially diabetic foot infections and leg ulcers caused by arterial insufficiency more than any other indication. They also outlined the diseases for which hyperbaric oxygen is currently being used (see Box 23-2).

Hyperbaric oxygen therapy can be administered in either a monoplace or multiplace hyperbaric chamber. A multiplace hyperbaric chamber will admit up to 12 ambulatory clients to breathe 100% oxygen by mask or hood while exposed to barometric pressure. The chamber is 7 feet in diameter and 26 feet long (eliminating claustrophobic effects for most people). It is equipped with bunks and fold-up seating, and the HBOT technician stays with the clients inside the chamber. A monoplace chamber is a one-man hyperbaric chamber that is most commonly used worldwide because of its portability, minimal personnel requirement, and relative low cost.

Once the door is closed, the client will feel a gradual increase in pressure and the rate of compression is adjusted toward the person's tolerance. The sensation one may feel is similar to driving down a mountain or flying. Toward the end of the treatment, the pressure is gradually decreased, and during this decompression stage a normal popping sensation may be experienced as one's ears adjust to the changing pressure. The duration of a single treatment varies from 45 minutes for carbon monoxide poisoning to an average of 90 minutes for each of 20–30 treatments of wounds that do not respond to antibiotic or debridement therapy.

Cases that are generally referred to HBOT are wounds that fail to improve after multiple treatments or therapies, slow nonhealing puncture wounds, lower leg ulcers with unknown causes, and radiation and thermal burns. Nonhealing pressure ulcers of the legs, as well as foot ulcers related to diabetes or peripheral vascular disease (PVD), are common conditions for which older adults need hyperbaric oxygen therapy. Hyperbaric medicine helps avoid hospital readmission and controls high cost of wound care services to an estimated 25 million people requiring costly therapeutic interventions every year. When used according to standard protocols, with oxygen pressures not exceeding three atmospheres and treatment time not to exceed 120 minutes, HBOT is safe, but like most treatments, although rare, there are possible adverse effects. "If used properly, HBOT has been reported to save money overall in gaping or ischemic wounds. The prevention of infection or preservation of a graft or flap with HBOT can vastly shorten hospitalization or need for reoperation" (Kindwall, 1992, p. 5365). One hyperbaric wound center in southwestern United States is staffed by a medical director, hyperbaric technicians, wound care nurses, and a nursing director.

BOX 23-2 Diseases for Which Hyperbaric Oxygen Is Currently Used

Diseases for which the weight of scientific evidence supports hyperbaric oxygen as effective therapy:

- Primary therapy—arterial gas embolism, decompression sickness, exceptional blood loss anemia, severe carbon monoxide poisoning

- Adjunctive therapy—clostridial myonecrosis, compromised skin grafts and flaps, osteoradionecrosis prevention

Diseases for which the weight of scientific evidence suggests hyperbaric oxygen may be helpful:

- Primary therapy—less severe carbon monoxide poisoning

- Adjunctive therapy—acute traumatic ischemic injury, osteoradionecrosis, refractory osteomyelitis, selected problem wounds, radiation-induced soft-tissue injury

Diseases for which the weight of scientific evidence does not support the use of hyperbaric oxygen but for which it may be helpful:

- Adjunctive therapy—necrotizing fasciitis, thermal burns

Source: *From "Hyperbaric oxygen therapy," by P. M. Tibbles and J. S. Edelsberg, 1996,* The New England Journal of Medicine, 334(25), pp. 1642–1648. Copyright © 1996 by the *Massachusetts Medical Society. All rights reserved. Reprinted with permission.*

CLINICAL ALERT

The following are possible adverse effects of HBOT:

- *Reversible myopia, a consequence of the direct toxic effects on the lens, is the most common side effect.*
- *Few clients may experience mild to severe pain from rupture of the middle ear, the cranial sinuses, and in rare cases, the teeth or lungs as a result of rapid pressure changes.*
- *Although rare and causes no permanent damage, inhalation of high concentrations of oxygen under pressure may precipitate generalized seizures.*
- *With repeated exposure to hyperbaric oxygen, some clients have reversible tracheobronchial symptoms, chest tightness, substernal burning sensation, and cough.*
- *Critically ill clients who have had high concentrations of normobaric oxygen for a prolonged period of time and then undergo hyperbaric oxygenation are at greater risk for toxic pulmonary effects.*
- *Claustrophia may be experienced in a monoplace chamber.*

Preventive Outpatient Services

Hospital administrators have recently become more and more conscious about their role in community health. They have made deliberate efforts to offer **preventive services** through health screenings and education because of Medicare hospital nonpayment of clients readmitted **(recidivism)** within 30 days of hospitalization. Diabetes and asthma education programs are now integral parts of hospital preventive outpatient services designed to help clients manage their diabetes effectively. Diabetes education classes focus on the management of diabetes through the balance of nutrition, medication, and exercise. These programs are interdisciplinary in nature and are conducted by Certified Diabetes Nurse Educators, registered dietitians, and medical **diabetitians.** Family caregivers of older adults are usually included and are often the only ones attending these classes. Diabetes edu-

---

BOX 23-3   Diabetes Education Program

- Definition of diabetes: types of diabetes, diabetes testing, blood sugar regulation
- Monitoring blood glucose: how to test for glucose, keeping an accurate record, long-term benefits, knowing the danger signals of hyperglycemia and hypoglycemia
- Diabetes medications, where they work
- Balancing diet, exercise, and medication
- Why diet is important: principles of diabetic diet, ideas for diabetes cooking, dining out for diabetics
- Rewards of exercise: guidelines for making food adjustments for exercise
- Preventing complications: foot care, dental care, eye care, avoiding neuropathy, avoiding heart and blood vessel diseases
- Diabetes and the kidneys
- Importance of family support
- Who is who on the health care team

cation programs start on an individual basis while clients are hospitalized for treatment of diabetes or diabetes-related complications. After discharge from acute care, diabetes education is offered in an ongoing outpatient area of the hospital. Classes offer content about the disease as well as techniques and skills to help control the disease. As clients continue these weekly classes, they attend supervised exercise classes and support groups. Some programs include telephone visits/contact to determine questions and potential problems of clients at home.

Box 23-3 presents contents of a diabetes education program of one hospital.

Cardiac Rehabilitation Services

"Cardiac **rehabilitation** [boldface added] is the process by which the patient and family system are restored to optimal physical, medical, psychological, and economic status" (Hall, 1993, p. 3). Its definition and objectives are evolving and it impacts program development as the population of those age 65 and older continues to grow. Older adults require highly skilled personnel because of their multiple medical conditions and complications that often require intensive care.

Cardiac rehabilitation is a holistic process in which all aspects of the older adult's life need to be considered and emphasis placed on the contributions of the client

BOX 23-4 Stages of a Cardiac Rehabilitation Program

- Initially, a noninvasive stress test is conducted to provide the staff with diagnostic information.

- As part of the client's weight management, a pre– and post–body composition measurement is done and education is provided.

- An admission lipid evaluation is done and is monitored throughout the program and reevaluated at the end of the program.

- Nutritional assessment and dietary counseling are performed. Nutrition education classes, cooking demonstrations, and a grocery store tour are provided. During this tour, the dietitian takes the class to the grocery store and teaches participants how to read labels, with particular attention to serving sizes; percentages of calories, carbohydrates, protein, and fat content; and the sugar and sodium content. The dietitian familiarizes clients with various types of sugar (or forms of sugar) in food labels and compares sodium content of frozen foods versus canned.

BOX 23-5 Conditions of Clients in Cardiac Rehabilitation Programs

- Arthritis
- Cancer
- Cardiac disease
- Deconditioned diabetes
- Hypertension
- Obesity
- Peripheral vascular disease
- Pulmonary disease
- Stroke

toward recovery. It is an interdisciplinary approach with the objective of improving recovery and making permanent lifestyle changes to prevent adverse risk factors.

Cardiac rehabilitation is very important to the older adult with cardiac problems. Its goals include the preservation of functions, strengthening, and coordination to provide mobility and self-sufficiency. A well-managed cardiac rehabilitation program needs to promote both physical and mental functional capacity as well as prevent anxiety and depression.

An integral part of cardiac rehabilitation is a well-structured inpatient component. A cardiac rehabilitation program may be designed for clients recovering from heart attacks, heart surgery, or cardiovascular disease and clients at high risk for developing heart problems. These programs are dedicated to meeting the needs of clients in every state of recovery and assisting in the recovery process. It consists of the stages shown in Box 23-4.

The outpatient phase of cardiac rehabilitation usually begins within 2 weeks to prevent a return to unhealthy habits such as smoking, not exercising, overeating, and eating high-fat foods. Home rehabilitation may be implemented through an organized **disease management program.**

The cardiac rehabilitation team consists of nurses, physicians, dietitians, social workers, and exercise physiologists who assist clients in lifestyle changes with emphasis on self-monitoring so that clients can assume responsibility for their own optimum health. Client and family education consists of lifestyle modifications, education about cardiovascular disease process and its treatment, proper nutrition, meal planning, methods of weight control, types and purposes of medications, exercise planning and programming, and strategies for reducing heart attacks.

Exercise regimens are prescribed for each client and are closely supervised by the cardiac rehabilitation team. Monitoring of the heart and closely watching blood pressure enables the team to identify potential problems. Classes last for 12 weeks; clients are reevaluated in the sixth week; and program reports are communicated to the attending physician.

The last phase of the rehabilitation program is the maintenance phase, which offers maintenance exercises to increase strength and endurance. This is a supervised program to increase or maintain endurance and strength but it is not monitored. It is designed to enhance that client's commitment to good health through exercise and education. Other conditions of clients in cardiac rehabilitation programs are listed in Box 23-5.

Sports Medicine and Rehabilitation Outpatient Services

The goal of rehabilitation is to improve human function through a comprehensive therapy plan provided by physical therapists, occupational therapists, speech-language pathologists, nutritionists, and athletic trainers. Rehabilitation helps individuals regain functioning that they may have lost through injury or disease. It may involve inability to speak, feed, dress, and groom oneself as well as bathe, transfer, and ambulate. Clients receive a comprehensive therapy plan specifically prescribed and

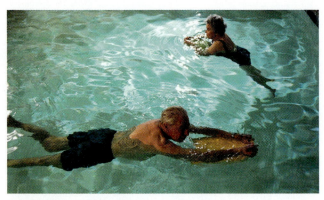

FIGURE 23-1 Aquatic therapy.

designed for their condition. Through detailed evaluation and individualized treatment plans, rehabilitation can help a client's recovery and beyond. Therapy services include physical therapy, occupational therapy, speech-language pathology, aquatic therapy, massage therapy, and specialty programs for clients with rheumatoid arthritis, osteoporosis, incontinence, pain management, and prostatic management (see Figure 23-1). Breast surgery rehabilitation programs consist of physical therapy to promote tissue healing, shoulder mobility, client education, and return to functional activities following a lumpectomy, quadrantectomy, or mastectomy.

Incontinence Program

Urinary incontinence (UI) is the frequent involuntary loss of urine that causes physical and psychosocial problems in some older adults (Glickstein, Smith, & Newman, 1990). It is treatable and is the second leading cause of nursing facility placement. According to Luft and Vriheas-Nichols (1998), "13 million Americans are incontinent of urine. The prevalence of UI among women 60 years and older has been estimated to be 40% for any urine loss and 7% to 17% for daily incontinence. UI is seen more frequently in women than in men at all ages but both men and women show an increase in the prevalence of UI with advancing age" (p. 66). The classification of UI is outlined in Box 23-6.

The risk factors associated with urinary incontinence include impaired cognition, medications, fecal impaction, immobility, inadequate fluid intake, environmental barriers, and medical conditions such as delirium, de-

---

BOX 23-6 Classification of Urinary Incontinence

- Transient or acute UI is of sudden onset, usually related to acute illness or an iatrogenic problem. It is potentially reversible and usually subsides once an illness or medical condition subsides.

- Chronic UI is urinary incontinence that persists over time. There are four types:

  - Stress UI—The involuntary leakage of small amounts of urine in response to intra-abdominal pressure. The individual leaks urine when sneezing, coughing, laughing, or lifting something heavy. It occurs predominantly in women and in 35% of incontinent elders. The causes of stress UI are weakened support of pubococcygeus muscle and other pelvic structures, sphincter weakness or damage, and the relaxation of the pelvic and periurethral musculature during childbirth, and it occurs in men who have undergone prostate surgery and have lost function of the urethral sphincter.

  - Urge incontinence—The leakage of larger amounts of urine that occurs when the individual is not able to reach the toilet after feeling the urge to void. It is the most common UI and

    occurs in 60%–70% of elders. It is caused by detrussor instability (sometimes called unstable bladder) and is associated with disorders of the lower urinary tract or neurological system by detrussor hyperflexia, tumor, stone, diverticula, and urological carcinoma.

  - Overflow incontinence—The leakage of urine when there is mechanical or functional obstruction of the urinary bladder outlet. The obstruction leads to overfill of the bladder and incontinence caused by detrussor contraction when a certain volume is reached. It accounts for 10%–15% of UI. Frequent dribbling is common, sensation of bladder fullness is diminished, and the stream of urine is weak.

  - Functional incontinence—Results when a person has difficulty moving from one place to another. It is very common when a client is admitted to an acute care hospital and accounts for 25% of UI seen. It can be caused by sensory problems, poor vision, poor hearing, poor speech, decreased cognition, lesser functional ability, or lack of motivation related to depression.

Source: *Adapted from "Urinary Incontinence in Older Adults Admitted to Acute Care," by C. Bradway, S. Hernly, and the NICHE faculty, 1998,* Geriatric Nursing, 19*(2), pp. 98–102.*

Nursing Tip

Urinary incontinence is *not* a normal part of aging. Some older adults believe that it is normal and that nothing can be done about it. Therefore, they may be reluctant to discuss the problem with a physician or a family member. The nurse should assess older individuals for this possible problem and discuss alternatives for treatment and make essential referrals for treatment and care.

BOX 23-7 Assessment of Urinary Incontinence

- Client interview while providing privacy
- Review of history and physical for medical conditions
- Review of client's medications
- Cognitive assessment
- Environmental evaluation
- Motivation determination
- Evaluation of bowel functions
- Functional evaluation
- Urological studies

---

pression, congestive heart failure, stroke, diabetes mellitus, bladder and prostate cancer, and **urinary tract infection (UTI).**

The continence care program is a conservative treatment program to combat pelvic floor muscle weakness and incontinence using therapeutic exercises, biofeedback, electrical muscle stimulation, and extensive client evaluation. Nurses play a key role in the evaluation and management of UI. Aspects of the assessment process are listed in Box 23-7.

During the assessment process, it is important that the nurse provide privacy for the client and is specific enough to get a positive response if the symptoms exist. The history and physical examination determine the medical factors contributing to the condition, and a review of the client's medications is crucial. The U.S. Department of Health and Human Services, Agency for Health Care Policy and Research, has outlined certain pharmaceuticals as potential causes of urinary incontinence. See Table 23-1.

Included in the assessment process are cognitive assessment, assessment of motivation factors that may necessitate assessment for depression, evaluation of environmental barriers to reaching the toilet, and mobility status, and it is important to determine bowel function and the presence of impaction. Other evaluations included are lumbar scan, trigger point palpation, and biofeedback evaluation. The treatment consists of determining causative factors, bladder habit training, therapeutic exercises with or without biofeedback, and electrical stimulation if needed (Bradway, Hernly, & NICHE faculty, 1998). In hospital-based continence clinics, the hospital bills for the nurse services and for the use of the hospital facilities. In this setting it is assumed that the hospital's medical staff is readily available if needed so that the ordering physician does not have to be on site. The physician may bill for the professional component (Krissovich, 1998).

Pain Clinic/Centers

Pain is both a physical and psychological experience and needs a **multidisciplinary management** approach. The first interdisciplinary pain clinic was established in Seattle, Washington. Since then, many pain clinics have opened around the world. The International Association for the Study of Pain recognizes four types of pain treatment facilities (see Box 23-8).

Who are the clients referred to these pain centers or clinics? They include those with persistent pain whose symptoms may or may not be consistent with physical findings. They may have progressive deterioration in function at work, home, and social activities and may show inability to cope emotionally. These clients may experience anger, hostility, and depression. Irving and Wallace (1997) cited that the prevalence of pain in older adults is between 73% and 80%. However, the rate of referral to pain centers is low. Among some of the suggested reasons are:

- High cost of therapy and poor insurance coverage.
- Ageism: Both physician and client believe that pain is a *normal consequence* of the aging process.
- The goal of treatment in pain centers focuses on return-to-work outcomes that are inconsistent with older adults who are retired.
- The high incidence of reported pain in older adults may be related to depression that is underdetected.

Sleep Laboratories

There is considerable interest in the effects of aging on sleep for two reasons: (a) there is a perception that older adults are sleepier during the day and (b) there is evidence that compared with wakeful (daytime) values, body functions are different during sleep and at night (Augustine-Gaspar, 1994).

TABLE 23-1   Pharmaceuticals as Potential Causes of Urinary Incontinence

Pharmaceuticals	Comment
Sedative hypnotics	Benzodiazepines, especially long-acting agents such as flurazepam and diazepam, may accumulate in older clients and cause confusion and secondary incontinence. Alcohol, frequently used as a sedative, can cloud the sensorium, impair mobility, and induce a diuresis, resulting in incontinence.
Diuretics	A brisk diuresis induced by loop diuretics can overwhelm bladder capacity and lead to polyuria, frequency, and urgency, thereby precipitating incontinence in an ill older person. The loop diuretics include furosemide, ethacrynic acid, and bumetanide.

Anticholinergic agents
  Antihistamines
  Antidepressants
  Antipsychotics
  Disopyramide
  Opiates
  Antispasmodics
    (dicyclomine and Donnatal)
  Anti-Parkinsonian agents
    (trihexyphenidyl and benztropine mesylate)
	Nonprescription (over-the-counter) agents with anticholinergic properties are taken commonly by older clients for insomnia, coryza, pruritus, and vertigo, and many prescription medications also have anticholinergic properties. Anticholinergic side effects include urinary retention with associated urinary frequency and overflow incontinence. Besides anticholinergic actions, antipsychotics such as thioridazine and haloperidol may cause sedation, rigidity, and immobility.

Alpha-adrenergic agents
  Sympathomimetics
  (decongestants)
  Sympatholytics (e.g., Prazosin, Terazosin, and Doxazosin)
	Sphincter tone in the proximal urethra can be decreased by alpha antagonists and increased by alpha agonists. An older woman, whose urethra is shortened and weakened with age, may develop stress incontinence when taking an alpha antagonist for hypertension. An older man with prostate enlargement may develop acute urinary retention and overflow incontinence when taking multicomponent "cold" capsules that contain alpha agonists and anticholinergic agents, especially if a nasal decongestant and a nonprescription hypnotic antihistamine are added.

Calcium channel blockers	Calcium channel blockers can reduce smooth muscle contractility in the bladder and occasionally can cause urinary retention and overflow incontinence.

Source: *From* Clinical practice guidelines: Urinary incontinence in adults, *1992, pp. 7–8, Washington, DC: Agency for Healthcare Policy and Research, U. S. Department of Health and Human Services.*

As people get older, several changes in sleep usually occur: There is less deep (delta) sleep and therefore more awakenings during the night, the periods of being awake are longer, and more early awakenings in the morning occur causing people to feel less rested (Merrin, 1996). Reasons for the increased number of awakenings include a higher incidence of indigestion, arthritic pains, restless leg syndrome, **sleep apnea,** and circulatory problems (irregular heartbeat). In addition, some individuals have more awakenings because of a decline in the capacity of the urinary bladder that requires them to void more often.

Sleep laboratories are making it easier for physicians to diagnose and treat sleep disorders. They are usually staffed by physicians certified by the American Board of Sleep Medicine and Registered Polysomnigraphic (sleep) technicians: "Physiologic measures of sleep are done by polysomnography performed in a laboratory controlled setting throughout the sleep cycle. It is performed by placing electrodes on the scalp and face to record EEG (brain waves), electrooculogram (extraocular movement), and electromyogram (chin and facial muscle movements) on a polygraph" (Beck-Little & Weinrick, 1998, p. 25).

Beck-Little and Weinrick (1998) pointed out that there is no consensus among researchers regarding the use of polysomnography. While some use polysomnog-

BOX 23-8 Types of Pain Treatment Facilities

- *Multidisciplinary pain centers:* Focus on research, teaching, and client care related to acute and chronic pain. It is the most comprehensive of the pain treatment facilities and usually coexists with a medical school or teaching hospital. The staff may include anesthesiologists, neurologists, neurosurgeons, psychologists, nurses, physical therapists, occupational therapists, and other specialized health care professionals.

- *Multidisciplinary pain clinic:* This type is almost identical to the multidisciplinary pain center and their services but it does not include research and teaching activities.

- *Pain clinic:* A health care facility that focuses on the diagnosis and management of clients with chronic pain. It may specialize in pain related to a specific region of the body, for example, headache.

- *Mortality-oriented clinic:* Offers a specific type of pain treatment, for example, nerve block clinics, acupuncture clinics, and biofeedback clinics. It does not provide comprehensive assessment and management.

BOX 23-9 Causes of Sleep Disorders in Older Adults

- Dyssomnias: obstructive sleep apnea syndrome, periodic limb movement disorder, restless leg syndrome

- Medical disorders: cardiovascular disease, diabetes, gastrointestinal reflux, arthritis

- Psychiatric disorders: anxiety disorder, depression, cognitive deficits

Source: *Adapted from "Assessment and Management of Sleep Disorders in the Elderly," by R. Beck-Little and S. Weinrick, 1998,* Journal of Gerontological Nursing, *24(4), pp. 21–29.*

raphy after a history and physical examination for the diagnosis and treatment of insomnia in older adults, others are reluctant to use it because of cost, availability, and the possible cause of increased confusion and agitation caused by change in sleeping environment. Still others believe that data obtained from polysomnography are helpful in delivering the best treatment for correction of sleep problems of older adults.

During a one-night sleep study, the laboratory screens for types of sleeping disorders by measuring the client's heart rate, brain waves, blood pressure, leg movement, and breathing. After the diagnosis, the client usually returns for a one-night treatment. Some of the possible underlying pathologies in sleep disorders of older adults are listed in Box 23-9.

The signs of sleep disorders are fatigue, snoring, high blood pressure, daytime drowsiness and aching muscles, and feeling paralyzed during sleep. Eighty percent of those who undergo sleep study have sleep apnea. Their throat muscles relax when they are asleep, restricting airflow, and the client wakes up to breathe as many as 100 times in one night. Sleep apnea decreases the oxygen level in the blood, and without

treatment it can cause brain damage. The most effective therapy for sleep apnea consists of a nasal **continuous positive airway pressure (CPAP)** device worn at night (see Figure 23-2). Room air is delivered through a mask at high pressure to maintain the airway open. The mask is worn over the nose and attached by a length of tubing to a small air compressor (Beck-Little & Weinrick, 1998).

> **Nursing Tip**
>
> Carefully observe your older clients during sleep. Listen for loud irregular breathing and snoring and observe skin color and movement (e.g., chest and legs).

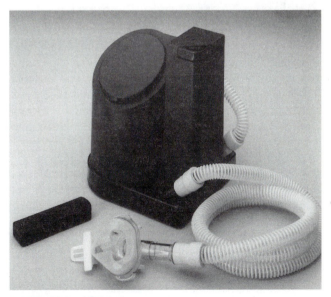

FIGURE 23-2 CPAP device.

Research Focus

Citation:

Gottlieb, D. J., Whitney, C. W., Bonekat, W. H., Iber, C., James, G. D., Lebowitz, M., Nieto, F. J., & Rosenberg, C. E. (1999). Relation of sleepiness to respiratory disturbance index: The Sleep Heart Health Study. *American Journal of Respiratory Critical Care Medicine, 159*(2), 502–507.

Purpose:

Examines whether there is a relationship between sleepiness and sleep-disordered breathing in community-dwelling individuals ($n = 1,824$; average age is 65). It is part of the larger longitudinal study called the Sleep Heart Health Study investigating cardiovascular health relative to sleep-disordered breathing.

Methods:

Measurement scales were used to quantify sleepiness and respiratory disturbance based on monitoring of in-home polysomnography.

Findings:

The scores for sleepiness and disturbed respiratory breathing demonstrated that high disturbance in breathing is correlated with excess sleepiness and not limited to only those with sleep apnea.

Implications:

This not-so-apparent disturbance may affect overall cardiovascular, respiratory, and functional health in community-dwelling, middle-aged, and older adults.

Ambulatory Care Centers

Because of the need for managing health care dollars more efficiently, hospitals have developed a wide range of outpatient ambulatory care services and centers. These centers that originally were designed to provide minor surgery and diagnostics are expanding the type of care they can provide. The changes in reimbursement for medical services on an inpatient basis have led to the expansion of services provided in an outpatient setting. For example, an inpatient stay of 3 days was considered reasonable and necessary for cataract extraction in the early 1980s. However, by the end of that decade cataract surgery was being routinely performed in an outpatient setting. By the late 1990s, clients were discharged from an outpatient surgery center less than 1 hour after the completion of the surgery. Improvements in surgical technology and changes in Medicare reimbursement were the factors that contributed to these changes.

Now, in the ambulatory care centers, in addition to surgery and diagnostics many other services are offered. Intravenous therapy for antibiotics and other medications is common. For example, dobutamine therapy for congestive heart failure is an option for some clients. Clients receive blood transfusions and chemotherapy in the ambulatory care setting. Hospitals have outpatient wound care programs. This type of care is preferable to most older people and their families because it offers an alternative to hospitalization. It is also more cost effective. However, it increases the need for discharge planning and teaching by the staff to prevent postoperative complications. The lack of safe reliable transportation to and from ambulatory care centers is a problem in some communities, especially if anesthesia and other medications have been used and family members are not available.

Other services have been developed by health care systems to complement and support the ambulatory care programs. Many hospitals have freestanding community-based pharmacies that offer medical supplies and durable medical equipment. These services not only add to the health system's net income but also offer a continuum of care to its clients.

Mobile Health Care Programs

Mobile health care programs are another example of a health care system's outreach to the people in their community. It is an effort to improve the health status of people in the community who may not have access to medical services. Mobile health units are frequently used in rural areas where there may be no medical clinic or hospital. While the programs are not specifically designed to serve any one age group, there exist many creative opportunities for serving older adults. Services that can be provided through mobile health units are listed in Box 23-10.

The advantage of using mobile health units to serve older adults is that health services can reach individuals who would not normally seek health care or lack access because of transportation difficulties or other factors. Mobile health units can be utilized at senior citizen centers, housing complexes, retirement communities, malls, and churches. This service provides a link between the health care system and older adults in the community.

Mobile health units are designed and customized to meet the health care provider's needs. They may be equipped with x-ray equipment, laboratory or pharmacy space, office equipment such as computer and fax, a defined office and waiting area, and examination rooms. They also may be equipped with television and video cassette recorders for playing educational tapes to clients. They are designed with wheelchair lifts and ramps to accommodate the needs of individuals with functional limitations.

Membership Programs

Many health care systems sponsor **membership programs** that focus on promoting wellness and healthy lifestyles for older adults. While the purpose of the health care system is marketing to the older population, these programs also support a positive attitude toward helping people live healthier lives.

Membership benefits include discounts for services and products such as pharmaceuticals, medical supplies, and optical and dental services. Travel discounts and group trips are social benefits offered. Workshops on health topics such as osteoporosis and stroke and health screenings for diabetes, cholesterol, and blood pressure are offered, usually at no charge to the members. Other programs offered are focused on educating older adults on Medicare options and changes, long-term care insurance, living wills, powers of attorney, and financial planning.

Because of the benefits of membership, these programs have become quite popular with older adults. Many of them have memberships in more than one program sponsored by different health systems. These programs indicate a positive attitude toward helping older adults lead healthier lives and have the potential for improving the health status of older adults in the community.

Caregiver Support Groups

In managing the care of ill older adults, health care systems should recognize the importance of the role of the family and/or other informal caregiver. The majority of all home care is provided by family members. The health and well-being of caregivers is important to the care of the client. Families need education and support on how to manage the care of a loved one, especially after hospital discharge for an acute illness.

Caregiver support groups vary in terms of membership and structure. Some groups are designed for specific issues such as Alzheimer's disease, stroke, and cancer. Other groups are structured to provide caregivers of older adults information on the aging process, effective communication with sensory-impaired individuals, community resources, and how to avoid caregiver burnout and maintain their own health. Caregiver support groups are set up to educate the members and share information, while others are designed to provide emotional support and counseling. Meeting times vary according to the needs of the group, as does the duration of the program. The greatest benefit to those attending support groups is the realization that their situation is not unique and that there are many others that face the same difficult issues and decisions.

Partial Hospitalization Day Programs

Partial hospitalization day programs are another example of hospitals creating new programs for individuals with psychiatric conditions who do not meet the criteria for inpatient hospitalization. Partial hospitalization day programs are designed for older adults who are experiencing anxiety, depression, or other mental health problems.

These programs are developed for individuals who do not require hospitalization but would benefit from an intensive outpatient psychiatric/mental health program. This type of program provides a continuum of care that allows individuals to remain in the community while receiving structured clinical services. This concept is sometimes more appealing to older clients than admission to an inpatient psychiatric unit.

Psychiatric/mental health services are provided under the direction of a geriatric psychiatrist with other services provided by gerontological nurses, social workers, licensed professional counselors, occupational and physical therapists, and recreational therapists. The programs offer a combination of group and individual therapy. Staff also can monitor the medication regimen to assess for effectiveness, side effects, and adherence. Program designs vary from half day to full day with meals and transportation provided in most programs. Partial hospitalization day programs for psychiatric/mental health care are reimbursable by Medicare Part B and some private and supplemental insurance plans.

Case Management Programs

Many health care systems have realized the benefits of providing a continuum of care for older people that extends beyond the hospital setting. By developing a case management or care coordination program for older clients, hospitals can decrease the cost of care for

---

BOX 23-10 Services in Mobile Health Units

- Health education and screening
- Immunizations (e.g., influenza and pneumonia)
- Respiratory therapy, physical therapy, and occupational therapy
- Dermatology screening
- Blood glucose monitoring
- Cholesterol screening
- Health fairs (e.g., blood pressure screening)
- Osteoporosis screening
- Mammography

chronic illness, decrease the risk of unnecessary hospitalizations, and promote wellness and independence

Case managers can care for and monitor high-risk older adults by coordinating medical and social services and providing clients and families information on disease and medication management, treatment options, and community resources. Many chronically ill older adults have difficulty following complex medication and dietary regimens and fail to recognize or act upon early signs of an impending medical crisis that leads to emergency room visits and hospitalizations. Older adults and their families may have difficulty accessing community resources and services and understanding what can be a confusing system of eligibility criteria and paperwork. By taking an assertive role in identifying high-risk older clients, case managers can facilitate access to community and medical services and ensure adherence to a plan of care through regular monitoring.

Care coordination is directed toward individuals with specific disease processes such as congestive heart failure, diabetes, chronic obstructive pulmonary disease (COPD), and stroke. These case managers are usually licensed nurses with expertise in clinical evaluation and treatment as well as availability of community resources.

Care coordination programs may take a more generalist approach with criteria focused on chronically ill older adults with a combination of medical and social needs. A care manager may be a licensed nurse or licensed social worker with geriatric expertise.

Care coordination programs are beneficial to health care systems and managed care organizations because of potential cost reduction benefits when taking care of chronically ill older adults. When managed effectively, the programs can better utilize health care services and funds. The benefit to older clients may be improved health status, greater quality of life even with chronic illness, and better access to services and resources that contribute to continued independence in the community (Evans, Yurkow, & Siegler, 1995).

PACE Programs

Health care systems continue to look for innovative programs to integrate the services they provide with community-based programs to provide comprehensive care for older adults. The Health Care Financing Administration (HCFA) began funding integrated care models in 1985 with the development of **Social Health Maintenance Organizations (SHMOs).** These programs were organized to utilize Medicare funding to deliver acute and chronic care services to older adults under an HMO model. These programs have not flourished because of the complexity of providing coordinated and integrated care cost effectively.

The Program of All-inclusive Care for the Elderly (PACE) is a replication of a fully integrated managed care demonstration project called On Lok that was developed in San Francisco in the 1970s. The PACE program differs from SHMOs in that PACE focuses on managing ill older adults with an individualized plan of care whereas the SHMO manages large groups of well and disabled older adults collectively. The major goals of the PACE program are to "stabilize chronic medical conditions and optimize functional status," thus preventing unnecessary use of hospital and nursing home care (Lee, Eng, Fox, & Etienne, 1998, p. 65).

These programs focus on the use of interdisciplinary teams providing community-based services to older adults who are at risk for nursing facility placement. Sources of funding for the program have come from private foundations, Medicare, and Medicaid. The Medicare reimbursement is a capitated monthly rate for each PACE client. The Medicaid capitated rate is based on a percentage of each individual state's daily reimbursement for nursing facility care.

The interdisciplinary team consists of physicians, dentists, nurses, social workers, physical, occupational, and recreational therapists, dietitians, personal care attendants in the centers, and representatives from home care and transportation services. The team works together to assess the participants' needs, develop treatment plans, and provide care. Because the same team members are responsible for assessment and provision of services, they are able to identify changes in the client's condition early. This program allows for modification of the treatment plan almost immediately. This approach often can prevent the client's condition from worsening to the point where more acute medical care would be needed.

All PACE programs provide their clients a comprehensive range of acute and chronic medical and social services. The service delivery site combines an adult day program with a primary care clinic. Clients attend the center on a regular basis, usually three to five times a week. At the center they receive skilled medical and rehabilitative care, personal care, and meals. They also participate in the recreational and social programs that are provided. At home the clients receive skilled care in addition to personal care, meals, and homemaker services. Transportation to and from the center is provided by the program. In addition, the program provides specialty services such as dental care, optometry and audiology services, durable medical equipment, and medications. The program provides hospital and nursing facility care as needed by the client. Regardless of the setting, the clients remain with the PACE network and receive the benefit of disciplinary approach to their care.

Funding for additional PACE sites has been approved by the federal Health Care Financing Administration; however, many health care systems are hesitant to assume the financial responsibility for comprehensive care for ill older adults. PACE sites bear the financial risk for the complete care of each client enrolled in the program. It is this amount of financial risk that makes the program difficult for many health care organizations to support. PACE programs are more financially viable in states that have a higher reimbursement rate for nursing facility care that helps offset the costs of client care (Eng, Pedulla, Eleazer, McCann, & Fox, 1997; Lee et al., 1998).

Think About It

What are other health care needs of older adults living independently in community settings that hospital systems should study, plan, and implement?

Implications for Nursing

Nurses function in any program described in this chapter. Because of the holistic perspective of nursing, nurses function as a clinician or direct caregiver; as a teacher and educator in wellness programs; as a counselor; as a facilitator in therapy and support groups; and as a case manager and source of referral for further care. As the health care delivery system continues to change, nurses will identify and fill new roles in a variety of settings. For example, advanced practice enterostomal therapy nurses function in the role of di-

rector of hyperbaric centers, and geriatric clinical nurse specialists are managers of continence clinics and coordinate the PACE program.

Nurses also need to be aware of all of these types of programs and services so that suggestions and referrals can be made for older adults and their families when indicated.

Summary

Hospital outpatient care is a major resource for those older adults who need some kind of specialized care but do not need to be hospitalized on an inpatient basis. Hospital lengths of stay have decreased because of new technology that can be used on an outpatient basis and reduced payments to hospitals for inpatient care. Some hospitals have changed their focus to provide a continuum of care from acute to rehabilitation to outpatient care and services (vertical integration).

Some of the major outpatient services provided by hospitals are wound healing centers, wellness education programs, cardiac rehabilitation services, incontinence programs, pain clinics, sleep laboratories, mobile health care programs, caregiver support groups, partial hospital day programs for mental and behavioral health problems, and case management.

Nurses can and do function in various roles in all of these programs, working with an interdisciplinary team to meet the holistic needs of older adults.

Review Questions and Activities

1. Why has hospital outpatient care increased in recent years?

2. Give an example of a hospital with vertical integration in your community.

3. What are conditions for which hyperbaric oxygen therapy is used?

4. What kinds of rehabilitation programs are offered by hospitals on an outpatient basis?

5. Where are mobile health screening programs and services provided in your community?

6. What kinds of services are provided in mobile health screening programs?

7. What are some sleep disorders common in older adults?

8. What are the services provided by a sleep center?

9. What is the PACE program?

10. What is the role of a nurse in a pain clinic?

References

Apple Extra: Adult prevention program for life enhancement. (1998, Fall). Fort Worth, TX: Apple Club, Osteopathic Medical Center of Texas.

A profile of older Americans. (1999). Washington, DC: American Association of Retired Persons, Administration on Aging, U.S. Department of Health and Human Services.

Ash, K. L., MacLeod, P., & Clark, L. (1998). A case control study of falls in the hospital setting. *Journal of Gerontological Nursing, 24*(12), 7–15.

Augustine-Gaspar, D. (1994). *Human aging: A biological perspective.* New York: McGraw-Hill.

Beck-Little, R., & Weinrick, S. (1998). Assessment and management of sleep disorders in the elderly. *Journal of Gerontological Nursing, 19*(2), 21–29.

Bradway, C., Hernly, S., & NICHE faculty. (1998). Urinary incontinence in older adults admitted to acute care. *Geriatric Nursing, 19*(2), 98–102.

Eng, C., Pedulla, J., Eleazer, G. P., McCann, R., & Fox, N. (1997). Program of all-inclusive care for the elderly (PACE): An innovative model of integrated geriatric care and financing. *Journal of the American Geriatrics Society, 45,* 223–232.

Evans, Yurkow, J., & Siegler, E. L. (1995). The CARE program: A nurse-managed collaborative outpatient program to improve functions of frail older people. *Journal of the American Geriatrics Society, 43*(10), 1155–1160.

Fihn, S., & McGee, S. (1992). *Outpatient medicine.* Philadelphia: Saunders.

Glickstein, J., Smith, D., & Newman, D. (Eds.). (1990, April). Urinary incontinence, a problem not often assessed and treated. *Focus on Geriatric Care and Rehabilitation, 3*(10).

Gottlieb, D. J., Whitney, C. W., Bonekat, W. H., Iber, C., James, G. D., Lebowitz, M., Nieto, F. J., & Rosenberg, C. E. (1999). Relation of sleepiness to respiratory disturbance index: The Sleep Heart Health Study. *American Journal of Respiratory Critical Care Medicine, 159*(2), 502–507.

Hall, L. K. (1993). *Developing and managing cardiac rehabilitation programs.* Pittsburgh, PA: Human Kinetics Publisher.

Irving, G., & Wallace, M. (1997). *Pain management for the practicing physician.* Philadelphia: Churchill Livingston.

Jacelon, C. S. (1999). Preventing cascade iatrogenesis in hospitalized elders. An important role for nurses. *Journal of Gerontological Nursing, 25*(1), 27–33.

Kindwall, E. (1992). Uses of hyperbaric oxygen therapy in the 1990s. *Cleveland Clinic Journal of Medicine, 59*(5), 517–528.

Krissovich, M. (1998). The financial side of continence promotion. *Geriatric Nursing, 19*(2), 91–94.

Lee, W., Eng, C., Fox, N., & Etienne, M. (1998). PACE: A model for integrated care of frail older patients. *Geriatrics, 53*(6), 62–74.

Luft, J., & Vriheas-Nichols, A. (1998). Identifying the risk factors for developing incontinence: Can we modify individual risk? *Geriatric Nursing, 19*(2), 66–72.

Merrin, E. L. (1996). Sleep disorders. In E. T. Lonergan (Ed.), *Geriatrics.* Stamford, CT: Appleton & Lange.

Sultz, H. A., & Young, K. M. (1999). *Health care USA* (2nd ed.). Gaithersburg, MD: Aspen.

Tibbles, P., & Edelsberg, J. (1996). Hyperbaric oxygen therapy. *The New England Journal of Medicine, 334*(25), 1642–1648.

Resources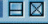

Healthzone (for information on wound healing): **www.healthzone.com**

National Guideline Clearinghouse (clinical practice guidelines for cardiac rehabilitation): **www.guideline.gov**

CHAPTER 24

Community Organizations and Services

Jacqueline M. Stolley, PhD, RN, CS
Beth Cameron, MS, RN, FNP
JoAnn Wedig, RN, MA

COMPETENCIES

After completing this chapter, the reader should be able to:

- Describe the National Aging Network and related programs for older adults.
- Discuss Area Agencies on Aging and programs and services provided.
- Describe at least 10 services provided by community organizations and other resources.
- Identify four types of access services.
- List five different community-based services and their role in promoting independence.
- Describe nutritional services and their role in supporting nutritional needs of older adults in the community.
- Differentiate among older adults' rights services provided in the community and in institutions.
- Describe other agencies that provide services in the community and their implications for older adults.
- Identify needs not met by the National Aging Network.
- Predict future community needs of older adults.

MAKING THE CONNECTION

Refer to the following chapters to increase your understanding of community organizations and services:

- **Chapter 9** Geriatric Nutrition
- **Chapter 10** Informal Support Systems
- **Chapter 20** Home Health Care
- **Chapter 26** End-of-Life Decisions and Choices
- **Chapter 27** Legal and Financial Issues

The Need for Community Organizations and Services

With changing demographics and economics of the aging population and projected increases in the twenty-first century, it is important that gerontological nurses and other health care providers utilize community organizations and services that will enable independent living, promote health, and ensure continued efforts toward healthy and productive aging. It is imperative for health care professionals and systems to understand that the character of the older population is changing and will continue to change. For example, life expectancy at age 65 was about 9 years when the Social Security program began in 1935. In 1997, life expectancy at age 65 was an additional 17.6 years (*A profile,* 1999). As a result, the need for organizations and services for older adults will continue to increase as the population ages. With the aging population, the prevalence of chronic disease will increase, resulting in the need for varied services in the community. However, with increased emphasis on disease prevention and health promotion, the older population may be healthier in the future. Because of the emphasis on health promotion and general improvements in living standards and health care in addition to longevity, definitions of aging are changing. Therefore, gerontological nurses and other health professionals will need to be aware of health trends in the older population.

A wide array of community organizations and services exist for older adults in a variety of environments. These services are available to older adults and their families and offer support and assistance in diverse settings, although the extent of services available may differ by region. This chapter presents a general overview of services that are available nationwide, along with directions for future demands for community organizations and services in the new century. When considering community organizations and services, the gerontological nurse should keep in mind national health promotion and disease prevention objectives for older adults as they relate to these services. Table 24-1 illustrates the priority areas and objectives of *Healthy People 2000* (U.S. Department, 1990) that are relevant to older adults and community organizations and services.

National Aging Network

One of the most significant developments in the creation of services for older adults resulted from the **Older Americans Act (OAA)** legislation in 1965. As a result of this congressional action and creation of the Administration on Aging (AOA), a national network of federal, state, and local agencies was developed to organize and administer services that enable families to "maintain and support older persons in their homes and communities to avoid unnecessary and costly institutionalization" (U.S. Senate, 1993, p. 313). In 1973, an amendment to the OAA resulted in the creation of local Area Agencies on Aging (AAAs). The purpose of the agencies is to plan and implement social service programs at the local level as well as serve as advocates for older people. Services available through AAAs include nutrition services, recreational opportunities, chore services, legal assistance, transportation, and information and assistance. Local AAAs attempt to provide services not already available and encourage communities to continue needed services without duplication. There is a priority to serve low-income and minority elders. The OAA was reauthorized in 2000.

Funding appropriated under Title III of the OAA is allocated annually based on the number of people 60 years and older living in a particular state or territory. The states or territories then award grants to AAAs to develop, execute, and oversee a range of services.

The **National Aging Network** consists of 57 state offices on aging at the state and territorial level and 661 AAAs at the community level. The Aging Network is directed by the U.S. Administration on Aging of the U.S. Department of Health and Human Services. Each AAA is required to have an advisory council to discuss and examine performance of programs and services funded. The 661 AAAs have an estimated 15,000 citizen advisory council members. In addition, special aging programs have been developed for more than 190 Native American tribal organizations under Title VI of OAA funding [**National Association of Area Agencies on Aging (NAAAA)**] (National Association, 1998). Figure 24-1 (page 506) illustrates the National Aging Network.

Area Agencies on Aging

Local AAAs are public or private nonprofit organizations that are charged with targeting needs and concerns of older adults on regional and local levels. Each AAA is responsible for a region, such as a large metropolitan area or several rural counties. Of the 661 AAAs across the country, 66% are public and 33% are private nonprofit organizations.

Three important functions of AAAs are to:

- Create multiyear plans for the development of comprehensive, **community-based services** that meet the needs of older adults in their communities.

- Provide information on available services, programs, and policies that affect older adults within their service areas and advocate for improved services for older Americans and their caregivers.

TABLE 24-1 Priority Areas for *Healthy People 2000* Relating to Older Adults

Priority Area	Objectives
Physical fitness and activity	• Reduce coronary heart disease deaths. • Reduce overweight prevalence in the population. • Increase the adoption of sound dietary habits combined with regular exercise to maintain appropriate body weight. • Reduce the number of older adults who have difficulty performing two or more personal care activities. • Reduce the number of older adults who engage in no regular physical activity. • Increase participation in regular light to moderate physical activity. • Increase participation in vigorous physical activity that promotes cardiovascular fitness. • Increase performance of regular physical activity that enhances and maintains muscular strength, muscular endurance, and flexibility. • Increase community availability and accessibility of physical activity and fitness facilities. • Increase the number of primary care providers who regularly counsel about the benefits of physical activity.
Nutrition	• Reduce the prevalence of overweight. • Reduce dietary fat intake to 30% of calories or less. • Increase complex carbohydrate and fiber intake. • Decrease salt and sodium intake. • Increase the adoption of sound dietary habits combined with regular exercise to maintain appropriate body weight. • Increase the proportion of the population utilizing food labels to make nutritious food choices. • Increase the receipt of home food services by those who need them. • Reduce blood cholesterol levels. • Reduce stroke deaths. • Reduce colorectal cancer deaths. • Reduce coronary heart disease deaths. • Reverse the rise in cancer. • Reduce diabetes incidence. • Increase proportion of those with hypertension whose blood pressure is under control. • Increase the proportion of primary providers who routinely provide nutrition assessment and counseling.
Tobacco	• Reduce cigarette smoking. • Slow the rise in lung cancer. • Slow the rise in chronic lung disease deaths. • Reduce coronary heart disease deaths. • Reduce deaths caused by oral cancer. • Reduce stroke deaths. • Enact comprehensive clean indoor air acts in all states. • Increase the average excise tax on cigarettes.

(continues)

TABLE 24-1 Priority Areas for *Healthy People 2000* Relating to Older Adults *continued*

Priority Area	Objectives
Tobacco—cont'd	• Increase the number of primary providers who routinely assess and counsel about tobacco use.
	• Increase the number of health plans that cover treatment of nicotine addiction.
Mental health and mental disorders	• Reduce the prevalence of mental disorders, including depression.
	• Increase the treatment of major depressive disorders.
	• Reduce adverse effects from stress.
	• Reduce the number of suicides.
	• Increase the use of community support services by those with severe, persistent mental disorders.
	• Establish a network of support, resources, and self-help activities for those experiencing emotional distress from mental or physical illness.
	• Increase the number of primary providers who routinely assess and counsel about cognitive, emotional, and behavioral functioning.
Violent and abusive behaviors	• Reduce physical abuse directed at women by male partners.
	• Encourage laws for proper storage of firearms.
	• Reduce firearm-related deaths.
	• Extend comprehensive violence prevention programs to more communities.
Education and community-based programs	• Increase years of healthy life.
	• Increase the number of older adults who have the opportunity to participate yearly in an organized health promotion program.
Unintentional injuries	• Reduce deaths from falls and fall-related injuries.
	• Reduce hip fractures.
	• Increase the use of safety belts.
	• Reduce deaths caused by motor vehicle accidents.
	• Reduce residential fire deaths.
	• Increase the prevalence of smoke detectors and fire suppression sprinkler systems.
	• Increase the use of design standards for highway markings and signs in all states.
	• Increase the number of primary providers who routinely counsel on safety precautions.
Oral health	• Reduce the proportion of the older adults who have lost all their teeth.
	• Reduce deaths caused by oral cancer.
	• Require all long-term care facilities to provide oral screening and services to clients.
Heart disease and stroke	• Reduce coronary heart disease deaths.
	• Increase the number of people who have had their blood pressure checked in the previous year.
	• Increase the proportion of people with hypertension who are taking steps to control it.
	• Increase the proportion of people who have their cholesterol checked and know their cholesterol levels.
	• Reduce mean serum cholesterol levels.
	• Reduce dietary fat intake.
	• Reduce overweight prevalence.
	• Increase participation in regular light to moderate physical activity.

(continues)

TABLE 24-1 Priority Areas for *Healthy People 2000* Relating to Older Adults *continued*

Priority Area	Objectives
Heart disease and stroke—cont'd	• Reduce cigarette smoking. • Slow the increase in incidence of end-stage renal disease. • Increase the number of women who have been counseled about the benefits and risks of estrogen replacement therapy. • Increase the number of primary care providers who initiate diet and, if necessary, drug therapy for cholesterol control.
Cancer	• Reduce the number of cancer deaths. • Reduce cigarette smoking. • Reduce dietary fat intake. • Increase intake of complex carbohydrates and fiber. • Increase the use of sun screen and limitation of sun exposure. • Increase the proportion of women who have annual breast exams and mammograms. • Increase the proportion of women who have Pap tests every 1–3 years. • Increase the proportion of older adults who receive fecal occult blood testing every 1–2 years. • Increase the proportion of older adults who have ever had a sigmoidoscopy. • Increase the proportion of older adults who receive oral, skin, and digital rectal exams yearly. • Increase the number of primary providers who routinely assess and counsel about tobacco cessation, diet modification, and cancer screening recommendations.
Diabetes and disabling conditions	• Increase years of healthy life. • Reduce the proportion of the population experiencing a limitation in major activity because of chronic conditions. • Reduce the proportion of the population that has difficulty performing two or more personal care activities. • Reduce significant hearing impairment. • Reduce significant visual impairment. • Reduce diabetes-related deaths. • Reduce the incidence of diabetes. • Increase the number of diabetics who receive annual eye examinations. • Reduce the most severe complications of diabetes. • Reduce the prevalence of overweight. • Increase participation in regular light to moderate physical activity. • Increase the proportion of the disabled who receive formal client education about community and self-help resources. • Increase the number of primary providers who routinely evaluate older adults for urinary incontinence and impairments in vision, hearing, cognition, and functional status.
Immunization and infectious diseases	• Reduce cases of vaccine-preventable diseases. • Reduce pneumonia-related days of restricted activity. • Increase immunization levels for pneumonia and influenza. • Increase the number of primary providers who routinely assess and counsel about immunizations.

(continues)

TABLE 24-1   Priority Areas for *Healthy People 2000* Relating to Older Adults   *continued*

Priority Area	Objectives
Clinical preventive services	• Increase years of healthy life. • Increase the proportion of the population having a specific source of on-going primary care. • Increase the proportion of primary providers who routinely provide screening, counseling, and immunization services.

Source: *Adapted from* Healthy People 2000: National Health Promotion and Disease Prevention Objectives, *1990, PHS Pub. No. 91-50213, U.S. Department of Health and Human Services.*

• Coordinate Older Americans Act funds and other funds that implement the service system. The AAAs administer these funds largely through contracts with local service providers furnishing these services at the community level as well as monitor and evaluate service providers for efficiency and effectiveness in delivering services. They work with providers to coordinate services and ensure that needed services are developed and provided in the community (National Association, 1996).

The primary aim of AAAs is to enhance the quality of life for older adults as well as their families. This aim is congruent with *Healthy People 2000* priority areas and objectives as given in Table 24-1. The AAAs accomplish their primary aim by furnishing information about services available in each locality. In this way, they serve as a "single point of information" (National Association, 1998, p. 2) about a variety of services that may otherwise be too complex or fragmented for easy accessibility.

Although AAAs coordinate and support a variety of services, it is important to note that not all services identified in this chapter, whether related to AAAs or not, are immediately available in every community. Nor do all services function in the same way nationally. Therefore, information on organizations and services identified in this chapter is general, and specific information may be obtained by contacting the local AAA or individual organization. See sample services available in one community in Figure 24-2. This type of information also can be found through the Eldercare Locator.

Priority services offered by AAAs are identified as access to services in local communities, supporting independent living through home and community-based care, meeting nutritional needs of older adults, and protecting the basic rights of the most vulnerable.

The Eldercare Locator

Services for older adults can be complex and fragmented. In addition, family members who live away from the older adult may be unfamiliar with services available in community where the individual lives. Therefore, the NAAAA and the U.S. AOA established a nationwide **Eldercare Locator** in 1993. This service provides information and access to over 4,800 state and local information and assistance service providers along with information about specialized services (e.g., Alzheimer's Associations, consumer fraud, and legal services) and methods of contacting these services in each locale. These services are identified by every ZIP code in the United States (National Association, 1998). Box 24-1 presents contact information for the Eldercare Locator.

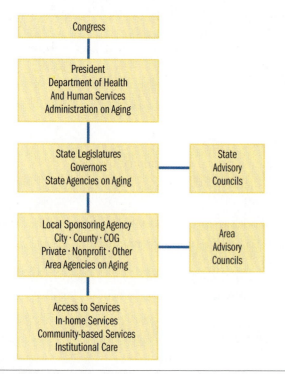

FIGURE 24-1   The National Aging Network. (Source: *National Association of Area Agencies on Aging (NAAAA), 1998, National Directory for Eldercare Information and Referral. Washington, DC: NAAAA.)*

New...Bilingual... Free...Confidential!

Telephone Information & Referral Service Specifically for Older Adults & Those Who Care for Them

- ►Older Adult Housing
- ►Home Health Care
- ►Benefits Counseling
- ►Nursing Home Care
- ►Utility Bill Assistance
- ►Recreation Opportunities
- ►Home Repair
- ►Supplemental Food
- ►Older Adult Education
- ►Supplemental Insurance
- ►Transportation

Aging Information Line
258-8180

SE HABLA ESPAÑOL
A service of Area Agency on Aging of Tarrant County and United Way's First Call

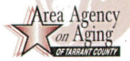 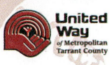

FIGURE 24-2 Aging Information Line. *(Courtesy of Area Agency and United Way of Metropolitan Tarrant County. Used with permission.)*

Eldercare Resources

Many types of services provided by organizations and agencies are available to older adults. Several of these are coordinated through AAAs as a response to their primary charge of promoting independence. These services include access resources, community-based programs, in-home assistance, nutritional services, **older adults' rights,** and institutional programs. Several of these resources will be discussed in depth in this section. It is important to remember that AAAs may either support these services or simply supply information and assistance. Much of the information contained in this section was obtained from the National Association of Area Agen-

cies on Aging (1998) Directory. However, because this chapter is limited to those services available in the community, the reader has been referred to other chapters in this book that address the information in more depth.

Access Services

The AAAs facilitate **access to services** by helping individuals and families identify specific needs, outlining eligibility criteria, and helping to evaluate the individual's ability to meet these criteria. Examples include service information and assistance, in which the agency provides information on specified services and makes referrals to appropriate services and agencies; assessment to determine eligibility; case management to enhance service coordination; and transportation services for those unable to drive or perhaps use public transportation. Information is available regarding organizations and services that are available so that older adults and their families can be informed and use the appropriate services.

Through access services, priority areas and objectives of *Healthy People 2000* can be achieved, depending on the needs of the older adults in the community. Priority areas target specific concepts with objectives that are relevant to access services. For example, information and assistance services can provide information that focuses on any of the priority areas and objectives. Client assessment and case management can promote quality of life, health promotion, and health protection in areas most needed, such as the physical fitness priority area objective: "Reduce the number of elderly who have difficulty performing two or more personal care activities" (National Center, 1996, p. 39). Transportation services may provide access to all services for those unable to drive or use public transportation, helping to achieve *Healthy People 2000* objectives that would otherwise be unattainable.

Information and Assistance

Information and assistance (I&A) services (formerly referred to as information and referral services) provide information to older adults about public, voluntary, and private services availability. In addition to this information, I&A also facilitates linkage to specific services to promote use and decrease barriers to access. The local AAA serves as I&A, and information about service locations nationwide are available through the Eldercare Locator (National Association, 1998).

Client Assessment

Client assessment elicits information regarding both the need for services and eligibility requirements. Usually, the AAA will perform this assessment. The assessment may include areas involving health, financial resources, environment, and safety. Along with this assessment, prenursing facility screenings can be completed, as well as screenings for various health conditions such as blood pressure, hearing, vision, and diabetes (National Association, 1998).

Care Management

With the accessibility and use of a variety of services, there is a danger of duplication and lack of communication among organizations and services providing resources for older adults. Care management provides review and analysis of information and data related to the individual's social, psychological, and physical health challenges and problems (National Association, 1998). Through care management, functional abilities are identified and needed support services can be organized. The care management process usually results in comprehensive treatment that flows from a written **plan of care,** which is coordinated by a member of the care management team. Many AAAs have a care or case manager for older people at risk or contract for this service with one of its service provider organizations.

Transportation

Transportation serves both human and economic needs. It enriches life by expanding opportunities for social interaction and community involvement and supports an individual's capacity for independent living by accessing necessary services (Administration on Aging, 1998a). Access to stores, social events, physicians' appointments, government offices, nutrition programs, and other community-based services is a problem for the many older Americans who have physical disabilities. Communities in the United States have undergone a restructuring in the last 50 years that has led to increased suburbanization—increased distances between homes, stores, and community services—which in turn has led to a greater dependence on automobiles for transportation. Public transportation services have had difficulty competing with the convenience of personal cars and so have decreased in number. Even in cities, those without cars must walk farther to get to fewer buses and trains. In rural areas, public transportation is limited because it is costly. Even among those well older adults who have cars, decreasing visual acuity with age may limit their ability to drive (see Figures 24-3 and 24-4). In addition, many have physical disabilities that impede their use of regular public transportation.

The Older Americans Act of 1965 authorized financial assistance for transportation services for older adults. State and local agency funding augmented these federal funds. Special transportation services for older adults and disabled became available, but only through a wide variety of agencies and providers, with varying requirements and eligibility for services. In some areas of the country, there are duplications of service, while in others, only limited services are available.

The **Americans with Disabilities Act (ADA),** passed in 1990, now requires all public transportation services to provide individuals with disabilities with a level of transportation service comparable to that provided individuals without disabilities on a fixed route system. This act has led to greater cooperation between public transportation authorities, the AAAs, and other services within the community. For those who live along a fixed public transportation route, there are now accommodations for wheelchairs and other assistance devices.

However, for older adults relying on the door-to-door transportation to and from local agencies, there are

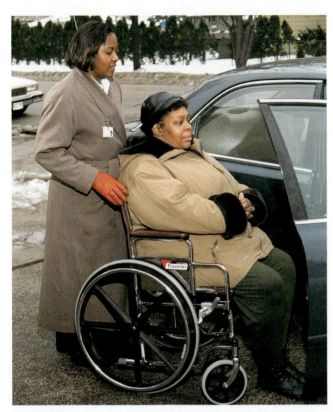

FIGURE 24-3 Physical disabilities may impede the use of public transportation.

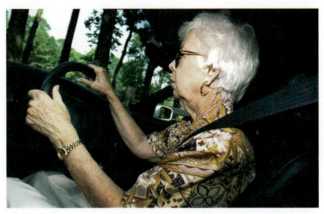

FIGURE 24-4 Driving ability may be limited because of decreasing visual acuity.

often 2-week advance notification requirements, limitations on the days of the week that the transportation is available, limits on the times of day the service is available, limits on the transportation of pets (to the veterinarian or elsewhere), and limits on the number of wheelchair passengers served in a day. In some areas, private cars are available with volunteers to escort older passengers, but in most areas, special transportation services must manage consumer requests, volunteer schedules, and client appointments to accommodate the passengers. Older riders who are transported by community vans to appointments or stores may first endure lengthy rides to pick up other special passengers, be taken to their appointments early or late, and then must wait for the van's return to get home. This not infrequently results in the passengers being gone from home for half a day or longer, a stress that many cannot endure. In rural areas, two or three counties may share the use of one special transportation vehicle, meaning even less accessibility to the service and longer rides for the passengers.

The OAA funding for transportation is directed to AAAs, which in turn give grants to agencies that provide direct services. In addition, federal dollars are allocated to each state's Department of Transportation (DOT), which contracts with cities to provide services through private agencies. The federal money is augmented by state and local funding and by voluntary contributions from pas-

sengers. Charging for the federal portion of the transportation costs is not allowed, but states and local groups can charge for all or part of their contribution to the total cost of the service. The practice of charging part of the cost to the passengers is called cost sharing and helps expand the availability of the transportation services.

Information about transportation for older adults is available from the local AAA, through the United Way (where available), and through the Eldercare Locator, operated by the Community Transportation Association of America and funded by the DOT and the Department of Health and Human Services (DHHS), which can provide names of local transit providers who receive federal money to provide services to older adults and people with disabilities. Nurses looking for services for specific clients within the community also should investigate local Veterans' Affairs offices (for veterans), medical centers' private transportation companies, churches, and voluntary agencies (such as the American Cancer Society and Lutheran Social Services) for potential sources of transportation. In some areas, groups of private physicians provide transportation to appointments at their offices. Updates on federal transportation programs for older adults are available in the *Transportation for the Elderly Fact Sheet,* through the National Aging Information Center, DHHS, Administration on Aging, 330 Independence Avenue, SW, Washington, D.C. 20201.

Community-Based Services

Several services are available in the community that enhance the well-being of older adults and contribute to their ability to live independently without facing financial distress and social isolation. Community-based services include such programs as employment resources, **senior center programs,** senior housing, **adult day services,** and alternative community-based living facilities. Many of these programs are funded through grants distributed through the AAA or the federal government.

Priority areas and objectives of *Healthy People 2000* can be addressed in a variety of ways through community-based services. For example, senior center programs have physical fitness and nutrition priorities to meet relevant objectives. Other priority areas can be targeted depending on the needs of each particular community and available resources (see Table 24-1).

Employment Services

Services exist that assist older individuals in securing employment in a meaningful job and supplementing income (National Association, 1998). The Senior Community Service Employment Program (SCSEP) is authorized under Title V of the OAA and is administered nationally by the U.S. Department of Labor. A portion of these monies are allocated to AAAs, which contract for employment service sites through national organizations (e.g., American Association of Retired Persons and Farmer's Union).

Employment services may include job placement, training, and demonstration of the effectiveness of older workers. Through this program, older individuals are employed in minimum wage positions for an average of 20 hours per week in subsidized positions with public agencies and private nonprofit corporations. The goal is to provide experience and training to place participants in jobs that are not subsidized outside of the SCSEP program. The program targets those individuals over age 55 whose incomes are 125% of poverty level or below. Employment services contribute to diminishing poverty in older adults.

Senior Center Programs

More than 12,000 senior centers exist across the United States that provide social, physical, religious, and recreational activities (National Association, 1998). Senior centers are funded by Title III of the OAA and are seen as a focal point for underserved older adults and furnish a gathering place for them. They may also serve as a source of information and referral. They provide linkage to the community to combat social isolation and may arrange a variety of recreation and social activities, depending on funding and the sophistication of the staff (Matteson, Bearon, & McConnell, 1997). Services offered by senior centers vary but may include meals, travel, education, exercise, health assessment, counseling, and other services (see Figure 24-5). Transportation services are usually available for those individuals who would otherwise be unable to attend. Some claim that older adults who use senior centers already have active social lives, although these lives may be enriched by the services offered.

Senior Housing

Senior housing includes rental apartments, group residence, and hotel-style housing designed for indepen-

dent older adults. They are usually designed with features that enhance functional abilities and promote a secure living environment. However, they do not provide nursing or personal care services (National Association, 1998). In addition to living facilities, senior housing centers may offer support services such as meals, transportation, and social and recreational programs. Subsidies for existing rental units or even substantial tax deductions for older adults holding mortgages may be available. Information about senior housing services options can be obtained through the local AAA.

Adult Day Services

Adult day service centers provide care for adults who cannot or choose not to be left alone during the day but do not require 24-hour institutional nursing care. A safe supportive environment within a group setting is provided for participants. Transportation service usually is provided to and from the center.

Adult day service centers provide the well spouse or caregiver some relief from the total responsibility of providing care for an older member. The services provided by adult day centers allow family members time to fulfill their various responsibilities such as work, school, shopping, and leisure time.

There are two primary models of adult day services, the social model and the health care model. The social model offers social and educational activities such as music, art, poetry, dancing, guest speakers, discussion groups, computer activities, nutrition, and exercise. This type of center provides a protective nurturing environment for older adults. The health care model offers many of the same services, in addition to health care services offered by interdisciplinary providers such as physicians, nurses, occupational and physical therapists, and speech pathologists. Both models use paid staff and volunteers, and some social models offer limited moni-

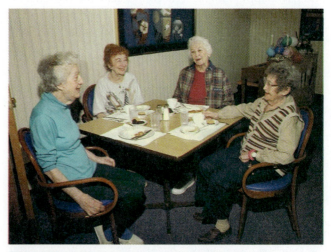

FIGURE 24-5 Many older adults enjoy a daily meal and the opportunity to socialize at their local senior center.

toring of general health and preventive health maintenance activities. Adult day services assist many families in postponing or avoiding institutionalization of an older loved one.

The goals of adult day services include:

- Improving participants' quality of life
- Delaying or preventing institutionalization
- Providing relief to family caregivers
- Enhancing participants' self-concept

Adult day service programs may be licensed and/or certified by the state. They are not federally regulated, but certification is required to receive federal funding. Sources of possible federal funding include Medicaid and Veterans' Affairs (VA) as well as Medicare. Some funding may be available on the state or regional level. However, most centers rely on grants, United Way contributions, fundraisers, and fees for service as their major revenue sources.

Alternative Community-Based Living Facilities

Several types of community-based living facilities exist that include adult foster care, board and care homes, residential care facilities, and assisted living. The intention of these facilities is to bridge the gap between totally independent living and nursing facility care (National Association, 1998). Through these living arrangements, which may or may not be supported by public monies, the independence of the older individual is enhanced and the need for more intense personal care delayed. Residents of these facilities may receive financial assistance through the Supplemental Security Income (SSI) program, depending on the state.

Home Services

Some services are available in the home of the older adult so that independent living is supported. As identified earlier, the primary aim of AAAs is to promote independence for older adults. This goal is accomplished by promoting the health, well-being, and independence of older adults by providing services that either complement or supplement services or care given by primary caregivers. In-home services can range from homemaking and personal care to weatherization assistance.

Healthy People 2000 priority areas and objectives can be met through home services that are congruent with AAAs' primary aim of independent living in the community. **Home services** [e.g., homemaker, chore service, **emergency response system (ERS)**] can also serve to prevent unintentional injuries by providing services for activities such as yard work that may not be safe for older adults. Food and drug safety priorities can be promoted through home health services and home care attendants (see Table 24-1).

Homemakers

Homemaker services assist individuals with household tasks that range from shopping for food and meal preparation to light housekeeping and laundry (National Association, 1998). Depending on the state or region, homemaker services are available on a fee-for-service basis, and costs may be based on income. See Figure 24-6.

Chore Services

Chore services consist of more heavy-duty tasks associated with maintaining a home. These services might include floor and window washing, minor home repairs, yard work, and other types of home maintenance (National Association, 1998). Many AAAs contract for chore services, subsidizing payment for those with lower incomes.

Home Health Services

Skilled nursing care, health monitoring and evaluation, medication administration, physical and other types of therapy, psychological counseling, and health care education are all part of home health services available in most communities. These services are usually provided under the supervision of a physician and/or nurse and

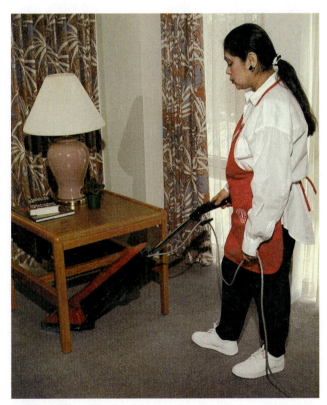

FIGURE 24-6 Homemaker services can help the older adult with a variety of tasks.

are offered through home health care agencies that are hospital based or community based.

Home Attendant or Aide Services

Services that are beyond the scope of homemaker responsibilities can be provided by a personal care attendant or nurse aide. Personal care attendant or nurse aide services provide assistance with activities of daily living, such as feeding, bathing, and walking. Home health aides usually have specialized training and quite often have certification through a local community college or health care agency. Because they provide personal care, services are supervised by a physician or nurse and are not covered by Medicare unless they are provided in conjunction with skilled nursing or therapy services. Some states or regions provide financial assistance to persons needing these services, and information can be obtained by contacting the local AAA.

Respite Care

Because caregiving for an older individual, particularly those with some form of dementia, can be challenging, many communities have respite care programs. These programs may be available in the home or in an institution that will admit the care recipient on a temporary basis so that the caregiver can have much needed relief. Availability of this service and funding to pay for it vary from community to community and may be accessed through special organizations such as the Alzheimer's Association.

CLINICAL ALERT

The caregiving process can lead to the following in the caregiver:

- *Physical health problems*
- *Emotional problems*
- *Social isolation*

Friendly Visiting

Another program that may be available to older adults in the home is a friendly visitor's program. The availability of this program varies with each community, but it offers social contact, human interaction, and reassurance to recipients (National Association, 1998).

Some agencies, volunteer services, and churches provide telephone reassurance to older adults through regular, prescheduled telephone calls to persons who are confined to the home. Through this service, a person who is socially isolated has contact with others. In addition, the service provides a sense of security for the older person (National Association, 1998). Volunteers, many times other

older adults, perform this service, fostering a sense of involvement and usefulness.

Energy Assistance and Weatherization

Most states offer some type of energy assistance and/or weatherization for low-income individuals. To support this assistance, federal dollars are allocated to various community action agencies. Included in this service is assistance in paying fuel bills or payment for weatherizing homes through activities such as insulation, caulking, and storm window application (National Association, 1998).

Emergency Response Systems

Emergency response systems (ERSs) usually consist of some type of electronic device that links the individual to the local fire department, hospital, or other health facility or social service agency (National Association, 1998) (see Figure 24-7). In general, individuals using this system wear the device, usually on a chain or tie around their neck, and can simply push a button when help is needed, such as when a fall occurs. This action sets in motion a system in which the response center is notified and emergency assistance is initiated (neighbor, relative, friend, or 911 as previously designated).

Nutritional Services

Frequently, AAAs oversee and/or fund nutritional services that enhance dietary needs of older adults who may not be financially, physically, or psychologically capable of providing their own balanced nutrition. Programs such as home-delivered meals and congregate meal sites are included in services aimed at meeting these needs.

The *Healthy People 2000* goals for nutrition of older people include many of the goals for the general population: balancing dietary intake, increasing the amount of dietary fiber, avoiding weight gain, ensuring adequate intake of fluids, and lowering the fat and salt content of the food consumed. *Healthy People 2000* goals specifically addressing nutrition for older people include increasing the availability of home food services and increasing the percentage of the population using the health care system each year (National Center, 1996).

Older adults are at increased risk for nutritional problems because of an increased incidence of both poverty and physical disability, which interfere with ability to obtain food from stores and prepare nutritious and appealing food at home. In addition, isolation and loneliness, which affect the desire to eat, and poor dentition, which affects the ability to eat, play a part in the development of malnutrition. The increased incidence of chronic diseases, such as chronic lung disease, heart disease, and diabetes, affects the nutritional needs of older adults. The medications used to treat these chronic dis-

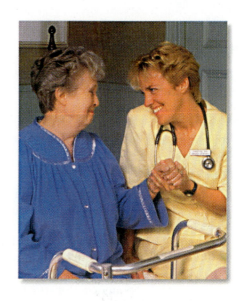
Lifeline Emergency Response System (ERS), Lifeline Systems, 111 Lawrence Street,

Framingham, MA 01702-8156. Used with permission.

FIGURE 24-7 Lifeline emergency response system (ERS) *(Courtesy of Lifeline Systems, 111 Lawrence St., Framingham, MA. Used with permission.)*

eases often affect their appetite. To further complicate matters, the signs of malnutrition are frequently confused with signs of aging, leading to under-recognition and undertreatment of the malnutrition.

> ### Nursing Tip
>
> Volunteer meal deliverers can assess the following during their brief visit:
> - Sanitation
> - Signs of abuse or neglect
> - Grooming
> - Mood/psychological status
> - Few social contacts
> - Decreasing functional ability
> - Potential safety problems (e.g., falls)
> - Decreasing nutritional status (weight loss)

Nutrition Programs

The nutrition program is administered through the AOA, state agencies, and local AAAs and provides grants to support nutritional services to older people. These federal funds, which are augmented by state, local, and private funds as well as donations and participant contributions, are intended to be used to improve the participants' dietary intake and offer opportunities for social interaction. The grants pay for both congregate meals and home-delivered meals. Federal dollars account for nearly 40% of congregate meal costs and about one-fourth of home-delivered meals. Voluntary personal contributions account for 20%–40% of meal costs (Administration on Aging, 1998b). Each meal served through this program must contain at least one-third of the daily recommended dietary allowance established by the Federal Nutrition Board of the National Academy of Sciences—National Research Council. In practice, most meals served contain 40%–50% of most of the participants' food intake for the day (Department, 1995). Some participants take part of the food home for their evening meal.

In some areas, the nutrition program funds individual nutrition screening and educational services to assist older adults in dealing with special health problems and/or in planning economical and nutritious meals (Administration on Aging, 1998b). There are no means tests (financial restrictions) for eligibility for the nutrition program, but the program is targeted to those with the greatest economic or social need, especially low-income minorities.

Congregate Meals

At meal sites, participants have the opportunity to socialize during their meals, and frequently health education and screening are offered before or after meals. This is an excellent opportunity for nurses to interact with the well older adults and provide health promotion information. For more information about the availability of these programs, contact the local AAA or the national Eldercare Locator.

Home-Delivered Meals

Home-delivered meals offered through this program include one hot midday or evening meal delivered 5 or more days a week for those who are unable to shop or prepare food at home. The OAA requires that particular attention be given to special diets, such as those for diabetics or those on low-sodium diets. Volunteers who deliver meals to homes are trained to spend time talking with the meal recipients and report any health problems or other problems noted during their visits. As a pilot program in 1997, 20 senior nutrition programs were chosen to deliver breakfasts to the doors of older people who were already receiving a second meal during the day. If successful, this program could ensure that they begin the day with a good meal.

Other Nutritional Programs

Other national resources for older adults' nutrition include the Food Stamp and the Commodities Supplemental Food Programs, which are accessed through local state welfare offices. Updated information about eligibility requirements, benefits, and applications to these programs are available through the U.S. Department of Agriculture (USDA) web site. Other federal nutrition programs for special populations are described at this web site.

Local nutrition programs in specific areas may include food banks (accessed through the United Way or other social service agencies), group meals offered through the Salvation Army or other charities, and nutrition, shopping, meal planning, and meal preparation instruction though state extension offices. Teaching materials for nurses to use in education of older adults are available through the National Dairy Council, the American Heart Association, the American Diabetes Association, and many other national organizations.

Older Adults' Rights

In addition to providing services to enhance physical independence in the community, AAAs are charged with overseeing and/or funding programs that protect rights of the most vulnerable older adults. Programs include legal assistance, prevention of older adult abuse, and the long-term care ombudsman program. *Healthy People 2000* priority areas of mental health and mental disorders and violent and abusive behaviors are examples that can be targeted through attention to older adults' rights.

Legal Services

In general, AAAs contract with local legal service organizations to provide legal assistance to older adults who may be unable to manage their own affairs appropriately. The Senior Citizens Law Project of HELP Legal Assistance is a publicly financed law resource that renders legal services at no cost to individuals 60 years of age and older in various civil (noncriminal) matters. The federal government also funds the Legal Service Corporation (LSC), which provides legal services to low-income individuals of all ages, although the type of services is the subject of ongoing debate in legislative bodies.

Legal services furnish guidance and instruction to persons age 60 and over and their families to help with concerns of a business or financial nature. The extent of services provided may vary by community, but in general, these services are designed to protect the rights and welfare of older persons and to shield them and/or their property from harm. Examples include power of attorney, guardianship, wills, living wills, government benefits and entitlements, and consumer services; landlord/tenant problems; pensions; age discrimination; and family law. In some cases, protective services can be initiated and implemented (National Association, 1998).

Abuse Prevention and Ombudsman Programs

State and community programs exist that provide adult protection and guardianship/conservatorship services that are aimed at preventing abuse, neglect, or self-neglect with regard to older adults. Examples of older adult abuse are material abuse (theft or misuse of property), physical abuse, psychological abuse, and medical abuse (National Association, 1998).

In addition to older adult abuse prevention, every state and many communities also have an ombudsman program that investigates potential abuse of older adults in institutions (National Association, 1998). The ombudsman monitors the implementation of federal, state, and local laws that govern long-term care facilities. They may target quality of care, the physical environment, finances, legal problems, and other factors that are important to protecting the rights of persons living in long-term care facilities.

Institutional Services

Although information about the provision of services in institutions is beyond the scope of this chapter, it is important to note that the Eldercare Locator can provide information that pertains to institutions, such as nursing facilities. For example, some states require preadmission screening of individuals to qualify for Medicaid programs that reimburse nursing facilities and some community-based services. The NAAAA may be able to provide information on local nursing facilities and the level of care provided (e.g., skilled, rehabilitation) as

well as information regarding continuing care retirement communities (CCRCs). Even though an older individual may live in an institution, *Healthy People 2000* priority areas are still relevant. For example, the priority areas of unintentional injuries and oral health are appropriate for persons living in institutions or in their own home.

Other Organizations and Services

Other organizations and resources exist that may be of benefit to older individuals but are not specifically for those age 60 and older. These organizations and services are usually driven by a particular need, such as a diagnosis of cancer or diabetes. The material that follows provides an overview of services that the gerontological nurse should be familiar with so that appropriate referrals may be made.

American Cancer Society

The American Cancer Society, founded in 1913, is a voluntary health organization dedicated to eliminating cancer as a major health problem by preventing cancer, saving lives, and diminishing complications from cancer (American Cancer Society, 1997). Among its many programs are research support, professional and consumer education, visitation programs, children's camps, publications, political advocacy on cancer-related issues, public service announcements about healthy lifestyle choices, and networks of volunteer drivers to help clients get to appointments. Twenty-four percent of the revenue raised by this organization goes to cancer research.

Cancer is the second leading cause of death among Americans age 65 and older. *Healthy People 2000* goals relating to cancer and older adults that are addressed by this agency include:

- Increasing the percentage of the population receiving recommended screening services

- Reducing the incidence and mortality from specific forms of cancer

- Decreasing the number of Americans who smoke

- Reducing the average dietary fat intake

- Increasing the dietary intake of complex carbohydrates and fiber

- Increasing the number of people who limit sun exposure and use sunscreen (National Center, 1996)

The American Cancer Society (ACS) operates through a network of 35 divisions and over 3,400 units that serve almost every community in the United States. Many ACS services are available nationally, such as Reach to

Recovery, a visitation program for women concerned about breast cancer, and Man to Man, a program that addresses prostate cancer. Individual units may have other services available, such as lodging assistance, discounted airline tickets, and assistance with home care. The organization has over two million volunteers.

American Heart Association

The American Heart Association, founded in 1924, supports research to investigate the causes and treatments of heart disease and stroke and provides community and professional education about the risk factors of cardiovascular disease and about emergency responses for heart attacks and choking. The goal of the American Heart Association is the prevention of disease and disability related to cardiovascular disease and stroke. As a nonprofit voluntary organization, it works primarily through volunteers to raise funds for its programs.

Heart disease is the leading cause of death among U.S. citizens 65 years of age and older, and stroke is the third leading cause of death. Many of the goals of *Healthy People 2000* aim to reduce the risk of heart disease and stroke by eliminating the controllable risk factors and improving life choices, as shown in Table 24-1 (National Center, 1996).

There are 56 affiliates within the American Heart Association, one for each state and the metropolitan areas of Chicago, Cleveland, Los Angeles, New York City, Philadelphia, and Washington, D.C. These affiliates are divided into over 2,250 smaller units, called divisions, that serve almost every community in the United States. Information available to nurses and to the public through the affiliates and divisions include catalogues of publications, statistics on the incidence of heart disease and stroke (nationally and within each affiliate), and classes on cardiovascular disease prevention and cardiopulmonary resuscitation. The American Heart Association web site offers access to the same materials as well as publications on the latest research findings and the direction of research efforts of the American Heart Association.

Nurses planning activities for promoting healthy life choices in the community will find many resources through the American Heart Association. These include books, pamphlets, posters, and videos for teaching about cholesterol, smoking cessation, dietary modifications, physical activity, weight and stress reduction, blood pressure monitoring and control, and the warning signs of heart attack and stroke. Pamphlets, notebooks, and videos about the major cardiovascular diagnoses, diagnostic tests, and treatments are available for clients who already have cardiovascular diseases. Cookbooks for low-cholesterol and low-salt diets are also available. Many of these resources are available in Spanish.

Arthritis Foundation

The Arthritis Foundation helps nearly 40 million U.S. citizens of all ages who have arthritis. The purpose of the organization is to support research to cure and prevent arthritis and provide resources to improve the quality of life for those affected by arthritis. In addition to all types of arthritis, the Arthritis Foundation provides support for research and services for persons with fibromyalgia, ankylosing spondylitis, and systemic lupus erythematosus. Several areas of *Healthy People 2000* can be addressed through programs administered by the Arthritis Foundation. For example, objectives associated with the priority areas of physical fitness and diabetes and disability are very appropriate. See Table 24-1 for other relevant priority areas.

Services offered by Arthritis Foundation chapters vary by region. They may offer exercise programs or contract with local facilities (e.g., YMCA) to provide aquatic programs. The national organization publishes a bimonthly magazine, *Arthritis Today*.

American Diabetes Association

The American Diabetes Association (ADA) is a voluntary, nonprofit organization founded in 1940. Its mission is to prevent and cure diabetes and to improve the lives of those who have the disease. It fulfills its mission through professional and consumer education, research support, publications, youth programs, counseling and support groups, advocacy services, and information and assistance services (American Diabetes, 1998).

Diabetes is one of the major chronic illnesses of older people. It is also a disease that often goes undetected until serious damage has occurred within the body and one that can positively be affected by changes in personal life choices. *Healthy People 2000* goals of this organization are included in Table 24-1.

The ADA has offices in over 800 communities within the United States. It has a monthly magazine for people with diabetes and publishes several professional journals on diabetic research and treatment.

Teaching tools and program assistance for nurses addressing these goals are available from the ADA. Information about the organization and its current publications, including brochures and tools for client education, can be obtained through the ADA web site (see Resources at the end of this chapter).

Alzheimer's Association

The Alzheimer's Association is a national organization with offices in Chicago and chapters throughout the United States. The purpose of the Alzheimer's Association is to support research and services for persons with Alzheimer's disease and related disorders (ADRDs) and their families. The national organization provides services related to research and education and has an annual meeting to update members and health care professionals on the latest developments regarding ADRDs.

Nearly all priority areas listed in Table 24-1 are relevant for older adults with dementia. Of particular note, however, are the priority areas addressing violent and abusive behavior, unintentional injuries, and food and drug safety. Persons with dementia and their families are vulnerable in all of these areas, the extent depending on each individual.

Local chapters offer a variety of services. The family counseling program offers extensive one-to-one help with daily problems and long-range planning. There is a telephone helpline that is available 24 hours per day in some locales that can provide callers with information and assistances at times when it is most needed. In addition, chapters conduct support groups for caregivers of persons with dementia, and many chapters offer support groups for persons who have dementia as well as for their children and grandchildren. Support group meetings provide an opportunity to talk about common problems, share caregiving strategies and ideas, and obtain information.

Local chapters offer educational programs for health care providers, family members, and law enforcement departments on the disease and ways to deal sensitively and suitably with the client. Nursing facilities that care for persons with dementia may request inservice training in their facility for a modest fee. In addition, chapters publish newsletters, maintain a chapter library, and promote advocacy on the local and national level.

The national organization sponsors a **Safe Return Program** for persons with dementia who may wander and become lost. The Safe Return Program provides an identification (ID) bracelet that contains an ID for the wearer, a statement that the person is memory impaired, and the phone number of the National Missing Persons Bureau in Washington, D.C. The Bureau maintains a database of all subscribers and is then able to contact the person or persons registered as responsible for the individual. In this way, the complete name and address of these vulnerable persons are protected, yet there is a mechanism in place for them to return home safely. This service can be accessed through local chapters at minimal cost. Some chapters have solicited funds to support the Safe Return Program from community organizations so that use of the program is at no cost.

The Alzheimer's Association is a nonprofit organization that relies on donations and grants for funding. Local chapters are managed by minimal staff and rely on volunteers to help implement many of the programs.

Widowed Persons

When one is widowed, one's overall health and life are disrupted. Widows and widowers often are not prepared to cope with the changes and decisions that may be nec-essary related to finances, legal issues, housing, family relations, and social demands. Society is very mobile, competitive, fast paced, and often impersonal. Workers are given 3 days bereavement leave from work if the deceased is a close relative or significant other. Subtle messages from well-meaning friends and relatives suggest that one should be over grieving in a relatively short period of time.

The literature validates that widows and widowers are at a higher risk for morbidity and mortality than their married peers. When reading Table 24-1, one can see that several of the priority areas are especially relevant to older widows and widowers. Three factors related to mortality from loss of a spouse are emotional stress and grief, loss of social support, and loss of material and task support. These findings suggest that bereavement leads to a weakening of a person's ability to resist and cope with disease (Martikainen & Valkonent, 1996). Bowling and Windsor (1995) found that lack of someone to telephone was a risk factor for mortality following bereavement. Higher levels of perceived social support were associated with lower levels of depression in both widows and widowers. Provision of social support should be a priority for this group of people (Martikainen & Valkonent, 1996).

Nurses in the community, extended-care facilities, and inpatient settings can be instrumental in facilitating and providing social support for bereaved widows and widowers. Nurses need to discuss the benefits of social support and encourage new widows and widowers to seek and accept support from family and friends. Because of the potentially large geographical distance between family members and possible smaller family networks, the nurse needs to be aware of community and organizational support services for new widows and widowers. Table 24-2 lists several national support services along with their functions and activities.

Support groups consist of people banding together to address a shared problem. Seeking help from people who have been there themselves and know how one feels unites, bonds, and comforts support group participants. Peer support groups differ from professional groups in that professional groups are grounded in theory, whereas peer support groups evolve from the members' collective experiences and shared concerns. Liberman (1996) found that members of support groups felt less depression and used less medication and alcohol to alter their feelings of sadness. The more active the new widows became in the groups, the greater their signs of recovery. They became less anxious, had a greater sense of well-being and higher self-esteem, and rated themselves as much improved.

One of the most profound losses experienced by humans is the death of a spouse. Studies support the

TABLE 24-2   Support Services for Widowed Persons

Support Services	Function/Activities
AARP's Widowed Person Service (WPS) 601 E. Street, NW Washington, DC 20049	• Offer support to recently widowed persons from trained, widowed volunteers; provide free assistance and resources to communities who wish to develop WPS programs • Provide outreach—trained widowed volunteer on a one-to-one basis • Telephone service—local telephone number is publicized • Mutual support group • Public education; sponsor an annual national conference; sponsor workshops, write articles, bring media attention to issues pertinent to widowed persons • Referral services—develops a directory or manual to facilitate local services and appropriate agencies for widowed persons in the community
Society of Military Widows (SMW) 5535 Hempstead Way Springfield, VA 22151	• Provide service and support to women whose husbands died while on active-duty military service or during retirement from the armed forces
They Help Each Other Spiritually 717 Liberty Avenue 1301 Clark Bldg Pittsburgh, PA 15222	• Provide mutual self-help for widowed persons of all ages and their families
To Live Again PO Box 415 Springfield, PA 19064	• Supports widowed persons through the grief cycle

concept that widowed persons who have made a satisfactory life adjustment can provide valuable support to newly widowed persons. The **Widowed Persons Service (WPS)** of the American Association of Retired Persons is one example of a support group using trained, experienced widowed volunteers to help the newly widowed. Nurses can be instrumental in facilitating and providing social support for newly bereaved widowed persons.

Retired and Senior Volunteer Program

The **Retired and Senior Volunteer Program (RSVP)** provides persons age 55 and over with the opportunities to use their knowledge, experience, and wisdom to contribute to the lives of persons in the local community. The program was established under the Domestic Volunteer Service Act of 1973. It is partially funded and administered nationally by the Corporation for National Service. Anyone age 55 and over may become an RSVP volunteer, and there are no membership dues.

The program orients, trains, and places volunteers with nonprofit and public agencies for a variety of jobs, such as tutoring, mentoring, and coaching. In addition to giving something to the community, RSVP volunteers receive a sense of purpose and meaning that may otherwise be untapped.

Summary

Community organizations and resources currently exist that are geared toward maintaining and/or improving the quality of life for older people. With the growing number of older adults projected in the twenty-first century, it is important that the health care community continue to assess this population and offer services that can meet their needs. Gerontological nurses are in a prime position to anticipate needs, assist older adults and their families to access services, and foster the development of future services based on social, cultural, and demographic trends of the community. Boxes 24-2 and 24-3 provide checklists for identifying and assessing available community resource services.

BOX 24-2 Checklist of Primary Intervention Community Resources

The following are community resources for healthier living:

Health care

- Medical centers
- Primary care practitioners
- Wellness centers
- Complemental therapies availability
- Informal health screening opportunities
- Dental services

Health information

- Disease-specific organizations (e.g., American Heart Association)
- State extension offices
- Medical centers' educational programs

General education

- Elderhostel
- Community colleges
- Internet access
- Television distance learning
- Books for the blind

Volunteering

- Retired Senior Volunteer Program
- Service Corps of Retired Volunteers
- Other, not age specific

Social activities

- Senior centers
- Senior groups
- Recreation opportunities

Transportation

- Public
- Disabled/older
- Car/van conversion availability

Financial assistance

- Social Security
- Medicaid
- Property tax relief
- Veterans' Affairs

Housing support

- Local health and human resources departments
- Living centers
- Home-rehabilitation groups

Legal services

- Publicly funded assistance
- Tax preparation assistance
- Protection services

Spiritual development

- Church programs
- Meditation centers
- Library resources

Nutrition services

- Meal sites
- Home-delivered meals
- Food pantries
- Education about nutrition and meal preparation

Emergency assistance

- Shelters
- Utilities
- Food

BOX 24-3 Checklist of Secondary and Tertiary Intervention Resources

The following are community resources for minimizing the effects of illness and disability:

Case management

- Medical centers
- Home care agencies
- Area Agency on Aging

Skilled professional home health care services

- Home care
- Mental health support
- Hospice

Monitoring services

- Social contact systems
- Emergency contact systems

Housekeeping/homemaker services

- Public programs
- Private agencies
- Lawn/yard services

Personal care assistance

- Publicly funded programs
- Private agencies

Family support services

- Publicly funded programs
- Private agencies

Disease-specific support groups

- American Cancer Society
- American Heart Association
- Arthritis Foundation

Assisted-living facilities/arrangements

- Adult day services
- Respite availability
- Congregate living facilities
- Personal care homes
- Skilled care facilities

Assistive equipment

- Private companies
- Equipment closets through local groups/clubs

Spiritual support

- Churches
- Nondenominational groups

Review Questions and Activities

1. What are current demographic facts and recent trends in health care that influence the need for more community services to support older adults?

2. What are three programs and related services provided by Area Agencies on Aging?

3. How does the National Aging Network promote the use of community organizations and services?

4. What are common nutritional problems that place older adults at risk?

5. How do support agencies provide services for widowed persons?

6. Explore the older adults' nutrition programs available in your community, investigating services provided, fees, and process of accessing the service.

7. Identify transportation services for older adults in your community and discuss access, constraints, and motivation issues related to use of these services.

8. Investigate and evaluate resources in your community that assist caregivers and families with the care of older members.

9. Visit a community center that provides adult day services. Discuss the services that are provided and relate the overall culture of the environment in which these services are provided.

10. Attend a support group for widowed persons. Discuss the value of support groups.

References

Administration on Aging (AOA). (1998a, February). *Fact sheet: Transportation and the elderly* (p. 25) [On-line]. Available: http://www.aoa.dhhs.gov.

Administration on Aging (AOA). (1998b, February). *Fact sheet: The elderly nutrition program* (p. 39) [On-line]. Available: http://www.aoa.dhhs.gov.

American Cancer Society. (1997). *Cancer facts & figures.* Atlanta, GA: American Cancer Society.

American Diabetes Association. (1998). *Learn about us* [On-line]. Available: http://diabetes.org.

A profile of older Americans 1999. (1999). Washington, DC: American Association of Retired Persons and the Administration on Aging, U.S. Department of Health and Human Services.

Bowling, A., & Windsor, J. (1995). Death after widow(er)hood: An analysis of mortality rates up to 13 years after bereavement. *Omega, 31,* 35–49.

Department of Health and Human Services (DHHS). (1995). *Evaluation of the Elderly Nutrition Program* [On-line]. Available: http://www.dhhs.gov.

Liberman, M. (1996). *Doors closed, doors open. Widows grieving and growing.* New York: Grosset/Putman.

Martikainen, P., & Valkonent. (1996). Mortality after the death of a spouse: Rates and causes of death in a large Finnish cohort. *American Journal of Public Health, 86*(8), 1087–1093.

Matteson, M. A., Bearon, L. B., & McConnell, E. S. (1997). Psychosocial problems associated with aging. In M. A. Matteson, E. S. McConnell, & A. D. Linton (Eds.), *Gerontological nursing, concepts and practice* (2nd ed.). Philadelphia: Saunders.

National Association of Area Agencies on Aging (NAAAA). (1998). *National directory for eldercare information and assistance.* Washington, DC: Author.

National Center for Health Statistics. (1996). *Healthy people 2000 review 1995–96.* Hyattsville, MD: Public Health Service.

U.S. Department of Health and Human Services. (1990). *Healthy people 2000: National health promotion and disease prevention objectives* (PHS Publication No. 91-50213). Washington, DC: U.S. Government Printing Office.

U.S. Senate. (1993). *Developments in aging, 1992* (Vol. 1). Washington, DC: U.S. Government Printing Office.

Resources

American Association of Retired People (AARP): **www.aarp.org**

American Association of Homes and Services for the Aging: **www.aahsa.org**

American Cancer Society: **www.cancer.org**

American Diabetes Association: **diabetes.org**

American Heart Association: **www.americanheart.org**

Arthritis Foundation: **www.arthritis.org**

Canadian Seniors Guide to Federal Programs and Services: **www.mbnet.mb.ca/crm**

Community resources—organizations: **www.fortnet.org/fortnet**

Elderhostel: **www.elderhostel.org**

Elder net: **www.eldernet.com**

Families USA Foundations: **www.familiesusa.org**

Grief recovery online widows and widowers (GROWW): **groww.com**

International parish nursing program: **www.advocatehealth.com/sites**

Maturity USA: **www.maturityusa.com**

National Senior Citizens Law Center: **www.nsclc.org**

Senior living alternatives: **www.senioralternatives.com**

Senior sites: **www.seniorsites.com**

U.S. Administration on Aging: **www.aoa.dhhs.gov/aoa**

U.S. Department of Agriculture (USDA): **www.usda.gov**

Widowed person service (AARP): **seniors-site.com**

WidowNet: **fortnet.org**

UNIT 7

Ethical, Legal, and Financial Issues

PERSPECTIVE . . .

"How should we handle our mother? She was always so independent and responsible and provided structure to our lives as we were growing up. It seems ever since she developed cancer and osteoarthritis and our Dad died, she has become more emotionally unstable. Sometimes she makes decisions that do not make sense and are unsafe. When we tell her she needs our help, she gets very angry!"

The three children of Mrs. Quann are facing difficult decisions related to the care of their mother. Mrs. Quann is an 84-year-old widow who was diagnosed with colon cancer and osteoarthritis approximately 5 years ago. Based upon a health care assessment and history, Mrs. Quann also was recently diagnosed with dementia when she was hospitalized several weeks ago. Yesterday she was readmitted with a diagnosis of dehydration and confusion. Upon questioning, her three children agree that they had noticed their mother becoming more confused over the past year. Despite concerns about their mother's ability to live independently, the children allowed her to stay in her home of 30 years. They live in the same community as their mother and have shared responsibilities for daily visits to their mother in her home.

After 2 days of intravenous therapy in the hospital, Mrs. Quann became more coherent but refused to eat when foods and fluids were offered. Her children, knowing that she had to eat to regain her strength and to return home, suggested to Mrs. Quann's physician that their mother be fed by inserting a nasogastric tube into her stomach to help her regain her strength. When told about this, Mrs. Quann became very upset and stated she just wants to "get this over with and go to heaven to be with my husband." Her children do not want to see her die like this and become emotionally distraught about their mother's behavior and decision. They are not really sure she can rationally make this decision based on her history of confusion and past behaviors that have influenced her safety.

CHAPTER 25

Ethical Theories and Principles

Carolyn Spence Cagle, PhD, RNC

COMPETENCIES

After completing this chapter, the reader should be able to:

- *Describe the ethical reasoning and ethical practice of health care professionals involved in the care of older people.*
- *Describe the basic premises of the ethical theories of utilitarianism, deontology, and the ethic of care.*
- *Delineate the four primary ethical principles and their relevancy to the three ethical theories discussed in this chapter.*
- *Define essential elements of informed consent and the influence of these elements on autonomy of older people.*
- *Utilize relevant ethical principles in developing a plan of care for an older individual or family composed of older adults.*
- *Discuss the influence of technology on defining the ethical practice of nurses of the future.*
- *Describe ethical decision-making models used to develop quality care approaches for older people in a variety of settings.*

MAKING THE CONNECTION

Refer to the following chapters to increase your understanding of ethical theories and principles related to aging:

- **Chapter 21** *Hospice and Palliative Care*
- **Chapter 26** *End-of-Life Decisions and Choices*
- **Chapter 27** *Legal and Financial Issues*

Ethical Dilemmas

With increasing numbers of persons living into old age, ethical approaches to their unique needs by nurses and other health care professionals have assumed critical importance. These care approaches should focus on meeting older persons' needs for independence, freedom, respect, and availability of health care regardless of condition or age. Provision of care to older people has recently become more challenging because of advances in technology, legal interpretations of needed health care, more complex health care, and control of costs implemented by changed health care delivery systems (managed care) (Low & Kaufman, 1999). Technology and medical advances in health care have allowed people to live longer with a variety of health care problems, and these advances may sustain life even when an older person's quality of life becomes limited. In the latter case, a health care professional faces an **ethical dilemma,** a situation involving a choice between equally undesirable alternatives. The dilemma involves deciding on the best health care treatment to benefit the person who may be ill without further decreasing the quality of life of that individual.

In resolving an ethical dilemma, a health care professional with a strong sense of ethical behavior will explore various actions deemed beneficial to the person based on the social, cultural, economic, and religious environment of that person. A total assessment of this person's life allows the professional as well as other members of the health care team to discuss an ethical decision defining an approach appropriate to meeting that person's needs for health care. Each person in the situation (client/resident, nurse, case manager, discharge planner, social worker, physician, family, legal system, etc.) has a personal perspective on effectively dealing with the situation based on their individual **values,** life experiences, education, and other factors. Each person also brings a set of **morals,** values used to identify right decisions from those that are wrong. The values of the participants, all reflecting different philosophical beliefs and disciplines, may oppose one another, create emotional responses among the participants, and require collaboration among the participants to engage in a critical thinking process to analyze possible resolutions for a person's health care problem. It is through consideration of possible resolutions from a variety of perspectives that participants realize they are involved in an ethical dilemma—a situation that involves making a choice between equally undesirable alternatives. For example, a nurse may value an older person's **autonomy** and, therefore, collaborate with an individual and his or her significant others to facilitate a peaceful dying process. On the other hand, his family may value nursing actions centered on doing *good* for the client, professional behav-iors that this family perceives as extending the person's life despite that individual's expressed desire to die peacefully without intervention. Through communicating their values, philosophies about life, and perception of their moral and legal roles, an interdisciplinary health care team can collaborate with the involved person and family to reach a resolution generally acceptable to everyone.

The purpose of this chapter will be to outline ethical **principles** and common ethical theories that consider ethical issues found in professional health care practice with older people. These ethical principles and theories will be discussed based on a foundation of values typically held by the predominant European-American culture in the United States. These values and ethical beliefs/actions will be compared with those of emerging diverse and minority groups in this country to define the ethical role of professionals in dealing with health care challenges of various groups of people. Although generically relevant to all people, the principles and theories addressed in this chapter apply well to the ethical care of older persons whose needs are often forgotten in the current health care delivery system. Providers of care frequently face ethical and legal issues arising from implementing care aimed at respecting the older adult's right for quality care based on state and national laws (e.g., Patient Self-Determination Act, 1991) and focusing on compliance with professional ethical codes of practice. This chapter will provide background information on some of these issues and provide guidelines for the reader in professional ethical decision making that involves both ethical reasoning and ethical practice with older people. According to several authors, ethical reasoning is a cognitive process used in solving an ethical dilemma, and ethical practice is behavior occurring after ethical reasoning and supports beneficial (good) decisions about care of another. Nurses and other health care professionals who critically reflect on their knowledge, skills, and caring approach to the needs of older people demonstrate both ethical reasoning and ethical practice and serve as moral agents in the health care delivery system (Dierckx de Casterlé, Grypdonck, & Vuylsteke-Wauters, 1997; Dierckx de Casterlé, Janssen, & Grypdonck, 1996; Smith, 1996).

An approach built on ethical reasoning and ethical practice to older persons seems particularly important because these individuals experience more disease and disability than other population groups (Figure 25-1), and these conditions may decrease older persons' freedom, self-respect, understanding, and overall ability to collaborate in their health care (Dierckx de Casterlé, 1998). Older persons also face loss of independence, fewer choices, and loss of individuality and often face unwanted situations because they have little power in the health care delivery system (Allert, Sponhotz, &

Baitsch, 1994; Copp, 1986). This chapter will also explore ways health care professionals can serve as advocates to protect, promote, and restore health and alleviate discomfort of older persons so that they may experience high quality and quantity of life.

CLINICAL ALERT

The nurse needs to be directly involved with the client, family members, and other health care providers when attempting to resolve a pressing ethical dilemma. The education, experience, and continued contact with the client give the nurse an opportunity to understand the total physical, emotional, social, cultural, economic, and spiritual dimensions of the client.

Ethical Theories

To understand the traditional theories of **ethics,** one must first understand the meaning of ethics. Ethics is a branch of philosophy utilizing a seasoned decision-making process that allows persons to choose the most appropriate life action relevant to a situation. For health care professionals, this action focuses on moral decision making on issues related to the health care of people, a philosophical approach called **bioethics.** According to Beauchamp and Childress (1994), a health care professional may use several types of ethics in the decision-making process. For example, normative ethics may be used to discuss standards of right or wrong and define what ought to exist. On the other hand, descriptive ethics may be used to describe people's beliefs and actions on ethical issues, and analytical ethics may be chosen to closely examine concepts and methods of ethics specified

in professional codes of practice. These latter two types of ethics are known as nonnormative ethics because they define what factually and conceptually exists rather than what ought to exist.

Regardless of the type of ethical approach, nurses and other health care professionals engage in daily ethical decision making as part of their professional role. They serve as moral agents by making judgments about the goodness of a proposed action, by choosing a just or appropriate course of action from a list of options, and by holding themselves accountable for the consequences of that choice. Such action mandates that nurses identify their personal and professional values, desirable beliefs that one holds in high esteem and that serve as guides for behavior. Professional and personal values may conflict with values of other health care professionals and people receiving health care based on a variety of factors previously discussed. Therefore, it is critical that nurses and those involved in providing or receiving health care openly communicate their values so that these can be used in a decision-making process essential for resolution of ethical dilemmas common in caring for persons in today's health care system. This decision-making process is somewhat similar to the steps used in the nursing process, according to one author (Miedema, 1991) (see Box 25-1).

Two traditional theories of ethics, **deontology** and **utilitarianism,** have been defined in most current ethical

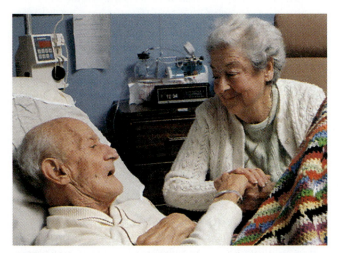

FIGURE 25-1   Illness and disability in the older population present many ethical challenges in the field of health care.

BOX 25-1   Steps of the Ethical Decision-making Process Related to the Nursing Process

Assessment
What are the medical facts?
What are the social facts?
What are the client's wishes?
What values are in conflict?

Planning
Determine the desired outcomes of the treatment.
Identify the decision makers (participants in decision).
List and rank options.

Implementation
Make a decision based on the above steps.
Act to implement the decision.

Evaluation
Maintain an ethical reflection on the decision.
Establish criteria for revision of goal or decision.

Adapted from "A Practical Approach to Ethical Decisions," by F. Miedema, 1991, American Journal of Nursing, 91*(12), pp. 20–25.*

literature. Deontology, the rule-oriented theory of ethics, was initially proposed by Immanuel Kant, who believed in the *categorical imperative,* a rule that one ought to apply to all people in similar circumstances when rendering an ethical decision (Beauchamp & Childress, 1994). In deontology, one acts as a moral agent in using ethically absolute and unchanging principles of ethics to make a moral decision. Deontology involves prioritizing the ethical principles of autonomy, **beneficence, nonmalificence,** and **justice** in resolving an ethical dilemma. Little consideration focuses on the consequences resulting from making choices based on these principles. In the deontological approach, a nurse or health care professional decides whether an ethical dilemma exists as part of professional practice. If so, the nurse identifies relevant ethical principles, relates facts of the case to these principles, and prioritizes principles based on a personal and professional value base (Brody, 1979; Gaul, 1989) (see Figure 25-2). The nurse may prioritize the principle of autonomy over the other principles of ethics. With this decision, the nurse would deliver care to a person that

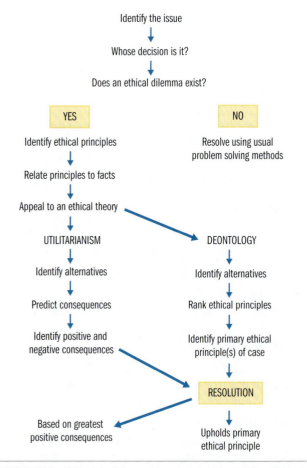

FIGURE 25-2   Ethical decision-making model. *(Adapted from* Ethical Decisions in Medicine, *by H. Brody, 1979, Boston: Little, Brown, & Co.; "Ethics Content in Baccalaureate Nursing Curricula," by A. L. Gaul, 1989,* Nursing Clinics of North America, 24, *pp. 475–483. Used with permission.)*

allowed that individual to freely make health care decisions based on that person's ability to do so and the ability not to infringe on the rights of others.

Think About It

Two months ago, Mr. Crupi and his wife were involved in a severe auto accident that caused the death of Mrs. Crupi. Mr. Crupi, an 80-year-old retired electrician, previously has stated to his three children that should he ever become seriously injured or ill and unable to live his life as he has in the past, he does not wish to be treated with extraordinary measures to continue his life. Currently, Mr. Crupi is in the intensive care unit on a ventilator because of a collapsed lung, serious internal bleeding caused by a lacerated liver, a closed head injury with a large intracranial hematoma, and abdominal trauma. He appears to be in a coma caused by the head injury and responds only to painful stimuli when assessed.

Two of the children agreed that their father would not want to live with the residual effects of his injuries should he recover. The third child, emotionally distant from her father until the last 6 months, desperately desires any relevant treatment for her father to allow him to possibly recover even if it means he has a decreased quality of life.

Consider the ethical principles and duties related to appropriate actions by the nurse and other health care professionals involved in this situation. Make a distinction between optional and obligatory care based on the facts of the case. Also, consider differences in resolution outcome if deontological and utilitarian theoretical approaches are used in an ethical decision-making process.

Utilitarianism, the second traditional ethical theory, is goal oriented and dictates that in all situations, one must morally act to produce the most good for the most people, according to its most famous proponent, John Stuart Mills. Here the end justifies the means, and consequences of actions assume primary significance in choosing the most appropriate action (Beauchamp & Childress, 1994). A nurse who values the utilitarian approach would identify the competing claims inherent in the ethical dilemma perceived in practice, consider the ethical principles, predict the positive and negative consequences of prioritizing each principle, and decide on a resolution that would meet the majority of the people's happiness or a resolution that would produce the greatest amount of value for those involved (Brody, 1979; Gaul, 1989) (see Figure 25-2).

With increasing acknowledgment that women may have different ethical values than do men, perhaps because of societal roles (Gilligan, 1982), a third theory of ethics, that of an **ethic of care,** has assumed more importance in the ethical literature. More common female values such as love, sympathy, trust, responsibility, interdependence, **fidelity,** and sensitivity to others' points of

nonMaleficence — not doing something that causes harm.
Hippocrates — "first do no harm"

view appear in the ethic-of-care theory. This theory, often referred to as relational ethics, supports that ethical dilemmas are best resolved by prioritizing interpersonal relationships of persons and relevant others, considering the ethical issue from the person's perspective, and by promoting basic acts of caring by a health care provider to the recipient of health care. This philosophy of ethics contrasts with both the deontological and utilitarianism models that use principles of ethics derived from intellectual and analytic processes; such processes appear to reflect rational ethics or a more male-centered approach to ethical decision making. Several critics of the ethic of care note that it does not sufficiently consider social issues in health care, may decrease the ability of the nurse to work in interdisciplinary ethical decision making, and may increase burnout in nurses who deliver care to persons but do not receive care in return (Nelson, 1992; Sherwin, 1992). However, the ethic-of-care theory appears consistent with nursing's commitment to ethical practice by prioritizing the nurse-patient relationship as the *instrument* that promotes the person's well-being by attempting to meet that individual's unique needs (Bishop & Scudder, 1990).

Ethical Principles

Ethical theories contain ethical principles, statements of fundamental beliefs or truths from which other ideas develop. The ethical practice of health care professionals involves application of these principles as part of an ethical theory in resolution of an ethical dilemma. In bioethics, four principles guide ethical deliberations and include principles of autonomy, beneficence, nonmalificence, and justice. Such discussions also involve moral duties as specified in a professional **code of ethics** such as in the American Nurses Association (ANA) Code for Nurses with Interpretive Statements (ANA, 1985). This code, currently under revision by the Congress on Nursing Practice of the ANA, summarizes the legal and ethical standards of professional nursing practice and defines ethical duties and moral conduct for the nursing profession (see Box 25-2). It is important to note that the Code contains statements of ethical practice based on European-American cultural values. Various interpretations

Ask Yourself

Which one of the ethical principles do you think is most important?
- Autonomy
- Beneficence
- Nonmalificence
- Justice

BOX 25-2 ANA Code for Nurses with Interpretive Statements (1985)

1. The nurse provides services with respect for human dignity and the uniqueness of the client, unrestricted by considerations of social or economic status, personal attributes, or the nature of health problems.

2. The nurse safeguards the client's right to privacy by judiciously protecting information of a confidential nature.

3. The nurse acts to safeguard the client and the public when health care and safety are affected by the incompetent, unethical, or illegal practice of any person.

4. The nurse assumes responsibility and accountability for individual nursing judgments and actions.

5. The nurse maintains competency in nursing.

6. The nurse exercises informed judgment and uses individual competence and qualifications as criteria in seeking consultation, accepting responsibilities, and delegating nursing activities to others.

7. The nurse participates in activities that contribute to the ongoing development of the profession's body of knowledge.

8. The nurse participates in the profession's efforts to implement and improve standards of nursing.

9. The nurse participates in the profession's efforts to establish and maintain conditions of employment conducive to high-quality nursing care.

10. The nurse participates in the profession's effort to protect the public from misinformation and misrepresentation and to maintain the integrity of nursing.

11. The nurse collaborates with members of the health professions and other citizens in promoting community and national efforts to meet the health needs of the public.

Reprinted with permission from Code for Nurses with Interpretive Statements, © 1985. American Nurses Publishing, American Nurses Foundation/American Nurses Association, Washington, DC.

BOX 25-3   Current Values Related to Selected Ethical Principles—Arab Americans

Principle of Autonomy

- With informed consent, it is important to use same-gender interpreters, particularly for sensitive material; family members may be used as interpreters for non-English-speaking family persons.

- A family spokesperson, generally a male but sometimes a grandmother, should be initially informed about the ill person's diagnosis and extent of health problem; this spokesperson may work with the health care team to decide the best way to tell the ill person about that person's health.

- Disclosure about an ill family member's health may take longer than usual because of the time needed by the family to decide the best way to inform the ill person of the illness and plans of care; the best approach for telling relates to the need to respect the older person's position in the family and in the culture.

- The spokesperson and family members may modify health care information received by the health care team to protect the ill family person (incomplete disclosure).

- Written consent is difficult to gain because of cultural value that verbal agreement is based on trust, a more acceptable form of consent than written consent.

- Many Arab Americans do not want to know about complications prior to implementation of a procedure; understanding complications is normally part of informed consent as process is defined.

Principle of Nonmalificence/Dying Rituals

- Generally there is little grieving by the family for the dying person before that person's death.

- Family spokesperson needs to be privately informed by the health care team about impending death and given sufficient time to decide the process of telling the dying person; it is important to provide a private room for family to make decisions about the dying process.

- Do-not-resuscitate orders are not usually acceptable; suggesting such orders may decrease trust between the family and health care providers.

- Males generally make funeral plans; women of the family care for the hospitalized ill person during the dying process and after death; children are expected to be at the bedside to provide support for the older person during the dying process; after death, rituals involve washing the body and all its orifices.

- Severely ill person may die in the hospital because of belief that Western medicine may delay death.

- Religious leaders (minister if Christian or Iman if Moslem) may be called after the death to help the family grieve.

Principle of Justice

- Generally do not believe in organ donation because of the need to respect the body and for body to be whole to meet the creator with integrity.

Adapted from "Arab Americans," by A. I. Meleis, 1996, in J. G. Lipson, S. L. Dibble, and P. A. Minarik (Eds.), Culture and Nursing Care: A Pocket Guide *(pp. 23–36), San Francisco, CA: UCSF Nursing Press. Used with permission.*

---

of the Code should occur as the nurse cares for older people of different cultures than the European-American culture to deliver culturally sensitive care. See Boxes 25-3 through 25-7 for examples.

Autonomy

The principle of autonomy conveys respect for a person's ability to govern self or to freely choose one's actions as long as these choices do not interfere with the autonomy or rights of other persons. This principle has been called self-governance or self-determinism. Ethical issues evolving from this principle frequently involve **informed consent** for or refusal of medical or research treatment. In the Western world, autonomy is often pri-

oritized above other ethical principles and considered supreme. However, in many Asian cultures, the family's or group's well-being is often prioritized above an individual's choice for well-being. According to one author, autonomy represents social, cultural, and historical influences; actions are not truly autonomous but represent a person's response to the social and cultural morality to which that person belongs (Castellucci, 1998).

An autonomous person freely acts after rationally and intentionally considering possible choices of action and then implementing the most appropriate action. During this process, no physical or psychological pressures are placed on the person, thus allowing that person to act autonomously. Autonomous individuals are physically and cognitively able to make sufficient decisions and to be

BOX 25-4   Cultural Values Related to Selected Ethical Principles—Vietnamese

Principle of Autonomy

- Oldest son is family spokesperson when family member is seriously ill; this person is privately consulted before telling the ill person about diagnosis; spokesperson and family may not want ill person to know information to decrease personal stress (lack of disclosure).

- Interpreter used for informed consent may be a family member; need to consider the gender of the interpreter when translating/involved in discussion of sensitive topics.

- Head nodding of ill person during informed consent may indicate knowledge has been heard but may not support information is understood.

Principle of Nonmalificence/Dying Rituals

- Males are generally the decision makers during times of crisis.

- Nursing facility or institutionalization of older person or ill person is considered disrespectful; older persons deeply respected in family and have valued social roles as caregivers of family.

- Preference is for dying person to be at home with close family and religious objects (medallions, spiritual objects) close by; family may pray during dying process, and Buddhist families may burn incense and conduct religious rituals throughout this process.

- Family may become uncontrollable with death of loved one and need extra time with loved one to increase their coping with the event; often family washes body based upon beliefs about body respect; spiritual rites take place in the room after death.

Principle of Justice

- Body highly respected and organ donation not generally accepted unless family well acculturated to America.

Adapted from "Vietnamese," by S. Ferrales, 1996, in J. G. Lipson, S. L. Dibble, and P. A. Minarik (Eds.), Culture and Nursing Care: A Pocket Guide *(pp. 280–290), San Francisco, CA: UCSF Nursing Press. Used with permission.*

BOX 25-5   Cultural Values Related to Selected Ethical Principles—Hispanic Americans

Principle of Autonomy

- Informed consent desired and ill person may ask health care provider's recommendation; it is important to assess the literacy level and understanding of migratory populations that may need health care while working in the United States.

- Use same-sex interpreter for informed consent; use person's language of choice for greater understanding of informed consent.

- Sensitive health care topics generally kept within family, and family may want to deny information to seriously ill family member based on belief of a strong body-mind connection and that worry will worsen ill person's health.

- Oldest son or daughter may serve as family spokesperson for ill family member, particularly for a highly respected older member of the family.

Principle of Nonmalificence/Dying Rituals

- Males are expected to be strong and provide for family during crisis of death.

- Extended family expected to be present and helpful during the dying process; dying in the hospital may be avoided because of concern that the ill person's spirit will have difficulty finding its way home; hospital environment may also be avoided because of belief that hospital personnel restrict family's involvement in dying process of family member.

- Death is a spiritual event involving much family prayer; relative may help with care of the body after death; religious medals/rosary beads expected to be near client; wailing a common response to show respect for deceased person.

Principle of Justice

- Organ donation not generally considered because of need to respect body and to be intact for burial.

Adapted from "Mexican Americans," by T. de Paula, K. Laganá, and L. Gonzalez-Ramirez, 1996, in J. G. Lipson, S. L. Dibble, and P. A. Minarik (Eds.), Culture and Nursing: A Pocket Guide *(pp. 203–221), San Francisco, CA: UCSF Nursing Press. Used with permission.*

BOX 25-6   Cultural Values Related to Selected Ethical Principles—American Indians

Principle of Autonomy

- Use a mature, same-gender interpreter for informed consent, addressing facts and not probabilities.

- Involve older person and family as desired by ill person; there may be some reluctance to sign consent form because of history of political and personal document misuse.

- Informed consent is a formal process of interpreting information and must emphasize personal autonomy of older persons, which is highly valued in this culture.

Principle of Nonmalificence/Dying Rituals

- Some tribes prefer not to discuss do-not-resuscitate codes because this may increase the rate of inevitable loss.

- Family meetings may be held to discuss prognosis and plans for treatment of ill family member and to make informed decisions.

- Men responsible for funeral plans of deceased, and women responsible for care of ill person in and out of hospital.

- Some tribes (Apache, Alaskan Native) avoid contact with/visiting the dying; relationship names (that is, sister) rather than deceased person's name may be used in conversation; individual mourning may occur away from dying person.

- Some tribes embrace intimate and extended family visiting rituals during the dying process of a loved one; positive attitude seen with some tribes during dying process while others openly emotionally grieve with death of a relative.

- Home care of older person generally the norm to allow person to maintain valued social roles of teacher, counselor, and grandparent.

Principle of Justice

- Generally do not support organ donation because of respect for the human body.

Adapted from "American Indians," by J. Kramer, 1996, In J. G. Lipson, S. L. Dibble, and P. A. Minarik (Eds.), Culture and Nursing Care: A Pocket Guide *(pp. 11–22), San Francisco, CA: UCSF Nursing Press. Used with permission.*

responsible for their decisions and actions. Based on these definitions of autonomy, an ill person may not be able to act autonomously during temporary times of pain or when medications have influenced one's ability to rationally consider choices of action. Likewise, older people may lack autonomy because of being judged as legally incapacitated or unable to make decisions with full knowledge of the consequences of those choices (Fellows, 1998). Most likely, all people have limited competency or intermittent competency in certain areas of their lives because of lack of knowledge or experience. In those situations, individuals cannot autonomously act because of those limitations (Beauchamp & Childress, 1994).

A major ethical issue arises in the case of older adults who have been diagnosed with dementia of some type such as Alzheimer's disease. It is often difficult to determine exactly when they lose the cognitive capacity to make independent, autonomous decisions or even if the diagnosis is correct. For example, in the early stages of Alzheimer's disease, some autonomous decisions can be made by clients with the help of a person who has the ability to communicate effectively with them. Also, the type and consequences of the decision to be made may be an important factor in the situation.

There may be internal and external constraints on an older person's autonomy. Internal constraints such as

physical or mental illness decrease an older person's ability to freely choose life decisions. According to one author, physical illness may cause loss of executional autonomy in which an individual may be able to make a decision but is unable physically to implement that decision. Decisional autonomy is also diminished when older people are cognitively impaired, thus creating the need for a moral surrogate to make the best choices for those individuals (Collopy, 1991). External constraints may arise when older persons change their living conditions, causing a loss of traditional support systems and an addition of new rules in the new environment. In order to prevent loss of autonomy of these individuals, the new environment must encourage individual choice by organizational changes that support a quality of life as defined by the older individual (Castellucci, 1998; Tolley, 1997). In one research study, when older people had a clear perspective on life goals and worked with health care providers to safely meet needs for independence, they did not perceive decreased autonomy, stress, or feelings of powerlessness, factors affecting perceived quality of life (McWilliam, Brown, Carmichael, & Lehman, 1994).

Inherent in the principle of autonomy is the concept of informed consent, a process of providing sufficient information to a competent person or research subject that

BOX 25-7   A Summary of European-American Cultural Values Related to Ethical Principles

Principle of Autonomy

- Informed consent is valued; same-gender interpreter recommended, especially for sensitive topics.

- Informed consent is desired from each individual involved in health care intervention or research study; age, maturity level, and physical and cognitive ability determine conditions under which individual informed consent honored; generally, one must be at least age 16 years to be legally allowed to give independent consent for medical procedures.

- A reasonable person standard is used to identify the amount of information disclosed in situations related to informed consent.

- In certain situations, paternalism is justified.

- Ethical principles of veracity, confidentiality, and privacy are honored as part of informed consent; in some situations, intentional deception or intentional nondisclosure is acceptable.

- Directives to physician support increasing numbers of people freely choosing end-of-life decisions.

Principle of Nonmalificence/Dying Rituals

- Accepted as the basis of social morality and reflected in laws that do not support killing of another (active euthanasia).

- Religious and health care policies influence acceptance of passive euthanasia.

- With high technology prolonging life, more persons are considering passive euthanasia and physician-assisted suicide to allow terminally ill persons a comfortable death; this process of dying may also be eased by palliative and hospice care processes, which for some is a more ethical approach to the dying process of a loved one.

- Do-not-resuscitate orders are completed while the client is able to give informed consent; these orders are frequently honored in the dying process of the client receiving hospice or nursing facility services.

- Family members are involved with funeral process and rely on prayer, religious faith, and spiritual beliefs to support the grieving process.

Principle of Justice

- Health care resources are focused toward those who have ability to pay; there is social belief among many that health care is a right and society needs to care for those who cannot afford to pay for care.

- Organ transplants are accepted by most persons if religious beliefs support this practice.

---

enables that person to freely choose to participate in a medical (treatment) or research intervention. Overall, informed consent demonstrates that information has been conveyed to the person involved in the research or medical intervention to meet that person's needs. Informed consent shows respect for persons by supporting autonomous choice, decreasing their anxiety about an intervention, encouraging health care providers and researchers to act responsibly, and increasing the willingness of the person to collaborate with health care providers based on a trusting relationship between the recipient of care and health care provider. Generally, a safeguards in human research committee must approve research involving human subjects to ensure protection of participant rights during the research. This type of approval has been intended to protect the **confidentiality** of the research participant and to prevent manipulation or coercion of the participant by the research team. See the sample informed consent form in Box 25-8.

Although similar elements of informed consent exist for both medical and research interventions, only the former will be discussed in this chapter. There are five

elements that must be present for informed consent for medical intervention to exist. The physician normally provides the first element—complete disclosure of known information about the person's health and any planned medical interventions to meet the health concern. Generally a *reasonable person* standard is used to identify the amount of information disclosed to an individual (what would a usual person need to know/understand to make a decision?). However, some ethicists argue that intentional nondisclosure might be justified (morally acceptable) in certain situations. These might include if the health care provider believes that the person might be harmed by knowing the information, telling would fail to protect the client's confidentiality or affect the outcome of the treatment, or telling would be burdensome to the person who might be severely ill or dying (Beauchamp & Childress, 1994). A health care provider who believes strongly in autonomous decision making may also face an ethical dilemma if an individual or individual's family expresses a wish to not know about a health diagnosis and relevant treatment. Forcing a person to receive information would be coercive and could negatively affect the

Research Focus

Citation:

Hui, E., Ho, S. C., Tsang, J., Lee, S. H., & Woo, J. (1997). Attitudes toward life-sustaining treatment of older persons in Hong Kong. *Journal of the American Geriatrics Society, 45*(10), 1232–1236.

Purpose:

To examine the attitudes of older Asians in Hong Kong on life-sustaining therapy such as cardiopulmonary resuscitation (CPR) and life support.

Methods:

A variety of instruments measuring sociodemographic, functional ability, perceived health, knowledge of life-sustaining procedures, and participant preferences for such procedures were used to examine the attitudes of older Asians. Qualitative measures to assess reasons to want or refuse CPR and a designated person to decide whether an older person should receive life-sustaining treatment also were completed by old-age home residents and geriatric ward clients.

Findings:

Approximately 80% of old-age home residents and 60% of clients in the hospital lacked knowledge about life-sustaining therapy. The CPR success rates were overrated by older clients, and most wanted to receive CPR, although 20% of these persons refused CPR once educated about its success rate. A variety of variables influenced clients' preferences for and refusal of CPR and life support, and a considerable number desired to be involved in the decision-making process related to life-sustaining treatment.

Implications:

Health care providers need to consider cultural differences in knowledge about and preferences for CPR and life-sustaining treatment among older persons. As desired, these people should participate in informed consent to honor the ethical principle of autonomy and to provide them control over decisions related to their quality of life.

Think About It

Is lying ever justified?

Mrs. Chu, a 75-year-old Chinese woman, was hospitalized recently for severe abdominal pain of several years duration. Based upon exploratory surgery, the physician discovers Mrs. Chu has a large and apparent metastatic cancerous tumor on her large intestine and liver. The physician talks to Mrs. Chu's children about the need for radiation and possible chemotherapy for their mother because of the surgical findings. The family, of Asian origin and values, believes it best not to tell their mother of the surgical findings and refuse the radiation and chemotherapy treatments. They request to take their mother home as soon as possible to spend her last remaining days with her family.

1. What ethical role does the health care team have in meeting this client and her family's needs?
2. What ethical principles are involved in this case; how would you prioritize the principles for a nurse's ethical practice?
3. Is the act of lying, as detailed above, morally justified?

Another form of incomplete disclosure occurs with intentional deception or providing untrue information to a person undergoing treatment. Intentional deception occurs in the use of **placebos** (interventions intended for psychological relief rather than an actual disorder). Although it seems ethically questionable to deny a person information used in making an informed decision, research has shown that placebos are quite effective in treating the same health problems (e.g., pain) perhaps related to the psychological belief that the real intervention has been given and will work.

The final four elements of informed consent include the voluntary action of the individual to participate, understanding of information by the individual, personal competency to consent to or refuse the treatment, and consent of the person to participate in the treatment. No coercive (real or imagined) influences should be directed toward the individual to meet the voluntary criterion. Any coercive action from the health care provider negates the autonomy of the person considering participation in a treatment. To meet the understanding criterion, there must be enough information to make a decision with adequate knowledge of any consequences. The person must also be deemed to have the mental/analytical ability to understand and then to choose a behavior with full knowledge of the consequences of that choice (to participate or not in the treatment). The last element of informed consent involves the individual agreeing to contribute to the treatment by signing an informed consent form. This form explains the proposed treatment, risks and benefits, alternatives to the treatment, and recommendations for care.

health care provider–person/family relationship. In situations where life is at risk, a physician may also exert therapeutic privilege and deliver an intervention without a person's receipt of information to save that person's life or to prevent client harm. For example, if an older individual is suicidal, a physician may not disclose information if it is believed that the client may cause harm to self if the information is known.

BOX 25-8 Example of Informed Consent as Participant in a Research Study

Title: Perception of Quality of Health Care by Medicare Recipients with Chronic Illness
Principal Investigator: Diane Sawyer, PhD, RN
Tel: 000-000-0123

I have been asked to take part in a research study conducted by Diane Sawyer, PhD, RN as part of her postdoctoral fellowship studies.

This research has been explained to me. I know that I will be one of about 50 Medicare recipients in this study. I am being asked to take part in the study because of my status as a Medicare recipient and because I have a chronic illness. This illness makes it necessary for me to have frequent medical care. I know the purpose of this study is to explore my thoughts and feelings about the quality of health care that I receive for my illness and about Medicare coverage for this illness.

I know being in the study will last about one hour. This time will be used to complete a private audio-taped talk between me and Dr. Sawyer. The exact time of the talk will depend on how much I want to talk about my perceptions of my health care and my Medicare insurance. I know that only Dr. Sawyer and the person writing the words from my talk onto a computer file will hear my tape. I know that Dr. Sawyer may need to contact me by phone or letter if she needs my help to complete the study. If I do not want her to contact me for this reason, I have signed my name here _____ .

I know that this study might make me uneasy by having me share personal parts of my life with someone else. In the event I become upset, Dr. Sawyer will help me find support services to assist me. I understand that Dr. Sawyer's job in this study will be to collect information from me and not to serve as a counselor to me. I know that the benefits of being in the study may include being able to share my feelings about my chronic illness and my Medicare coverage in a private talk. My sharing may also provide information that can be used in programs to help other older people like me.

I know that every effort will be made to protect my identity in the study. I know that my name will not be used in any report or its results. I know that my being in the study will not result in any money costs to me, but that I will receive a gift once I have completed my talk.

I have freely chosen to be part of this study. However, I may refuse to start or to be in this study if I choose. If I decide to do either of these things, I will not lose benefits I have been promised. My refusal to be part of the study will not affect my present or future health care. I know that Dr. Sawyer has the right to stop my being in the study at any time if the needs of the study change.

I have had a chance to ask, and have had answered, all my questions about this research. If I have any questions or a research-related injury occurs, I will call Dr. Sawyer at 000-000-0123. If I have questions Dr. Sawyer cannot answer or I believe my rights in this research have been violated, I can contact the chair of the Research in Human Rights Committee at 000-123-0000 (Dr. Sawyer's place of employment).

I have read the information provided above. I freely choose to be part of this study. After it is signed, I understand that I will receive a copy of this consent form.

_____   _____
Signature of participant   Date

_____   _____
Signature of person obtaining consent   Date

The nurse should be particularly concerned about providing informed consent to older people needing medical interventions. Although the physician is legally responsible to explain any proposed medical or surgical treatment, the nurse often becomes responsible for re-emphasizing and clarifying the information initially provided and in gaining the person's signature on the informed consent form. Sufficient time should be spent with the older client and family to ensure understanding of the proposed treatment, alternatives to participation, risks and benefits, and in the case of illness, the relationship of the illness, prognosis, and planned intervention.

As part of the informed consent process, the nurse needs to encourage the older individual's questions and collaborate with that person/family in making an autonomous decision. Factors such as illness, information overload, cultural values, language, and anxiety of the person may provide barriers to full understanding, and informed consent cannot be obtained until these factors are considered. By evaluating these barriers to full understanding, the nurse facilitates the older person's continued introspection about the meaning of life in the later years. The older individual has developed the need, ability, and desire based on life experiences to act autonomously in later years to meet a sense of fulfillment in life (Castellucci, 1998). This goal of fulfillment directs an older individual's expectations and desired choices for health care, and when the health care provider meets

> ### *Nursing Tip*
>
> Keep these questions in mind when involved with informed consent:
>
> Has the nurse provided the essential components of informed consent and met the older person's right to autonomy?
>
> *Does the person have the cognitive capacity needed to understand the request?*
>
> - Does the person possess the mental and analytical ability to understand and to decide all the options presented for care?
> - Does the person understand the plan of care, give authorization for the care, and foresee the potential results of a choice for care?
>
> *Has the person been given complete disclosure of the proposed care?*
>
> - Has the person received enough information to meet the *usual person* standard—both the quality and quantity of information that a usual person would need and want to know to make a choice for care?
> - Does the use of intentional nondisclosure or therapeutic privilege seem ethically justified in denying full disclosure to the person to allow a choice to be made?
>
> *Has the person voluntarily agreed to the plan of care?*
>
> - Has there been physical or mental coercion perceived by the person that has led to that person's agreement to a plan of care?
> - Have there been threats, lies, or emotional appeals perceived by the person that oppose that person's autonomy to freely choose?
>
> *Has the person given consent?*
>
> - Has the person made a decision in favor of the plan of care?
> - Has the person authorized a personal willingness to contribute to the plan of care?
>
> *Has the person complete understanding of the proposed plan of care?*
>
> - Has the person received sufficient quality and quantity of information to make a choice?
> - Has the person received sufficient quality and quantity of information to make a choice with full knowledge of the consequences?

these expectations, the older individual perceives autonomy and a sense of well-being. Other researchers have found that older people who were given more choices in health care outcomes felt less socially isolated and had more energy than did those not given such choices (Brandreit, Lyons, & Bentley, 1994) and had less depression after a stroke (Castellucci, 1996).

Ethical Duties

Many ethicists believe the ethical duties of **veracity,** confidentiality, and **privacy** derive from the principle of autonomy. Ethical duties are those nursing behaviors based on a nurse's knowledge of ethical principles that may or may not be supported by law. The nurse demonstrates these behaviors in meeting a definition of ethical practice. According to Beauchamp and Childress (1994), an ethical duty is established when a physician or nurse and client, institution, or other health care provider initiate a relationship. This duty has been called fidelity, the duty to keep a promise and honor commitments and contracts. According to this duty, a nurse fails in her ethical duty to hospitalized clients if that health care provider engages in a collective bargaining dispute and, thereby, abandons those clients who need her care.

The ethical duty of veracity defines the duty to be truthful in client interactions. This duty, also part of the medical Hippocratic Code, shows respect for a client's autonomy and fidelity and helps build a relationship of trust between the health care provider and the person receiving health care (Beauchamp & Childress, 1994). This trust relationship may be harmed if benevolent deception occurs. The health care provider may decide not to tell a client the whole truth or may misconstrue the truth because the provider believes the client will be harmed by knowing the real truth. Many discussions have occurred over whether benevolent deception is ever ethically justified, and nurses must fully consider the entire situation to determine the answer. Other factors relevant to withholding the truth involve the idea that no one probably ever knows the full truth and the fact that different cultures support *editing* of the truth in some situations. Perhaps one way of dealing with these factors is to have the health care provider ask the individual/family at the onset of a person's illness and early in the hospitalization course the extent of information desired and the preferred transmission of information, particularly in situations of terminal illness.

A third ethical duty, confidentiality, implies that the health care professional keeps client or relevant other information safe from the knowledge of others. This information may not be communicated to others without the client's consent. This duty supports that one has a right to protect oneself by decreasing access of personal information by others. The **Human Genome Project,** a federally funded project focusing on the mapping of genetic structures that could potentially predict disease, will have significant impact on the ethical duty of confidentiality. Could information on individuals at risk for cancer because of their genetic history be denied health insurance if information available from the Genome Project was shared with employers who might then use it to decrease employee health care costs?

A final duty, that of privacy, also is derived from the principle of autonomy. This duty obligates the ethically acting health care provider to control information about self and others. With massive computer networks that contain personal information, some of which may be highly sensitive, the potential of a health care provider failing to honor the duty of privacy exists at the pressing of a computer key or the click of a computer mouse.

Beneficence

The ethical principle of beneficence defines *doing good* or participating in behavior that benefits a recipient of care. This principle is the foundation for many professional codes of ethical practice, and for many, this principle overrides the ethical principle of autonomy. For example, in the earlier situation in which the physician chose not to disclose information to a suicidal person, the principle of beneficence assumed prominence over the person's right to know to self-govern. In an ethical dilemma, one must weigh the *good* and the *bad* of each considered action and then render a decision based on which action would be the most beneficial to the person/family and, thus, meet nursing goals for high-quality care of that person and family.

Much of the discussion evolving from beneficence centers on the concept of **paternalism.** One author has noted that paternalism results when the ethical principles of beneficence and autonomy conflict (Breeze, 1998). Paternalism involves having another more powerful or knowledgeable person make health care decisions on a less powerful or less knowledgeable person's behalf. For example, paternalistic acts may occur when an older individual delegates decisions to a personal physician because that provider "knows what is best for me." In many health care situations, a health care provider may have an ethical conflict between a duty to benefit a recipient of care by supporting paternalism and a duty to respect that recipient's right to autonomy. Paternalism may be justified (morally acceptable) if the harm prevented exceeds the loss of the person's autonomy or if a person's condition severely limits the ability to act autonomously, such as after a stroke. Much like therapeutic privilege, paternalism may be justified in emergency situations until a person is capable of making free choices about health care decisions.

Nonmalificence

The ethical principle of nonmalificence involves *above all, do no harm* and includes not killing or intentionally or through lack of understanding causing pain or suffering to another person (Beauchamp & Childress, 1994). This principle is the basis of social morality and has been reflected in laws that exert punishment for those who kill or harm other people. Overall, the principle acknowledges the importance of each person's life and the need to honor the human dignity and choices of each person.

Ethical issues related to maintenance of life revolve around both the principles of beneficence and nonmalifi-

Research Focus

Citation:
Robertson, D. W. (1996). Ethical theory, ethnography, and differences between doctors and nurses in approaches to patient care. *Journal of Medical Ethics, 22*(5), 292–299.

Purpose:
To delineate in a research study focused on practice the ethical theory that British physicians and nurses use in older client care in a psychiatric facility.

Methods:
Ethnography involving participant (physician and nurse) observation and interviews, both of which were used to identify themes of ethical approaches to care.

Findings:
Physicians and nurses tended to differ in their prioritization of the ethical principles of autonomy and beneficence. Although both groups valued a utilitarian ethical theory approach to care, nurses placed greater reliance in their practice than did doctors on maintaining interpersonal relationships and preservation of client autonomy. Physicians prioritized the principle of beneficence if autonomy conflicted with the former.

Implications:
Health care providers, to provide quality care to older people with psychiatric illness, need to communicate clearly with one another about their values of care and their beliefs about ethical professional practice. Based on an understanding of these foundational beliefs, providers of care can collaborate to improve their own work environments and the environments of care for older people.

cence. Many ethical dilemmas directly involve these principles and require a critical thinking process to reach an ethical resolution for all participants in an ethical dilemma situation. For example, in the giving of a pain medication to a dying individual in pain, the nurse may unintentionally contribute to a slower respiratory rate of the person, thus causing that person's death. The beneficent act was to comfort the client, but in the process of alleviating pain, the nurse contributed to the client's death, an act considered by some to be malicious. To overrule nonmalificence, Beauchamp and Childress (1994) noted four conditions must exist in the *rule of double effect* often found in situations involving nomalificence: the action alone must be morally good or indifferent; the person acting must intend only the good outcome; the bad effect cannot be the means to the good outcome; and there must be a balance between the good and bad outcomes of the action (the most important condition).

Discussions of active and passive euthanasia involve the principle of nonmalificence. Active euthanasia, actively *committing* a killing act of an ill person by another, is not morally acceptable in most societies. However, passive euthanasia, letting a person die by *omitting* treatment to maintain life and letting the disease or injury cause the death, is practiced in this country and other societies. Beauchamp and Childress noted that in cases of requested euthanasia, one must consider the actor's (person committing the act) motive, the individual's request, and consequences of the act to justify the euthanasia act. For those who support euthanasia in some form, any medical treatment prevents a natural death, a passing that many consider as part of the continuum of life and one that should be handled with dignity and respect.

Some ethicists note there are sufficient moral reasons to justify **mercy killing** or **euthanasia** in some cases, but these reasons are not sufficient to support changes to professional codes of practice or implementation of legislation that would support euthanasia. Concerns about implementing euthanasia, even in some instances of severe illness, have been expressed by many people who believe a society that allows killing of persons who meet certain criteria might initiate killing of others who fail to meet those criteria (the **slippery slope** or wedge argument). This argument seems to be stronger when one considers the reality of scarce health care resources in the current health care delivery system. For example, would persons needing high-cost care or difficult-to-access services to maintain life be coerced into finalizing their lives much like those individuals who state they wish to die because of intolerable pain? Or, if a society accepts passive euthanasia, would this lead to euthanasia of persons who are not able to make an informed choice to die (mentally ill or challenged individuals) or persons who have cognitive capacity but do not wish to die (persons with views different from the caregivers)?

With significant medical technology maintaining life functions of severely ill people, health care providers are increasingly faced with ethical dilemmas when these people have expressed a wish to die to end their pain. Health care providers may be faced with the following dilemmas: Is it a beneficent act to maintain someone's life when that individual has expressed a wish to die? Is maintaining that life coercive and does it negate that person's autonomy to choose the quality of life? Is maintaining a person's life when it increases that individual's pain a malicious act? If a person is judged to have cognitive capacity, should that person have the right to die or to engage a health care practitioner to assist in that

dying process? Why cannot an individual choose to die much like choices made earlier in life related to contraceptive practices, marriage, and lifestyle choices? If a person has the cognitive capacity and the right to decide to participate in treatment, why should that person not also have the right to decide about conditions for continued existence? These questions are difficult to answer for ill and dying individuals, their families, and health care providers. A comprehensive assessment, open communication process, and an ethical decision-making approach involving all relevant participants can help define an acceptable resolution for participants. In many health care agencies, interdisciplinary ethical review boards assist participants in this process by offering an interdisciplinary and global view that has been structured along an ethical decision-making model. Overall, these boards explore all options to meet the ethical principles of beneficence and nonmalificence as well as the principle of autonomy to support personal and family choices with end-of-life decisions.

Although 37 states have passed legislation opposing physician-assisted suicide and 3 additional states (California, Hawaii, and Maryland) are currently debating this issue, support for physician-assisted suicide for terminally ill people continues in this country (American Health Consultants, 1999b). Of the Americans polled, 69% favor physician-assisted suicide, and even more people oppose federal laws that would prevent such suicide (American Health Consultants, 1999a). Increasing popular press coverage of terminally ill people depicting their powerful stories of choices for a self-directive death also has affected American views on this topic (Barcott, 1999; Branegan, 1997).

Several countries (Australia, the Netherlands) and at least one state (Oregon) in this country have laws that support ill individual and health care provider interdependence to support a person's request to be allowed to die. In the Netherlands, legal guidelines exist for voluntary euthanasia in which a physician helps a client who has requested help in facilitating the dying process (Branegan, 1997). In Australia, physician-assisted suicide is legal. The physician helps a person requesting death to achieve a comfortable death, although the individual has the final say about the timing of the lethal medication that causes death (Muller, Kimsma, & van der Wal, 1998). There are strict criteria in most countries for the client to meet to justify consideration of an ill person's request for dying. These include the person having less than 6 months to live; the person having the cognitive capacity to make the dying decision; a confirmation by a second physician that the requesting person has only 6 months to live and is cognitively alert; perception that the person is experiencing unacceptable pain; consistent requests for assistance with dying; nonacceptance of alternatives to the dying choice; and a long-term relationship with a primary provider who will assist with the dying process (Branegan, 1997). Several researchers have found that fewer severely ill people request help in ending their lives if they can maintain their bodily functions and remain autonomous in their life decisions (Chin, Hedberg, Higginson, & Fleming, 1999) or if they can receive prompt treatment for pain or symptoms of distress (Valente & Trainor, 1998). Other researchers have found fear of pain and finances do not appear to be significant factors in choice of physician-assisted suicide (Chin et al., 1999). The ANA Code for Nurses prohibits intentional ending of another's life, but there are examples in the media that support medical personnel practicing at least passive euthanasia.

Also relevant to nonmalificence are those discussions on withholding and withdrawing care from severely ill or dying people. Ethicists vary on whether either action is morally justified. Bishop and Scudder (1990) noted that the client-nurse relationship, based on a caring attitude of the nurse, promotes the person's well-being; withholding or withdrawing care would be perceived as opposing the ethical principle of nonmalificence and, thus, would be unethical professional behavior. If one believes that the nurse-client relationship commences with health care of the person, then withdrawing of care despite a person's positive response to treatment negates the contract established between client and nurse, a salient part of the Code for Nurses (ANA, 1985). Others might argue that in cases where the severely ill person is not expected to improve quality of life or is irreversibly dying, withholding care might be most appropriate. On the other hand, initiating treatment may improve the quality of life of this individual and, if treatment was initially withheld, the health care professional would never know the positive effect of treatment. Overall, in reaching decisions on these situations, health care providers must work with a cognitively alert client and family to evaluate the burdens versus the benefits of various actions and act on solutions that seem to benefit the individual and family. For example, a nurse may assist a severely ill or dying individual to refuse personal nutrition and hydration to hasten the dying process, particularly if this person has validated this request in a living will (ANA, 1992b). It would be morally justified in this instance for the nurse to respect the person's request for a dignified death by providing comfort measures, privacy, and palliative care (care that supports the dying process) (ANA, 1985, 1991).

Futility of treatment also relates to the principle of nonmalificence. Futility, the idea that regardless of intervention, the person's life will not improve, involves considering personal, religious, economic, and medical meanings of continuing the life of a person. A physician and recipient of care may define a treatment or regimen of care as futile if it is not medically effective in stabilizing

Research Focus

Citation:
Sullivan, M., Ormel, J., Kempen, G. I., & Tymstra, T. (1998). Beliefs concerning death, dying, and hastening death among older, functionally impaired Dutch adults: A one-year longitudinal study. *Journal of the American Geriatrics Society, 46*(10), 1251–1257.

Purpose:
To define older functionally impaired Dutch individuals' views on death, dying, and hastened death (euthanasia and assisted suicide) and to relate these views to sociocultural and health status factors.

Methods:
Six hundred thirty-two community-dwelling older persons in 1994 and 575 of the same group in 1995 completed interviews and questionnaires. Independent variables related to sociocultural factors such as age, sex, income, education, strength of religious belief, religious affiliation, and physical and mental health status. Outcome variables included preoccupation with and fear of death, fears of the dying process, and attitudes toward hastened death.

Findings:
Low and stable rates of preoccupation with death and fear of death over the year assessment period of time were found; even those with decreased functional impairment or increased anxiety and depression over the time assessed showed no significant change. Fears of death and dying related most closely with health status and most directly to mental health status. Beliefs about euthanasia and assisted suicide related most closely to religious affiliation and beliefs.

Implications:
A complete assessment of an older person's life including mental status and religious beliefs is important in helping both health care providers and older people collaborate in decisions affecting the person's health care during the final years of life.

or improving a client's already compromised health. It is important to understand who has defined the treatment as futile to prevent problems in the client/family/health care provider relationship. If the physician believes the treatment is futile but the ill person and/or family disagrees, this could provoke distrust by the involved person/family of the physician and a negatively affected physician-client relationship (Low & Kaufman, 1999). It is important to acknowledge that language barriers to full understanding of a futile diagnosis may influence acceptance of a diagnosis by a person and family. Also, ethnic and sociocultural differences between provider of care and recipient of care may prevent full understanding of the treatment or lack of treatment by the involved individual and family. Religious orientation or belief that the right and loving thing to do for a severely ill person is to continue treatment until God or a spiritual being makes the decision to end that life must also be considered by the health care team in considering treatment options when the situation seems futile. Open communication between all participants in the situation about choices to be made if no options exist to improve an ill person's health status also assists participants in structuring a plan to meet the involved person and family's needs when the person is irreversibly dying. This plan may have been specified in the client's advance directive and/or living will and, therefore, will provide legal support for a similar plan implemented in an acute care facility.

In cases where treatment has been determined as futile for an ill person, nurses and other members of the health care team must assist the person and his or her support system with a comfortable process toward death. Such care has been defined as a palliative approach to the dying process. According to the ANA Position Statement on Promotion of Comfort and Relief of Pain of Dying Patients (ANA, 1991), the ethical behavior of nurses includes medicating clients to manage their pain and control their symptoms even though this action may hasten the death of the client. Nurses, who have the most frequent contact with clients, have a primary obligation to comfort them by decreasing sleeplessness, depression, and loss of morale in persons who are dying (Melzack, 1990). Nurses also have an obligation to educate the family about the dying process and to provide support with that process. By understanding the client's/family's culture, personality, coping style, spiritual, emotional, and physical needs, the nurse can meet a professional goal of alleviating suffering and serving as a moral agent for the client and family in the dying process of a loved one.

A final ethical issue relevant to the principle of nonmalificence involves confusing or conflicting do-not-resuscitate (DNR) orders of ill clients under a nurse's care. To decrease this confusion and conflict, all hospitalized are asked if they have a document on file that specifies their wishes for resuscitation in a format congruent with agency policy. Validation of individual choice on DNR orders also decreases recent concern that the technique may have been overused in clients who might have desired to die because of their low quality of life (Lo, 1991). Much like conversations relevant to futility of treatment, health care providers and client and family need to prioritize discussions about DNR orders early in the hospitalization course and educate the client and family about DNR and treatment decisions throughout the care cycle

(ANA, 1992a). Ideally, DNR decisions should be made before hospital admission in a directive to physician. If not, these discussions should occur early in the hospital course if the client does not have a directive to physician that would describe personal preferences for resuscitation. Because a person's condition may change during hospitalization, a DNR order should be reviewed and updated periodically to meet the individual's and family's needs and to honor their decisions on this matter (ANA, 1992a).

To summarize the principle of nonmalificence, a distinction might be drawn between extraordinary (optional) and ordinary (obligatory) care of hospitalized persons by health care providers. Care that is extraordinary or optional usually is costly and unusual, creates little good (is futile), and involves more burdens than benefits in the process and outcome of care. Even if optional care was delivered, the outcome might be severe pain or minimal existence for the recipient of care. In this case, it might be morally unacceptable to treat the person with those predicted outcomes. For example, long-term use of an expensive high-frequency ventilator for one with a severe and continuing intracranial bleed might be defined as optional treatment. An important point is that recipients of care must define their meaning of quality of life, not observers who have lacked the lived experience of the ill person contemplating the burdens or benefits of a treatment. Ordinary or obligatory care, on the other hand, is morally required and offers a reasonable chance of benefit to the person, is inexpensive, does not cause excess pain or suffering if given to the person, and is often simple, noninvasive, or routine (Beauchamp & Childress, 1994). For example, urinary catherization to treat urinary retention would be defined as an obligatory treatment.

Principle of Justice

The principle of justice supports fair allocation of resources to individuals or the provision of an equal share of available resources to each person. Justice involves giving resources to an individual that are due to that person. Ethical issues that arise from this principle involve distribution of health care resources at local and national levels, concepts known as microallocation and macroallocation. Consistent with this principle are discussions on whether health care is a right for all persons, a value belief accepted by several countries (e.g., Germany, Great Britain, Canada) that have implemented national insurance programs as part of their public health policy.

According to Beauchamp and Childress (1994), justice can be examined according to various perspectives. In the **libertarian** approach, health care resources are distributed through actions of a free marketplace; this makes health resources more available to those who have money to pay for health care services or those who arrive first to access those resources. An **equalitarian** approach focuses on equally distributing health care resources essential to life to all people. This approach also favors providing more resources to those who initially were disadvantaged—these consumers of health care may actually get more health care resources to make up for their initial disadvantaged position relevant to other groups. Medicare is an equalitarian approach with its provision of basic coverage for all those meeting criteria for that governmental program. A third approach, that of utilitarianism, favors equal distribution of resources to most people for the most good (a pubic health approach and one supported by most nurses). An ethical issue evolving from the latter approach is how to meet individual rights (and prioritize the principle of autonomy) with a focus on the majority. Other questions arising from all three approaches involve:

- To each person an equal share but on what basis and on what scheme to distribute

- How to distribute resources equitably with the constraints of today's scarce health care resources

- How to deal with the health needs of a large proportion of the American population that cannot afford health insurance

- How to equitably spread health care resources to everyone within the constraints of managed care that was instituted to save health care costs

The high rate of persons insured under managed care programs has influenced both the quality and quantity of health care delivered to clients. In some geographical sectors, older people have found health care programs no longer willing to cover their health care costs because of more frequent and more expensive health care needs of this population. This has meant that these people have had to reestablish a physician-client relationship and to become familiar with a different health care plan that may not meet their health care needs. Additionally, increasing premiums for health care coverage in the future may affect many older people's ability to access and participate in programs intended to maximize their health, an example of limited support for the ethical principle of justice.

Decisions about choosing which persons will receive transplanted organs directly relate to the principle of justice. Because of the high costs of transplanted organs, transplant agencies use various criteria to choose persons who will receive donated human organs. For example, the likelihood of success of the transplant in one person versus another, life expectancy, family role, and existence of a strong family support system have been proposed as factors used to determine which persons receive organs. Severity of need, age, and lifestyle as well as the relative health of the potential recipient are also considered in determining organ placement.

Research Focus

Citation:
Gerad, M. J., & Frank-Stromborg, M. (1998). Screening for prostate cancer in asymptomatic men: Clinical, legal, and ethical implications. *Oncology Nursing Forum, 25*(9), 1561–1569.

Purpose:
To describe the often conflicting recommendations for prostate cancer screening for asymptomatic men of major medical organizations that influence advanced practice nurses (APN) roles.

Methods:
Examining published medical, legal, and economic articles, published legal statements and settlements, case law, and news reports generated data.

Findings:
National recommendations for prostate screening for asymptomatic men vary and produce legal, ethical, and economic considerations for health care providers of primary care. Currently available early diagnostic tests and expected ranges of prostate specific antigen (PSA) levels that are age and race specific create confusion about treatment, as does lack of coverage by some managed care plans for early detection of prostate cancer. The APNs who do not screen at-risk men, however, may face legal charges of negligence despite reimbursement and inconsistencies in treatment protocols.

Implications:
Using their knowledge, skills, and caring approaches to health care consumers, APNs need to individualize their care approaches to older males to assist them to make informed decisions about screening for prostate cancer despite social and economic barriers to such screening.

Use of these criteria implies that rationing of health care and resources exists in an effort to provide an organ to a person perceived to most successfully respond to the new organ. Overall, health care decisions such as these reflect political, social, economic, and cultural values that determine present health care policy and decisions related to organ transplantation.

Other issues of justice refer to deciding when or how to withdraw a treatment from one person and to give it to another person to meet an ethical commitment to practice. For example, the charge nurse in an intensive care unit may be faced with a decision to transfer an older person, who is believed to be stable after a heart attack, out of an intensive care unit to have an available bed for a younger uninsured person who has experienced a traumatic auto accident. Should the older person who worked and contributed employment monies to develop technologies to save lives and to support public health care have a greater right to have that bed than the younger person who has not worked at all? As in other ethical dilemmas, a decision-making process will provide a structured format to allow both health care professionals and the involved family to make a decision that appears morally justified.

Summary

Overall, older people make significant contributions to American society based on their educational preparation, political activity, and value base that supports working for societal benefit. However, for some older people, aging may be a time of decreased abilities, personal resources, and physical activities that place vulnerable older persons at risk for receiving care that does not meet their unique needs. Older persons, particularly those with illness and disability, may demonstrate behaviors that are different than those behaviors valued by American society, those for personal independence and a strong involvement with life activities. Because of their vulnerability, health care professionals have an ethical duty to older persons to provide high-quality care that meets the physical and social needs of this population group. Some research has supported that nursing values and perceptions of appropriate ethical behavior may conflict with institutional policy, physician beliefs and behavior, available time and resources needed for critical decision making, and beliefs of the older person and/or family (Corley & Selig, 1994; Erlen & Frost, 1991; Kelly, 1991; Leners & Beardslee, 1997). These contextual factors, which influence health care provider implementation of ethical practice, need to be discussed to meet older persons' needs for quality care based on ethical principles contained in various codes of professional practice. By demonstrating skills, knowledge, and a caring approach built on an ethical model of care, nurses can improve their own workplace and the quality of life and health of older adults.

Review Questions and Activities

1. You are caring for a 75-year-old woman who has fallen several times during the past month outside her home. She denies this behavior, although she has bruises and wounds on both elbows and legs and her neighbors have reported to you that she has fallen several times. The woman has lived alone since her husband died 1 year ago. Prior to his death, she effectively cared for him and herself and functioned independently to meet her family's needs. Her children remain concerned about the recent falls and their mother's denial of the frequency of the falls. What would you do as a health care provider to allow this woman to maintain her autonomy but also honor the ethical principles of beneficence and nonmalificence?

2. Compare and contrast the ethical principles of beneficence and nonmalificence as used in the ethical practice with older individuals.

3. Read a research article in which the subjects were older adults. Identify the process used to ensure informed consent and honoring of ethical principles of professional nursing care for the study sample.

4. Compare and contrast the concepts of therapeutic privilege, paternalism, and intentional nondisclosure as part of the ethical principle of autonomy. How might these concepts operate differently in older people than in younger people?

5. Consider the ethical practice of a nurse in caring for an 80-year-old Arab American man with metastatic liver cancer. How might the care delivered to this older individual differ from the care delivered to a Mexican American man of the same diagnosis and age?

6. Visit two older persons who reflect diversity from the European American culture. Interview these people with questions that will provide insight into their cultural beliefs about individual freedom, purpose in life, and the role of health professionals in the dying process.

7. Provide an example of how the current American society responds to the needs for care of older people according to the following ethical approaches: analytical, descriptive, and normative ethics.

8. Discuss the questions posed under the section on nonmalificence specific to issues related to dying choices. How might the nurse respond to these questions based on personal values and philosophical beliefs?

References

Allert, G., Sponhotz, G., & Baitsch, H. (1994). Chronic disease and the meaning of old age. *Hastings Center Report, 24,* 11–13.

American Health Consultants. (1999a). Americans say, "keep your laws off my body." *Medical Ethics Advisor, 15*(5), 52.

American Health Consultants. (1999b). Increase in debates, state bans don't change central fact: It's coming. *Medical Ethics Advisor, 15*(5), 49.

American Nurses Association (ANA). (1985). *Code for nurses with interpretative statements.* Kansas City, MO: Author.

American Nurses Association (ANA), Task Force on the Nurse's Role in End of Life Decisions. (1992a). *Nursing care and do-not-resuscitate decisions.* Washington, DC: Author.

American Nurses Association (ANA), Task Force on the Nurse's Role in End of Life Decisions. (1992b). *Position statement: Foregoing nutrition and hydration.* Washington, DC: Author.

American Nurses Association (ANA), Task Force on the Nurse's Role in End of Life Decisions. (1991). *Promotion of comfort and relief of pain in dying patients.* Washington, DC: Author.

Barcott, B. (1999, September). Dale's dilemma. *Life,* pp. 73–76, 78, 81–82.

Beauchamp, T. L., & Childress, J. E. (1994). *Principles of biomedical ethics* (4th ed.) (pp. 4–6, 47–56, 120–170, 189–231, 336–341, 395–406). New York: Oxford University Press.

Bishop, A. H., & Scudder, J. R. (1990). *The practical, moral, and personal sense of nursing: A phenomenological philosophy of practice.* New York: State University of New York Press.

Brandreit, L. M., Lyons, M., & Bentley, J. (1994). Perceived needs of post-stroke following termination. *Nursing and Health Care, 15,* 514–520.

Branegan, J. (1997, March 17). I want to draw the line myself. *Time, 149*(11), 30–31.

Breeze, J. (1998). Can paternalism ever be justified in mental health care? *Journal of Advanced Nursing, 28,* 260–265.

Brody, H. (1979). *Ethical decisions in medicine.* Boston: Little, Brown and Company.

Castellucci, D. (1996). *The relationship and differences between depression and perceived enactment of autonomous scores among post-stroke elderly.* Unpublished doctoral dissertation, University of Maryland, College Park.

Castellucci, D. T. (1998). Issues for nurses regarding elder autonomy. *Nursing Clinics of North America, 33,* 265–274.

Chin, A. E., Hedberg, K., Higginson, G. K., & Fleming, D. W. (1999). Legalized physician-assisted suicide in Oregon—the first year's experience. *New England Journal of Medicine, 340*(7), 577–583.

Collopy, B. J. (1991). Health care decision making. In N. Jecker (Ed.), *Aging and ethics* (pp. 177–178). Clifton, NJ: Humana Press.

Copp, L. A. (1986). The nurse as advocate for vulnerable populations. *Journal of Advanced Nursing, 11,* 255–263.

Corley, M. C., & Selig, P. M. (1994). Nurse moral reasoning using the Nursing Dilemma Test. *Western Journal of Nursing Research, 14,* 380–388.

Dierckx de Casterlé, B. D. (1998). Supporting nurses in ethical decision making. *Nursing Clinics of North America, 33,* 543–555.

Dierckx de Casterlé, B., Grypdonck, M., & Vuylsteke-Wauters, M. (1997). Development, reliability, validity testing of the Ethical Behavior Test: A measure for nurses' ethical behavior. *Journal of Nursing Measurement, 5,* 87–112.

Dierckx de Casterlé, B., Janssen, P. J., & Grypdonck, M. (1996). The relationship between education and ethical behavior of nursing students. *Western Journal of Nursing Research, 18,* 330–350.

Erlen, J. A., & Frost, B. (1991). Nurses' perceptions of powerlessness in influencing ethical decisions. *Western Journal of Nursing Research, 13,* 387–407.

Fellows, L. K. (1998). Competency and consent in dementia. *Journal of the American Geriatrics Society, 46,* 922–926.

Gaul, A. L. (1989). Ethics content in baccalaureate degree curricula: Clarifying the issues. *Nursing Clinics of North America, 24,* 475–483.

Gilligan, C. (1982). *In a different voice: Psychological theory and women's development.* Cambridge, MA: Harvard University Press.

Kelly, B. (1991). The professional values of English nursing undergraduates. *Journal of Advanced Nursing, 16,* 867–872.

Leners, D., & Beardslee, N. Q. (1997). Suffering and ethical caring: Incompatible entities. *Nursing Ethics, 4,* 361–369.

Lo, B. (1991). Unanswered questions about DNR orders (editorial). *Journal of the American Medical Association, 265,* 1874–1876.

Low, L. L., & Kaufman, L. J. (1999). Medical futility and the critically ill patient. *Hawaii Medical Journal, 58*(3), 58–62.

McWilliam, C. L., Brown, J. B., Carmichael, J. L., & Lehman, J. M. (1994). A new perspective on threatened autonomy in elderly persons: The disempowering process. *Social Science & Medicine, 38,* 327–338.

Melzack, R. (1990). The tragedy of needless pain. *Scientific American, 262,* 27–33.

Miedema, F. (1991). A practical approach to ethical decisions. *American Journal of Nursing, 91*(12), 20–25.

Muller, M. T., Kimsma, G. K., & van der Wal, G. (1998). Euthanasia and assisted suicide: Facts, figures, and fancies with special regard to old age. *Drugs and Aging, 13,* 185–191.

Nelson, H. (1992). Against caring. *Journal of Clinical Ethics, 3*(1), 8–15.

Sherwin, S. (1992). *No longer patient.* Philadelphia: Temple University Press.

Smith, K. V. (1996). Ethical decision making by staff nurses. *Nursing Ethics, 3,* 17–25.

Tolley, M. (1997). Power to the patient. *Journal of Gerontological Nursing, 23*(10), 7–12.

Valente, S. M., & Trainor, D. (1998). Rational suicide among patients who are terminally ill. *AORN Journal, 68,* 252–258, 260–264.

Resources

4MedicalEthics.com: **www.4medicalethics.4anything.com**

Journal of Clinical Ethics: **www.clinicalethics.com**

CHAPTER 26

End-of-Life Decisions and Choices

Kay Weiler, BSN, RN, MA, JD

COMPETENCIES

After completing this chapter, the reader should be able to:

- *Relate the right of autonomy to the nursing care of older adults.*
- *Identify four constitutional rights of all citizens of the United States.*
- *Discuss the right to privacy related to client care.*
- *State examples of assault and battery in giving nursing care.*
- *Differentiate euthanasia from assisted suicide.*
- *Discuss the American Nurses Association position on assisted suicide.*
- *Describe the major provisions of the Patient Self Determination Act.*
- *Differentiate a living will from a durable power of attorney for health care.*
- *Discuss the role of the nurse in ensuring clients' autonomy and individual rights.*
- *Relate the American Nurses Association Code for Nurses to your own nursing care.*

MAKING THE CONNECTION

Refer to the following chapters to increase your understanding of end-of-life decisions and choices:

- **Chapter 21** *Hospice and Palliative Care*
- **Chapter 25** *Ethical Theories and Principles*
- **Chapter 27** *Legal and Financial Issues*

Autonomy

An adult's common law right to autonomy or **self-determination** regarding decisions about one's own health and welfare has been firmly established. The individual's right to make decisions regarding bodily integrity were succinctly stated by Justice Cardozo as "every human being of adult years and sound mind has a right to determine what shall be done with his own body" (*Schloendorff v. Society of New York Hospital,* 1914, p. 93). This right also has been described as "no right is held more sacred, or is more carefully guarded by the common law, than the right of every individual to the possession and control of his own person, free from all restraint or interference of others, unless by clear and unquestionable authority of law" (*Matter of Conroy,* 1985, p. 1221).

This principle has been directly applied to health care treatment decisions and the subsequent actions. If health care providers proceed with care, even after the client has indicated that he or she does not want the treatment or procedure, the care providers may be liable for **assault** and **battery** upon the client (*Schloendorff v. Society of New York Hospital,* 1914). Assault, in the health care environment, may be characterized as a client who is threatened with potential harm, believes that the threatening person is capable of creating the harm, and is fearful that the harm will occur (Brent, 1997). Examples of a nurse's assault upon a client are unusual. However, assault could occur if a nurse used a syringe in a threatening manner toward a client before giving an injection or threatened to make any other procedure (e.g., bath, nasogastric tube placement, enema) more painful or uncomfortable than necessary. The client could conclude that the nurse has threatened harm and is capable of creating the harm, and the client may experience fear that the harm will occur.

Assault may or may not be accompanied by battery. Battery occurs if the client has refused physical contact or care and the health care provider continues the treatment and actually touches the client (Brent,

1997). If a physician performs a medical procedure without valid consent, then a battery against the person has occurred (*Schloendorff v. Society of New York Hospital,* 1914).

An adult's primary expression of autonomy within the health care system is the requirement that adults must give **informed consent** (Figure 26-1) before any treatment is initiated (*Schloendorff v. Society of New York Hospital,* 1914). Each state has the authority to determine what criteria must be met in that state to establish that the client was appropriately informed about the anticipated intervention. Even though the state statutes vary, "there are three basic prerequisites for informed consent: the client must have the capacity to reason and make judgments, the decision must be made voluntarily and without coercion, and the client must have a clear understanding of the risks and benefits of the proposed treatment alternatives or nontreatment, along with a full understanding of the nature of the disease and the prognosis" (Council on Ethical and Judicial Affairs, American Medical Association, 1992).

"In the absence of these three elements, neither consent nor refusal can be informed. Thus, it is definitionally impossible for a person to make an informed decision—either to consent or to refuse—under hypothetical circumstances; under such circumstances, neither the benefits nor the risks of treatment can be properly weighed or fully appreciated" (*Cruzan v. Harmon,* 1988, p. 417).

If an individual has the right to consent to treatment, then it follows that a person may also refuse unwanted treatment: "The patient's ability to control his bodily integrity through informed consent is significant only when one recognizes that this right also encompasses a right to **informed refusal**" (*Matter of Conroy,* 1985, p. 1222, emphasis added).

CLINICAL ALERT

Remember that the nurse cannot force a client to take a specific medication or participate in an ordered treatment. If the client refuses, the nurse must document the refusal in the medical record and notify the physician. Developing a good relationship with the client and family through effective communication early may prevent these problems from occurring. Perhaps the client does not understand the need, process, or desired results of the treatment and a clear timely explanation will help.

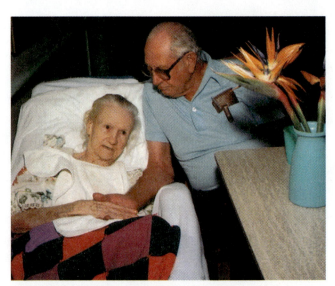

FIGURE 26-1 Cooperation with treatment can be facilitated by developing a good relationship with client and family.

The New Jersey Supreme Court considered if a nasogastric feeding tube could be removed from an **incapacitated** 84-year-old nursing facility resident (*Matter of Conroy,* 1985). In reference to this decision, the U.S. Supreme Court later noted, "While recognizing that a federal right of privacy might apply in the case, the court [New Jersey Supreme Court] . . . decided to base its decision on the common-law right to self-determination and informed consent. On balance, the right to self-determination ordinarily outweighs any countervailing state interests, and competent persons generally are permitted to refuse medical treatment, even at the risk of death. Most of the cases that have held otherwise, unless they involved the interest in protecting innocent third parties, have concerned the patient's competency to make a rational and considered choice of treatment" (*Cruzan v. Director, Missouri Department of Health,* 1990, pp. 272–273; citing *Matter of Conroy,* 1985, p. 1225).

> ### Nursing Tip
>
> Remember that every individual, regardless of age and/or diagnosis, has a right to autonomy. Ask for, carefully listen to, and document your clients' concerns, needs, and choices.

Constitutional Rights

In addition to the historical common law tradition of self-determination and informed consent, the right to self-determination in health care treatment decisions also has received constitutional protection (*Jacobson v. Massachusetts,* 1905). The breadth of the constitutional right to self-determination and specific aspects of the right, as related to health care treatment decisions, have been litigated (*Brophy v. New England Sinai Hospital, Inc.,* 1986; *Cruzan v. Director, Missouri Department of Health,* 1990; *Griswold v. Connecticut,* 1965; *Matter of Conroy;* 1985; *Roe v. Wade,* 1973; *Superintendent of Belchertown v. Saikewicz,* 1977). The basis of the constitutional right to self-determination has been examined from the perspective of the constitutional rights to (a) privacy, (b) religion, (c) liberty, and (d) **equal protection.**

Right to Privacy

While the Constitution does not explicitly state the **right to privacy,** the Supreme Court has determined that this right is implied in the intent and wording of the Constitution (*Brophy v. New England Sinai Hospital, Inc.,* 1986; *Griswold v. Connecticut,* 1965; *Superintendent of Belchertown v. Saikewicz* 1977). This implication of the

right to privacy has been referred to as the penumbra or zone of rights in the Ninth (*Griswold v. Connecticut,* 1965) and Fourteenth (*Roe v. Wade,* 1973) Amendments. The right to privacy has specifically been applied to health care treatment decisions. In *Griswold v. Connecticut* (1965), the executive director of the Planned Parenthood League of Connecticut (Estelle Griswold) opened a birth control clinic and was arrested for violating a Connecticut statute that prohibited the use of contraceptives, even by married couples. Upon appeal, the case was heard by the U.S. Supreme Court. In *Griswold v. Connecticut,* the Supreme Court clearly described the right to privacy as applicable to the Connecticut statute. The Court stated, "The present case, then, concerns a relationship lying within the zone of privacy created by several fundamental constitutional guarantees. And it concerns a law which, in forbidding the *use* of contraceptives rather than regulating their manufacture or sale, seeks to achieve its goals by having a maximum destructive impact upon that relationship" (*Griswold v. Connecticut,* 1965, p. 485, emphasis in original).

"We deal with a right of privacy older than the Bill of Rights—older than our political parties, older than our school system. Marriage is a coming together for better or worse, hopefully enduring, and intimate to the degree of being sacred. It is an association that promotes a way of life, not causes; a harmony in living, not political faiths; a bilateral loyalty, not commercial or social projects. Yet it is an association for as noble a purpose as any involved in our prior decisions" (*Griswold v. Connecticut,* 1965, p. 486).

After *Griswold v. Connecticut,* one of the questions that remained was, What other behaviors or actions were protected by this constitutional right of privacy? The next application of the right to privacy in health care treatment arose in the landmark Quinlan decision (*Matter of Quinlan,* 1976), in which the New Jersey Supreme Court found that the constitutional right to privacy was "broad enough to encompass a patient's decision to decline medical treatment under certain circumstances" even if that personal decision would foreseeably result in death (*Matter of Quinlan,* 1976, p. 663). Karen Quinlan's parents, as her substitute decision makers, were able to assert Karen's right to privacy and refused the use of a ventilator.

One possible extension of the right to privacy in health care treatment was presented to the Supreme Court by the parents of Nancy Cruzan (*Cruzan v. Director, Missouri Department of Health,* 1990). Nancy's parents, as her legal guardians, requested that artificial feeding and hydration be removed from Nancy. They asserted that Nancy had a protected *right to die* within the context of the constitutional right to privacy: "On the night of January 11, 1983, Nancy Cruzan lost control of her car . . . The vehicle overturned, and Cruzan was discovered lying face down in a ditch without detectable respiratory or cardiac function. Paramedics were able to restore her breathing and heartbeat at the accident site, and she was transported to a hospital in an unconscious state" (*Cruzan v. Director, Missouri Department of Health,* 1990, p. 266). She was in "what is commonly referred to as a persistent vegetative state: generally, a condition in which a person exhibits motor reflexes but evinces no indications of significant cognitive function" (*Cruzan v. Director, Missouri Department of Health,* 1990, p. 266). "After it had become apparent that Nancy Cruzan had virtually no chance of regaining her mental faculties, her parents asked hospital employees to terminate the artificial nutrition and hydration procedures. All agreed that such a removal would cause her death. The employees refused to honor the request without court approval. The parents then sought and received authorization from the state trial court for termination" (*Cruzan v. Director, Missouri Department of Health,* 1990, pp. 267–268). The trial court's decision was appealed and the Supreme Court of Missouri reversed on a divided vote. "We granted **certiorari** to consider the question whether Cruzan has a right under the United States Constitution which would require the hospital to withdraw **life-sustaining treatment** from her under these circumstances" (*Cruzan v. Director, Missouri Department of Health,* 1990, p. 269, emphasis added). The Court reviewed the history of the right to privacy and other constitutional rights that were asserted by Nancy's parents on her behalf. The Court also reviewed the requirements of the State of Missouri that required clear and convincing evidence of an incompetent person's previously expressed wishes for the removal of life-sustaining treatment.

The Supreme Court concluded that the State of Missouri had a significant interest in the preservation of all human life. The Missouri statute provided for the removal of life-sustaining treatment from an incompetent person if there was clear and convincing evidence of that person's previously stated wishes. Therefore, even though Nancy Cruzan had a constitutionally protected right of privacy in requesting the removal of the artificial feedings and hydration, her surrogate decision makers (parents) could not assert her right under Missouri law. Her parents were not able to present clear and convincing evidence of what Nancy would have chosen if she were to have made the decision.

Right of Freedom of Religion

The First amendment of the Constitution protects the individual's **freedom of religion:** "Congress shall make no law respecting an establishment of religion, or prohibiting the free exercise thereof" (U.S. Constitution, Amendment I, 1791). The amendment has two distinct components. The first phrase, the establishment clause, prohibits Congress from establishing a mandatory religion. The second phrase protects the individual's right to the free exercise of his or her own religion. The establishment clause has not been applicable to cases involving health care treatment decisions. The free-exercise clause, however, has been examined when a person has refused life-sustaining treatment based upon a religious conviction that the treatment violates his or her religious beliefs (Figure 26-2). In *Norwood Hospital v. Munoz* (1991), Norwood Hospital sought court approval to administer blood or blood products to Mrs. Munoz, a 38-year-old, competent adult who had refused consent for a blood or blood products transfusion. Mrs. Munoz had a history of stomach ulcers. A week before her hospitalization, Mrs. Munoz had taken two aspirin every 4 hours for a pain in her arm. The aspirin apparently caused her ulcers to bleed and Mrs. Munoz began vomiting blood and collapsed in her home. Upon admission to the hospital, Mrs. Munoz stopped bleeding; however her hematocrit was 17%. The physician assigned to care for Mrs. Munoz feared that if Mrs. Munoz had another episode of bleeding, without consenting to transfusions, she would most probably die. Mrs. Munoz refused consent for the administration of blood or blood products based upon her religious convictions as a Jehovah's Witness. Mrs. Munoz and her husband had become members of this religious group 16 years prior to her hospitalization and she attended three religious meetings every week. A principal belief of the Jehovah's Witness religion is that receipt of blood or blood products would preclude an individual's resurrection and everlasting life after death (*Norwood Hospital v. Munoz,* 1991). The Court in *Norwood Hospital v. Munoz* readily identified that Mrs. Munoz had common law rights to accept or refuse health care treatment and to privacy. After confirming her right to refuse treatment, the court did need to consider her claim of right to refuse treatment based upon her free exercise of religion (*Norwood Hospital v. Munoz,* 1991).

Right to Liberty

The Fourteenth Amendment states, no state shall "deprive any person of life, liberty, or property, without due process of law" (U.S. Constitution, Amendment XIV, 1868). Historically the **right to liberty** included within the due process clause have included the right to marry, (*Loving v. Virginia,* 1967); have children (*Skinner v. Oklahoma ex rel. Williamson, Attorney General,* 1942); direct the education and upbringing of one's children (*Meyer v. Nebraska,* 1923; *Pierce v. Society of Sisters,* 1925); marital privacy and the use of contraception (*Griswold v. Connecticut,* 1965); bodily integrity (*Rochin v. California,* 1952); and abortion (*Planned Parenthood of Southeastern Pennsylvania v. Casey,* 1992). The Court has also strongly suggested that the right also included the right to refuse unwanted lifesaving medical treatment (*Cruzan v. Director, Missouri Department of Health,* 1990).

In analyzing the Cruzan case, the Supreme Court reviewed the history of its own cases regarding whether a person's right to liberty encompassed the right to refuse unwanted medical care. In *Jacobson v. Massachusetts* (1905), the court considered whether a competent adult had a right to liberty that protected his right to refuse an unwanted smallpox vaccine. In *Washington v. Harper* (1990) the question involved whether a nonconsenting adult's liberty interest was violated by the forcible injection of medication. In *Viteck v. Jones* (1980) the plaintiff asserted that a transfer from a state prison to a state mental hospital for mandatory behavior modification treatment violated his liberty interest. The Supreme Court concluded, "the principle that a competent person has a constitutionally protected liberty interest in refusing unwanted medical treatment may be inferred from our prior decisions" (*Cruzan v. Director, Missouri Department of Health,* 1990, p. 278). Therefore, for purposes of the Cruzan case the Court assumed that the U.S. Constitution would grant a competent person a constitutionally protected right to refuse life-saving hydration and nutrition (*Cruzan v. Director, Missouri Department of Health,* 1990).

The most recent examination of the right to liberty in relation to health care issues was the question of whether the right to liberty in refusal of health care extended to the right to **assisted suicide** (*Washington v. Glucksberg,* 1997). The plaintiffs in *Washington v. Glucksberg* were terminally ill clients and physicians who asserted that they would assist their clients with suicide, except for Washington's ban on assisted suicide. The terminally ill clients died prior to the Supreme Court hearing. However, the physicians persisted in claiming that the liberty interest protected by the Fourteenth Amendment extended to a mentally competent, terminally ill adult's choice to commit physician-assisted suicide (*Washington v. Glucksberg,* 1997).

In *Washington v. Glucksberg* the plaintiffs asserted that the request for withdrawal or withholding of life-sustaining treatment, which hastens a client's death, was the same as the client's request for physician-assisted suicide. The Supreme Court did not agree and stated, "The decision to commit suicide with the assistance of another may be just as personal and profound as the decision to refuse unwanted medical treatment, but it has never enjoyed similar legal protection. Indeed, the two acts are widely and reasonably regarded as quite distinct. In Cruzan itself, we recognized that most States outlawed assisted suicide—and even more do today— and we certainly gave no intimation that the right to refuse unwanted medical treatment could be somehow transmuted into a right to assistance in committing suicide" (*Washington v. Glucksberg,* 1997, p. 21).

Equal Protection

On the same day that the Glucksberg decision regarding the constitutionality of the Washington statute was published, the Supreme Court issued another decision that applied to the New York statute banning physician-assisted suicide. The question raised by the New York statute was whether a competent, terminally ill client had a constitutionally protected right to assisted suicide under the Fourteenth Amendment Equal Protection Clause (*Vacco v. Quill,* 1997). The plaintiffs were physicians who asserted that it was consistent with their standards of medical practice to prescribe lethal doses of medications for "mentally competent, terminally ill patients" (*Vacco v. Quill,* 1997, p. 2). They were prohibited from prescribing these medications by the New York statute prohibiting assisted suicide (*Vacco v. Quill,* 1997, p. 2). The plaintiffs argued that "New York permits a competent person to refuse life-sustaining medical treatment, and because the refusal of such treatment is 'essentially the same thing' as physician-assisted suicide, New York's assisted suicide ban violates the Equal Protection Clause" (*Vacco v. Quill,* 1997, p. 2).

The Fourteenth Amendment Equal Protection Clause commands that no state shall "deny to any person within its jurisdiction the equal protection of the laws" (U.S. Constitution, Amendment XIV, 1868). This provision does not create any substantive rights; instead it embodies a general rule that states must treat like cases alike but may treat unlike cases accordingly (*Plyler v. Doe,* 1982).

In examining New York's ban on assisted suicide and New York's advance directive legislation, the Supreme Court concluded, "On their faces, neither New York's ban on assisting suicide nor its statutes permitting clients to medical treatment treat anyone differently than anyone else or draw any distinctions between persons. *Everyone,*

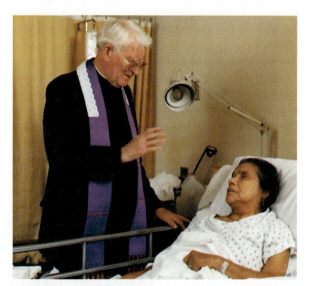

FIGURE 26-2 Religious convictions are protected by the First Amendment of the Constitution.

regardless of physical condition, is entitled, if competent, to refuse unwanted lifesaving medical treatment; *no one* is permitted to assist a suicide" (*Vacco v. Quill,* 1997, p. 4).

The legal principles of causation and intent were used to demonstrate the distinction between the two statutes. The cause of the client's death differs between the use of refusal of life-sustaining treatment and assisted suicide. If a client refuses life-sustaining treatment and dies, the death results from the underlying disease or pathology. However, if a client consumes or receives a lethal quantity of medication, the client's death is a direct result of the lethal medication.

In examining the intent of the client and physician, the Court stated, "a physician who withdraws, or honors a patient's refusal to begin, life-sustaining medical treatment purposefully intends, or may so intend, only to respect his patient's wishes and to cease doing useless and futile or degrading things to the patient when (the patient) no longer stands to benefit from them" (*Vacco v. Quill,* 1997, p. 6). Conversely, a physician who assists a suicide "must, necessarily and indubitably, intend primarily that the patient be made dead" (*Vacco v. Quill,* 1997, p. 7).

A client "who commits suicide with a doctor's aid necessarily has the specific intent to end his or her own life, while a patient who refuses or discontinues treatment might not" (*Vacco v. Quill,* 1997, p. 7). Clients who refuse life-sustaining treatment may "fervently wish to live, but to do so free of unwanted medical technology, surgery, or drugs" (*Matter of Conroy,* 1985, p. 1224).

State Legislative Actions

In *Washington v. Glucksberg* (1997) and *Vacco v. Quill* (1997) presented above, the U.S. Supreme Court refused to recognize a constitutional right to assisted suicide. However, the Court did identify that individual states could have legislative initiatives that would permit assisted suicide within the state's defined parameters.

The Supreme Court's rulings in both assisted suicide cases gave the voters in Oregon an opportunity to pursue an assisted suicide measure that would be included in the state statutes. In November 1994, the Oregon voters narrowly passed the Oregon Death with Dignity Act (1995). This ballot initiative provided that physicians could legally prescribe lethal doses of medications to a competent terminally ill client and the client could administer the lethal dose to himself or herself with the intent of ending his or her own life. Even though the ballot passed, a lawsuit was brought that successfully challenged the constitutionality of the statute (*Lee v. State of Oregon,* 1995).

The *Washington v. Glucksberg* (1997) and the *Vacco v. Quill* (1997) decisions suggested that if there were

a legitimate state interest in providing assisted suicide for terminally ill clients, that state interest should be explored and created through the state legislative system. The assisted suicide initiative in Oregon was placed on the ballot again and was passed for the second time.

Societal Interests

In each of the cases discussed and cited above, the decisions that the client had a protected right to accept or refuse health care treatment were not determinative. After identifying the right to refuse care, the court did a balancing test to determine if the individual's right to refuse care outweighed all of the societal interests involved in maintaining the client's treatment. The right to refuse life-sustaining treatment, and by analogy the right to assisted suicide, must be balanced against societal or state's interests in preserving that life. The counterbalancing state interests were to (a) preserve life; (b) prevent suicide; (c) avoid the involvement of third parties who may use arbitrary, unfair, or undue influence; (d) protect family members and loved ones; (e) protect the integrity of the medical profession; and (f) avoid future movement toward euthanasia and other abuses (*Compassion in Dying v. State of Washington* (1996). These state interests are of particular relevance to older adults who may be vulnerable to influence by others.

Preservation of Life

The state's interest in **preservation of life** has two separate facets: concern for the individual life of the client and an interest in the sanctity of all human life (*Cruzan v. Harmon,* 1988). "The concern for preservation of the life of the patient normally involves an interest in the prolongation of life. Thus, the State's interest in preserving life is very high when human life [can] be saved where the affliction is curable" (*Superintendent of Belchertown v. Saikewicz,* 1977, pp. 425–426). That interest wanes when the underlying affliction is incurable and "would soon cause death regardless of any medical treatment." The strength of the state's interest shifts when the "issue is not, whether, but when, for how long, and at what cost to the individual that life may be briefly extended" (*Superintendent of Belchertown v. Saikewicz,* 1977, p. 426).

In the Brophy decision, the court found that statements made by the client before his onset of incapacity were sufficient information to identify that the client's wishes for removal of treatment outweighed the states' interest in the preservation of human life (*Brophy v. New England Sinai Hospital, Inc.,* 1986). In *Bouvia v. Superior*

Court (1986), the California Superior Court determined that a competent adult who wanted life-sustaining treatment removed had a more compelling interest in the preservation of her own life than the state's interest in that same life.

The difficulty for the court, health care providers, and family has been to identify if a specific adult who cannot participate in the treatment decision would choose to accept or reject the life-sustaining treatment. This identification of the adult's preferences may be simplified if the adult has written a **living will (LW)** or a **durable power of attorney for health care (DPAHC)** (discussed later in this chapter). However, if these documents have not been written, there may be limited or no information about the incapacitated adult's preferences. Nurses in all settings can discuss and clearly inform older adults of their options that may aid in their decisions.

In reviewing the state's interest in the sanctity of all human life, the court in *Cruzan v. Harmon* identified that Nancy was alive; the life-sustaining treatments had not been characterized as burdensome for her; she did not have a terminal illness with a shortened life expectancy; nor did she express pain. Given those facts, the Missouri Supreme Court concluded that Nancy's right to refuse treatment, as expressed by her guardians, was outweighed by the state's clear interest in the sanctity of her life (*Cruzan v. Harmon,* 1988).

Prevention of Suicide

An additional state interest that was asserted by Washington State was the **prevention of suicide** of its residents. The legislative and judicial actions of the State of Washington, historically, had insisted that "all persons' lives, from beginning to end, regardless of physical or mental condition, are under the full protection of the law" (*Washington v. Glucksberg,* 1997, p. 25).

Avoiding Involvement of Third Parties

This state interest generated a considerable amount of controversy during the judicial appeals process. The first appeal of this case to the Circuit Court was decided by a panel of three circuit judges (*Compassion in Dying v. State of Washington,* 1995). However, upon review, the Justices of the Ninth Circuit Court of Appeals decided to rehear the same case with the entire judicial panel (*Compassion in Dying v. State of Washington,* 1996).

The judicial panel decision identified that Washington State had valid state interests in protecting older adults or infirm from potential psychological harm from physicians related to consent to their own deaths. If physician-assisted suicide was permitted, then physicians could determine who would be the best candidates for treatment and who would be the best candidates for assisted suicide (*Compassion in Dying v. State of Washington,* 1995). The panel also identified that the poor and minorities were vulnerable to coercion in the assisted suicide decision. The poor and minorities have historically received less attention for pain management strategies and were also more likely to have received public assistance. The need for cutting health care costs could become a factor in bedside treatment decisions regarding assisted suicide (*Compassion in Dying v. State of Washington,* 1995). The panel also was concerned that handicapped and disabled persons were potentially vulnerable to coercion in assisted suicide decisions. The panel was specifically concerned that all vulnerable populations would be confronted with the burden of explaining why each of them had chosen to live, and consume health care resources, and had not chosen assisted suicide (*Compassion in Dying v. State of Washington,* 1995).

During the second examination of this case, by all of the justices of the Ninth Circuit Court, the question regarding the vulnerability of specific groups to coerced assisted suicide was addressed. In examining whether vulnerable populations might be coerced into physician-assisted suicide, the court identified that this concern was "ludicrous on its face" (*Washington v. Glucksberg,* 1997; citing *Compassion in Dying v. State of Washington,* 1996, p. 825).

However, the U.S. Supreme Court, upon hearing an appeal of the case, did not summarily dismiss the potential vulnerability of selected groups and recognized "the real risk of subtle coercion and undue influence in end-of-life situations," (*Washington v. Glucksberg,* 1997, p. 28). The Supreme Court identified that "the risk of harm is greatest for the many individuals in our society whose autonomy and well-being are already compromised by poverty, lack of access to good medical care, advanced age, or membership in a stigmatized social group" (*Washington v. Glucksberg,* 1997, p. 28).

Protecting Family Members and Loved Ones

The state has a legitimate interest in protecting innocent third parties, such as minor children, who may be dependent upon adults who request assisted suicide. This interest, however, may have negligible weight when the adult requesting the assisted suicide is terminally ill and death is "imminent and inevitable" (*Compassion in Dying v. State of Washington,* 1996, p. 827).

This state interest in protecting innocent and vulnerable third parties has been valuable in balancing individual and state interests regarding the refusal of life-sustaining treatment. However, this state interest has not been critical to any of the current court decisions regarding providing or banning assisted suicide.

Protecting the Integrity of the Medical Profession

The state's interest in protecting the integrity and ethics of the medical profession has been defined as "physician-assisted suicide is fundamentally incompatible with the physician's role as healer" (*Washington v. Glucksberg*, 1997, p. 27). Also, concern was expressed that the establishment of "physician-assisted suicide could . . . undermine the trust that is essential to the doctor-patient relationship by blurring the time-honored line between healing and harming" (*Washington v. Glucksberg*, 1997, p. 27).

Ask Yourself

Would you consider helping a physician with the process of physician-assisted suicide?

Avoiding Future Movement Toward Euthanasia and Other Abuses

The Washington statute banned assisted suicide for competent, terminally ill adults who wish to hasten their deaths by obtaining medication prescribed by their doctors (*Compassion in Dying v. State of Washington*, 1996). However, Washington State was concerned that if competent, terminally ill adults could request assisted suicide, then any adult could request assisted suicide, and, by analogy, substitute decision makers could request assisted suicide for incapacitated adults (*Compassion in Dying v. State of Washington*, 1996).

After enumerating and discussing the validity of the various state interests, the Supreme Court identified that it did not need to weigh or measure the magnitude of each interest in relation to Washington State's legislative ban on assisted suicide. The Court concluded that the interests were important and legitimate and that the ban on assisted suicide was reasonably related to the protection and promotion of those state interests. Therefore, the Court held that the Washington ban on assisted suicide did not violate the Due Process Clause of the Fourteenth Amendment and the ban would remain in place (*Washington v. Glucksberg*, 1997)

The Patient Self Determination Act

In response to the multiple issues raised by the various court cases in the 1980s, the federal legislature passed the **Patient Self Determination Act (PSDA)** (1990). Each state has the authority to conclude if the citizens of that state would benefit from advance directive legislation. Therefore, the federal legislature could not impose the requirement that each state adopt advance directives legislation, nor could the federal legislature compel the states to include specific language in the state advance directives. However, the U.S. legislature does control the disbursement of Medicare funds. Therefore, in order to promote the distribution of information about advance directives, increase all adult's knowledge about advance directives, and decrease the number of uninformed families who experienced end-of-life decisions for their loved one, the federal legislature passed the Patient Self Determination Act (1990).

The Patient Self Determination Act (1990) requires every health care institution to maintain specific policies and procedures for every adult who receives health care in that institution. Failure to comply with the act may result in a facility's loss of Medicare and Medicaid payments. The major policies are listed in Box 26-1.

Advance Directives for Health Care Treatment Decisions

The advance directives addressed by the Patient Self Determination Act were developed by the various states to assist individuals in communicating their potential health care treatment preferences through a variety of means. Verbal comments, a living will, and a durable power of attorney for health care have been recognized as valid advance directives for future health care treatment decisions. One method of communicating treatment preferences is the use of oral statements made by the older person in relation to potential health care problems and possible treatment decisions. Verbal comments, indicating a thoughtful and consistent approach

BOX 26-1 Patient Self Determination Act

- To provide written information to each such individual concerning:

  - An individual's rights under state law (whether statutory or as recognized by the courts of the state) to make decisions concerning such medical care, including the right to accept or refuse medical or surgical treatment and the right to formulate advance directives . . .

  - The written policies of the provider or organization respecting the implementation of such rights.

- To document in the individual's medical record whether or not the individual has executed an advance directive.

(Figure 26-3), have been recognized as valid indicators of the person's preferred approach to potential treatment alternatives (*In re Storar,* 1981).

There are legal relations that may be established in which one adult may make a substitute or surrogate decision for another adult in need of care. In essence, the surrogate decision maker exercises the impaired adult's right to self-determination by making substituted decisions on behalf of the impaired adult. The title and purpose of the surrogate decision maker will vary according to who has initiated the appointment of the substitute decision maker and the scope of authority that has been delegated to the substitute decision maker. Specifically, there are some situations in which an adult who retains competency and capacity may make a current designation of another person to make financial, health care, or personal care decisions if the declaring adult becomes incapacitated in the future (Hall, 1996). If these delegations of authority are specifically for future health care treatment decisions, they are referred to as advance directives and are generally classified as a living will (LW) or a durable power of attorney for health care (DPAHC) (Hall, 1996; Teno et al., 1997).

Living Wills

The LW provides adults the opportunity to describe any life-sustaining treatment they wish to accept or reject if they experience a terminal condition or permanent state of unconsciousness and are not able to participate in health care treatment decisions. This document is the individual's statement of preferences for future health care. All 50 states have legislation recognizing either LW or DPAHC options (*Choice in dying,* 1994). Each state has the authority to draft legislation applicable only to the residents of that particular state; however, the legal

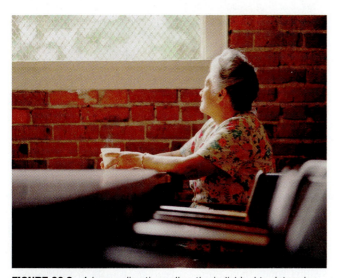

FIGURE 26-3   Advance directives allow the individual to determine potential treatment choices.

Research Focus

Citation:

Teno, J. M., Licks, S., Lynn, J., Wenger, N., Conners, A., Phillips, R. S., O'Connor, M. A., Murphy, D. P., Fulkerson, W. J., Desbiens, N., & Knaus, W. A. (1997). Do advance directives provide instructions that direct care? *Journal of the American Geriatrics Society, 45,* 508–512.

Purpose:

To evaluate whether the lack of effect of advance directives (Ads) on decision making in SUPPORT might arise from the content of the documents.

Methods:

Advance directives placed in the medical records were abstracted for date of completion and content of additional written instructions in five teaching hospitals in the United States. Directives were examined with instructions to forego life-sustaining treatment in the current state of health to determine whether care given was consistent with preferences noted in those directives. A total of 4,804 clients with at least one of nine serious illnesses were admitted to five teaching hospitals in the 2 years following implementation of the Patient Self Determination Act. Clients were part of a randomized controlled trial to improve decision making and outcomes.

Findings:

From the medical records of 4,804 clients, a total of 688 directives were collected from 569 clients. The majority of these directives (66%) were durable powers of attorney; in addition, 31% were standard living wills or other forms of written instructions (3%). Only 90 documents (13%) provided additional instructions for medical care beyond naming a proxy or stating the preferences of a standard living will. Only 36 contained specific instructions about the use of life-sustaining medical treatment, and only 22 of these directed foregoing life-sustaining treatment in the client's current situation. For these, the treatment course was consistent with the instruction for nine clients. In two cases, clients may have changed an inconsistent directive after discussion with hospital staff.

Implications:

Advance directives placed in the medical records of seriously ill clients often did not guide medical decision making beyond naming a health care proxy or documenting general preferences in a standard living will format. Even when specific instructions were present, care was potentially inconsistent in half of the cases.

and ethical principles of personal autonomy are the premise of each statute (Krauskopf, Brown, & Tokarz, 1996, Supplement §13.32). Typical criteria for LW statutes include that the individual (a) is an adult; (b) has lost the capacity to participate in the necessary health care treatment decision; (c) has a terminal illness or a condition that is not considered curable (e.g., persistent vegetative state); and (d) requires life-sustaining treatment (Uniform Rights of the Terminally Ill Act, 1985).

The LW is usually a written statement regarding the adult's preferences for life-sustaining treatment. Because the LW is a written form generally filed with the adult's medical record, the usefulness of the LW in conveying the individual's wishes or preferences for care depends upon health care personnel, especially physicians and nurses, to assess and carry out the decisions (Cohn, 1983).

Ask Yourself

Should you and members of your family have a living will and/or durable power of attorney for health care?

Durable Power of Attorney for Health Care

A DPAHC is a private legal relationship that is created by a document in which one person (the principal) grants another person (the agent, surrogate, proxy, or attorney-in-fact) the authority to act for him or her in making personal or health care treatment decisions. This delegation of authority continues even if the principal becomes **cognitively incapacitated.** This relationship has the advantage of authorizing a designated person to receive pertinent diagnostic information, analyze potential treatment options, act as an advocate for the client, and give consent for or refusal of care. Some states call this document a Medical Power of Attorney. See Figure 26-4.

This legal advance directive offers greater flexibility than a living will. The document is not limited to life-sustaining measures but may apply to nursing facility placement, surgery, or other forms of nonemergency treatment. The greatest limitation of the Durable Power of Attorney for Health Care is the requirement of having a person who is willing to serve in the role of substitute decision maker. If older adults have outlived all of their significant others and do not have anyone to serve as a surrogate decision maker, they are not able to benefit from the flexibility offered by a durable power of attorney for health care.

Implications for Nurses

Attention in the nursing profession to the entire concept of self-determination has increased greatly since the pas-

Think About It

Mr. Bartling was 70 years old and had emphysema, chronic respiratory failure, arteriosclerosis, an abdominal aneurysm (abnormal ballooning of the main artery passing through the abdomen to the legs), and a malignant tumor of the lung.

The tumor on his lung was discovered when a routine chest x-ray was done. Mr. Bartling had a biopsy performed to examine the tumor and subsequently the lung collapsed. Mr. Bartling was then placed on a ventilator and efforts to wean him were unsuccessful.

Mr. Bartling was considered competent in the legal sense to decide whether he wanted to have the ventilator disconnected. On several occasions, Mr. Bartling tried to remove the ventilator tubes. Despite requests from Mr. and Mrs. Bartling, the hospital and Mr. Bartling's treating physicians refused to remove the ventilator or the restraints that prevented him from pulling out the ventilator tube on his own.

Mr. Bartling had a signed and witnessed living will that stated, in part, "If at such time the situation should arise in which there is no reasonable expectation of my recovery from extreme physical or mental disability, I direct that I be allowed to die and not be kept alive by medications, artificial means, or heroic measures."

Mr. Bartling also had a signed and witnessed durable power of attorney for health care that named his wife as his attorney-in-fact. The DPAHC stated, "My desires concerning future medical and supportive care, which I direct my attorney-in-fact to follow, are . . . I am totally unable to care for myself, and believe that I am dependent on a mechanical ventilator to support and sustain my respiration and life. I continuously suffer agonizing discomfort, pain, and humiliating indignity of having to have my every bodily need and function tended to by others. I do not wish to continue to live under these circumstances."

The hospital and his physicians continued to refuse Mr. Bartling's request to have the ventilator removed. Mr. Bartling and his family sought an injunction to prevent the hospital from forcing his acceptance of the ventilator for respiratory function. The trial court refused Mr. Bartling's request. The appeals court determined that Mr. Bartling, as a competent adult, had the right to refuse respiratory support. This decision was, however, reached after Mr. Bartling had died while still receiving respiratory support from the ventilator.

Adapted from Bartling v. Superior Court, *209 Cal. Rep. 220,* *(1984).*

sage of the Patient Self Determination Act (PSDA) in 1990 (Public Law 101-508). Articles on the important issue of use of advance directives after passage of the PSDA have emerged. The use of advance directives in home health (Davitt & Kaye, 1996; Gates, Schins & Smith, 1996), in long-term care (Cohen-Mansfield et al., 1991; Walker & Blechner, 1995–1996), and in various

MEDICAL POWER OF ATTORNEY

THIS IS AN IMPORTANT LEGAL DOCUMENT. BEFORE SIGNING THIS DOCUMENT, YOU SHOULD KNOW THESE IMPORTANT FACTS.

Except to the extent you state otherwise, this document gives the person you name as your agent the authority to make any and all health care decisions for you in accordance with your wishes, including your religious and moral beliefs, when you are no longer capable of making them yourself. Because "health care" means any treatment, service, or procedure to maintain, diagnose, or treat your physical or mental condition, your agent has the power to make a broad range of health care decisions for you. Your agent may consent, refuse to consent, or withdraw consent to medical treatment and may make decisions about withdrawing or withholding life-sustaining treatment. Your agent may not consent to voluntary inpatient mental health services, convulsive treatment, psychosurgery, or abortion. A physician must comply with your agent's instructions or allow you to be transferred to another physician.

Your agent's authority begins when your doctor certifies that you lack the capacity to make health care decisions.

Your agent is obligated to follow your instructions when making decisions on your behalf. Unless you state otherwise, your agent has the same authority to make decisions about your health care as you would have had.

It is important that you discuss this document with your physician or other health care provider before you sign it to make sure that you understand the nature and range of decisions that may be made on your behalf. If you do not have a physician, you should talk with someone else who is knowledgeable about these issues and can answer your questions. You do not need a lawyer's assistance to complete this document, but if there is anything in this document that you do not understand, you should ask a lawyer to explain it to you.

The person you appoint as agent should be someone you know and trust. The person must be 18 years of age or older or a person under 18 years of age who has had the disabilities of minority removed. If you appoint your health or residential care provider (for example, your physician or an employee of a home health agency, hospital, nursing facility, or residential care home, other than a relative), that person has to choose between acting as your agent or as your health or residential care provider; the law does not permit a person to do both at the same time.

You should inform the person you appoint that you want the person to be your health care agent. You should discuss this document with your agent and your physician and give each a signed copy. You should indicate on the document itself the people and institutions who have signed copies. Your agent is not liable for health care decisions made in good faith on your behalf.

Even after you have signed this document, you have the right to make health care decisions for yourself as long as you are able to do so and treatment cannot be given to you or stopped over your objection. You have the right to revoke the authority granted to your agent by informing your agent or your health or residential care provider orally or in writing or by your execution of a subsequent medical power of attorney. Unless you state otherwise, your appointment of a spouse dissolves on divorce.

This document may not be changed or modified. If you want to make changes in the document, you must make an entirely new one.

You may wish to designate an alternate agent in the event that your agent is unwilling, unable, or ineligible to act as your agent. Any alternate agent you designate has the same authority to make health care decisions for you.

THIS POWER OF ATTORNEY IS NOT VALID UNLESS IT IS SIGNED IN THE PRESENCE OF TWO COMPETENT ADULT WITNESSES. THE FOLLOWING PERSONS MAY NOT ACT AS ONE OF THE WITNESSES:

(1) the person you have designated as your agent;

(2) a person related to you by blood or marriage;

(3) a person entitled to any part of your estate after your death under a will or codicil executed by you or by operation of law;

(4) your attending physician;

(5) an employee of your attending physician;

(6) an employee of a health care facility in which you are a patient if the employee is providing direct patient care to you or is an officer, director, partner, or business office employee of the health care facility or of any parent organization of the health care facility; or

(7) a person who, at the time this power of attorney is executed, has a claim against any part of your estate after your death.

MEDICAL POWER OF ATTORNEY
DESIGNATION OF HEALTH CARE AGENT

STATE OF TEXAS   §

           §

COUNTY OF TARRANT   §

I, _____ of _____, appoint _____ of _____ as my agent to make any and all health care decisions for me, except to the extent I state otherwise in this document. This medical power of attorney takes effect if I become unable to make my own health care decisions and this fact is certified in writing by my physician.

LIMITATIONS ON THE DECISION-MAKING AUTHORITY OF MY AGENT ARE AS FOLLOWS: _____

FIGURE 26-4 Sample Durable Power of Attorney for Health Care. *(Courtesy of Steven E. Katten, Attorney at Law, Fort Worth Texas. Used with permission.)*

(continued)

DESIGNATION OF ALTERNATE AGENT

(You are not required to designate an alternate agent but you may do so. An alternate agent may make the same health care decisions as the designated agent if the designated agent is unable or unwilling to act as your agent. If the agent designated is your spouse, the designation is automatically revoked by law if your marriage is dissolved.)

If the person designated as my agent is unable or unwilling to make health care decisions for me, I designate the following persons to serve as my agent to make health care decisions for me as authorized by this document, who serve in the following order:

A. First Alternate Agent

Name: _____

Address: _____

_____

Phone: ( ) _____

B. Second Alternate Agent

Name: _____

Address: _____

_____

Phone: ( ) _____

The original of this document is kept at _____

The following individuals or institutions have signed copies:

Name: _____

Address: _____

Name: _____

Address: _____

DURATION

I understand that this power of attorney exists indefinitely from the date I execute this document unless I establish a shorter time or revoke the power of attorney. If I am unable to make health care decisions for myself when this power of attorney expires, the authority I have granted my agent continues to exist until the time I become able to make health care decisions for myself.

(IF APPLICABLE) This power of attorney ends on the following date: _____

PRIOR DESIGNATIONS REVOKED

I revoke any prior medical power of attorney.

ACKNOWLEDGMENT OF DISCLOSURE STATEMENT

I have been provided with a disclosure statement explaining the effect of this document. I have read and understand that information contained in the disclosure statement.

(YOU MUST DATE AND SIGN THIS POWER OF ATTORNEY.)

I sign my name to this medical power of attorney on this _____ day of _____, 20_____.

_____

—Printed name—

—address—

—city/state—

FIGURE 26-4 *(continued)*

STATEMENT OF WITNESSES

I am not the person appointed as agent by this document. I am not related to the principal by blood or marriage. I would not be entitled to any portion of the principal's estate on the principal's death. I am not the attending physician of the principal or an employee of the attending physician. I have no claim against any portion of the principal's estate on the principal's death. Furthermore, if I am an employee of a health care facility in which the principal is a patient, I am not involved in providing direct patient care to the principal and am not an officer, director, partner, or business office employee of the health care facility or of any parent organization of the health care facility.

Witness _____

(Printed name) _____

Address _____

_____

Telephone number _____

Date: _____

Witness _____

(Printed name) _____

Address _____

_____

Telephone number _____

Date: _____

FIGURE 26-4 *(continued)*

hospital medical/surgical units (Collins & Mozdzierz, 1996; Kolcaba & Fisher, 1996; Rein, Harshman, Frick, Phillips, Lewis, & Nolan, 1996) has been explored.

In addition, the use of advance directives with specific client populations has been investigated. The use of advance directives among clients with cancer (Collins & Mozdzierz, 1996; Schonwetter, Walker, Solomon, Indurkhya, & Robinson, 1996), Alzheimer's disease (Mezey, Kluger, Maislin, & Mittelman, 1996), acquired immunodeficiency syndrome (AIDS) (Klaus, 1995), and renal failure (Perry, Nicholas, Molzahn, & Dossetor, 1995) has been examined.

Additional issues associated with advance directives have also been investigated. Lack of client knowledge about advance directives (Gamble, McDonald, & Lichstein, 1991; Ott & Hardie, 1997; Sabino, 1996; Schonwetter, Walker, & Robinson, 1995), vague or conflicting directions within an advance directive (Campbell, 1995), recognition of advance directives across care settings (Meier, Fuss, O'Rourke, Baskin, Lewis, & Morrison, 1996), and ethical issues (Ferdinand, 1996; Hepburn & Reed, 1995; Mouton, Johnson, & Cole, 1995) have been included in discussions regarding advance directives. Finally, some studies discuss nurses' knowledge of advance directives (Weiler, Eland, & Buckwalter, 1996) and the role of the nurse (American Nurses Association, 1991; Huth, 1995; Johns, 1996).

Maintaining the integrity of the medical profession was discussed above as one of the societal interests that must be considered in any debate regarding an adult's right to refuse life-sustaining treatment or request assisted suicide. In this section, the integrity of the nursing profession will be explored. While the court analyses

have limited their consideration to physicians, nurses know that if assisted suicide is initiated, nurses will be at the bedside. The nurse's role may be to administer the lethal medication, assist with physical care of the client, or assist families to say their good-byes (Johnson & Weiler, 1990).

The American Nurses Association (ANA) Code for Nurses explicitly identifies the nurse's role in client autonomy (ANA, 1985). The interpretive statements support that position (ANA, 1985). The ANA also has issued a statement regarding the profession's position regarding participating in assisted suicide. The ANA Position on Assisted Suicide was published in 1994 after extensive reflection, research, and debate. The first paragraph of the Position Statement states (ANA, 1994):

Nurses, individually and collectively, have an obligation to provide comprehensive and compassionate end-of-life care which includes the promotion of comfort and the relief of pain, and at times, foregoing life-sustaining treatments. The American Nurses Association (ANA) believes that the nurse should not participate in assisted suicide. Such an act is in violation of the Code for Nurses with Interpretive Statements (Code for Nurses) and the ethical traditions of the profession.

The Position Statement offers definitions for assisted suicide and withholding, withdrawing, and refusal of treatment. According to the Position Statement,

"suicide is traditionally understood as the act of taking one's own life. Assisting in suicide entails making a means of suicide (for example, providing pills or a weapon) available to a client with knowledge of the client's intention. The client who is physically capable of suicide subsequently acts to end his or her own life. Assisted suicide is distinguished from active euthanasia. In assisted suicide, someone makes the means of death available, but does not act as the direct agent of death."

Regarding withholding, withdrawing, and refusal of treatment, the Position Statement says,

Honoring the refusal of treatments that a patient does not desire, that are disproportionately burdensome to the patient, or that will not benefit the client is ethically and legally permissible. Within this context, withholding or withdrawing life-sustaining therapies or risking the hastening of death through treatments aimed at alleviating suffering and/or controlling symptoms are ethically acceptable and do not constitute assisted suicide. There is no ethical or legal distinction between withholding or withdrawing treatments, though the latter may create more emotional distress for the nurse and others involved.

The background portion of the position statement relies on the ANA Code for Nurses and reiterates that nurses traditionally have had the role of health care provider to "promote, preserve and protect human life" (ANA, 1994). Historically, the code has reaffirmed that "the nurse does not act deliberately to terminate the life of any person" (ANA, 1994).

The rationale offered by the position statement on assisted suicide identifies two major points. First, the nursing profession is grounded in the goals of the profession and the profession's covenant with society. Second, assisted suicide could have potential serious consequences for the profession and society including accompanying potential abuses (ANA, 1994).

The goals of the profession and the profession's covenant with society are identified by three elements. The first element is that the nursing profession has an obligation to do no harm and a repeatedly expressed strong moral opposition to killing another human being. The second element that supports the profession's position is the profession's covenant to respect and preserve human life. The third element that supports this position on assisted suicide is that, although the profession supports an individual's right to self-determination in health care treatment decisions, that right to autonomy has limitations. Those limitations do not extend to the nurse's expectation or obligation to comply with client or family requests for assisted suicide (ANA, 1994).

Some people who support physician-assisted suicide frequently stress that it is essential to relieve clients of continuing severe pain. However, hospice is an excellent option, and multiple new types of medications and dosages are available to relieve such severe pain.

Nurses need to be strong advocates for older adults and their families by providing correct information on end-of-life issues, recognizing that the decision must be made by the client. Nurses also need to assist older clients who are in special circumstances (e.g., have no family, have various religious beliefs and cultural values, and/or are physically or cognitively incapacitated) so that appropriate referrals (e.g., legal guardianship) can be made.

Summary

End-of-life decisions are complex and frequently agonizing for the client, family, and health care providers. The adult's right to determine personal bodily integrity has been recognized since the late 1800s (*Union Pacific Railroad Co. v. Botsford,* 1891). The legal basis of this right has been identified within the common law and constitutional law. The legitimate state's interests that may limit the adult's personal right to self-determination have been presented, discussed, and expanded. Finally, all of the potential state interests and personal rights of self-determination have been applied to several Supreme Court decisions regarding the right to assisted suicide.

After a great deal of legal analysis, the right to assisted suicide only exists in Oregon, and the limits of that right are defined by that state's statute. Currently, the ANA has taken the position that a nurse's participation in assisted suicide is not acceptable. There are many questions about end-of-life decisions that remain unanswered.

Think About It

Will the Oregon statute serve as the model for other states? Will the nursing profession stand firm in its conviction that assisted suicide is not acceptable nursing practice or will nursing serve as a role model for the assessment and evaluation of potential clients who have requested assisted suicide? Will nurses develop skills to assist clients and their loved ones to plan and execute a peaceful death? Or will this issue disappear and merely be identified in the future as an historic footnote?

Regardless of the future of assisted suicide, it is clear that adults who contemplate assisted suicide will look to health care professionals for information, advice, and, perhaps, the critical means of carrying out the suicide. Nurses, individually and collectively, must recognize the advancement of the assisted suicide movement and actively participate in defining the future of this movement. If assisted suicide becomes legally acceptable, nurses will be involved. The challenge for nursing is either to continue to assert and define its role in assisted suicide or have the lay public, judiciary, or other health care professionals define nursing's role.

Review Questions and Activities

1. What are the common law bases for an adult individual's right to self-determination in health care treatment decisions?

2. What are the constitutional law bases for an adult individual's right to self-determination in health care treatment decisions?

3. What is the rationale or analysis that has extended the individual's right to self-determination in health care treatment decisions to the individual's right to refuse unwanted health care treatment?

4. How has the rationale for refusal of health care treatment been extended to the right to assisted suicide?

5. What is the nurses' role in caring for or advocating for an adult who requests (a) information about proposed health care treatment; (b) that unwanted health care treatment be removed; (c) that he or she wants assistance with suicide?

6. Compare the state advance directives with hypothetical advance directives drafted from sample advance directives found in medical records.

7. Compare and contrast the state advance directives with the Uniform Rights of the Terminally Ill Act and the Uniform Rights of the Durable Power of Attorney Act.

References

American Nurses Association (ANA). (1985). *Code for nurses with interpretive statements*. Kansas City: Author.

American Nurses Association (ANA). (1991). *Position statement on nursing and the patient self-determination act*. Kansas City: Author.

American Nurses Association (ANA). (1994). *Position statement on assisted suicide*. Kansas City: Author.

Bouvia v. Superior Court, 225 Calif. 297 (1986).

Brent, N. J. (1997). *Nurses and the law: A guide to principles and applications*. Philadelphia: Saunders.

Brophy v. New England Sinai Hospital, Inc., 497 N.E.2d 626 (1986).

Campbell, M. L. (1995). Interpretation of an ambiguous advance directive. *Dimensions of Critical Care Nursing, 14*(5), 226–233.

Choice in dying. (1994). New York: The National Council for the Right to Die.

Cohen-Mansfield, J., Rabinovich, B., Lipson, S. Fein, A. Gerber, B., Weisman, S., & Pawlson, G. (1991). The decision to execute a durable power of attorney for health care and preferences regarding the utilization of life-sustaining treatments in nursing home residents. *Archives of Internal Medicine, 151,* 289–294.

Cohn, S. D. (1983). The living will from the nurse's perspective. *Law, Medicine & Health Care, 11*(3), 121–124, 136.

Collins, E., & Mozdzierz, G. (1996). Ethical considerations in treating oncology patients in the intensive care unit. *Critical Care Nursing Quarterly, 18*(4), 44–53.

Compassion in Dying v. State of Washington 49 F. 3d 586 (1995).

Compassion in Dying v. State of Washington 79 F. 3d 816 (1996).

Council on Ethical and Judicial Affairs, American Medical Association. (1992). Decisions near the end of life. *Journal of the American Medical Association, 267*(16), 2229.

Cruzan v. Director, Missouri Department of Health, 497 U.S. 261 (1990).

Cruzan v. Harmon, 760 S.W. 2d 408 (1988).

Davitt, J. K., & Kaye, L. W. (1996). Supporting patient autonomy: Decision making in home health care. *Social Work: Journal of the National Association of Social Workers, 41*(1), 41–50.

Ferdinand, R. (1996). Ethical dilemmas. Jehovah's Witness and advance directives. *American Journal of Nursing, 96*(3), 64.

Gamble, E., McDonald, P., & Lichstein, P. (1991). Knowledge, attitudes, and behavior of elderly persons regarding living wills. *Archives of Internal Medicine, 151,* 277–280.

Gates, M. F., Schins, I., & Smith, A. S. (1996). Applying advanced directive regulations in home health agencies. *Home Health Care Nurse, 14*(2), 127–133.

Griswold v Connecticut, 381 U.S. 479 (1965).

Hall, J.K. (1996). *Nursing ethics and law.* Philadelphia: Saunders.

Hepburn, K., & Reed, R. (1995). Ethical and clinical issues with Native-American elders: End-of-life decision making. *Clinics in Geriatric Medicine, 11*(1), 97–111.

Huth, J. (1995). Practical points. Advanced directives and the patient self determination act: What is a nurse to do? *Journal of Post Anesthesia Nursing, 10*(6), 336–339.

In re Storar, 420 N.E.2d 64 (1981).

Jacobson v. Massachusetts,197 U.S. 11 (1905).

Johns, J. L. (1996). Advance directives and opportunities for nurses. *Image: The Journal of Nursing Scholarship, 28*(2), 149–153.

Johnson, R.A., & Weiler, K. (1990). Aid-in dying. *Journal of Professional Nursing, 6*(5), 258–264.

Klaus, B. D. (1995). Advance directives: Matters of life and death. *Nurse Practitioner: American Journal of Primary Health Care, 20*(10), 88, 90.

Kolcaba, K. Y., & Fisher, E. M. (1996). A holistic perspective on comfort care as an advance directive. *Critical Care Nursing Quarterly, 18*(4), 66–76.

Krauskopf, J. M., Brown, R. N. & Tokarz, K. L. (1996). *Elderlaw: Advocacy for the aging* (2nd ed.). St. Paul, West.

Lee v. State of Oregon, 891 F. Supp. 1429 (1995).

Loving v. Virginia, 388 U.S. 1 (1967).

Matter of Conroy, 486 A.2d 1209 (1985).

Matter of Quinlan, 355 A.2d 647 (1976).

Meier, D. E., Fuss, B. R., O'Rourke, D., Baskin, S. A., Lewis, M., & Morrison, R. S. (1996). Marked improvement in recognition and completion of health care proxies. A randomized controlled trial of counseling by hospital patient representatives. *Archives of Internal Medicine, 156*(11), 1227–1232.

Meyer v. Nebraska, 262 U.S. 390 (1923).

Mezey, M., Kluger, M., Maislin, G., & Mittelman, M. (1996). Life sustaining treatment decisions by spouses of patients with Alzheimer's disease. *Journal of the American Geriatrics Society, 44*(2), 144–150.

Mouton, C. P., Johnson, M. S., & Cole D. R. (1995). Ethical considerations with African-American elders. *Clinics in Geriatric Medicine, 11*(1), 113–129.

Norwood Hospital v. Munoz, 409 Mass. 116 (1991).

Oregon Death with Dignity Act. (1995). Oregon Revised Statutes, Chapter 127.800.

Ott, B. B., & Hardie, T. L. (1997). Readability of advance directive documents. *Image: The Journal of Nursing Scholarship, 29*(1), 53–57.

Patient Self Determination Act (PSDA). (1990). (Public Law 101-508). Codified at 42 U.S.C.A. §§1395cc(a)(1)(Q), 1395mm©(8), 1395(f); 42 U.S.C.A. §§1396a(a)(57), (58), 1396a(w).

Perry, L. D., Nicholas, D., Molzahn, A. E., & Dossetor, J. B. (1995). Attitudes of dialysis patients and caregivers regarding advance directives. *ANNA Journal, 22*(5), 457–463, 481.

Pierce v. Society of Sisters, 268 U.S. 510 (1925).

Planned Parenthood of Southeastern Pennsylvania v. Casey, 505 U.S. 833 (1992).

Plyler v. Doe, 457 U.S. 202 (1982).

Rein, A. J., Harshman, D. L., Frick, T., Phillips, J. M., Lewis, S., & Nolan, M. T. (1996). Advance directive decision making among medical patients. *Journal of Professional Nursing, 12*(1), 39–46.

Rochin v. California, 342 U.S. 165 (1952).

Roe v. Wade, 410 U.S. 113 (1973).

Sabino, C. P. (1996). Ten legal myths about advance directives. *Journal of Nursing Law, 3*(1), 35–41.

Schloendorff v. Society of New York Hospital, 105 N.E. 92 (1914).

Schonwetter, R. S., Walker, R. M., & Robinson, B. E. (1996). The lack of advance directives among hospice patients. *Hospice Journal: Physical, Psychological, & Pastoral Care of the Dying, 10*(3), 1–11.

Skinner v. Oklahoma ex rel. Williamson, Attorney General, 316 U.S. 535 (1942).

Superintendent of Belchertown v. Saikewicz, 370 N.E.2d 417 (1977).

Teno, J. M., Licks, S., Lynn, J., Wenger, N., Connors, A. F. Jr., Phillips, R. S., Oconnor, M. A., Murphy, D. P., Fulkerson, W. J., Desbiens, N., & Knaus, W.A., (1997). Do advance directives provide instructions that direct care? *Journal of the American Geriatrics Society, 45*(4), 508–512.

Uniform Rights of the Terminally Ill Act (U.L.A.). (1985). St. Paul: West Group.

Union Pacific Railroad Co. v. Botsford, 141 U.S. 250 (1891).

U.S. Constitution, Amendment I. (1791).

U.S. Constitution, Amendment XIV. (1868).

Vacco v. Quill, No. 95-1858, slip op. (U.S. June 26, 1997).

Viteck v. Jones, 445 U.S. 480 (1980).

Walker, L., & Blechner, B. (1995-6). Continuing implementation of the Patient Self Determination Act in nursing homes: Challenges, opportunities, and expectations. *Generations, 19*(4), 73–77.

Washington v. Glucksberg, No. 96-110, slip op. (U.S. June 26, 1997).

Washington v. Harper, 494 U.S. 210 (1990).

Weiler, K., Eland, J., & Buckwalter, K. C. (1996). Iowa nurses' knowledge of living wills and perceptions of patient autonomy. *Journal of Professional Nursing, 12*(4), 245–252.

Resources

American Nurses Association: **www.ana.org**

CHAPTER 27

Legal and Financial Issues

Kay Weiler, BSN, RN, MA, JD
Perle Slavik Cowen, PhD, RN

COMPETENCIES

After completing this chapter, the reader should be able to:

- *Discuss the concept of decision-making capacity.*
- *Identify some reasons for decreased decision-making capacity in older adults.*
- *Differentiate a power of attorney from a durable power of attorney.*
- *Describe the role of a legal agent.*
- *Clarify the difference between a durable power of attorney and a durable power of attorney for health care.*
- *Discuss advantages and disadvantages of joint tenancy accounts.*
- *Identify the key concepts of a trust.*
- *Discuss common features of a will.*
- *Explore reasons why older people are frequent targets for consumer fraud and mistreatment.*
- *Summarize the role of the nurse related to the legal and financial issues of older adults.*

MAKING THE CONNECTION

Refer to the following chapters to increase your understanding of legal and financial issues:

Options Regarding Financial Issues Available for Adults with Decision-Making Capacity

Many of the changes associated with aging are accompanied by legal issues that elders and those who care for them must consider. To exercise autonomy, individuals must have the **decision-making capacity** to make decisions, voluntarily act, and choose the option(s) that they prefer. Within the legal domain, decision-making ability is generally referred to as **competency.** The determination regarding whether or not an individual has legal competency is generally easily determined—all adults are presumed competent. The concept of competency, however, is not useful if an individual retains the status of an adult but has never had, has experienced decreased, or has lost decision-making capacity (Willis, 1996).

The term decision-making capacity is frequently used by health care professionals because it is a more useful measure of decision-making ability than the legal term of competency. Decision-making capacity may be described as the ability "to understand the nature and effects of one's acts" (Aiken & Catalano, 1994, p. 102). Another definition of decision-making capacity is (1) a set of personal values or goals, (2) the ability to communicate and understand information, and (3) the ability to consider and decide upon the available options (Northrop & Kelly, 1987). An absence of decision-making capacity in an adult may be demonstrated by the lack of ability to make and communicate cognitive decision-making processes, an inability to meet personal essential needs, or personal endangerment because of the lack of decision-making capacity (Smyer, Schaie, & Kapp, 1996).

There are several options that may be useful in planning for future financial needs. Some of the options have limitations, such as a **trust,** which is limited to those who have significant financial assets, and **joint tenancy,** which is limited to those who have a trusted friend or family member. However, even with these limitations, the options are extremely helpful for many older adults who have or anticipate having the need for assistance with financial affairs (see Table 27-1).

Power of Attorney

A **power of attorney** is a delegation of authority to an **agent** and must be written while the **principal** has decision-making capacity. The delegation of authority is only valid until the defined transaction has taken place or the principal (the person who granted the agent authority) no longer has decision-making capacity. The power of attorney may be useful for the sale of property, negotiation of a loan, or transfer of property (Strauss &

Lederman, 1996). The power of attorney may also be helpful in filing income taxes for the older adult with the Internal Revenue Service (IRS) (Power of Attorney, 1998). Or, the power of attorney may be used in seeking the resolution of problems with the IRS (Problem Resolution Program, 1997).

Durable Power of Attorney

The **durable power of attorney** is one legal mechanism that may be written to provide a very limited or extensive delegation of financial decision-making authority. A durable power of attorney is a private written document in which the older adult who is requesting assistance (the principal) has granted another person (the agent or **attorney-in-fact**) the authority to act for him or her. The primary difference between a power of attorney and a durable power of attorney is that with the durable form the delegation of authority continues even if the principal loses decision-making capacity. The durable power of attorney may be especially important for older adults who anticipate decreasing decision-making capacity (e.g., Alzheimer's disease or progressive organ failure).

As with the agent in the power of attorney, the person who serves as an agent for a durable power of attorney does not need to be an attorney. The agent should, however, be a person that the principal respects and trusts with his or her financial resources. It is important to recognize that the durable power of attorney may be very limited, such as the delegation of authority for the sale of a home. Or the delegation of authority may be very extensive and encompass authority over all of an older adult's financial property, such as sale of real estate, management of savings and checking accounts, and investment of stocks.

It is very important to recognize that the durable power of attorney is similar to but not the same as the durable power of attorney for health care. The durable power of attorney does not grant the agent authority to make personal or health care treatment decisions for the principal (Strauss & Lederman, 1996).

While the traditional or durable power of attorney offers many advantages to the older adult who is delegating the authority, there is a major disadvantage to this relationship. There is very limited protection for the principal or older adult. If the agent is not acting in the principal's best interests or is misappropriating the principal's funds, the principal may revoke the agreement. However, if the principal has become incapacitated and is not able to demand or understand an accounting, the agent may exert extensive financial control over the principal's property without any fiscal accountability (Weiler, 1989). If the principal is not able to request or demand an accounting, friends or relatives do not have the authority to intervene. The durable power of attorney is a private relationship and is not open to the scrutiny of concerned third parties. See Figure 27-1 for a sample durable power of attorney. These forms will differ from state to state based on state laws and regulations, so it is essential to obtain and use the appropriate form.

Joint Tenancy Accounts

If two or more persons open an account at a financial institution, the parties are required to stipulate the legal relationship that the parties will have in relationship to the money in the account. If the account is held as a joint tenancy, one party is *not* an agent for the other party. All of the parties are equal co-owners of the account. The owners of the joint tenancy account share in all the benefits and responsibilities of the account. In addition, upon the death of one co-owner, the remainder of the account immediately becomes the undisputed property of the surviving co-owner(s) (Krauskopf, Brown, Tokarz, & Bogutz, 1999, Supplement §8.51).

The use of the joint tenancy is extremely useful for many adults who wish to give another adult unlimited access to the funds in the account (such as spouse or adult child). The primary disadvantage of a joint tenancy account, however, is that the co-owners have no obligation to use the assets for the benefit of the other co-owners. Therefore, one co-owner (parent) may have automatic deposits made to the account, become incapacitated, and the other co-owner (child) may use the assets for the adult child's own benefit (such as a new car). Upon the death of one co-owner (parent), the surviving co-owner (child) has no legal obligation to share the balance of the account with others not listed on the account (e.g., siblings or a spouse still living but not named on the account) (Krauskopf et al., 1999, Supplement §8.51).

An additional disadvantage to the joint tenancy account may arise if one of the owners needs access to a governmental or community benefit that has income restrictions or is "needs based" (Arnason, Rosenzweig, & Koski, 1995, p. 214). Each owner of the joint tenancy account is considered to have total unrestricted access to the entire account. Therefore, when a disclosure of financial assets is required to apply for the community benefit, the entire balance of the account is assumed to be the entire property of the applicant. This assumption by the governmental or community agency may not reflect the intent of the co-owners in the establishment of the joint tenancy account. However, the legal status of a joint tenant account dictates the inclusion of that account (Arnason et al., 1995).

Trusts

The establishment of a trust offers the maximum opportunity to maintain control of financial assets while transferring the management responsibilities usually associated with the ownership of property. A trust is a written document with defined property to be managed in a

TABLE 27-1 Financial Options Available for Adults with or without Decision-Making Capacity

Adult with Decision-Making Capacity	Adult without Decision-Making Capacity
Handle own transactions	Not capable of handling own transactions
Power of attorney	Cannot write or sign a power of attorney
Durable power of attorney	Durable power of attorney continues
Joint tenancy	Cannot create a joint tenancy
Write will for use upon death	Conservator/Guardian
Trust	Cannot create or sign a trust

The terms *conservator* and *guardian* may have separate and distinct meanings within a state or may be used interchangeably. The terms are used here to identify the court-appointed substitute decision maker for financial decisions.

specified manner by an identified party (trustee) for the benefit of specific party(ies) (**beneficiaries,** e.g., parents, grandchildren). All trusts contain the following elements: restrictions identified for the property held by the trust; a named representative who is required to follow the dictates of the trust; and requirements for record keeping of the transactions involving the trust property. This option provides continued ownership (not co-ownership) of the financial assets. However, the long-term expenses associated with maintaining the trust limit this option to individuals with significant financial resources (Krauskopf, Brown, Tokarz, & Bogutz, 1993, §8.41).

Wills

A **will** is a written document that provides for the distribution of financial assets upon the death of the person who has written the will (**testator**). The specific requirements for having a valid will are determined by state law. For example, some states allow **holographic** (handwritten) **wills** and accept verbal videotaped wills. Common features generally include that the testator must (a) be an adult (usually 18 years or older); (b) understand the purpose of the will; (c) know the assets that are being distributed; (d) know who is receiving a portion of the assets; (e) indicate that the will is the last statement regarding the distribution of financial assets; and (f) voluntarily sign the will (Strauss & Lederman, 1996).

NOTICE: THE POWERS GRANTED BY THIS DOCUMENT ARE BROAD AND SWEEPING. THEY ARE EXPLAINED IN THE DURABLE POWER OF ATTORNEY ACT, CHAPTER XII, TEXAS PROBATE CODE. IF YOU HAVE ANY QUESTIONS ABOUT THESE POWERS, OBTAIN COMPETENT LEGAL ADVICE. THIS DOCUMENT DOES NOT AUTHORIZE ANYONE TO MAKE MEDICAL AND OTHER HEALTH CARE DECISIONS FOR YOU. YOU MAY REVOKE THIS POWER OF ATTORNEY IF YOU LATER WISH TO DO SO.

I, _____ (principal) of _____ , Texas, appoint _____ (agent) of
　　　(name)　　　　　　　　　　　　　　(city)　　　　　　　　　　　　　　　　(name)

_____ , Texas, as my agent (attorney-in-fact) to act for me in any lawful way with respect to all
　　　(city)

of the following powers except for a power that I have crossed out below.

TO WITHHOLD A POWER, YOU MUST CROSS OUT EACH POWER WITHHELD.

　　Real property transactions, including but not limited to the real property, described on Exhibit "A" (if such Exhibit is attached hereto);

　　Tangible personal property transactions;

　　Stock and bond transactions;

　　Commodity and option transactions;

　　Banking and other financial institution transactions;

　　Business operating transactions;

　　Insurance and annuity transactions;

　　Estate, trust, and other beneficiary transactions, including the power to create trusts, whether revocable or irrevocable, on behalf of the principal, and to fund such trusts on behalf of the principal or to make transfers and additions to any trust(s) already in existence;

　　Claims and litigation;

　　Personal and family maintenance;

　　Benefits from Social Security, Medicare, Medicaid, or other governmental programs or civil or military service;

　　Retirement plan transactions;

　　Tax matters; gifting powers, including but not limited to, the power to make gifts (either outright or in trust) either to or for the benefit of my spouse (if any), my children, my grandchildren, and any more remote descendants, or any charitable organization that I have supported, for gift, estate, generation skipping, or income tax planning purposes.

IF NO POWER LISTED ABOVE IS CROSSED OUT, THIS DOCUMENT SHALL BE CONSTRUED AND INTERPRETED AS A GENERAL POWER OF ATTORNEY AND MY AGENT (ATTORNEY-IN-FACT) SHALL HAVE THE POWER AND AUTHORITY TO PERFORM OR UNDERTAKE ANY ACTION I COULD PERFORM OR UNDERTAKE IF I WERE PERSONALLY PRESENT.

SPECIAL INSTRUCTIONS:

　　Special instructions applicable to gifts (initial in front of the following sentence to have it apply):

_____ I grant my agent (attorney-in-fact) the power to apply my property to make gifts, except that the amount of a gift to an individual may not exceed the amount of annual exclusions allowed from the federal gift tax for the calendar year of the gift.

　　ON THE FOLLOWING LINES YOU MAY GIVE SPECIAL INSTRUCTIONS LIMITING OR EXTENDING THE POWERS GRANTED TO YOUR AGENT.

_____

_____

_____

　　UNLESS YOU DIRECT OTHERWISE ABOVE, THIS POWER OF ATTORNEY IS EFFECTIVE IMMEDIATELY AND WILL CONTINUE UNTIL IT IS REVOKED.

FIGURE 27-1   Sample Statutory Durable Power of Attorney. *(Courtesy of Steven E. Katten, Attorney at Law, Fort Worth, Texas. Used with permission.)*

CHOOSE ONE OF THE FOLLOWING ALTERNATIVES BY CROSSING OUT THE ALTERNATIVE NOT CHOSEN:
(A) This power of attorney is not affected by my subsequent disability or incapacity.
(B) This power of attorney becomes effective upon my disability or incapacity.
YOU SHOULD CHOOSE ALTERNATIVE (A) IF THIS POWER OF ATTORNEY IS TO BECOME EFFECTIVE ON THE DATE IT IS EXECUTED.
IF NEITHER (A) NOR (B) IS CROSSED OUT, IT WILL BE ASSUMED THAT YOU CHOSE ALTERNATIVE (A).

If alternative (B) is chosen and a definition of my disability or incapacity is not contained in this power of attorney, I shall be considered disabled or incapacitated for purposes of this power of attorney if a physician certifies in writing at a date later than the date this power of attorney is executed that, based on the physician's medical examination of me, I am mentally incapable of managing my financial affairs. I authorize the physician who examines me for this purpose to disclose my physical or mental condition to another person for purposes of this power of attorney. A third party who accepts this power of attorney is fully protected from any action taken under this power of attorney that is based on the determination made by a physician of my disability or incapacity.

I agree that any third party who receives a copy of this document may act under it. Revocation of the durable power of attorney is not effective as to a third party until the third party receives actual notice of the revocation. I agree to indemnify the third party for any claims that arise against the third party because of reliance on this power of attorney.

If any agent named by me dies, becomes legally disabled, resigns, or refuses to act, I name _____ (agent)
                                                                                              (name)
as successor to that agent.

Signed this _____ day of _____ , 2000.

_____
(signature of principal)

STATE OF TEXAS   §

                           §

COUNTY OF TARRANT   §

This document was acknowledged before me on this _____ day of _____ , 2000, by _____ .
                                                                                                   (name of principal)

_____
Notary Public / State of Texas

My Commission expires:

_____

THE ATTORNEY-IN-FACT OR AGENT, BY ACCEPTING OR ACTING UNDER THE APPOINTMENT, ASSUMES THE FIDUCIARY AND OTHER LEGAL RESPONSIBILITIES OF AN AGENT.

FIGURE 27-1 *(continued)*

Think About It

As a nurse in a health care facility or agency, can you act as a witness to your client's signing of a will or other legal document? Why or why not?

Consumer Protection

Unfortunately, older people are frequently a target for **consumer fraud** schemes. Telephone solicitation, credit card scams, door-to-door sales, and home improvement contracts are several of the typical forms of consumer fraud that may lure the older adult into sending money or authorizing payment for a nonexistent or worthless item. To protect themselves from consumer fraud, older adults

should not provide a credit card number to anyone over the telephone unless that buyer initiated the call to the seller. An additional protection is that the older adult should not provide a checking account number or authorization for a transfer out of a bank account without a signed withdrawal or transfer slip. Finally, the older adult

Nursing Tip

If your older client in the home receives numerous telephone calls from strangers and letters in the mail for ordering trinkets or requesting donations, discuss the possible issue of financial abuse.

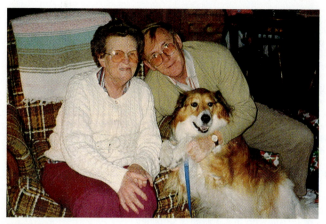

FIGURE 27-2　Many older adults live in their own homes or apartments and may be vulnerable to door-to-door fraud.

should not provide a credit card number if a caller requests the number for verification of the adult's identity (American Bar Association, 1998).

Older people may be particularly vulnerable to door-to-door salesmen and to promotions for home improvement contracts that are fraudulent. Older adults are more likely to be at home (Figure 27-2) than adults who are employed in the work force and may be lonely and believe the salesperson is very friendly and kind. Therefore, the older adult is more likely to answer the door and be pressured by a salesperson to make a purchase immediately. To protect against fraud, the older adult should not make an immediate decision regarding the purchase and should ask for all materials in writing with clear descriptions of what is, or is not, provided in the cost (e.g., delivery, installation). The older adult should also know, and be told by the salesperson, that the buyer has the right to cancel the contract or agreement within 3 days after the contract is signed. The salesperson should provide a cancellation form and a mailing address for the cancellation form. The buyer should only need to sign the cancellation form and mail it for the cancellation to be effective. However, for the consumer's protection, the older adult may choose to mail the cancellation form via certified mail so that there is a signed receipt indicating that the company received the cancellation notice (American Bar Association, 1998).

Options Available for Financial Decisions after Loss of Decision-Making Capacity

For older adults who have experienced loss of decision-making capacity, states have developed judicial structures that provide for the appointment of a legal surrogate decision maker. The surrogate decision maker is empow-

BOX 27-1　Elements of State Older Adult Mistreatment Statutes

- Define who is protected by the statute.
- Describe the behavior that is classified as abusive.
- Identify which settings provide protection from potential abuse (e.g. institutional or home care).
- Determine if nurses and other health care providers are mandatory or voluntary reporters of suspected abuse.
- Impose penalties for health care providers if suspected abuse is not reported.
- Provide protections from liability if the nurse makes a good faith reporting of suspected abuse.
- Determine which agency has the responsibility to investigate suspected abuse.
- Create criminal sanctions for the abuser if the suspected abuse is confirmed.

Source: *Adapted from "Elder Abuse, Neglect and Mistreatment," by G. R. Hall and K. Weiler, 1996, in C. W. Bradway (Ed.), Nursing Care of Geriatric Emergencies (pp. 225–251), New York: Springer.*

ered and monitored, by the court, to make decisions regarding the incapacitated adult's personal, health care, and financial interests (Smyer et al., 1996).

The terms used by the states to designate judicially appointed substitute decision makers may vary. Some states use the term *guardian*. For clarity in this chapter, the term **conservator** will be identified as a court-appointed substitute decision maker for the incapacitated adult's financial decision-making needs. Once the conservatorship has been established, the incapacitated person is frequently referred to as the **ward** (Krauskopf et al., 1993, §9.5).

A conservatorship is a court-authorized relationship in which the conservator assumes control of the financial assets of the ward. This relationship is not designed to authorize substitute or surrogate decision making for personal or health care treatment decisions. A conservatorship is limited to decisions regarding the ward's financial assets. The property controlled by the conservator is identified and monitored by the court. The conservator is responsible for filing a regular financial report with the court. The report generally must indicate how the conservator has protected the ward's financial assets. Also, the conservator must record how the assets have been dispersed to provide for the ward's benefit or to protect the ward's long- or short-term financial needs (Krauskopf et al., 1993, §9.5).

BOX 27-2 Types of Older Adult Mistreatment Caused by a Caregiver

- Physical abuse
- Physical neglect
- Psychological abuse
- Psychological neglect
- Financial exploitation
- Sexual abuse
- Violation of personal rights

Protective Statutes

Protective statutes to safeguard vulnerable older adults have been passed in all fifty states (Hunzeker, 1990). The statutes may be categorized as older adult abuse, **older adult mistreatment,** or adult protective service legislation. Each state has the responsibility and authority to create statutes that meet the criteria identified in Box 27-1.

Generally, older adult mistreatment is defined in terms of acts of commission (intentional infliction of harm) or acts of omission (harm occurring through **neglect**) by a caregiver. The definition of a caregiver may vary among states. However, a typical definition includes "a related or nonrelated person who has the responsibility for the protection, care or custody of a dependent adult as a result of assuming the responsibility, voluntarily, or by contract, through employment, or by order of the court" (Iowa Code, 1996). Many older adults may exhibit characteristics of multiple types of mistreatment with a wide range of severity (Box 27-2).

Physical neglect is often the most difficult form of older adult mistreatment to evaluate because of the varying etiological factors related to the older adult and the **perpetrator** (the person who causes or allows victim to be harmed). Major considerations in assessing and intervening in cases of caregiver-initiated neglect are the physical and cognitive abilities and the intent of the caregiver. This problem is particularly important if the caregiver, and suspected perpetrator, is also older and not physically or cognitively capable of caring for his or her mate. Active physical neglect arises from the purposeful withholding of necessities, whereas passive neglect results from the caregiver's inability to identify the older adult's needs or to perform the tasks essential to meet the older adult's needs (Bristowe, 1989). The term neglect implies a failure to perform an obligation and, therefore, raises questions regarding whether a family does have an obligation to provide care for an older adult (Lachs & Fulmer, 1993; Phillips, 1988).

The incidence of older adult mistreatment is difficult to determine and has been estimated to range from 4% (Block & Sinnott, 1979) to 10% (Fulmer, 1992; Lau & Kosberg, 1979) of the older population. This means that

Research Focus

Citation:
Weiler, K., & Buckwalter, K. C. (1992). Abuse among rural mentally ill. *Journal of Psychosocial Nursing and Mental Health Services, 30*(9), 32–36.

Purpose:
To determine if a rural mental health outreach program identified incidents of abuse, characteristics of those abused, types of abuse experienced, and nature of the relationship between the abuser and the victim.

Methods:
Three hundred thirty-five medical records of older rural clients receiving active mental health care were reviewed.

Findings:
Twenty-four percent of the records indicated some form of abuse. Victims were most likely women (70%) between the ages of 65 and 84 (71%) who were widowed (48%), divorced or separated (13%), and living alone (62%). The most frequent forms of abuse were self-neglect (47%), psychological abuse (19%), and physical and financial abuse (16%). The most frequent abusers were the client (49%), spouse (22%), children (15%), and grandchildren (4%).

Implications:
Older people needing mental health care may be in an abusive situation. Nurses need to identify such abusive situations and take appropriate action, including mandatory reporting.

between 700,000 and 2.5 million older adults are affected by mistreatment each year (Fulmer, McMahon, Baer-Hines, & Forget, 1992; Iowa Department of Elder Affairs, 1992). The differences in the reported rates have been attributed to differences in various state definitions of older adult mistreatment, the methodological limitations of the studies, and extrapolation of the results from

CLINICAL ALERT

Nurses should be alert to signs and symptoms of physical violence of older adults. Some of these are:

- *Bruises about the face, eyes, trunk, and legs*
- *Fractures of the jaw and arms*
- *Silence and withdrawal of the client in the presence of the abuser*

small sample sizes to the total older population of the United States (Pillemer & Suitor, 1988). The number of older Americans is expected to increase and correspondingly, the incidence of older adult mistreatment is also expected to increase (Figure 27-3).

Physical violence was the most common form of mistreatment in one study of community-dwelling older adults (Pillemer & Finkelhor, 1988). However, in a study of hospital-based older adults the referrals for neglect occurred approximately five times more frequently than referrals for physical abuse (Carr et al., 1986). Another review of older adult mistreatment reports found that financial exploitation was the most frequently reported abuse (49%), followed by emotional abuse (36%) and neglect (33%) (Neale, Hwalek, Goodrich, & Quinn, 1996). One study noted that financial exploitation is a common type of older adult mistreatment, particularly among those with dementia (Rowe, Davies, Baburaj, & Sinha, 1993).

The greatest potential for reducing or preventing the occurrence of older adult mistreatment is early identification and intervention. However, identification of older adult mistreatment is difficult because older victims often do not tell health care providers about the violence. Victims may feel dependent upon the perpetrator and fear reprisal if they report the mistreatment. In addition to the victims' reluctance to report the mistreatment, barriers to detection also include the older adult's impaired memory, cognitive impairments, impaired ability to communicate, or confounding variables such as interactions of multiple medications, falls, dehydration, and malnutrition (Haviland & O'Brian, 1989; Hogstel & Curry, 1999).

It is estimated that family members provide approximately 80% of the care for older adults (Baines & Oglesby, 1992). Unfortunately, it has also been repeatedly reported that family caregivers are the primary abusers of older adults (Anetzberger, 1987; Baines & Oglesby, 1992; Council on Scientific Affairs, 1987; Fulmer & Cahill, 1984; Gelles & Cornell, 1982; Homer & Gilleard, 1990; Kosberg, 1988; Pillemer & Finkelhor, 1988; Pillemer & Finkelhor, 1989; Tomita, 1982; Wolf, 1990). In 86% of reported mistreatment cases the abuser was a relative who lived with the older adult (O'Malley, Everitt, & O'Malley, 1983). The relationship of the abuser to the victim may be an older adult's adult child (Hirst & Miller, 1986; Mildenberger & Wessman, 1986) or the spouse (Hagebock & Brandt, 1981; Pillemer & Finkelhor, 1988; Wolf, 1986).

The caregiver's role and responsibilities may create stress that is situational, acute, or chronic in nature. Other variables associated with that stress are sociocultural issues, family dynamics, attributes of the caregiver, and individual characteristics of the older adult. These factors are not determinative of older adult mistreatment; however, the identification of these risk factors may provide an opportunity for intervention during stressful interpersonal relationship and volatile environmental circumstances (Committee on the Assessment of Family Violence Interventions, 1998).

The advances in technology combined with shorter hospital stays often result in placement decisions that must be made rapidly with limited time or information available. The time limitations may result in placement decisions that fail to consider the older adult's need for complex physical care, the family's lack of experience in providing care, and the family's lack of understanding regarding the long-term consequences of caring for a family member (Boland & Sims, 1996; Sims, Boland, & O'Neill, 1992). Additionally, the trend toward smaller family size often results in a decreasing pool of relatives to provide care for the expanding group of vulnerable older adults (Steinmetz, 1990).

Family risk factors frequently reported with older adult mistreatment are a lack of family support, isolation, economic pressures, history of family violence, and a lack of awareness or eligibility for government or community assistance programs (Fulmer, 1989; Grafstrom, Nordberg, & Wimbald, 1992; Straus, Gelles, & Steinmetz, 1981). The at-risk family caregiver may demonstrate signs of being overwhelmed and stressed in the caregiver role (Lachs & Fulmer, 1993) and frustrated with continued financial dependency on the older adult (Hwalek & Sengstock, 1986). The caregiver may also have a history of emotional illness or substance abuse (Pillemer & Finkelhor, 1989), poor health, or physical frailty (Lachs &

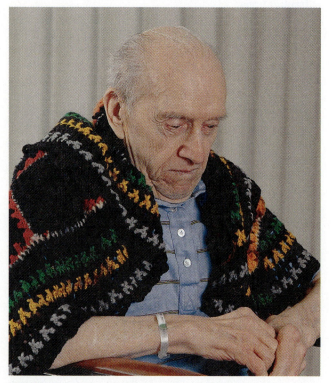

FIGURE 27-3 Behavior changes, such as withdrawal, may indicate mistreatment or abuse.

Fulmer, 1993). In addition, the caregiver may demonstrate unrealistic expectations of the older adult's abilities (Quinn & Tomita, 1986) or a lack of concern for the older adult (Sengstock & Hwalek, 1985).

Characteristics of the older adult that places that person at risk for mistreatment include being 75 years or older (O'Malley et al., 1983), multiple health problems that decrease the older adult's ability to function without assistance (Rounds, 1992), loss of cognitive decision making or dementia (Coyne, Reichman, & Berbig, 1993), substance abuse (Quinn & Tomita, 1986), and overly demanding behavior of the older adult (Kosberg & Cail, 1986).

Important elements to detection and intervention of older adult mistreatment are the health care professionals' knowledge of the mistreatment and recognition of mistreatment as a possible diagnosis. Tilden, Schmidt, Limandri, Chiodo, Garland, and Loveless (1994) reported that 75% of the health care professionals surveyed had not received any education on older adult mistreatment. Additionally, the health care professionals who received education regarding older adult mistreatment were more likely to report older adult abuse than those who did not receive information in family violence (Committee on the Assessment of Family Violence Interventions, 1998). Clinicians are also affected in their judgment of older adult mistreatment by the severity of the situation, the personalities of the older adult and caregiver, and the degree of effort that clinicians perceive the caregiver as expending (Phillips & Rempusheski, 1985).

In evaluating older clients for potential mistreatment, nurses in all care settings must know the state's protective statutes regarding vulnerable older adults. Nurses must know the state's definition of older adult mistreatment. Specifically, the nurse must know if abuse and neglect are defined separately; if psychological mistreatment and financial exploitation are described in the state's statute; if the nurse is a voluntary or mandatory reporter; and what the channels of communication are for notifying the appropriate state agency of suspected older adult mistreatment. Without this information, the nurse will be severely hampered in any attempts to assist a suspected victim of older adult mistreatment (Hall & Weiler, 1996) and in some cases may not even consider the possibility that mistreatment is occurring.

Implications for Nurses

The legal and financial issues of older adults are often not discussed in nursing textbooks. However, these elements are frequently intertwined with providing direct nursing care. If the older client or the client's family is concerned about potential diminishing decision-making capacity, the nurse may identify for the family the potential need for a power of attorney, a durable power of attorney, or a joint tenancy agreement. If the client has already progressed to the stage of diminished or absence of decision-making capacity, the nurse may identify options that the family can pursue with the assistance of an attorney. A judicially appointed conservator may be the best, and perhaps only, avenue available to assist the older client with financial issues.

Think About It

How can you become aware of legal and financial problems that the family members of your clients are experiencing? Would you be prepared to assist them with information and other resources for legal assistance? How can you get prepared?

While recognizing that many families express genuine concern about their older family members, nurses must be alert for signs of older adult mistreatment. The nurse needs to assess for signs or symptoms of physical or psychological mistreatment. Nurses must recognize that physical or psychological harm may be initiated by the staff, friends, family members, or caregivers in the home or institutional setting. The nurse must also recognize that family discussions about the older client's financial holdings may be the family's attempt to determine what financial assets the older adult may have disclosed to the nurse or the nurse's employment agency.

Summary

It is essential that nurses be aware of some of the legal and financial issues that are crucial to an older adult's everyday routine. Many older adults have scarce financial resources to pay for their needs (e.g., food, shelter, or clothing). The older adult must be able to have access to those limited resources (e.g., transportation to the bank) or the older adult must have a surrogate who is willing to assist with financial matters.

For some older adults the primary financial resource that they have is their home. If the older adult lives alone, he or she may not be able to provide for the essential needs even if there is available money. If the older adult is not able to purchase food, cook meals, or spend the money to pay the utility bills, mistreatment may be self-induced. The older adult may need someone to provide assistance (e.g., helping with housework, meals, or writing and mailing checks). The presence of a caregiver may provide the necessary assistance; however, the nurse must recognize that the caregiver may also be a potential source of older adult mistreatment. It is the continuous interaction of many different daily responsibilities that indicates the need for nurses to be familiar with basic legal and financial options and obstacles for older adults.

Review Questions and Activities

1. What are the planning options for financial assets that are available to an adult with decision-making capacity?

2. What are the planning options for financial assets that are available to an adult without decision-making capacity?

3. What are differences between the durable power of attorney and the durable power of attorney for health care? Are they interchangeable?

4. If you were in community or home health nursing, what are some suggestions that you could give to older clients to help protect them against consumer fraud?

5. What are the various forms of older adult mistreatment? Where could such mistreatment occur (e.g., home, long-term care facility)? What types of abuse should the nurse be aware of when caring for an older client?

6. If a nurse does not have any information about older adult mistreatment, what is the most important strategy the nurse could use to assist in protecting older clients?

7. Visit a bank and a credit union. Ask for blank forms for the various forms of joint bank accounts. Compare the terms of the various accounts. If an older adult and another adult were listed on the account, identify who could claim the money in the account if the older adult (a) loses decision-making capacity; (b) dies; (c) dies and has heirs not listed on the account; or (d) retains decision-making capacity and the other adult dies.

8. Monitor the news media for several weeks and identify the various forms of consumer fraud that are identified. Are older adults at heightened risk for any of the forms of consumer fraud? How could the nurse help protect the older client from consumer fraud?

9. Select a home setting (e.g., independent, long-term care, assisted living) and identify a combination of physical, psychological, and social impairments (e.g., diabetes, intermittently confused, no living relatives). Identify different combinations of settings and impairments, and then identify how each older person could be vulnerable to mistreatment.

References

Aiken, T. D., & Catalano, J. T. (1994). *Legal, ethical, and political issues in nursing.* Philadelphia: Davis.

American Bar Association. (1998). *The American Bar Association legal guide for older Americans: The law every American over fifty needs to know.* New York: Random House.

Anetzberger, G. J. (1987). *The etiology of elder abuse by adult offspring.* Springfield, MO: Thomas Publishing.

Arnason, S., Rosenzweig, E., & Koski, A. (1995). *The legal rights of the elderly.* New York: Practicing Law Institute.

Baines, E., & Oglesby, M. (1992). The elderly as caregivers of the elderly. *Holistic Nurse Practitioner, 7*(4), 61–69.

Block, M. R., & Sinnott, J. D. E. (1979). *The battered elder syndrome: An exploratory study.* College Park, MD: University of Maryland Center on Aging.

Boland, D., & Sims, S. (1996). Family care giving at home as a solitary journey. *Image, 26*(1), 55–58.

Bristowe, E. (1989). Family mediated abuse of noninstitutionalized frail elderly men and women living in British Columbia. *Journal of Elder Abuse and Neglect, 1*(1), 45–64.

Carr, K., Dix, G., Fulmer, T., Kaulsh, B., Dravitz, L., Matlaw, J., Mayer, J., Minaher, K., Wetle, T., & Zarle, N. (1986). An elder abuse assessment team in acute hospital setting. *The Gerontologist, 35,* 115–118.

Committee on the Assessment of Family Violence Interventions. (1998). *Violence in families: Assessing prevention and treatment programs.* National Research Council. Washington, DC: National Academy Press.

Council on Scientific Affairs. (1987). Elder abuse and neglect. *Journal of the American Medical Association, 257,* 966–971.

Coyne, A. C., Reichman, W. E., & Berbig, L. J. (1993). The relationship between dementia and elder abuse. *American Journal of Psychiatry, 150,* 643–646.

Fulmer, T. (1992). Clinical outlook: Elder mistreatment assessment as a part of everyday practice. *Journal of Gerontological Nursing, 18*(3), 42–45.

Fulmer, T. T. (1989). Mistreatment of elders. Assessment, diagnosis, and intervention. *Nursing Clinics of North America, 24*(3), 707–716.

Fulmer, T. T., & Cahill, V. M. (1984). Assessing elder abuse: A study. *Journal of Gerontological Nursing, 10*(12), 16–20.

Fulmer, T., McMahon, D., Baer-Hines, M., & Forget, B. (1992). Abuse, neglect, abandonment, violence, and exploitation: An analysis of all elderly patients seen in one emergency department during a six-month period. *Journal of Emergency Nursing, 18,* 505–510.

Gelles, R. J., & Cornell, C. P. (1982, July). Elder abuse: The status of current knowledge. *Family relations, 31,* 457–465.

Grafstrom, M., Nordberg, A., & Wimbald, B. (1992). Abuse is in the eye of the beholder: Reports by family members about age of demented persons in home care: A total population based study. *Scandinavian Journal of Social Medicine, 21*(4), 247–255.

Hagebock, H., & Brandt, K. (1981). *Characteristics of elder abuse.* Unpublished manuscript, University of Iowa Gerontological Center.

Hall, G. R., & Weiler, K. (1996). Elder abuse, neglect and mistreatment. In C. W. Bradway (Ed.), *Nursing care of geriatric emergencies* (pp. 225–251). New York: Springer.

Haviland, S., & O'Brian, J. (1989). Physical abuse and neglect of the elderly: Assessment and intervention. *Orthopaedic Nursing, 8*(4), 11–19.

Hirst, S., & Miller, J. (1986). The abused elderly. *Journal of Psychosocial Nursing, 24*(10), 28–34.

Hogstel, M. O., & Curry, L. C. (1999). Elder abuse revisited. *Journal of Gerontological Nursing, 25*(7), 10–18.

Homer, A. C., & Gilleard, C. (1990). Abuse of elderly people by their carers. *British Medical Journal, 301*(6765), 1359–1362.

Hunzeker, D. (1990). *State legislative response to crimes against the elderly.* Paper presented at the National Conference of State Legislatures, Denver, CO.

Hwalek, M. A., & Sengstock, M. C. (1986). Assessing the probability of abuse of the elderly: Toward development of a clinical screening instrument. *Journal of Applied Gerontology, 5,* 153–173.

Iowa Code, Chapter 235B, §2(1), 1996.

Iowa Department of Elder Affairs. (1992). *Iowa Aging Information* (Memo 92-72). Des Moines, IA: Author.

Kosberg, J. I. (1988). Preventing elder abuse: Identification of high risk factors prior to placement decisions. *The Gerontologist, 28*(1), 43–50.

Kosberg, J., & Cail, R. (1986). The cost of care index: A case management tool for screening informal care providers. *The Gerontologist, 26,* 273–278

Krauskopf, J. M., Brown, R. N., & Tokarz, K. L. (1999, Supplement). *Elderlaw: Advocacy for the aging* (2nd ed.). St. Paul: West Publishing.

Krauskopf, J. M., Brown, R. N., Tokarz, K. L., & Bogutz, A. D. (1993). *Elderlaw: Advocacy for the aging* (2nd ed.). St. Paul: West Publishing.

Lachs, M., & Fulmer, T. (1993). Recognizing elder abuse and neglect. *Clinics in Geriatric Medicine, 9,* 665–681.

Lau, E., & Kosberg, J. (1979). Abuse of the elderly by informal care providers. *Aging, 12,* 10–15.

Mildenberger, C., & Wessman, H. (1986). Abuse and neglect of elderly persons by family members. *Physical Therapy, 66*(4), 537–539.

Neale, A., Hwalek, M., Goodrich, C., & Quinn, K. (1996). The Illinois elder abuse system: Program description and administrative findings. *The Gerontologist, 36*(4), 502–511.

Northrop, C. E., & Kelly, M. E. (1987). *Legal issues in nursing.* St. Louis: Mosby.

O'Malley, T., Everitt, D., & O'Malley, H. (1983). Identifying and preventing family mediated abuse and neglect of elderly persons. *Annals of Internal Medicine, 98,* 998–1005.

Phillips, L. R. (1988). The fit of elder abuse with the family violence paradigm, and the implications of a paradigm shift for clinical practice. *Public Health Nursing, 5*(4), 222–229.

Phillips, L. R., & Rempusheski, V. F. (1985). A decision-making model for diagnosing and intervening in elder abuse and neglect. *Nursing Research, 34*(3), 134–139.

Pillemer, K., & Finkelhor, D. (1988). The prevalence of elder abuse: A random sample survey. *The Gerontologist, 28*(1), 51–57.

Pillemer, K., & Finkelhor, D. (1989). Causes of elder abuse: Caregiver stress versus problem relatives. *American Journal of Orthopsychiatry, 59*(2), 179–187.

Pillemer, K., & Suitor, J. J. (1988). Elder abuse. In R. L. M. V. B. Van Hasselt, A.S. Bellack, & M. Hersen (Eds.), *Handbook of family violence* (pp. 247–270). New York: Plenum Press.

Power of Attorney: Everything you need to know and more . . . about filing Form 2848 at IRS Service Centers. (1998). Department of the Treasury, Internal Revenue Service, Publication 2036.

Problem Resolution Program of the Internal Revenue Service: A guide for taxpayers who have unresolved tax problems with IRS. (1997). Department of the Treasury, Internal Revenue Service, Publication 1546.

Quinn, M. J., & Tomita, S. K. (1986). *Elder abuse and neglect: Causes, diagnosis and intervention strategies.* New York: Springer.

Rounds, L. (1992). Elder abuse and neglect: A relationship to health characteristics. *Journal of the American Academy of Nurse Practitioners, 4*(2), 47–52.

Rowe, J., Davies, K., Baburaj, V., & Sinha, R. (1993). F.A.D.E.A.W.A.Y: The financial affairs of dementing elders and who is the attorney. *Journal of Elder Abuse and Neglect, 5*(2), 73–79.

Sengstock, M., & Hwalek, M. (1985). *Comprehensive index of elder abuse* (2nd ed.). Detroit, MI: SPEC Associates.

Sims, S. L., Boland, D. L., & O'Neill, C. (1992). Decision-making in home health care. *Western Journal of Nursing Research, 14,* 186–200.

Smyer, M., Schaie, K.W., & Kapp, M. B. (1996). *Older adults' decision-making and the law.* New York: Springer.

Steinmetz, S. K. (1990). Elder abuse by adult offspring: The relationship of actual vs. perceived dependency. *Journal of Health and Human Resources Administration, 12*(4), 434–463.

Straus, M., Gelles, R., & Steinmetz, S. (1981). *Behind closed doors: Violence in the American family.* New York: Doubleday.

Strauss, P. J., & Lederman, N. M. (1996). *The elder law handbook: A legal and financial survival guide for caregivers and seniors.* New York: Facts on File.

Tilden, V., Schmidt, T., Limandri, B., Chiodo, G., Garland, M., & Loveless, P. (1994). Factors that influence clinician's assessment and management of family violence. *American Journal of Public Health, 84*(4), 628–633.

Tomita, S. K. (1982). Detection and treatment of elderly abuse and neglect: A protocol for health care professionals. *Physical and Occupational Therapy in Geriatrics, 2,* 37–51.

Weiler, K. (1989). Financial abuse of the elderly: Recognizing and acting on it. *Journal of Gerontological Nursing, 15*(8), 10–15.

Weiler, K., & Buckwalter, K. C. (1992). Abuse among rural mentally ill. *Journal of Psychosocial Nursing and Mental Health Services, 30*(9), 32–36.

Willis, S. L. (1996). Assessing everyday competence in the cognitively challenged elderly. In M. Smyer, K. W. Schaie, & M. B. Kapp (Eds.), *Older adults' decision-making and the law.* New York: Springer.

Wolf, R. (1986). *Major findings from three model projects on elder abuse.* Dover, MA: Auburn House.

Wolf, R. S. (1990). Elder abuse: Scope, characteristics, and treatment. *Nurse Practitioner Forum, 1*(2), 102–108.

Resources

Administration on Aging: `www.aoa.dhhs.gov`

American Association of Retired People (AARP): `www.aarp.org`

UNIT 8

The Future

PERSPECTIVE...

Health care in the future will offer many rewarding, challenging, and innovative roles for nurses. In the year 2015 a gerontological nurse practitioner (GNP) with a master's degree in care coordination (case management) has so many offers of employment that she has difficulty deciding whether to work in a new geriatric medical technology business, a continuum of care health system or a geriatric managed health care organization or join a group of other nurse practitioners in an independent private nurse-owned clinic. All of the positions offer income over $300,000 annually. Geographic location, degree of autonomy, and/or administrative structure of the position will help her decide.

KEY TERMS

aging in place

baby-boom generation

compressed morbidity

generation X

geriatric case managers

geriatrics

gerontologist

personal care attendants (PCAs)

public policy

subacute care units

Supplemental Security Income (SSI)

translocation

CHAPTER 28

Trends and Future Needs

Mildred O. Hogstel, PhD, RN, C

COMPETENCIES

After completing this chapter, the reader should be able to:

- *Discuss the effects of the baby-boom generation on society and health care.*
- *Evaluate the continuum of health care and housing needs for older adults.*
- *Identify future trends in community resources for older adults.*
- *Discuss translocation issues.*
- *Identify the major types of human resources in geriatric health care.*
- *Evaluate medical technology evolving in geriatric health care.*
- *Discuss how legislation affects public policy in health care.*
- *Identify research needs in gerontology health care.*
- *Evaluate trends and predictors for the future that will affect the health, life, and care of older adults.*
- *Describe the evolving role of the nurse in geriatric health care.*

MAKING THE CONNECTION

Refer to the following chapters to increase your understanding trends and future needs:

- **Chapter 1**   Aging Yesterday, Today, and Tomorrow
- **Chapter 2**   Gerontological Nursing
- **Chapter 3**   Changes in the Health Care Delivery System Affecting Older Adults
- **Chapter 8**   Successful Aging
- **Chapter 12**   Health Education
- **Chapter 20**   Home Health Care
- **Chapter 22**   Primary Care Centers
- **Chapter 23**   Hospital Outpatient Care and Services
- **Chapter 24**   Community Organizations and Services
- **Chapter 25**   Ethical Theories and Principles

Evolving Demographics

As a new century begins in the year 2000, predictions for an ever-increasing number of older people age 65 and over will probably be confirmed and updated. The greatest increase will be "between the years 2010 and 2030 when the '**baby boom' generation** reaches age 65" and the percentage of those age 65 and older will increase from 13% in the year 2000 to 20% by 2030 (*A profile,* 1999, p. 2, emphasis added). The baby boomers (76 million born between 1946 and 1964) had a major effect on society when they were born, growing up, starting public school, attending college, and buying homes and starting families. It is difficult to know exactly how they will affect society when they are in their sixties, seventies, eighties, and nineties. Dychtwald (1999) predicted that the twenty-first century will be ruled by the new old, those formerly known as baby boomers. He noted that because of their numbers they grew up in a world of competition (space in schools, club membership, sports, college entrance, jobs, and homes). As they age, the same thing will occur in health care, technology, financial services, work/leisure activities, lifestyle support, housing, and transportation.

Not only will there be more people age 65 and older in the future, but there will be more of the oldest-old category (those age 90–110). In 1998 a 90-year-old surgeon was still performing open-heart surgery and a 77-year-old former astronaut and senator spent 9 days in space. In 1999 an 89-year-old woman was walking from the west coast to the east coast of the United States to protest a political issue in Washington, D.C. There will be more older people accomplishing similar activities in the twenty-first century. In early 2000 the Area Agency

on Aging in one area planned special recognition for all those people who had lived in three centuries, 1800, 1900, and 2000, which is the first time such an event has occurred in the history of mankind. A public reception, personal visit if unable to attend, and other events were planned to honor those special people. More than 100 people age 100 and older lived in the area at the time. Predictions for the future are difficult but challenging. This chapter will attempt to predict future issues and concerns as well as resources and services needed for an increasing aging population (Figure 28-1).

Continuum of Care

The health care delivery system in the United States is changing every day. Change is good and needed. However, often change simply evolves based on needs as they emerge rather on a specific planning process. While it is anticipated that not only will older people live longer in the future (possibly 110–140 years), they will also live healthier longer. Because all life must have an end, the ideal is to live healthy, happy, and content until the day or week before death, thus avoiding many years of chronic debilitating expensive illnesses. A major future goal is **compressed morbidity,** fewer chronic diseases occurring later in life shortly before death. For example, a great-grandmother living in her own home made cookies for her great-grandchildren in the morning, which she enjoyed greatly, and she died later that same night. Perhaps the goal of longer independence and wellness can be accomplished for more people with an increasing emphasis on health promotion, exercise, good nutrition, and improvements in medical technology.

Because older people in the future will be healthier as well as much older (the fastest growing segment of the U.S. population are people age 100 and older), a wide variety of choices will be available to them (Cowley, 1997). In the past, when an older person developed multiple chronic physical and/or mental problems requiring health care, the primary and sometimes first option was a nursing facility if family members could not provide the essential physical care (e.g., bath, gastric tube feedings, and/or urinary catheter care) and supervision in the home on a 24-hour basis. Now there are many other options. In fact, nursing facility census is decreasing (Bectel & Tucker, 1998) because of alternative options. Many long-term care residents in nursing facilities probably do not need to be there and could function just as well in a different kind of setting. Older people, family members, and health care providers need to become familiar with all of the current and emerging community health care and housing options available.

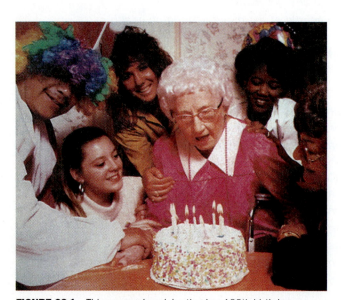

FIGURE 28-1 This woman is celebrating her 100th birthday, surrounded by family and friends.

There is a great need for nurses prepared and interested in gerontological nursing, either as clinical nurse specialists or nurse practitioners, to coordinate and guide older people through the continuum of care in a complex health care delivery system. Hospital stays are short, and some discharge planners may not recognize all of the immediate and long-term care needs of older clients. When a client who has had a cerebrovascular accident (CVA) has to leave the hospital a few days after an acute incident with only a few hours notice, it is dangerous for the client and extremely difficult for the family. They may have to make arrangements for needed medical equipment and supplies for the home and perhaps adjustments in living arrangements for all family members. Discharge planning is supposed to begin at the time of admission to the hospital, but neither client nor family may be ready to make such decisions so soon after a major life-threatening event.

Think About It

A 92-year-old woman had a fractured wrist and was taken to the hospital to have a cast applied. She was taken home shortly after. She lived alone and used a walker frequently. The next day a church visitor found that she slept in her clothes all night because she could not take them off with the cast on her arm. Also, she could not prepare her breakfast so she had not eaten. How could this situation have been prevented?

Community Resources Needed

A wide variety of community resources have been presented in this text. Some of these services are decreasing in availability and cost (e.g., home health care because of 1997 Medicare legislation changes) and some are increasing (such as assisted-living facilities that provide personal care and 24-hour supervision). In fact, one of the fastest growing types of care and housing is assisted living (Figure 28-2). Controversy exists about exactly what role these services should fulfill related to the residents' status and needs. There is a focus on **aging in place**, meaning that when a person moves to a facility from a private home, that individual may live there for the rest of his or her life. That is an excellent concept, but can such a facility meet all of the basic needs, social activities, and health care, including hospice care when it becomes essential? For example, can and should assisted-living facilities (ALFs) care for residents who are primarily confined to bed, those who have difficulty ambulating independently, and those who have urinary retention catheters and/or gastric tube feedings? What are the qualifications and abilities of the employees in these facilities to meet those needs? Many are **personal care attendants (PCAs)**, a type of unlicensed assistive

personnel (UAP), who usually have no specific required standard education, certification, and/or inservice education for what they are doing.

States differ in terms of names, licensing laws, regulations, and staffing of ALFs. Federal regulations do not generally apply because most of these types of homes do not qualify for Medicare and/or Medicaid funding. However, the increasing emphasis on long-term care insurance will provide more financial assistance to residents of ALFs. A few predicted changes in the continuum of care for older adults in the twenty-first century are listed in Box 28-1.

Unfortunately, those older people who do not have adequate financial resources, through pensions, lifelong savings, or investments, may have difficulty finding housing and health care to meet their needs in the future. Although the baby boomers have probably had higher average salaries and incomes than their parents and grandparents, their savings may not be as good as people who lived through the Great Depression of the 1930s and learned to manage with less and save more. Some baby boomers have accumulated debt with multiple high-cost purchases and will have less guaranteed pensions on retirement (Dychtwald, 1999). Decreasing federal and state financing of Medicare and Medicaid also are predicted, thus perhaps decreasing coverage of health care needs for older people in the future.

Translocation Issues

When an older person who may have had an acute illness and several preexisting chronic diseases moves

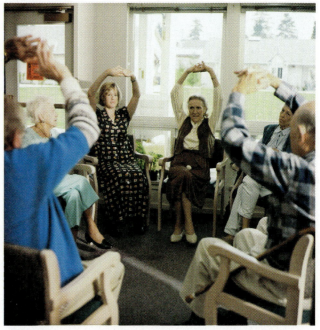

FIGURE 28-2 An exercise class in an assisted-living facility.

BOX 28-1 Health and Housing Options and Needs in the Twenty-First Century

- Increase in shared housing, expenses, and support by family members and friends

- Increase in governmental benefits and payments for home health skilled care services

- Decrease in number of nursing facilities (NFs) that provide long-term custodial care because of increases in ALFs

- Increase in ALFs offering supervised personal (touching) assistance 24 hours a day

- Increase in continuing care retirement communities (CCRCs) or similar concepts without a large initial investment for aging in place

- Increase in inner city high-rise retirement communities close to medical, cultural, and recreational activities

- Increased options for care and assistance in the home with special education and support for family caregivers

from one environment to another, there may be difficulties in orientation and adjustment. When a person of any age takes a vacation trip and sleeps in several locations, that person may be temporarily disoriented when getting up to go to the bathroom at 3:00 AM. An older person also may have some difficulty adjusting to different locations in a short period of time. The person may think that a door to the hall or closet is the bathroom door and feel lost or possibly urinate there and then fall on a wet slippery floor when attempting to go back to bed. If any kind of dementia is a diagnosis, the problems can be worse because of the sundown syndrome (Merrin, 1996). A safe, secure, and stable environment is one of the factors most important in the treatment and care of people with dementia.

The nurse and other health care providers need to be aware of the issue of translocation and orient clients to new environments and facilities. What happens the first few hours and days in a new environment may affect the person's physical and mental status as well as ultimate adjustment to the move. In the absence of short-term delirium caused by a physical problem or dementia related to an organic disease, older people can learn just as well as any other age group. It is the nurses' responsibility to assess the clients' needs and determine adjustments in orienting and teaching a client about a new environment. Effective, sensitive communication is essential and probably the most important continuing

nursing function in any setting. Allowing time for older people to adapt to a new environment also is important.

Geriatric Health Care

Geriatric health care has improved greatly in the last few decades in the United States, but it still has a long way to go, probably more in the area of human resources than in research and technology.

Human Resources

Robert Butler, a physician, **gerontologist**, and psychiatrist, founded and is the former chairman of the Department of Geriatrics and Adult Development at the Mount Sinai Medical Center in New York. It was the first department of **geriatrics** in a medical school in the United States. In 1975 Butler also served as the founding director of the National Institute of Aging of the National Institutes of Health. He received a Lifetime Achievement Award in the field of Living with Chronic Health Conditions from the American Association of Retired Persons Andrus Foundation in 1998 (AARP Andrus Foundation, 1998).

Although not all medical schools have a separate department of geriatrics, more are beginning to require student rotations in areas of clinical geriatrics. In 1997, a 95-year-old physician (Irving Wright) noted that "every medical school should have a program involving aging" (Reinemer, 1997a, p. 4). The number of fellowship-trained and board-certified specialists in geriatric medicine is still low in most areas. For example, in one large urban area there are only four fellowship-trained geriatricians and three geriatric psychiatrists among the 2,400 licensed physicians in the area. Managed care insurance plans should consider a geriatrician as a primary care provider (PCP) and not a specialist, just as a pediatrician is a PCP or gatekeeper for children (Figure 28-3). However, when asked about this issue, insurance salespersons often do not even know what a geriatrician is. Medicare health maintenance organization (HMOs) also should employ geriatricians and **geriatric case managers** such as gerontological clinical nurse specialists to ensure that a continuum of quality holistic care is provided.

Think About It

The baby boomers will increase the need for geriatricians after 2011 as they did for pediatricians after 1946.

Although gerontological nursing content is included in most basic nursing programs in some way, not all programs have a required course in gerontological nursing.

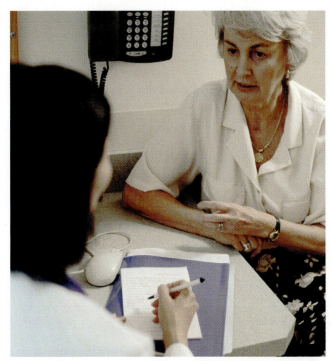

FIGURE 28-3   Insurance companies should consider a geriatrician as a primary care provider.

The number of schools requiring a separate course in gerontological nursing has increased in recent years. However, one study found that still only 23% of baccalaureate degree nursing programs in the United States had a specific course in gerontology (Rosenfeld, Bottrell, Fulmer, & Mezey, 1999). Gerontology content may be integrated in several courses, including clinical experiences in the community such as in senior centers (Schneiderman, Jordan-Marsh, & Bates-Jensen, 1998). It is important that these experiences be positive and rewarding for students so that they will consider employment in areas of gerontology after graduation.

Only 7% of the working registered nurse population in the United States specialize in gerontological nursing (Institute of Medicine, 1996). The demand for such nurses will increase in the future as various types of long-term care facilities expand and acute care hospitals' occupancy rates decrease. Hospitals added skilled nursing units (SNUs), rehabilitation units, and community

---

Research Focus

Citation:
Schneiderman, J. U., Jordan-Marsh, M. A., & Bates-Jensen, B. (1998). Senior centers: Shifting student paradigms. *Journal of Gerontological Nursing, 24*(10), 24–30.

Purpose:
To evaluate an innovative community learning experience for new nursing students with older adults.

Methods:
One hundred twenty-eight junior nursing students were assigned to one of five centers for 5 weeks. Questionnaires were designed and given after the 5-week rotation to the students, teaching assistants, center directors, and sample older adult recipients.

Findings:
All four groups reported the experience as positive. However, the students had difficulty applying some classroom content such as the nursing process and health assessment skills. They were more likely to be able to apply teaching-learning content. The teaching assistants reported that the students needed better preparation in the areas of communication and gerontology.

Implications:
The best placement and objectives for this type of experience must be evaluated carefully so that students do not develop a negative attitude about caring for older adults.

Ask Yourself

- Does the curriculum in your nursing program include a specific, separate, and required course in gerontological nursing? If the answer is "no," why not?
- To what extent do other nursing courses such as growth and development, adult nursing, mental health nursing, and community nursing include specific information related to older adults?

---

health care clinics especially for older adults in an attempt to regain customers lost when hospital reimbursements and lengths of stay were decreased. However, they are also being closed because of decreased Medicare funding.

The number of nurses interested in and with special education and experience in the care of older adults is continuing to expand as society, especially the baby boomers, expect to receive more specialized health and nursing care as they age. See Table 28-1 for the categories and numbers of nurses certified by the American Nurses Credentialing Center (ANCC) in the three special areas of gerontology.

Gerontological nurse practitioners (GNPs) and geriatric case managers are especially increasing in numbers in many areas of health care. Nurses with these types of preparation who can assess needs and provide and/ or arrange for holistic care for older adults will have

TABLE 28-1 **American Nurses Credentialing Center Gerontological Nurses Certified, 1997–2000**

Category	1997			Total Number, 2000
	Number Taking Exam	Number Passing	Percent Passing Rate	
Gerontological nurse generalist	4,721	3,469	73.5	18,338
Gerontological clinical nurse specialist	100	55	55.0	847
Gerontological nurse practitioner	492	332	67.5	3,380

Sources: *American Nurses Credentialing Center. (Spring, 1999).* Credentialing News, *2(1), 5; American Nurses Credentialing Center. (2000, November 9).* Personal correspondence.

numerous choices for employment in the twenty-first century. Current and emerging sites of practice for GNPs and case managers are listed in Box 28-2.

Although not new, community nursing organizations (CNOs) continue to provide nurse-managed care that specifically benefits older people on Medicare. Four pilot programs, funded by the Health Care Financing Administration (HCFA), continue to provide comprehensive services, including a focus on "health promotion and disease prevention" as well as some of the newer "alternative and complementary therapies such as therapeutic touch, biofeedback, and visualization therapy to promote comfort" (Burtt, 1998, p. 54). Nurses have a tremendous opportunity to meet the needs of older people in community settings. Nurses are well respected and develop good continuing relationships with their clients, who respond well to their services and special care.

Nursing Tip

Encourage your older clients and their family members to be more assertive when receiving care from a physician, nurse, or other health care provider. They have a right to have the best treatment and care that are available regardless of their age or condition.

Medical Technology

Scientific technology is one of the most effective components of the health care delivery system in the United States. New electronic monitors, artificial organs, all kinds of medications and similar substances, and computerized devices and medical records improve the quality of life for people and make treatment and care easier for health care providers. Much of the new technology has con-

BOX 28-2 **Current and Emerging Practice Sites for Gerontological Nurses**

- Hospitals (acute and rehabilitation)
- Utilization review and quality management in institutions and health insurance plans
- Discharge planning and health education
- Telephone medical case managers for health care institutions and health insurance companies
- Legal nurse consulting focusing on quality of care issues
- Health insurance plans including HMOs
- Clinics (physician groups, community neighborhood centers, malls)
- Home health care agencies
- Medical product companies
- Independent practice
- Skilled nursing facilities (SNFs)
- Subacute care units in SNFs
- Hospital skilled nursing units (SNUs)
- Assisted-living facilities
- Continuing care retirement communities

Adapted from "Case Management: A Training Ground for LNCs," 1998, Journal of Legal Nurse Consulting, *9(3), 25.*

tributed to the increasing life expectancy throughout the world. The creative and discovery potential of the human mind is endless. Questions related to many of these "medical miracles" primarily relate to cost and possibly ethics.

Ask Yourself

- Can society afford to provide *every* woman age 40 and over a mammogram *every* year as recommended by the American Cancer Society?
- Should a 75-year-old woman receive a heart transplant?
- Should a 90-year-old man receive kidney dialysis?

An ever-increasing aging population also increases a business focus on new technology that will improve and enhance the quality and quantity of life (Fagerstrom, 1998). Some emerging technologies specifically related to geriatric health care are listed in Table 28-2.

Legislation and Public Policy

Nurses can and must be directly involved in advocating strongly for both state and federal legislation that will initiate and/or strengthen **public policy** to improve the health and life of older adults. Nurses have the knowledge, experience, and communication skills to influence health care, nursing, and aging legislation. Advocacy includes such activities as listed in Box 28-3.

Health care, housing, finances, and transportation are topics that are of vital interest to older people and organizations such as the American Association of Retired Persons (AARP). Two of the most important concerns are Social Security and Medicare. For example, should Social Security funds be invested in the stock market? Some believe that it would mean higher benefits and others think it would be too risky (Aaron & Myers, 1999). Some federal legislators want to privatize Medicare completely, but how would that affect choices, costs, and benefits?

Some of the specific issues that will likely require legislative action in the future are listed in Box 28-4.

Think About It

Will Social Security and Medicare be there when you need them?

Research Needs

As more students and health care providers in all disciplines become involved and interested in the field of gerontology, more research in their fields of interest and specialties will be generated. There is a special need to study issues related to the health care needs of people in their 90s and 100s as these age groups increase in numbers. There is also a need to study the aging process and health care needs in subgroups of older people based on culture and ethnicity. How do their needs differ? How can nurses learn to assess and meet their needs in a sensitive manner? Some of these issues relate to direct care and others affect the way health care delivery is evolving. See Box 28-5 for a list of suggested ideas for research related to both issues.

Burggraff and Barry (1998) and Gueldner et al. (1995) proposed the following needs for research:

- Evaluation of clinical interventions
- Quality of life
- Healthy lifestyles
- New theories of aging
- Phenomena of aging redefined
- Culture-sensitive instruments
- Innovation in education of nurses
- Analysis of new systems of health care delivery

TABLE 28-2 Emerging Technology in Geriatric Health Care	
Technology	**Uses**
Tiny devices implanted in the body that send out signals to the nervous system	Relieve pain, prevent tremors, prevent incontinence, Parkinson's disease
New types of hip, knee, and shoulder joint implants	Osteoarthritis pain, traumatic injuries
Lightweight flexible extremity prostheses	Diabetes gangrene, peripheral vascular disease (PVD), ulcers causing amputation of a lower extremity
Low-pressure mattresses and other alternating air beds	Prevent pressure ulcers and other skin problems

Adapted from "Companies Catering to Needs of Aging Populace Stand to Benefit," by S. Fagerstrom, July 19, 1998, *Fort Worth Star-Telegram, p. F-2.*

BOX 28-3   Keys to Effective Legislative Advocacy

- Study the issues and the legislative process.

- Decide what needs to be changed.

- Become active and encourage others to do the same.

- Identify the key contacts (legislators, committee members, staff members).

- Know the legislators.

- Establish a relationship with the legislator and his or her staff.

- Work in candidates' campaigns.

- Contribute to candidates' campaigns and Political Action Commitees (e.g., American Nurses Association).

- Write to the legislators:
  - Be concise, to the point, raising only one issue on one page.
  - Use proper title and correct spelling of names.
  - State purpose in first paragraph.
  - Use a personal letterhead.
  - Use your own words in a personal letter.
  - Discuss timely content—current issues, identify by bill number and name.
  - Provide accurate, relevant, compelling, and timely information and facts.
  - Give related personal experiences (if appropriate).
  - Discuss how proposed action affects you, family members, or friends.
  - Ask for a response.
  - Type and sign personally.
  - Do not be a pen pal (write too often).
  - Send a handwritten note only if clearly written.
  - Write for self (officers write for organizations).
  - Do not send petitions as they are not very effective.
  - Write a thank you note, or if a note is unfavorable, write a polite note expressing disappointment.

- Telephone, fax, or e-mail legislators if action is to be taken in 24–48 hours.
  - Try to find out which is preferred by the legislator (fax is better than e-mail).
  - Leave a message with the appropriate staff member.

- Organize a telephone tree:
  - Be sure all people called know what facts to discuss.

- Visit the legislators' offices:
  - Tell what you want.
  - Be brief.
  - Be polite.
  - Be open to negotiation.

- Testify at public hearings:
  - Check agenda, time limits, and room set-up early.
  - Provide multiple copies of the presentation to members and media.
  - Be brief and to the point.
  - Encourage others to present, but do not duplicate content.

- Don'ts: Do's:
  - Make demands.   - Be polite, honest, and courteous.
  - Threaten.
  - Harass.   - Send thank you letters.
  - Get angry.
  - Stay too long in the office.

- Write a draft of a bill and discuss with a legislator's aide first:
  - Only certain bills can be introduced after the first 60 days.
  - Get a strong group to support it (e.g., American Nurses Association, American Association of Retired Persons).
  - Get media coverage (TV and newspaper).
  - Have a rally of the public at the capitol to increase public awareness and education.

BOX 28-3 Keys to Effective Legislative Advocacy *continued*

- Keep up with status of current legislative proposals:
  - Call, fax, or e-mail the office of your senator or representative.
- Thank legislators for their efforts when appropriate.
- For congressional information go to www.house.gov or www.senate.gov.
- For Medicare reform information go to www.medicare.gov.

- Summary:
  - Set goals and organize.
  - Determine groups to help.
  - Determine groups that are against and why.
  - Determine tactics.
  - Be strong advocates.

Appreciation is expressed to Alma Burnam, Senior Political Action Committee of Tarrant County, Texas, and Reed Bilz and Margaret De Moss of the League of Women Voters of Tarrant County for their suggestions.

Trends

As discussed throughout this book, several issues emerge as future trends. Some of the most important ones include:

- Care for increasing numbers of those in their 90s and 100s
- Need for more geriatric care (case) managers in the community

- Need for more emphasis on health promotion and wellness in community centers and assisted-living and long-term care facilities
- Evaluation of quality of care for nursing facility residents on Medicaid in HMOs
- Development of more diverse housing options available with several categories of personal care assistance

BOX 28-4 Possible Future Federal and State Legislation Affecting Older Adults

- Medicare—Will there be more or less coverage? How high will the premiums go? Will the total structure change?
- Medicaid—Will there be block grants to states? How will states allocate those funds?
- HMOs—Will they become the only choice for Medicare recipients? Will there be other choices? Will there be more client protection legislation?
- Social Security—Will there be decreased payments? Will it be means tested based on income?
- Nursing facility regulations—Will there be more or fewer federal and/or state regulations?
- Assisted-living facilities—Will they continue to increase in number? How will they change?
- Availability of health care—Can society afford what is needed for all age groups?

- Caregiving—Will there be increased tax deductions for family members who care for an older member in the home?
- Transportation—What kind of local affordable accessible transportation can be provided to those oldest-old who cannot or do not want to drive?
- Quality of health care—What should be the legal requirements for assistant technicians in health care (hospitals, home health care, assisted-living facilities, pharmacies)?
- Federally funded housing—Where will indigent, older people live?
- Home health care—How should it be regulated and paid for?
- Long-term chronic and custodial health care—Where will it be provided, how will it be funded, and who will provide it?

BOX 28-5   Suggested Ideas for Research

Direct Care

- Do older people perceive, react to, and respond to pain differently than other adults? How do older people respond (react) to acute and chronic pain?

- How do older people define quality health care and quality of life? How can their health care and lives be improved?

- Are falls in health care facilities (hospitals, nursing facilities, assisted-living facilities) accidental or a result of negligence? How can they be prevented and still provide as much freedom of movement as possible?

- What are the essential resources that a 95-year-old widower needs to live at home alone?

- Which generic medications are not safe or act differently than trade name medications in older people?

- What is the average number of routine and as-needed medications given in nursing facilities? What are the implications in terms of adverse effects and costs?

- How does sleep differ for older people?

- What are the major cultural, ethnic, and racial differences in physiological, psychological, and social aging?

- What are health education needs of different cultural groups?

- Will the trend to alternative therapies be accepted and ordered by traditional medical practitioners?

Health Care Delivery

- To what extent is preventive health care emphasized in nursing facilities (e.g., annual mammograms)? How can it be improved?

- How much do Medicare recipients pay for prescription and over-the-counter (OTC) medications? Medicare only? Medicare and Medigap? HMOs? To what extent is this a problem? What is the best proposed policy to help meet this need?

- What are the primary concerns, conflicts, problems, and needs of certified nurse aides (CNAs) in nursing facilities?

- What percentage of home health agencies are accredited by Joint Commission on the Accreditation of Healthcare Organizations (JCAHO)?

- How does home health care differ in benefits for Medicare HMOs and original Medicare?

- How does the quantity and quality of health care for older people differ in private not-for-profit and for-profit hospitals, nursing facilities, and home health agencies?

- What are the primary needs of informal/family caregivers of older people?

- What are the primary methods of transportation for older people to obtain health care? How can this need be met?

- What is the best environment for older people who have multiple chronic health problems and require supervised living?

- Increasing optional surgery (e.g., knee replacements) common for those in their 90s and 100s

- Eligibility age for Social Security and Medicare increased to 67, 70, or beyond

- More people age 65 and older employed longer in full- or part-time jobs based on personal preference and not economic needs

- Increasing use of alternative medicine such as herbs and acupuncture by older adults

- More medical students interested in geriatric medicine because of effects of the baby-boom generation, more emphasis on primary care, and more research scholarships, clinical programs, and incentives to specialize in the care of older adults (Willingham, 1997)

Predictions for the Future

It is difficult and dangerous but challenging and rewarding to attempt to look into the future. Gerontology is one field in health care and social services that will affect public policy in the next 50 years. Some of these challenging predictions are:

- Safer, more comfortable, and faster group transportation will be available for older adults in community settings as well as for greater distances.

- Six-generation families living will be common, although they will live in diverse settings, making care of the oldest-old more difficult.

- There will be fewer family caregivers for the oldest-old because the baby boomers and their children married later and had fewer children (Figure 28-4).

- **Generation X** will need to learn how to assist their baby boomer parents as they age.

- With later retirement, there will be an aging work force and more focus on wellness and health education provided by employers.

- Assessment of health care needs, management of care, and health education will increasingly be available by way of telephones, computers, and television (telephonic nursing and telemedicine).

- Medicare HMOs will continue to decrease in numbers and benefits, leaving older people with the problem of having to change physicians they have had for a long time and with no or limited coverage of prescription medications for a time.

- Original Medicare Part B will add a limited prescription medication benefit and cover more preventive services.

- Baby boomers will demand changes in the organization of the health care delivery system and will "have the ability and desire to share medical decisions with their providers" (Grosel, Hamilton, Koyana, & Eastwood, 2000, p. 132).

- More health care information, advice, and services (e.g., ordering medications) will be available on the Internet.

- Prevention, cure, and effective treatment for Alzheimer's disease will occur in the early part of the twenty-first century.

- More focus and assistance will be provided on the issue of informal/family caregiving of older people, especially as more people in their 70s are caring for people in their 90s and 100s. Universities will develop caregiver centers for the purpose of support and education of caregivers and research on their needs and resources (Carter, 1997).

- Women will continue to live longer than men (Cowley, 1997) (Figure 28-5).

John Rother, Director of Legislation and Public Policy for the AARP, predicted that there will be more income and ethnic diversity among the baby boomers as they age and that the wealthy boomers in the future will have a "loud voice" politically (Reinemer, 1997b, p. 10). They will have more focus on individual responsibility and want more choice in health care. Some members of Congress (baby boomers) will not want to continue social safety nets such as welfare, **Supplemental Security Income (SSI)**, and benefits for immigrants. However, that leaves the other segment of baby boomers (those who are not saving for retirement are estimated at 50%, and 15% of them have no health insurance) who will have economic and health care needs. This group is not very politically active, and baby boomers in general have no organized voice or leaders.

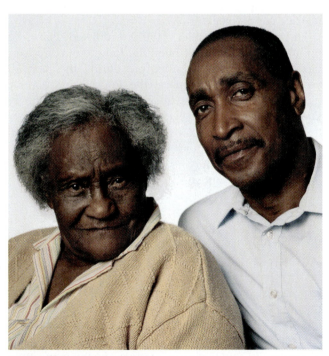

FIGURE 28-4 Smaller family size directly impacts the availability of caregivers for the older adult.

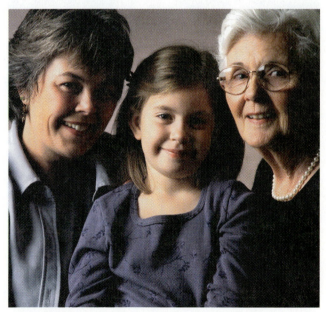

FIGURE 28-5 Women will continue to live longer than men.

Rother also predicted that "the biggest threat to boomers as a group is the rising cost of health care" (Reinemer, 1997b, p. 13), especially the cost of chronic illness and long-term care. He also noted that baby boomers had fewer children and more divorces, so that there will be fewer children to care for them when they get old (Reinemer, 1997b).

Irving Wright, a 95-year-old physician (Reinemer, 1997b, p. 3), has suggested that:

- Older people should continue their education.

- People should continue to be active mentally and physically (Figure 28-6).

- People should not retire as early as 55 or 60 because it is detrimental to their health and to the future health of the country.

- Because of health care advancements, diseases common in the aging process are occurring later in life.

- Medical professionals should continue to research a variety of diseases and there may be progress on Alzheimer's disease.

Ask Yourself

Will the children of generation X, those born between 1984 and 2004, have more or fewer children than their parents? Do you think birth rates will continue to decrease worldwide? Why?

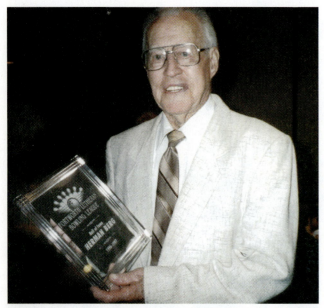

FIGURE 28-6 This 95-year-old man has just won an award from his bowling league.

Burggraf and Barry (1998) predicted that current nurses will need to rely on continuing education programs to learn more about aging issues because most of them did not have formal education in the specialty; more electronic technology including the Internet will be used in the classroom; a master's degree in nursing will eventually be the entry level into nursing; nurses will become architects, controllers, and marketing directors; and community colleges will offer various types of degrees in gerontology. They also predicted more gerontological nurses in the workplace because of an aging workforce; more education and supervision of unlicensed assistive personnel (UAP) who will be certified in all settings; more nurse positions in businesses where older people travel and eat; increased support and care for family caregivers of older people; development of geriatric hospitals; and a return to private duty nurses for affluent older people. They also see more advanced practice nurses (APNs) as managed care providers; the decline of nursing facilities; more hospice care; and respite care coverage by health care plans (Burggraff & Barry, 1998).

Dychtwald (1999) predicted an increase in anti-aging-related research projects that will continue to increase longevity; specialty treatment centers for specific body parts such as eyes and bones within an Internet-based health system; cloned body parts (e.g., kidneys) for replacement purposes; new tissue and organs created to be transplanted; and robotic home care nurses and aides to help people with chronic health problems to remain independent at home. The possibilities are endless as researchers and health care providers test out new ways to manage old problems.

Beck and Chambler (1997) predicted that "the number of consumers needing long-term care services . . . will more than triple during the next 30 years" (p. 12). In summary, the injured and acutely ill will be cared for in hospitals and/or community **subacute care units** (Levenson, 1998), and the chronically ill, who will decrease in number with more emphasis on wellness and health promotion, will live with minimal assistance as needed in a variety of community settings until shortly before death.

Gerontological Nursing: Where to Go from Here

The role of the gerontological nurse will be vital in the twenty-first century, especially in the areas of management, supervision, leadership, advocacy, and public policy. Baby boomers will be better educated than most older people traditionally have been in the past, probably will have more income, and they will be more assertive in demanding quality health care. Most of them were probably in some type of MCO (managed care organization) while they were employed so they should know how to maneuver the system. However, nurses in the future have to understand the evolving health care delivery system so that they can educate and be strong advocates for their clients and families who need information and assistance, especially those who are acutely or chronically ill and those who need a strong safety net and support.

Nurses also need to take the lead in focusing more on interdisciplinary planning and care so that older people will receive the holistic care they need in whatever setting is appropriate. When there are gaps in care and services, nurses should be strong advocates by working for changes in health care institution and agency philosophy and policies as well as in public policy through legislative efforts when needed.

> ### Nursing Tip
>
> Nurses—Speak up and out for your patients!

Summary

No one can predict the future, but it is stimulating to try to look into the twenty-first century. Some facts are known, such as the increasing number of older people, especially those in their late 80s, 90s, and 100s. Many questions arise when considering the needs of the baby boomers beginning in 2011. For example, where will they live and receive health care? What new community resources will evolve to meet their needs? To what extent will geriatric health care providers such as geriatricians and gerontological nurse practitioners be available to them? What new medical technology and alternative therapies will be needed and available? What new vaccinations and cures for diseases will be discovered? What diseases will be eliminated in the twenty-first century (such as smallpox and poliomyelitis were in the twentieth century)?

Most of all, what will be the role of nurses when most of their clients, residents, and customers will be age 65 and older? All nurses need to be more active in initiating and pursuing federal and state legislation to impact public policy that will improve the health care and quality of life for older people. Nurses must be active and speak up for quality of health care for older people in all settings. If nurses do not, who will?

Review Questions and Activities

1. Who are the baby boomers and what effects will they have on society as they age?

2. Where do most older people live?

3. Describe the continuum of care in your community and discuss examples of each type of care.

4. What are major community resources older adults are lacking in your local community?

5. Why are more medical students becoming interested in the field of geriatric medicine?

6. Where will gerontological nurses be employed in the future?

7. Why is there an increasing emphasis on alternative therapies among older adults?

8. What are the legislative and public policy priorities for aging in the early twenty-first century?

9. Of the research needs listed, which ones do you think are most important?

10. Identify several predictions for the future of aging and health care.

11. Visit an American Association of Retired Persons or a nursing political action committee meeting.

12. What is the most important future role of the gerontological nurse?

References

Aaron, H., & Myers, R. J. (1999, March). Should a portion of Social Security funds be invested in the stock market? *AARP Bulletin*, pp. 29–30.

AARP Andrus Foundation. (1998, September 23). 30th anniversary year donor recognition and awards gala. Washington, DC.

A profile of older Americans: 1999. (1999). Washington, DC: American Association of Retired Persons and Administration on Aging, U.S. Department of Health and Human Resources.

Beck, C., & Chambler, N. (1997). Planning for the future of long-term care: Consumers, providers, and purchasers. *Journal of Gerontological Nursing, 23*(8), 6–13.

Bectel, R. W., & Tucker, N. G. (Eds.). (1998). *Across the states. Profiles of long-term care systems* (3rd ed.). Washington, DC: American Association of Retired Persons.

Burggraf, V., & Barry, R. (1998). Gerontological nursing in the 21st century. *Journal of Gerontological Nursing, 24*(6), 29–35.

Burtt, K. (1998). Nurses step to forefront of elder care. *American Journal of Nursing, 98*(6), 52–57.

Carter, R. (1997, Spring). Building a strong future for caregivers. *Innovations in Aging.* Washington, DC: National Council on the Aging.

Cowley, G. (1997, June 30). How to live to be 100. *Newsweek,* pp. 56–65.

Dychtwald, K. (1999). *Age power.* New York: Jeremy P. Tarcher/Putnam.

Fagerstrom, S. (1998, July 19). Companies catering to needs of aging populace stand to benefit. *Fort Worth Star-Telegram,* F2.

Grosel, C., Hamilton, M., Koyana, J., & Eastwood, S. (Eds.). (2000). *Health and health care 2010. The forecast, the challenge.* San Francisco: Jossey-Bass.

Gueldner, S., Brant, B., Joyce-Nagata, B., Kaeser, L., Kitchen, E. K., LoMonaco, M., Paul, P., Thatcher Winger, R., & Dye, C. A. (1995). Gerontological nursing issues and demands beyond the year 2000. *Journal of Gerontological Nursing, 21*(6), 6–8.

Institute of Medicine. (1996). *Nursing staff in hospitals and nursing homes: Is it adequate?* Washington, DC: National Academy Press.

Levenson, S. A. (1998). Sub-acute settings: Making the most of a new model of care. *Geriatrics, 53*(7), 69–75.

Levin, J. (1998, Spring). Alternative health care. *NCGNP Newsletter, 59,* 1–2.

Merrin, E. L. (1996). Sleep disorders. In E. T. Lonergan (Ed.), *Geriatrics.* Stamford, CT: Appleton and Lange.

Passing scores and rates, ANCC Certification Examinations, October 1997. (1999, Spring). *ANCC Credentialing News, 1*(1), 8.

Reinemer, M. (1997a, Summer). A pioneer looks to the future. *Innovations in Aging* (pp. 3–5). Washington, DC: National Council on the Aging.

Reinemer, M. (1997b). Boomers and the politics of aging. *Innovations in Aging* (pp. 10–13). Washington, DC: National Council on the Aging.

Rosenfeld, P., Bottre, II, M., Fulmer, T., & Mezey, M. (1999). Gerontological nursing content in baccalaureate nursing programs: Findings from a national survey. *Journal of Professional Nursing, 15*(3), 84–94.

Schneiderman, J. U., Jordan-Marsh, M. A., & Bates-Jensen, B. (1998). Senior centers: Shifting student paradigms. *Journal of Gerontological Nursing, 24*(10), 24–30.

Willingham, T. (1997, Spring). The promise of a new era for geriatrics. *Innovations in Aging.* Washington, DC: National Council on the Aging.

Resources

Administration on Aging: **www.aoa.dhhs.gov**

Alzheimer's Association: **www.alz.org**

American Association of Retired People: **www.aarp.org**

American Geriatrics Society: **www.americangeriatrics.org**

Gerontological Society of America: **http://www.geron.org**

MedWeb: Geriatrics: **www.medweb.emory.edu/medweb**

National Council on the Aging: **http://www.ncoa.org**

GLOSSARY

access to services. Community services made available to older adults.

accreditation. Voluntary standards usually set by a national organization.

acrochordons. Small flesh-colored skin tags on neck, trunk, axilla, and groin.

activities. Physical, mental, and social functions that contribute to successful aging.

acupuncture. A method of producing analgesia by inserting thin, wirelike needles at specific body sites.

addiction. Compulsive, uncontrollable dependence on a substance or habit to the point where this becomes a major or life-controlling function.

adherence. Following a treatment/medication regimen prescribed by a health care provider.

Administration on Aging (AOA). Federal agency responsible for the Older Americans Act of 1965 and funding for certain state and local aging services.

adult day services. A place where older adults can stay during the day and receive medical and social services.

advanced cardiac life support (ACLS). An American Heart Association designation for the latter end of a continuum of efforts to restore cardiovascular/cardiopulmonary function and includes defibrillation, advanced airway management, and arrhythmia intravenous medication.

advance directive. Written legal documents (e.g., living will) stating a person's preference for life-sustaining treatments.

Advanced Practice Nurse (APN). Nurses with advanced education and experience as a nurse practitioner, clinical nurse specialist, nurse midwife, or nurse anesthetist.

adverse drug events. Medication side effects that can be dangerous.

advocate. A person who takes action for the needs of older adults.

affective. A domain of learning that relates to emotions, attitudes, and personal values; it occurs when the learner exhibits awareness, interest, attention, concern, responsibility, interaction, or acceptance of the subject matter.

affective assessment. Evaluation of mood.

age conflict. Opposition of the social, political, or economic interests of different age groups.

age-integrated social structure. A social structure in which the roles, norms, and values for age-appropriate behaviors are the same throughout the life course.

ageism. Negative actions, terms, and labels for older adults based on poor attitudes and lack of adequate information and knowledge about aging.

age normative. Those causes of developmental change that are highly correlated with age; they may be biological, social, or behavioral in nature.

age norms. Shared expectations of appropriate age-related behaviors for different age groups.

agent. Someone who officially and legally acts for another person.

age roles. The activities, rights, and responsibilities that accompany a particular position for people in different age groups in society.

age-segregated social structure. A social structure in which the roles, norms, and values for age-appropriate behaviors are strictly tied to age strata.

age structure. The roles, norms, and values for age-appropriate behavior within the basic social institutions, including the economy, family, educational system, political system, religion, leisure institutions, and the community.

age values. The values of individuals based on age.

aging in place. Continuing to live in one place despite changes in condition and needs.

Alcoholics Anonymous (AA). A national self-help organization for the treatment of alcoholism based on a 12-step program to maintain sobriety.

alendronate (Fosamax). Bone resorption inhibitor. Medication used to prevent and/or treat osteoporosis in women after menopause.

alternative therapies. Herbs, vitamins, and touch and music therapy not usually used in traditional medicine.

Alzheimer's and Related Disorders Association. A voluntary national organization that sponsors public education programs and provides services to clients and families.

Alzheimer's disease (AD). A chronic, progressive, irreversible form of dementia.

American Association for Geriatric Psychiatry. A professional organization of psychiatrists whose special interest is the mental health care of older adults.

American Association of Retired Persons (AARP). National active organization for persons age 50 and older that focuses on helping older Americans to live independently with dignity and purpose.

American Cancer Society (ACS). A national, voluntary organization that focuses on research, education, and services related to cancer.

American Geriatrics Society (AGS). A national organization of health care providers concerned with providing quality health care for older adults.

American Nurses Association (ANA). National association for registered nurses.

American Nurses' Credentialing Center (ANCC). National organization that certifies various types of nursing specialists based on experience and education.

Americans with Disabilities Act (ADA). Federal law that requires certain institutions and businesses to provide for access and mobility of people with disabilities.

andragogy. The art and science of teaching adults where the student is placed at the center of the learning environment; learning, rather than teaching, is emphasized and collaborative relationships among students and between the student and the instructor are promoted.

andropause. Male stage of life similar to menopause, usually more psychological than physical symptoms.

aneurysm. Localized abnormal weakening or dilitation of a blood vessel, usually an artery.

ankle-brachial index. An index derived by dividing pressure in the brachial and posterior tibial artery and used to determine the adequacy of peripheral arterial circulation.

antagonist. A medication that has an opposite action to another medication.

aphasia. Impaired ability to communicate.
  expressive. Impaired ability to communicate verbally.
  receptive. Impaired ability to understand.
  global. Impaired ability to speak or understand.

appeals process. The sequence of individuals, institutions, and agencies to which one can appeal an action and/or decision by a health care provider or an insurance company.

appraisal. That process by which evaluation and interpretation occur.

arcus senilis. A white deposit of fat around the outer surface of the iris that does not normally interfere with vision.

Area Agency on Aging (AAA). Local agency that monitors services for older adults through Older Americans Act funding.

arrhythmia. Irregularity of the heart rhythm.

arthritis. Many types of diseases that affect the bones, joints, and/or muscles.

Arthritis Foundation (AF). Provides general information and referral services for people with arthritis.

As People Grow Older (APGO). A 12-hour educational course for informal caregivers of older adults.

aspiration. The inhaling of a substance other than air.

assault. Threatening a person with bodily harm or injury or fearful that bodily harm will occur.

assertiveness. Being active in speaking out and seeking answers and solutions to concerns and problems.

assignment. Health care provider accepts the amount Medicare allows for 80% of the cost.

assisted-living facility (ALF). A facility that provides 24-hour supervision. May or may not provide personal care assistance such as bathing, dressing, and eating to those who are unable to live alone.

assisted suicide. Assisting a person to commit suicide, perhaps by providing a lethal dose of medication.

atelectasis. Abnormal collapse of a segment of lung tissue.

attention. That aspect of cognition that refers to the act of devoting mental effort and concentration to a task.

attitude. Behavior shown toward others, objects, or situations.

attorney-in-fact. Person granted the authority to act for another person.

autonomic dysfunction. Abnormal function of the autonomic nervous system, which controls involuntary bodily functions.

autonomy or self-determination. A principle of ethics that defines self-governance or self-determinism.

baby boomers/baby-boom generation. Those individuals born between 1946 and 1964. Will become 65 in 2011.

bacteriuria. Bacteria in the urine.

basal energy expenditure (BEE). The Harris-Benedict equation is one way to determine BEE. It is used in the older population because it has a factor for age, which other formulas do not. BEE can also be calculated using 30 kcals/kg or by indirect calorimetry.

battery. Being touched by another person without consent.

behaviorist. A school of psychology that concentrates on methods of strengthening or weakening new habits through the presence or absence of stimuli intended to produce a response.

behavior therapy. A means by which behavior can be changed by altering positive and negative consequences associated with particular behaviors, thus increasing their frequency, duration, and intensity.

bends. Decompression sickness that occurs with hyperbaric oxygen therapy.

beneficence. A principle of ethics that dictates a health care professional to do good or participate in behavior that benefits a recipient of care.

beneficiary. Those who would gain from a will or trust (e.g., a spouse or child).

benefits. What the insurance plan will cover and pay for.

benign prostatic hyperplasia (BPH). Increase in the number of cells in the prostate often causing dysuria.

bereavement. Period of mourning following the death of a loved one.

bioethics. A branch of ethics dealing with moral decision making on issues related to health care of people.

biofeedback. A process of using equipment to provide visual or auditory information regarding body activities or processes.

birth cohorts. Groups of people born during the same time period.

body mass index (BMI). An index determined by dividing measured body weight in kilograms by the height in meters squared. The National Institutes of Health divides obesity into three levels based on this index.

body transcendence versus body preoccupation. One of three psychological developmental tasks of old age described by Robert Peck: emphasis on cognitive and social skills to allow compensation for physical limitations that are part of everyday life with aging.

bone mineral density (BMD). X-rays for determining density of bones and aids in the diagnosis of osteoporosis.

bradykinesia. Extreme slowness of movement.

bruit. A turbulent sound heard on auscultation of a vessel.

burdens. The stress that results from caring for an older family member over a period of time.

Butler, Robert. Psychiatrist, early leader in geriatric medicine.

calcitonin. A peptide hormone that increases deposition of calcium and phosphate in bone.

calorie. A unit of heat measurement.

cancer. A major chronic disease in which abnormal cells multiply and destroy an organ system.

cardiac cripple. A disabling condition caused by a sedentary lifestyle resulting in severe muscle and cardiac deconditioning. Individuals are unable to tolerate normal levels of activity.

care coordination. A more individualistic and humane concept of case management.

care recipient. A patient, client, consumer, or customer.

carotenoid. Yellow-red pigment widely distributed in plants; precursor of vitamin A.

carotid angiography. A radiographic study of the carotid arteries using dye.

case management. A term that is used in many ways but classically involves the concept of coordinating care and resources to individualize care and maximize wellness and function of the client and family.

case manager. A health care provider who manages the continuum of care for a client.

catatonic. A state of schizophrenia marked by a severe psychomotor retardation requiring assistance with all activities of daily living.

centenarian. A person age 100 or more.

Centers for Disease Control and Prevention (CDCP). A federal agency concerned with the epidemiology and prevention of disease.

cerebral angiography. Radiological test of blood vessels in the brain.

cerebral vascular accident (CVA, stroke). The obstruction of blood and oxygen supply to a segment of the brain caused by a thrombus, an embolus, or bleeding.

certification. The completion of a specific course of study and the attainment of a certificate.

certified hospice palliative nurse (CHPN). A registered nurse who has been certified by the National Board for Certification of Hospice Nurses and who specializes in end-of-life care.

certified medication aide (CMA). A certified nurse aide who has had specific education that allows that person to administer certain medications under the direct supervision of a registered nurse.

certified nurse assistant (CNA). A technical caregiver who has had specific training and certification to perform certain kinds of direct client care under the supervision of a registered nurse.

certiorari. A legal order from a superior court calling for the record of an inferior court proceeding for review.

chief executive officer (CEO). The administrative officer at the top of an organizational chart in a business or system.

Children of Aging Parents (CAPs). Support group for children of aging parents.

chronic illness/health problems. Chronic illnesses last for 3 to 6 months or more but a healthy lifestyle can prevent or delay many of the negative effects of such chronic illnesses.

chronic pain. Pain that extends past the normally expected time of healing. Pain that extends 3 months is commonly accepted as chronic within a clinical context, whereas 6 months is preferred for research purposes.

chronologically gifted. Those who live into their 90s and 100s.

clinical pathway. A written time line for specific care of a client by an interdisciplinary team that focuses on evaluating outcomes based on goals.

code of ethics. A written statement of moral conduct for a profession.

coenzyme. A substance that enhances or is necessary for the action of enzymes.

cognition. The mental capacity characterized by recognition, memory, processing, learning, and judgment.

cognitive. A school of psychology that recognizes learning as discontinuous and sudden, with behavior changing when insight occurs.

cognitive assessment. Evaluation of ability to think, reason, remember, and make judgments.

cognitive behavioral perspective. Management perspective that recognizes and incorporates the connections between cognition, affect, and behavior.

cognitively incapacitated. Decreased ability to think, reason, and make personal health care decisions.

cognitive therapy. A means by which the relationship between one's thoughts, emotions, and behaviors can be changed. It assumes that the manner in which one thinks about events affects the resulting emotional reaction to them and consequently behavior.

cohort effects. The extent to which cultural change makes persons different from those whose birth either precedes or follows them in time. Each generation or cohort grows up in a unique context that influences what they experience and when they experience it.

cohort norm formation. New patterns of behavior and norms formed by a large number of individuals reacting independently but in similar fashion to societal changes.

comorbidity. Many diseases occurring in one person at the same time.

community-based services. Those services that are provided to individuals in free-standing agencies outside of institutional care.

Community Based Alternative (CBA). A program that allows people on Medicaid to remain in the home or assisted-living facility rather than move to a nursing facility.

community nursing organization (CNO). Health care nurse-managed organizations reimbursed by Medicare on a capitated (set-fee-per-member) basis.

community rating. The cost of health insurance premiums are based on the average expected use of health care services of *all* categories of people (e.g., all ages and lifestyles).

competency. Ability to make independent decisions.

comprehensive. Total holistic care involving all the needed health care disciplines.

compressed morbidity. More people living healthier longer until shortly before death.

computerized axial tomography (CAT) scan. A radiological study using computer tomography for diagnostic purposes.

confidentiality. The ethical duty to keep other's personal information safe from the knowledge of others.

conservator. Court-appointed decision maker for the incapacitated adult's financial decision-making needs.

constructivist. An educational approach based on the premise that learning is influenced by beliefs, attitudes, and the context in which an idea is taught and that cognition results when students apply new information to what they already know.

consumer fraud. Acts that lure older adults into sending money or authorizing payment for a nonexistent or worthless item.

consumers. People who buy goods and services.

Continuing Care Retirement Community (CCRC). Provides a continuum of care from independent living to hospice care.

continuity focus. The central concentration of spirituality for a given individual, whether primarily intellectual (inner continuity focus) or primarily related to geographic location, external aspects of worship, ceremony, music, and religious symbols (external continuity focus).

continuous positive airway pressure (CPAP). A relatively low level of back pressure to keep the airway from closing during expiration. It can be delivered via a mask that is tightly strapped to the face or via a mechanical ventilator.

continuum of care. Coordinated care from emergency and acute care services to recovery or hospice care.

contracture. Usually permanent flexion and fixation of a joint into an abnormal and often nonfunctional position.

copayment. Amount the client has to pay for specific services provided by an insurance plan.

coronary artery bypass graft (CABG). Using a segment of the mammary artery to allow blood flow to an area of the heart where blood supply is obstructed.

cor pulmonale. Right-sided heart failure, usually secondary to chronic osbstructive lung disease or another condition of chronic hypoxia.

crackles. A snapping sound heard on lung auscultation in the person who has atelectasis or other situations of alveolar closure. Formerly called rales. A similar sound can be obtained by twisting and rubbing your hair right behind the ear.

crystallized intelligence. That ability that is linked to the accumulation of experience over time, which for the most part remains stable over the adult years.

curative care. Care that aims to eliminate the symptoms and problem.

decision-making capacity. To make decisions, voluntarily act, and choose preferred options.

decompensation. Failure of the heart to maintain a circulation that is sufficient to sustain life.

deconditioning. Loss of muscle strength and stamina, usually because of disease.

decrement with compensation. A view of adult development and aging that states that declines in functioning are not inevitable and can be compensated for by the use of experience, wisdom, the development of new skills, or environmental redesign.

deductible. Amount the client has to pay before the insurance pays anything.

dehydration. Excessive loss of water from body tissues.

delirium. A rapid-onset state of confusion, disorientation, delusions, and sometimes hallucinations that is usually reversible with prompt appropriate treatment.

delirium tremens (DTs). A type of frenzy, agitation, disorientation, and impaired judgment related to alcohol withdrawal.

dementia. A slow-onset irreversible state of cognitive defects that can be the result of a medical condition or disease (such as Alzheimer's) or substance reaction (such as long-term alcoholism) or a combination of these.

dementia special care unit (DSCU). A specific section of a nursing facility designated for the care of residents with various types of dementia.

deontology. An ethical theory that prioritizes ethical principles in the resolution of an ethical dilemma.

Department of Veterans' Affairs. Federal government agency that provides benefits to veterans of military service and their dependents.

dependence. The adjustment of the body to consistent use of drugs or alcohol, so that withdrawal symptoms occur if the substance is withdrawn.

depression. Various degrees of feeling sad, helpless, hopeless, and perhaps suicidal.

developmental task. A growth responsibility that occurs at a particular time in life.

diabetitian. A health care provider that specializes in the care of clients with diabetes.

diagnosis-related group (DRG). Federal law passed in 1983 that attempted to reduce hospital costs by setting specific payment amounts from Medicare for each diagnosis of clients admitted to hospitals.

diagnostic tests. Tests that determine a specific disease (as opposed to a screening test).

diaphoresis. Excessive perspiration.

dietary approaches to stop hypertension (DASH). A specific diet designed to reduce the effects of risk factors on cardiovascular disease.

discharge planning. The systematic assessment of client and family needs for education, care, resources, and supplies. The act of providing optional education and resources for the purpose of maximizing quality of life and care in the noninstitutionalized setting.

disease management program. A specific plan of goals and services aimed toward the management of specific diseases (e.g., diabetes).

disengagement. A 1960s social theory that proposed that older adults withdraw from society and that the action is of mutual benefit to society.

disorganized. A type of schizophrenia characterized by the inability to speak properly (the words come out in the wrong order), to carry out activities of daily living (unable to do the steps of brushing teeth or bathing in order), and to react with appropriate behaviors to situations as they arise.

diverticulosis. The presence of sacs or pouches in the walls of an organ (e.g., large intestine).

Drug Enforcement Agency (DEA). A U.S. Department of Justice agency that enforces controlled substances and regulations, including those associated with distributing and dispensing controlled substances.

drug formulary. A list of specific medications that can be prescribed to particular constituents (i.e., insurance plan enrollees, hospital clientele).

durable medical equipment (DME). Medical equipment that may be partially covered by insurance (e.g., wheelchairs).

durable power of attorney. Document by which the principal has granted another person (agent or attorney-in-fact) to act for him or her in financial matters after the loss of decision-making capacity.

durable power of attorney for health care (DPAHC). A legal document whereby a person (principal) grants another person (agent) the ability to make personal health and treatment decisions.

dying well. Relief of symptoms and having met life goals.

dyspareunia. Difficult painful intercourse.

dysphagia. Difficulty in swallowing.

dyspnea. Subjective difficulty in breathing.

echo home. A small house or apartment next to a larger home where an older family member lives to be close to other family members for assistance when needed.

ectropion. Eversion of the eyelids.

Eden alternative. Bringing the community (e.g., animals, birds, fish, and children) into the nursing facility to provide a more normal homelike environment.

edentulous. Being without natural teeth.

education. Formal or informal learning opportunities.

ego differentiation versus work and role preoccupation. One of three psychological developmental tasks of old age described by Robert Peck: the development of valued alternatives in addition to one's work role, acting to reaffirm self-worth.

ego integrity versus despair. The eighth stage of development described by Eric Erikson as self-acceptance (ego integrity) versus dissatisfaction with life (despair).

ego transcendence versus ego preoccupation. One of three psychological developmental tasks of old age described by Robert Peck: development of the ability to devote energies to the welfare of future generations without preoccupation with one's own death.

Eldercare Locator. A national phone number to help people locate resources for older adult care throughout the country.

eldercare programs. Community programs (e.g., in churches) that focus on identifying and meeting the needs of older adults.

elderhostel. An international educational network providing opportunities for older adults to participate in educational activities on college campuses and in other educational settings.

electroconvulsive therapy (ECT). An effective treatment for clients with treatment-resistant depression in which an electrical current is sent through the brain, causing a grand mal seizure. It is particularly effective in older adults or in those clients with acute suicidal ideation who have not responded to traditional antidepressant treatment.

electroencephalogram (EEG). Diagnostic test to assess electrical activity of the brain.

elite old. Those age 95 and older.

elopement. Resident leaving a nursing or assisted-living facility without the knowledge of staff, which could result in injury.

emergency response system (ERS). A device that is worn by an older adult who lives alone that can be used to notify neighbors and/or relatives of an emergency requiring immediate assistance.

empty calories. Foods that contain kilocalories but little nutritive value; lacking in vitamins, minerals, and fiber.

encoding. The assigning of meaning to a stimulus so that it can be identified and recalled later in time.

endarterectomy. Surgery to remove placque from the interior of an artery.

end-of-life care. Care during the final days and hours of life.

end-stage renal disease (ESRD). Kidney failure.

enterostomal therapist (ET). A person that specializes in ostomy care.

entropion. Eyelids that turn in, causing the possibility of infection in the eye.

epigenetic. Development produced by the cumulative effect of experience. Resolution of each developmental crisis helps to define later crises and form the individual.

equal protection. All people should have equal protection based on laws.

equianalgesic. The use of a formula to compute equivalent doses of analgesic medications.

erectile dysfunction. Inability to attain and maintain an erection sufficient for intercourse (impotence).

estrogen replacement therapy (ERT). Estrogen hormone given after menopause when the natural production of estrogen decreases.

ethical dilemma. A situation involving a choice between equally undesirable alternatives.

ethic of care. An ethical theory that prioritizes honoring interpersonal relationships in the resolution of an ethical dilemma.

ethics. A branch of philosphy utilizing a seasoned decision-making process that allows persons to choose the most appropriate life action relevant to a situation.

euthanasia. Act of facilitating someone's death as painlessly as possible to end that person's discomfort. Allowing (passive) or assisting (active) a person to die.

exacerbation. A worsening of the symptoms of a chronic disease.

exercise. Sustained or periodic movement of muscles and joints.

experience rating. The cost of health insurance premiums are based on the health care experiences of a specific group (e.g., when a few have major medical expenses, the costs for premiums go up for all in that group).

failure to thrive (FTT). A syndrome depicting the presence of malnutrition in combination with a diminished will to live in older adults.

family therapy. An approach to treating dysfunctional family interactions by emphasizing the relationship of each family member to the entire family system.

fatigue. Feeling tired. Could be many causes, including medications.

fat-soluble vitamins. Those vitamins soluble in fat solvents and insoluble in water, specifically vitamins A, D, E, and K. Excessive amounts of fat-soluble vitamins can cause damage to the liver (where they are stored).

federally qualified health center (FQHC). A federally designated health care center that provides the infrastructure to primary health care of the indigent. Care is funded primarily through Medicaid.

fee-for-service. The health care provider gives the service and later bills the insurance company for that service.

fibrinogen. A plasma protein that is essential for blood clotting.

fibromyalgia. A myofascial syndrome classified as a rheumatic disease that may include such symptoms as headache, generalized muscle pain, nonrestorative sleep, and fatigue. There are identifiable tender points that are helpful in making a diagnosis.

fidelity. The ethical duty to keep a promise and honor commitments and contracts.

field (in) dependence. The extent to which the individual relies on cues from the environment as a means of making judgments.

filial maturity. An adult one-to-one relationship between an adult child and older parent.

financial limitations. Difficulty meeting financial obligations.

fiscal intermediary (FI). Organization responsible for arranging insurance payments to health care providers.

five-factor model of personality. A five-factor analytically based approach to personality that emphasizes neuroticism, openness to experience, extroversion, agreeableness, and conscientiousness.

flashes. Sudden light flashes in the eyes.

floaters. Particles of cells that are free floating in the vitreous humor of the eyes and can be seen by the person.

fluid intelligence. An ability whose levels are dependent on the immediate learning situation that may decline with increasing age.

Food and Drug Administration. A federal agency that monitors and approves the safety and effectiveness of food, drugs, and medical devices.

Food Stamp Program. A government program that provides stamps for the purchase of food for those who qualify financially.

formative. A type of evaluation in which an assessment is made during the course of a program, with suggestions used to modify and improve the remaining endeavor.

freedom of religion. There can be no mandatory religion, and individuals are free to exercise their own personal religious beliefs.

functional assessment. To determine ability to perform physical activities of daily living (PADL).

functional limitations. Inability to perform one or more physical activities of daily living (PADL).

functions. The special action or physiological property of one organ or part of the body of a person in the course of activity.

gag reflex. A normal reflex elicited by touching the back of the palate.

gastroesophageal reflux disease (GERD). Persistent reflux of the stomach contents into the esophagus.

gatekeeper. The primary care provider (PCP) in a health maintenance organization. All health care must be provided by or through the PCP.

generational equity. The idea that differing cohorts should be treated similarly with respect to benefits over the life course.

generation X. Those people born after the baby boomers (1964 and later).

generic medications. Non–brand name drugs that are not protected by a trademark.

genotypic continuity. The stability of underlying personality type or structure over time.

geragogy. A process of education distinct from andragogy and pedagogy that is used with older learners and utilizes a humanist, developmental approach; it refers to issues and practices that are relevant to aging.

geriatrician. A physician who has special postgraduate education and experience in the medical care of older adults.

geriatric nursing. The specialty of caring for ill older adults.

geriatric psychopharmacology. Medications used to treat mental, mood, and emotional problems in older adults.

geriatrics. The medical care of older adults who have health problems.

gerofriendly. Environmental conditions favorable to the health, safety, and comfort of older adults.

gerontological case manager. A person who manages the continuum of care for older adults.

gerontological clinical nurse specialist (GCNS). A registered nurse with specific graduate-level education and experience in the care of older adults.

gerontological nurse practitioner (GNP). A nurse prepared at the graduate level who has special assessment, diagnostic, and treatment skills in the care of older adults.

gerontological nursing. The holistic nursing care of sick and well older adults.

gerontologist. An individual who studies the process of aging.

gerontology. An interdisciplinary study of the process of aging.

gerontophilia. Exalting and/or venerating aging persons.

gerontophobia. Fear and aversion of aging.

gerontic nursing. Nursing care pertaining to older adults, a compromise between geriatric nursing (nursing care primarily for older adults who are ill) and gerontological nursing (a more holistic view of the nursing care of older adults).

geropsychiatric nursing. Nursing care of older adults with mental and behavioral problems.

glaucoma. An eye disease that is characterized by increased intraocular pressure and can cause blindness without treatment.

good death. This varies by personal desire and belief, but in general, it refers to an expected death in which the client's symptoms are relieved, emotional and spiritual support are provided to the client and family, the client has as much control as possible of the setting and care, and quality of life is as good as it can possibly be throughout the dying process.

goodness of fit. The extent to which the needs, aspirations, and abilities of individuals mesh with the expectations and opportunities that are available to them in the social structure.

grandparent caregiving. Grandparents having the major responsibility for caring for grandchildren.

grandparenthood. The social role that one enters when one's children give birth or adopt their first child.

gross national product (GNP). The amount spent on all goods and services in the United States in one year.

group activities. Activities planned for a group and usually led or monitored by a facilitator.

group therapy. A therapeutic approach that emphasizes support from others. The sharing of experiences with other group members under the guidance of a group leader.

group work. Eight to 10 people who meet, share, and work together to meet specific goals.

guardian. Court-appointed substitute decision maker for the incapacitated adult's financial decision-making needs.

Guillain-Barré syndrome. A peripheral polyneuritis that usually spreads upward from the feet and legs and can result in paralysis or paresis at various levels of the body.

half-life. The amount of time it takes the body to metabolize one-half of a medication taken.

hazards of immobility. The various physiological results of having a sedentary lifestyle in bed or chair.

Health Care Financing Administration (HCFA). The part of the U.S. Department of Health and Human Services responsible for administering the Medicare and Medicaid programs.

health care providers. Professional people who are physicians, nurses, social workers, dietitians, psychologists, and others in the health care field.

health maintenance organization (HMO). A method of health insurance payment that attempts to provide quality care at an affordable cost with a focus on maintaining wellness.

health professional shortage area (HPSA). A geographical designation of an area that is underserved by health professionals.

health status assessment. A total assessment of current status and needs.

Healthy People 2000. 1990 report on needs for health promotion and health education by the year 2000.

hemodynamic. Relating to the circulation of blood through the body.

hiatal hernia. Protrusion of a portion of the stomach through the diaphragm.

hierarchy of needs. A hierarchical framework consisting of five levels developed by Abraham Maslow to explain a person's level of functioning.

high-density lipoproteins (HDLs). Good cholesterol that helps to get rid of low-density lipoproteins (bad cholesterol) in the blood.

history normative. A causal factor in development that emphasizes historical change; persons growing up during a common historical era are assumed to share common experiences.

holistic approach. Assessing and treating the whole person.

holographic will. A will that is handwritten by the principal.

home health aide (HHA). A nurse assistant that provides some types of health services in the home under the supervision of a registered nurse.

home health services. A variety of health care services provided in the home from skilled care to personal care.

hormone replacement therapy (HRT). The use of hormones such as estrogen and progestin to supplement and eventually replace the natural ones that decline with menopause. HRT is believed to prevent osteoporosis and menopausal symptoms, and possibly reduce the incidence of other diseases in postmenopausal women.

hospice. Alternative end-of-life care in which the emphasis is on acceptance of death, control of pain, making peace with and saying goodbye to loved ones, and social support for the survivors.

human genome project. Mapping of genetic structures that could potentially predict specific diseases.

human insight. The act of intuitive perception or seeing the inner nature of things.

hyperbaric oxygen therapy (HBOT). A comprehensive medical therapy in which clients breathe 100% oxygen at increased pressure. By increasing the amount of oxygen in cells, this therapy removes carbon monoxide and nitrogen from the circulatory system and helps destroy certain bacteria sensitive to high oxygen concentrations. It promotes red blood cell growth and speeds healing, especially in chronic wounds.

hyperkalemia. High serum potassium level.

hypnosis. An induced passive, trancelike state.

hypokalemia. Low serum potassium level.

hyponatremia. Decreased sodium in the blood.

hypotension. Low blood pressure.

hypoxemia. Deficiency of oxygen in the arterial blood.

iatrogenesis. The process of inducing unfavorable response to medical and surgical treatments.

iatrogenic. Complication caused by medical treatment and/or health care providers.

identify style. Whitbourne's notion that personality and adaptation to aging can be understood in terms of accommodative, assimilative, or balanced personality styles.

incapacitated. Legal term to identify loss of thought process, reasoning, judgment, and memory.

Independent Practice Association (IPA). A group of physicians who organize to negotiate with various health insurance plans.

informal caregiving. Care for another person without pay such as a family member or friend.

informed consent. Requires the capacity to reason and make judgments, make decisions voluntarily, and understand the risks and benefits of decisions.

informed refusal. Refusing a specific treatment or care after having been fully informed of the benefits and risks and having the capacity to reason and make judgments.

Institutes for Learning in Retirement (ILR). An organization of retirement-age learners dedicated to meeting the educational needs of its members.

instrumental activities of daily living (IADL). Managing money, shopping, housekeeping, preparing meals, and taking medications correctly.

interdisciplinary team (IDT). Health care providers that utilize an accepted traditional care of geriatric clients requiring complex systems of care that involve numerous services and therapies. Usually health care providers are responsible for different aspects of care.

International Unit (IU). A unit of measure assigned to labeling the trans-retinol content of vitamin A supplements. One IU equals 0.300 μg of all trans-retinol. This has recently been changed to retinol equivalents (RE).

isolated systolic hypertension. Periodic high systolic (contraction of heart) blood pressure.

job displacement. The loss of employment due to plant closure or layoff, in which the worker had been employed for at least 3 years.

Joint Commission on the Accreditation of Healthcare Organizations (JCAHO). An Illinois nonprofit corporation, formed in 1951 to conduct voluntary accreditation of hospitals; the commission later expanded its accreditation programs to other health care organizations.

joint tenancy. All of the parties are equal co-owners of an asset such as a bank account.

justice. A principle of ethics that supports fair allocation of resources to persons or the provision of an equal share of available resources to each person.

Kegel exercises. Contracting exercises of the perineum to help treat urinary incontinence.

keratosis. A brownish pigmented area on the skin commonly found on the trunk and sometimes face of older people. Three types are actinic, senilis, and seborrheic.

kilocalorie. A unit of heat content or energy. The amount of energy required to raise the temperature of one kilogram of water one degree Celsius (from 15°C to 16°C).

lean body mass. That portion of the body made up of muscle and bones excluding adipose tissue.

learner directed. The teacher takes the cues for goals and experiences of clients.

learning. The change in behavior as a function of the accumulation of experience over time.

left ventricular hypertrophy (LVF). Enlargement of the left ventricle of the heart.

lethality (high, moderate, low). The probability that a person with suicidal ideation will commit suicide based on the plan, method, and availability of the means. (A person with plans to kill himself with an available gun at a set time is considered of high lethality whereas a person who is physically weak who thinks about suffocating herself but with no specific time or means on hand is considered of low lethality.)

libertarian. Ethical concept that health care resources are distributed through actions of a free marketplace with those who have money to pay for services being the first to access those services.

licensure. The legal ability to practice a specific profession based on education, other credentials, and testing.

life expectancy. The average number of years one can be expected to live based on a specific year of birth or age.

life review. Systematically evaluating one's successes and failures in life, with professional help, to resolve conflicts and prepare for death. Butler's concept states that it is the awareness of one's own death that elicits an evaluation of one's life and how one has lived it.

life span. The maximum length of life that is biologically possible.

life span development. A view of aging that assumes that later life is best understood in terms of the entirety of the life span; factors that both precede and follow an experience are necessary to understand that experience.

lifestyle. Life practices and habits.

life-sustaining treatment. Medical treatment designed to prolong life, especially when prognosis is poor.

limitations. What the health insurance plan will not cover or pay for.

lipofuscin. Fatty pigments in the cells of adults.

litigation. Legal action by one party against another party.

living will. Directive to physician stating whether or not life-sustaining treatment is desired if in a terminal state.

locus of control. That aspect of personality referring to whether one feels in control of events or is controlled by them.

longevity. The long lived, for example, 90s and 100s.

long-term care. Care usually needed for 3 or more months.

long-term care insurance. A special kind of private insurance that pays for care in the home, nursing facility, and assisted-living facility for months or years.

low-density lipoproteins (LDLs). Bad cholesterol that contributes to blockage of arteries and cardiovascular disease.

lumbar puncture. A diagnostic test that involves inserting a needle into the spinal canal.

malnutrition. Inadequate amount and quality of food intake.

mammogram. An x-ray of breast tissue to detect abnormal conditions such as cancer.

managed care organization (MCO). The category of health insurance plans whereby all care must be given or approved by a primary care provider (PCP).

managed service organization (MSO). An agency that provides basic practice supports services (i.e., billing, collection, electronic data exchange) to physicians. The providers can usually remain independent and do not have to exclusively use the services of this agency.

Masters in Social Work (MSW). A graduate-level program at the masters level in social work.

McBurney's point. A point in the right lower quadrant of the abdomen situated in the area of the appendix.

Meals-on-Wheels. A federally funded program that provides at least one hot home-delivered meal 5 days a week for those who qualify.

mean arterial pressure (MAP). A calculated value related to blood pressures.

mediated learning. Learning that depends upon a mediator to link a stimulus and a response. May be verbal or visual in nature.

Medicaid. A federal and state program that pays for health care of indigent people of all ages who meet financial criteria.

medical alert bracelet. A bracelet (or necklace) that contains vital medical information and a telephone number where more registered information may be obtained.

medical assistant (MA). An unlicensed person who assists health care professionals in caring for clients. Most gain experience through specific training programs. The job functions vary among organizations.

medically underserved area/population (MUA/MAP). A geographic or population classification of medical resource availability. For example, rural areas are both geographically underserved and have specific populations (e.g., children) underserved. A medically underserved area can exist within a large city (e.g., the inner city).

medical malpractice. A health care provider doing something that should not have been done or failing to do what should have been done.

medical neglect. Lack of needed health care because of ageism, lack of knowledge, or lack of money.

medical savings account (MSA). A two-part plan that is a tax-free investment. The person pays up front for all minor health care costs and purchases a health insurance plan with a high deductible to cover major health care expenses.

Medicare. A federal health insurance program for those who are 65 years of age and older, those who have paid into the Social Security program and become disabled, and those who have end-stage renal disease (renal failure).

Medicare Conditions of Participation (MCOP). Federal regulations that a health care facility must meet to receive Medicare funds.

Medicare reimbursement. Payments from the Health Care Financing Administration to health care providers.

Medicare Risk HMO. Health Care Financing Administration contracts with health maintenance organizations to provide health care to older people eligible for Medicare. Persons who enroll in these plans must receive all of their health care through the HMO network of providers.

medicolegal. Legal issues in health care.

Medigap. A private health insurance plan that is purchased to cover what Medicare does not pay, such as the deductibles and copays.

membership programs. Special social and activity programs for older adults that some health systems provide.

memory. The ability to retain and recall information at some later time that one has learned. Memory also includes the ability to remember events that are yet to occur.

   immediate. Recalling events of a few seconds or minutes ago.

   recent. Recalling events of a few hours or days ago.

   remote. Recalling events of many years ago.

   old. Recalling distant events not recently recalled.

memory processes. Those dynamic skills that determine how one transforms new information so that it can be recalled later: registration, encoding, storage, and retrieval.

memory structures. Hypothetical entities that help people process and store information for varying lengths of time: the sensory, short-term, and long-term stores.

menopause. The point in a woman's life when the hormone estrogen decreases and the ovaries no longer produce ova (average age is 50).

mental health. Feelings of personal wellness and successful adaptation to the environment.

mercy killing. Another term for euthanasia. It implies that the client is perceived to be in so much distress that it is more merciful to assist him or her to die than it is to allow the dying process to take its natural course or to attempt to relieve symptoms and suffering.

method of loci. A particular memory enhancement skill where one associates things to be remembered with points along a journey (loci) one travels often.

minimum data set (MDS). Assessment data to be completed by the registered nurse and others within the first 14 days after admission to a nursing facility.

mitosis. Cell division.

mobility. One of the major problems with a sedentary life is the decreased use of muscle groups and joints. Lack of movement reduces the functioning of all organs in the body system and affects both the mind and body.

monoamine oxidase inhibitor (MAOI). A seldom used class of antidepressants that work by blocking various subtypes of monoamine oxidase. Clients must stick to a strict diet low in tyramines or they can have a hypertensive crisis that can be potentially fatal.

morals. Values that people use to identify right decisions from those that are wrong.

morbidity rates. The number or incidence of a particular disease or disorder out of a given base (e.g., 1,000, 100,000) in the population in a given time period.

mortality rates. The number of deaths per 1,000 in a population in a given time period.

motor time. That aspect of reaction time referring to the speed with which a physical movement can be made.

multidimensionality. The fact that developmental change needs to be described in terms of many factors.

multidirectionality. The fact that different dimensions of development display diverse paths of growth and decline.

multidisciplinary. Many different health care providers and others involved with a specific client plan and care.

multiple intelligence theory. A theory based on cognitive research that documents the extent to which students learn, remember, perform, and understand in different ways (i.e., through language, logical-mathematical analysis, spatial representation, musical thinking, the use of the body to solve problems or make things, an understanding of other individuals, and an understanding of ourselves).

myoclonus. Spasm of a muscle or group of muscles.

Narcotics Anonymous (NA). A national self-help organization for the treatment of drug abuse based on the Alcoholics Anonymous 12-step program to maintain sobriety.

National Aging Network. All of those organizations and agencies devoted to improving the health and life of older adults.

National Association for Home Care (NAHC). Organization of agencies that provide home health care, hospice care, and homemaker services.

National Association of Area Agencies on Aging (NAAAA). Represents the interests of local area agencies on aging across the country.

National Conference of Gerontological Nurse Practitioners, Inc. A national organization of gerontological nurse practitioners.

National Council on the Aging (NCOA). A national resource for information, technical assistance, training, and research related to the field of aging.

National Gerontological Nursing Association. A national organization of nurses who work in the field of gerontological nursing.

National Institute of Mental Health (NIMH). Federal agency that conducts and supports research to learn more about the causes, prevention, and treatment of mental and emotional illnesses.

National Institute on Aging (NIA). Federal agency that supports research on the aging process and diseases common to older people.

necrosis. Death of areas of tissue or bone.

neglect. Failure to provide assistance to meet basic needs; failing to perform an obligation.

neuroleptic malignant syndrome (NMS). A rare and potentially fatal reaction to treatment with neuroleptic drugs. This reaction might occur days, weeks, or even many months after beginning treatment. Symptoms include sudden high fever, muscle rigidity, tachycardia, diaphoresis, and rapid deterioration of cognition. Emergency medical treatment is imperative.

nonmalificence. A principle of ethics that supports a health care professional to avoid harm in caring for a person.

nonmodifiable risk factors. Risk factors for disease that cannot be changed, such as genes.

nonnormative. Referring to the fact that some causes of developmental change are unique to individuals and cannot be understood in either age-related or historical terms.

nonpharmacological pain management. Approaches that do not use medicine for the relief of pain, but rather assist the individual in modulating pain over time. These represent such techniques as relaxation, distraction, positive self-talk, and balancing activities to avoid overexertion.

normal aging. Common aging-related physical and psychological changes that occur in the absence of disease.

nurse practitioner. A registered nurse who has advanced education and experience in a health care specialty. May function independently based on legal state limits.

nursing facility (NF). Nursing facility that provides custodial care 24 hours a day.

nutrition. Food and fluids required to sustain life.

Office of Technology Assessment (OTA). A federal agency that utilizes resources from the private sector to provide Congress with analysis of technical issues.

older adult mistreatment. Acts of commission (intentional infliction of harm) or acts of omission (harm occurring through neglect) by a caregiver.

older adults' rights. Individual rights and freedom of older adults.

Older Americans Act (OAA). Passed in 1965 and provides funds to states for services for older people.

ombudsman. An agency staff member or volunteer who is trained to be an advocate for older people in nursing facilities and assisted-living facilities by investigating complaints and reporting abuses.

Omnibus Budget Reconciliation Act (OBRA) of 1997. A federal law that set up specific guidelines and regulations for nursing facilities that receive Medicare and/or Medicaid funding.

onychomycosis. Parasitic fungal condition causing a thick scaly substance to collect between the top of the toe nail and the skin in older persons.

opioids (opiates). A narcotic drug that contains opium or a synthetic with opiumlike activity.

optimal aging. Aging that occurs under optimally supportive environments; it reflects what persons are capable of under ideal conditions.

organizational resources. Disease-specific organizations that provide education and research such as the Arthritis Foundation and the American Cancer Society.

orthopnea. A respiratory symptom in which the person breathes most comfortably when in an upright position.

orthostatic hypotension. Condition in which the blood pressure falls when changing from a sitting or lying position to standing and that can cause dizziness or fainting.

osteoarthritis. Degeneration of joints related to wear and tear.

osteomalacia. Softening of bones causing weakness and fractures.

osteoporosis. Thin, weak bones.

outcome assessment information sets (OASIS). A group of data sets designed to measure client outcomes in home health care.

outpatient. One who receives care from a health care facility for periods of time during the day only.

outpatient hospital services. All those hospital activities and services that are provided on an outpatient (hourly or daily) basis.

over-the-counter (OTC) medications. Medications that a person can legally buy without a prescription.

pacemaker. An electrical apparatus that maintains normal heart rate and rhythm.

pain. Various degrees of discomfort that affects functional abilities.

pain assessment. Assessment that includes measures of pain intensity and pain experience, a combination that is important in evaluating chronic pain.

pain experience. One's response to living with persistent pain. Underlying dimensions of this experience include the individual's perceived effects of pain on function, distress, and feelings of helplessness.

pain intensity. The perceived intensity of pain; while it is generally thought to represent the sensory component of pain, it is likely influenced by the affective and cognitive components as well.

pain management. Assessment, interventions, and evaluation of the outcome of pain relief measures.

palliative care. Care that provides support and comfort rather than treatment aimed for cure.

pallidotomy. Surgery on the globus pallidus (part of brain's communication center) to decrease rigidity and bradykinesia and partly reduce tremors of Parkinson's disease.

Papanicolaou testing. A diagnostic test of the cervix to determine abnormal conditions such as cancer.

paranoid. Suspicious thoughts and delusions characterized by intense feelings of persecution and threatening hallucinations.

parish nursing. A registered nurse employed by a church to do health education, counseling, and referrals.

Parkinson's disease. A neurological deficiency of dopamine that results in a variety of symptoms, primarily tremor, muscle rigidity, and slow movement.

paroxysmal nocturnal dyspnea (PND). Severe respiratory distress at night while sleeping flat, relieved by sitting up, and caused by left-sided heart failure.

partial hospitalization day programs. A hospital-based program that provides treatment, care, and support (e.g., mental health care) on a daily basis.

participating physician. A physician who accepts Medicare assignment (the amount allowed by Medicare).

paternalism. A more powerful or knowledgeable person makes health care decisions for a less powerful or knowledgeable person.

pathological aging. Age-related changes that are primarily a function of underlying disease states and are therefore not normal.

Patient Self Determination Act (PSDA). National legislation passed in 1990 requiring that all clients being admitted to a health care facility receiving Medicare or Medicaid funds must be asked if they have signed an advance directive and be given information about their rights to do so if desired.

pedagogy. The art and science of teaching children; the traditional approach in formal education.

peer review organization (PRO). A state organization that is mandated by federal law to monitor the quality of care received by Medicare patients.

penumbra. Zone of privacy rights in the Ninth and Fourteenth Amendments.

perceptual/cognitive style. An individual's characteristic manner of responding to the stimuli in the environment.

percutaneous transluminal coronary angioplasty (PTCA). A technique using flouroscopy, a catheter and a balloon, to open up coronary arteries by flattening plaque against the vessel.

periodontal disease. Disease of the gums and alveolar bones of the mouth. The common cause of tooth loss in older people. Can be prevented with proper consistent care.

peripherally inserted central catheter (PICC). A long, thin intravenous catheter that is inserted into the superior vena cava, usually via the antecubital vein.

per member, per month (PMPM). The process of capitation in which a health care provider is paid each month for each client in a specific plan even if no care is given in that month.

perpetrator. The person who causes or allows the victim to be harmed.

personal care attendant. A person who assists an older adult with the physical activities of daily living in a home or institutional setting. Neither licensure nor certification is usually required.

personal care home. A facility that provides supervision and assistance with physical activities of daily living (PADL) 24 hours a day excluding skilled care.

personality types. A characteristic style or mode of responding to the environment and others in it that is formed early in life and maintained thereafter. Some personality types are more adaptive than are others.

person-environment interaction. A view of development that states the behavior can be understood in terms of the relationship between the individual's skills and the demands of the environment.

pharmacodynamics. The effect of drugs at the receptor level.

pharmacogeriatrics. Medications safe and useful in older adults.

pharmacokinetics. Study of the absorption, distribution, metabolism, and excretion of drugs in the body.

pharmacotherapy. Medications used in the treatment of disease.

phenotypic persistence. The stability of specific personality characteristics over time.

physical abuse. Causing physical harm such as hitting a person.

physical activities of daily living (PADL). Eating, bathing, dressing, toileting, grooming, and walking.

physical dependence. Needing another person to assist in or perform basic activities of daily living; unable to care for oneself.

physical therapy assistant (PTA). Works under the supervision of a physical therapist after completing a training program and/or examination.

physician's assistant (PA). A person who assists a physician by performing assessments and visiting clients and may write some medical orders requiring a physician's signature. A baccalaureate degree and state licensure may be required.

physician-assisted suicide. A physician provides and prepares a lethal dose of medication that the consenting client then injects.

placebo. A medication lacking a therapeutic effect but having a psychological effect on a person with symptoms.

plan of care (POC). A written interdisciplinary identification of the client's problems and specific plans for helping to resolve them.

plan of treatment (POT). A comprehensive interdisciplinary written plan to meet the needs of clients based on the history, physical examination, and other assessment data.

plasticity. The malleability of behavior in an individual and the resulting capacity of persons to develop new skills irrespective of age.

pluralism. A characteristic of life span development that generally states that there is no one true or best course of development. Development and aging are best viewed as having many possibilities and trajectories rather than in unitary or single terms.

podiatrist. A doctor licensed to treat foot disorders.

point of service (POS). A health insurance plan that pays based on where and by whom the service is provided. A health maintenance organization may have a point-of-service option that provides more choice at a higher cost.

policy changes. Change created by the deliberate actions of policymakers through the use of political and legislative processes.

polypharmacy. The administration of multiple prescription and nonprescription medications simultaneously, often seen with older persons and resulting in increased adverse effects.

postural hypotension. Synonymous with orthostatic hypotension—a condition in which the blood pressure falls when changing to an upright position, resulting in dizziness or fainting.

power of attorney. Delegation of authority to an agent for financial decisions while the principal still has decision-making capacity.

practical memory. Memory for everyday events that involves both the development and maintenance of one's memory skills.

preexisting condition. Medical problem or illness a person has before applying for health insurance.

preferred provider organization (PPO). A type of managed care organization that provides more choice at a higher cost.

premium. Cost of health insurance (e.g., monthly, quarterly).

premotor time. That aspect of reaction time that involves interpreting what one must respond to and selecting a response.

presbycusis. Decreased ability to hear high-pitched voices as one ages.

presbyopia. Increased farsightedness in later middle age.

preservation of life. Concern for the individual's life and interest and the sanctity of all human life.

prevention of suicide. Assessing for suicide risk and implementing suicide precautions.

preventive services. Care that prevents the development or progression of disease.

primary care physician (PCP). The gatekeeper in a health maintenance organization. All health care must be given by or approved by the PCP.

primary care provider (PCP). The provider who is responsible for helping the client meet her or his health care needs by either providing them or referring the client to other providers.

primary health care clinic/center. The location where the client and primary care provider meet, assess, plan, and implement treatment regimens to meet health care goals and evaluate their effectiveness.

primary memory. Memory for stimuli that involves immediate storage and recall of information whose capacity is limited.

primary mental abilities. A view of human intelligence that states that one's abilities are limited to a select number of basic skills, such as those that are verbal, spatial, or numerical in nature. Each ability shows a distinct pattern of age-related change.

primary prevention. Services that prevent a disease or illness from occurring.

principal. Person who grants an agent authority to act for him or her.

principle. A fundamental truth or belief from which other ideas evolve.

privacy. The ethical duty to control personal information about self and others.

program of all-inclusive care for the elderly (PACE). A model of integrated geriatric care to prevent unnecessary use of hospital and nursing facility care.

prospective payment system (PPS). Health care providers know before treatment and care how much they will be paid for a specific service.

prostate specific antigen (PSA). A screening blood test that indicates an abnormal condition of the prostate, especially cancer.

proteinuria. The presence of unusual amounts of protein in the urine.

provider-sponsored organization (PSO). A health maintenance organization that is owned and operated by physicians and/or hospitals rather than insurance companies.

pseudoaddiction. The term for a situation when a person is seeking additional narcotics because pain has been inadequately treated.

pseudodementia. Some of the same symptoms as dementia, such as confusion, but usually treatable, temporary, and reversible.

pseudohypertension. A condition in which the blood pressure appears high because of stiffening of the vascular walls rather than true hypertension.

psychoanalysis. Freud's theory of personality and psychotherapy that emphasizes interactions between the ego, superego, and id, wherein the demands of the latter are influenced by defense mechanisms to reduce conflict and anxiety within the person.

psychological abuse. Talking to and/or yelling at an older person in a demeaning and disrespectful manner.

psychopharmacology. The study of medications that are used to treat psychomotor behavior and emotional problems.

psychosocial crises. Erikson's series of biosocial choices and conflicts with which every individual must cope. Psychosocial crises may be resolved positively or negatively, and the consequences of this process accumulate over time.

psychosociospiritual assessment. A holistic assessment of the psychological, social, and spiritual needs of clients.

psychomotor. A domain of learning concerned with fine or gross motor skills and demonstrated by physical skills, coordination, dexterity, strength, or speed.

public policy. Policy that results from governmental legislation and/or regulation.

pulmonary edema. The accumulation of fluid in the lung tissues, usually caused by left-sided heart failure.

pulmonary emboli. The blockage of a pulmonary artery by foreign matter, usually plaque migrating from vessels in the hips and legs.

pulse oximetry. Indirect measurement of oxygenation via a sensor on the outside of the body, often one ear lobe or finger.

pursed-lip breathing. Exhaling through lips brought close together to gain control of respiratory distress or breathing during activity; usually used by clients with chronic obstructive pulmonary disease (COPD).

quality of life. What the individual determines is quality.

raloxifene (Evista). Medication used to prevent thinning of bones in postmenopausal women. It is one of the new selective estrogen receptor modulators.

Raloxifene works like an estrogen to stop bone loss without stimulating the breast or uterus, thus reducing the risk of breast or endometrial cancer.

rapid eye movement (REM) sleep. The deepest level of sleep when the muscles are most relaxed, the eyes move, and dreams occur. The amount of REM sleep time is decreased in older adults.

reaction time. The time between the onset of a stimulus and one's response to it.

reality orientation. Orienting a person who is confused to place, person, time, and other current facts.

recidivism. Rehospitalization possibly because of too early discharge.

recommended dietary allowances (RDAs). National recommendations for the daily intake of certain vitamins and minerals by age groups.

registration. The initial memory process that requires that in order for a stimulus to be further processed, it must exceed that person's sensory threshold.

rehabilitation. Activity and therapy to return the client to as near normal as possible.

reimbursement. Method of paying for a service provided.

relocation. Movement from one place to another, such as home to hospital to nursing home. May cause confusion and other symptoms.

reminiscence therapy. Remembering and talking about mostly pleasant memories from the past.

Resident Bill of Rights. Part of the Omnibus Budget Reconciliation Act of 1997 that gives residents in nursing facilities the full rights of any citizen.

resource-based relative value scale (RBRVS). Federal regulations from 1992 that set a scale for determining fair Medicare payments to certain types of physicians before treatment and care.

respite care. Relief care for a caregiver responsible for home or other care of a dependent older adult.

restraints. Any of many devices used to immobilize or prevent movement. Could include physical (bed rails) or chemical (medications).

retinal detachment. The retina separates from the choroid in the eye, possibly causing blindness without immediate treatment.

retinol equivalents (RE). Unit of measure used to express both preformed vitamin A and B-carotene equivalents as a single nutritive value. One microgram RE is equal of 1 μg of all-trans retinol in food or to 6 μg of all-trans B-carotene in food or 12 μg of other provitamin A carotenoid in foods.

Retired Senior Volunteer Program (RSVP). An initiative sponsored by ACTION (the federal agency that coordinates volunteer activities) and authorized by the 1969 amendments to the Older Americans Act that coordinates community volunteer service opportunities.

retirement. Leaving a specific job or type of employment to pursue other types of activities.

retrieval. Recalling information in memory that has been encoded and stored.

rheumatoid arthritis (RA). A chronic disease that causes inflammation, swelling, and deforming of joints.

riboflavin. B vitamin (vitamin B_2); helps break down carbohydrates, proteins, and fats. Found in dairy products, fish, meats, green leafy vegetables, and whole-grain/enriched cereals and breads.

right to liberty. A person shall not be deprived of life, liberty, or property without due process of law.

right to privacy. All clients have a right to privacy in any health care facility.

risk factors. A factor that causes a person or group of people to be especially vulnerable to an unwanted health event.

rote learning. Learning that is dependent on repetition.

rural health center (RHC). A federally designated classification of health centers in rural areas. Because rural areas are underserved, they often receive incentive Medicare/Medicaid reimbursement consideration, and laws and procedures are modified to account for the unavailable health care providers in the area.

Safe Return Program. A program of the Alzheimer's Association that assists in the location of persons with dementia who may wander from home.

sandwich generation syndrome. Family members who are caring for parents and grandparents as well as children and grandchildren.

screening test. A relatively simple test that may show that further testing is needed to make a definite diagnosis.

secondary condition. Problems and/or other diagnoses that develop as a result of a primary diagnosis.

secondary memory. That memory store into which information is deposited when it exceeds the capacity of primary memory.

secondary prevention. Treatment and activities to prevent progression of a specific disease process.

selective serotonin reuptake inhibitors (SSRIs). A relatively new class of antidepressants that work by inhibiting the reuptake of serotonin, thus increasing its concentration in the neuroleptic synapse. Because of the side effect of insomnia, SSRIs are usually given in the morning to give the client a boost to start the day.

self-actualization. The highest level of personal growth as defined by Abraham Maslow.

self-care. Ability to meet one's own daily needs.

self-concept. That aspect of personality that reflects how one views oneself and the feelings attached to this self-view.

self-determination. The process of making one's own choices without outside influence.

self-efficacy. A feeling, thought, or belief that one is capable and can use one's skills to perform a behavior.

senescence. The process of aging; the biological, physiological, sociological, and psychological changes that accompany the aging process.

senior center programs. A community center open during the day where older people eat, socialize, learn, and participate in other group activities.

sensory impairment. Decrease in one or more of the five senses (sight, hearing, taste, smell, touch).

sensory memory. A memory store where stimuli can be recalled for a period of seconds after which they must be processed further or they will be lost.

sigmoidscopy. The procedure for examining the lower colon by way of a lighted instrument.

silent killer. A health condition such as high blood pressure that can cause death but is often asymptomatic until a major stroke or death occurs.

skilled nursing facility (SNF). Nursing facility that provides skilled care 24 hours a day.

skilled nursing inpatient facility (SNIF). A skilled nursing facility within a hospital.

skilled nursing unit (SNU). A skilled nursing facility within a hospital.

sleep apnea. Loss of respiration during sleep.

sleep disturbance. Any activity that keeps one from sleeping, such as apnea, depression, pain, or urinary frequency.

sleep hygiene. Activities and procedures that aid in achieving normal sleep patterns.

slippery slope. A concept used to describe the phenomenon of a society allowing the increased use of a practice such as euthanasia without some regulation or control.

social health maintenance organization (SHMO). A managed care organization that focuses on meeting the social rather than medical needs of clients.

social limitations. Factors that prevent one from usual or normal social contacts. These opportunities to interact with others are often influenced by the physical limitations that one experiences related to a chronic condition such as arthritis or cardiovascular disease.

social roles. The activities, rights, and responsibilities that accompany a particular position in society.

Social Security. A federal program started in 1935 that provides a basic income to retirees that starts at ages 62–65.

social support. A person, agency, or organization from which one receives individual assistance and support when needed.

somnolence. A condition of sleepiness or drowsiness that can also be characterized by disorientation or excitability.

special care unit (SCU). One unit in a hospital or nursing facility that specializes in the care of clients with a specific diagnosis.

speech/language pathologist. A professional who specializes in diagnosis and treatment of speech and language abnormalities.

spirituality. Belief in a higher being.

spiritual activity. Reflective action that one undertakes to meet the needs of the human spirit; these actions may or may not be connected with an organized religious institution or group.

spiritual journey. The quest throughout the life course to meet the needs of the spirit.

spiritual need. Inner needs for relief from anxieties and fears, preparation for death, personality integration, personal dignity, and a philosophy of life.

spiritual well-being. The affirmation of life in a relationship with a God, self, community, and environment that nurtures and celebrates wholeness.

Stephen ministry. A church ministry by volunteers that helps members with short-term crises in their lives.

storage. That memory process where information that has been encoded is organized so that it can later be retrieved.

structural lag. A mismatch between older adults' needs and desires and the social structural opportunities for them.

subacute care unit. A unit in a nursing facility that is equipped and staffed to care for clients needing more skilled care such as ventilators.

substance abuse. Using a substance to the point of not only neglecting major role obligations but also causing major problems in one's life.

substance dependence. Behavioral, cognitive, and physiological symptoms of requiring a substance despite having no medical need to continue its use.

successful aging. A state of mind and body dedicated to a disciplined lifestyle for a more healthy and productive life to promote and maintain optimal life status for older adults.

summative. A type of evaluation that provides a summary of the assessment of results at the conclusion of a program.

sundown syndrome. Increased degree of confusion and disorientation that occurs in older persons with dementia in the late afternoon or early evening.

sunrise syndrome. Decreased cognitive functioning early in the morning.

Supplemental Security Income (SSI). Additional benefits provided based on resources and income level. Qualifies recipients for Medicaid.

support systems. Those people, programs, agencies, and organizations to whom one can turn when a need arises.

symptom management. Preventing, treating, and relieving specific symptoms of a disease.

syncope. A transient symptom of dizziness, light-headedness, or fainting.

synergistic. One substance or activity enhances the activity of another one.

tardive dyskinesia. Abnormal movements of the tongue, neck, fingers, trunk, and legs exhibited as side effects of some antipsychotic medications.

target pulse rate. The pulse rate that is calculated as optimal for a person to achieve during exercise. For example, 220 minus age times 80%.

teacher directed. Educational experiences planned and directed by the teacher.

teleshopping. Selecting and purchasing products via technology-based sources (e.g., television, telephone, and Internet).

terminally ill. Those who are expected to live 6 months or less.

tertiary memory. That memory store whose capacity is unlimited and in which information is stored for long periods of time.

tertiary prevention. A period of rehabilitation after treatment to return the client to as near normal as possible.

testator. Person who has a will prepared.

thalamotomy. Surgical destruction of a portion of the thalamus to reduce the tremor of Parkinson's disease.

therapy. The treatment of disease by various methods.

time-of-measurement effects. Short-term environmental factors that have an influence on development and aging.

tissue plasminogen activator (tPA). A drug that destroys vascular thrombi; a clot-buster (Activaser).

tocopherol. Vitamin E; fat-soluble vitamin important in the function of nerves and muscles; one of the antioxidant vitamins. Found in significant quantity in vegetable oils, margarine, shortening, wheat germ, and green, leafy vegetables.

trajectory. A path or process driven by a specific force (e.g., the course of the dying process over time and what happens along the way).

transactional model. A model of development and aging that stresses the individual's ongoing interactions with the environment, which can be either adaptive or maladaptive in nature.

transcutaneous electrical stimulation (TENS units). A method of pain control by the application of low-level electrical impulses to specific areas of the skin.

transient ischemic attack (TIA). A "little" stroke; symptoms of a stroke that usually last 20 minutes to 24 hours and can be a predictor of a major stroke.

translocation syndrome. The effects, including temporary confusion, of being moved from one environment to others over a short period of time (e.g., from home to hospital to nursing facility).

tremor. Rhythmic, purposeless, quivering movements of the skeletal muscle groups.

tricyclic antidepressants (TCAs). An early class of antidepressants that work by blocking the reuptake of various neurotransmitters that allow chemicals to remain in the synaptic junction for a longer period of time. TCAs have many side effects, including anticholinergic effects.

trust. Document with defined property to be managed in a specific manner by a trustee for the benefit of a specific party.

unbundled. Each service/product that is used in care (e.g., dressings) is identified and billed in addition to the procedure in which the product is used.

University of the Third Age (U3A). An educational program founded in France in 1973 that emphasized personal development for well older adults; the program subsequently spread through Europe, Britain, Australia, Canada, and the United States.

unlicensed assistive personnel (UAP). A category of assistants and technicians who have no legally required education, licensure, or certification and assist health care providers such as physicians and nurses in a variety of settings.

urgent care center. A center where timely care that is considered to be necessary to prevent a threat to well-being is provided. The care does not require hospitalization or emergency interventions (airway or cardiovascular support). The event that precipitates the need for urgent care is unforeseen (e.g., asthmatic attack, infection, traumatic wound).

urinary incontinence (UI). Leakage of urine from the bladder.

urinary tract infection (UTI). Bacterial infection of the bladder, ureter, and/or kidneys.

usual, customary, and reasonable (UCR). The amount Medicare pays for a specific service in a geographic region.

utilitarianism. An ethical theory that prioritizes actions that will produce the most good for the most people in the resolution of an ethical dilemma.

validation therapy. Accepting and supporting persons with dementia as they are without attempting to change them.

values. Desirable beliefs that one holds in high esteem and that serve as guidelines for personal behavior.

veracity. The ethical duty to be truthful.

vigilance. One's ability to monitor events in the environment for a sustained period of time.

wandering behavior. Constantly walking around or trying to walk away from a place because of boredom, agitation, or seeking someone or something (often seen in clients with dementia).

ward. The person who is incapacitated and represented by a conservator/guardian in financial matters.

wellness in dying. This is closely related to "good death" and involves the client feeling as well as possible and either functioning as well as possible or being able to do the things that are personally considered most important up to the end of the dying process.

white coat hypertension. A high blood pressure reading in the physician's office because of anxiety and/or stress.

Widowed Persons Service (WPS). An organization that provides group support and activities to widowed persons.

widowhood. A state of losing a spouse.

will. Legal document that provides for the distribution of financial assets upon the death of the person.

withdrawal. The unpleasant symptoms that occur when a drug (legal or illegal) is tapered and/or stopped.

working memory. That aspect of memory that holds information in temporary form so that it can be actively processed by the individual.

xerophthalmia. A sequence of abnormalities such as loss of visual acuity in dim light (night blindness) and drying of the surface of the conjunctiva and cornea of the eye caused by vitamin A deficiency. Rare in the United States but common in southeastern Asia and parts of Africa and South America.

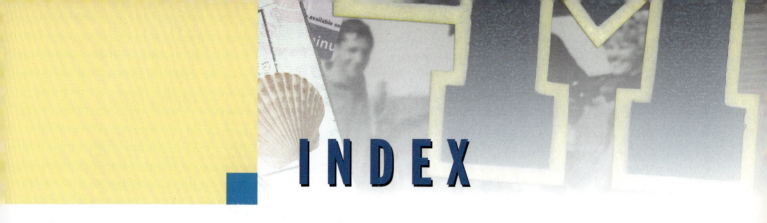

INDEX

('b' indicates boxed material; 'i' indicates an illustration; 't' indicates a table)